# INVASIVE CARDIOVASCULAR THERAPY

# DEVELOPMENTS IN CARDIOVASCULAR MEDICINE

**Recent volumes**

Hanrath P, Bleifeld W, Souquet, J. eds: Cardiovascular diagnosis by ultrasound. Transesophageal, computerized, contrast, Doppler echocardiography. 1982. ISBN 90-247-2692-1.

Roelandt J, ed: The practice of M-mode and two-dimensional echocardiography. 1983. ISBN 90-247-2745-6.

Meyer J, Schweizer P, Erbel R, eds: Advances in noninvasive cardiology. 1983. ISBN 0-89838-576-8.

Morganroth J, Moore EN, eds: Sudden cardiac death and congestive heart failure: Diagnosis and treatment. 1983. ISBN 0-89838-580-6.

Perry HM, ed: Lifelong management of hypertension. 1983. ISBN 0-89838-582-2.

Jaffe EA, ed: Biology of endothelial cells. 1984. ISBN 0-89838-587-3.

Surawicz B, Reddy CP, Prystowsky EN, eds: Tachycardias. 1984. ISBN 0-89838-588-1.

Spencer MP, ed: Cardiac Doppler diagnosis. 1983. ISBN 0-89838-591-1.

Villarreal H, Sambhi MP, eds: Topics in pathophysiology of hypertension. 1984. ISBN 0-89838-595-4.

Messerli FH, ed: Cardiovascular disease in the elderly. 1984. ISBN 0-89838-596-2.

Simoons ML, Reiber JHC, eds: Nuclear imaging in clinical cardiology. 1984. ISBN 0-89838-599-7.

Ter Keurs HEDJ, Schipperheyn JJ, eds: Cardiac left ventricular hypertrophy. 1983. ISBN 0-89838-612-8.

Sperelakis N, ed: Physiology and pathophysiology of the heart. 1984. ISBN 0-89838-615-2.

Messerli FH, ed: Kidney in essential hypertension. 1984. ISBN 0-89838-616-0.

Sambhi MP, ed: Fundamental fault in hypertension. 1984. ISBN 0-89838-638-1.

Marchesi C, ed: Ambulatory monitoring: Cardiovascular system and allied applications. 1984. ISBN 0-89838-642-X.

Kupper W, MacAlpin RN, Bleifeld W, eds: Coronary tone in ischemic heart disease. 1984. ISBN 0-89838-646-2.

Sperelakis N, Caulfield JB, eds: Calcium antagonists: Mechanisms of action on cardiac muscle and vascular smooth muscle. 1984. ISBN 0-89838-655-1.

Godfraind T, Herman AS, Wellens D, eds: Calcium entry blockers in cardiovascular and cerebral dysfunctions. 1984. ISBN 0-89838-658-6.

Morganroth J, Moore EN, eds: Interventions in the acute phase of myocardial infarction. 1984. ISBN 0-89838-659-4.

Abel FL, Newman WH, eds: Functional aspects of the normal, hypertrophied, and failing heart. 1984. ISBN 0-89838-665-9.

Sideman S, Beyar R, eds: Simulation and imaging of the cardiac system. 1985. ISBN 0-89838-687-X.

Van der Wall E, Lie KI, eds: Recent views on hypertrophic cardiomyopathy. 1985. ISBN 0-89838-694-2.

Beamish RE, Singal PK, Dhalla NS, eds: Stress and heart disease. 1985. ISBN 0-89838-709-4.

Beamish RE, Panagio V, Dhalla NS, eds: Pathogenesis of stress-induced heart disease. 1985. ISBN 0-89838-710-8.

Morganroth J, Moore EN, eds: Cardiac arrhythmias. 1985. ISBN 0-89838-716-7.

Mathes E, ed: Secondary prevention in coronary artery disease and myocardial infarction. 1985. ISBN 0-89838-736-1.

Lowell Stone H, Weglicki WB, eds: Pathology of cardiovascular injury. 1985. ISBN 0-89838-743-4.

Meyer J, Erbel R, Rupprecht HJ, eds: Improvement of myocardial perfusion. 1985. ISBN 0-89838-748-5.

Reiber JHC, Serruys PW, Slager CJ: Quantitative coronary and left ventricular cineangiography. 1986. ISBN 0-89838-760-4.

Fagard RH, Bekaert IE, eds: Sports cardiology. 1986. ISBN 0-89838-782-5.

Reiber JHC, Serruys PW, eds: State of the art in quantitative coronary arteriography. 1986. ISBN 0-89838-804-X.

Roelandt J, ed: Color Doppler Flow Imaging. 1986. ISBN 0-89838-806-6.

Van der Wall EE, ed: Noninvasive imaging of cardiac metabolism. 1986. ISBN 0-89838-812-0.

Liebman J, Plonsey R, Rudy Y, eds: Pediatric and fundamental electrocardiography. 1986. ISBN 0-89838-815-5.

Hilger HH, Hombach V, Rashkind WJ, eds: Invasive cardiovascular therapy. 1987. ISBN 0-89838-818-X

Serruys PW, Meester GT, eds: Coronary angioplasty: a controlled model for ischemia. 1986. ISBN 0-89838-819-8.

Tooke JE, Smaje LH: Clinical investigation of the microcirculation. 1986. ISBN 0-89838-819-8.

Van Dam RTh, Van Oosterom A, eds: Electrocardiographic body surface mapping. 1986. ISBN 0-89838-834-1.

Spencer MP, ed: Ultrasonic diagnosis of cerebrovascular disease. 1987. ISBN 0-89838-836-8.

Legato MJ, ed: The stressed heart. 1987. ISBN 0-89838-849-X.

# INVASIVE CARDIOVASCULAR THERAPY

*edited by*

## H.H. HILGER and V. HOMBACH
*Medical Clinic III, Department of Cardiology, University of Cologne*
*Cologne, Federal Republic of Germany*

## W.J. RASHKIND
*Cardiovascular Laboratories, The Children's Hospital of Philadelphia*
*One Children's Center, Philadelphia, U.S.A.*

1987 **MARTINUS NIJHOFF PUBLISHERS**
a member of the KLUWER ACADEMIC PUBLISHERS GROUP
DORDRECHT / BOSTON / LANCASTER

**Distributors**

*for the United States and Canada*: Kluwer Academic Publishers, P.O. Box 358, Accord Station, Hingham, MA 02018-0358, USA
*for the UK and Ireland*: Kluwer Academic Publishers, MTP Press Limited, Falcon House, Queen Square, Lancaster LA1 1RN, UK
*for all other countries*: Kluwer Academic Publishers Group, Distribution Center, P.O. Box 322, 3300 AH Dordrecht, The Netherlands

**Library of Congress Cataloging in Publication Data**

```
Invasive cardiovascular therapy.

   (Developments in cardiovascular medicine ; 57)
   Based on the oral presentations given at an inter-
national symposium held in Cologne on 5-8 May 1985.
   Includes index.
   1. Heart--Surgery--Congresses.  2. Transluminal
angioplasty--Congresses.  3. Cardiac catheterization--
Congresses.  4. Pacemaker, Artificial (Heart)--
Congresses.  5. Heart valve prosthesis--Congresses.
I. Hilger, H. H.  II. Hombach, V. (Vinzenz)
III. Rashkind, William J.  IV. Series: Developments
in cardiovascular medicine ; v. 57.  [DNLM:
1. Angioplasty, Transluminal--congresses.  2. Cardiac
Pacing, Artificial--congresses.  3. Cardiovascular
Diseases--therapy--congresses.  4. Heart Catheteriza-
tion--congresses.  5. Heart Valve Prosthesis--
congresses.  6. Streptokinase--therapeutic use--
congresses.  W1 DE997VME v.57 / WG 166 I62 1985]
RD598.I55  1986          617'.412          86-12394
```

ISBN-13:978-94-010-8408-6     e-ISBN-13:978-94-009-4293-6
DOI: 10.1007/978-94-009-4293-6

**Copyright**

# Preface

In recent years considerable progress and new developments in diagnostic and interventional cardiology have been observed, such as balloon angioplasty of coronary artery stenoses, reperfusion techniques in acute myocardial infarction, new pacing, and cardioversion-defibrillation techniques in ventricular tachyarrhythmias. On 5–8 May, 1985, an international symposium on 'Invasive Cardiovascular Therapy' was held in Cologne, which provided a survey on the experimental and routine therapeutic measures presently available and practiced in cardiovascular medicine.

This volume is based on the oral presentations given during the symposium. In five chapters the most important traditional and new interventional techniques are discussed by experts in the field.

Chapter I contains a description of results from catheter palliation of congenital shunt disorders or relief of congenital pulmonary or aortic valve stenoses as well as the recent experience with surgical repair of single ventricle, Fallot's tetralogy and tricuspid atresia.

Chapter II presents the surgical results of valve replacement with different valve prostheses in acquired valvular disease, the surgical management of bacterial endocarditis, as well as the various techniques of partial transient left heart support devices and of cardiac transplantation.

In chapter III, the invasive management of chronic coronary heart disease, peripheral vascular disease by balloon catheter or laser techniques, and the surgical approach to coronary heart disease are discussed.

In chapter IV aspects of immediate recanalization of occluded coronary vessels by intravenous or intracoronary Streptokinase are described, and the role of the mechanical recanalization and balloon angioplasty in acute myocardial infarction is discussed, regarding patient selection, time limits and choice of treatment schedules.

In the last chapter, chapter V, the most recent developments in electrical and surgical treatment of brady- and particular tachyarrhythmias are discussed. These include the various types of pacing in bradycardias, chronic antitachycardia pacing in supraventricular tachycardias, endocardial catheter ablation in chronic drug resistant supraventricular tachyarrhythmias, chronic antitachycardia pacing in recurrent sustained ventricular tachycardias, endocardial cardioversion, automatic epicardial defibrillation, endocardial ablation and surgical stabilization in ventricular tachyarrhythmias.

Many of the techniques described have become routine measures, some are in an experimental stage and have to be further developed to improve their effectiveness and increase their safety. We do hope that this book will offer important new information to the interested reader, who either may translate this information to his daily diagnostic and therapeutic practice, or may be stimulated for further research activities when engaged in one of the particular fields described. We would like to express our sincere thanks to Mrs. A.D.E. Greeven and Mr. B.F. Commandeur for their extremely valuable assistance in publishing this book, and to Martinus Nijhoff Publishers for their high quality design and printing.

V. Hombach
H.H. Hilger
W.J. Rashkind
Cologne and Baltimore, Spring 1986

# List of contributors

Altieri, P.I.
Cardiovascular Laboratories, Medical Science Campus, University of Puerto
Rico, P.O. Box 23134, U.P.R. Station, Rio Piedras, PR 00931, U.S.A.
Co-authors: E. Defendini, J.M. Toro, H. Banchs, I. Llado

Baldwin, J.C.
Department of Cardiovascular Surgery, Stanford University School of
Medicine, Stanford, CA 94305, U.S.A.
Co-author: N.E. Shumway

Bleifeld, W.
Department of Cardiology, Medical Clinic II, University Hospital
Eppendorf, Martinistrasse 52, 2000 Hamburg 20, F.R.G.
Co-authors: D.G. Mathey, J. Schofer

Busquet, J.
Cardiological Hospital, Avenue de Magellan, F-33604 Bordeaux-Pessac,
France
Co-authors: G. Fernandez, F. Fontan

Buxton, A.E.
Clinical Electophysiology Laboratory, Hospital of the University of
Pennsylvania, Room 656A Ravdin Building, 3400 Spruce Street,
Philadelphia, PA 1910, U.S.A.
Co-authors: J.M. Miller, W.C. Hargrove, F.E. Marchlinski, J.U. Doherty,
A.H. Harken, M.E. Josephson

Camm, A.J.
Department of Cardiology, St. Bartholomew's Hospital, West Smithfield,
London ECIA 7BE, United Kingdom

Cohen, M.
  Division of Interventional Cardiology, Mount Sinai Medical Center, One
  Gustave Levy Place, New York, NY 10029, U.S.A.
  Co-author: K.P. Rentrop

Dalichau, H.
  Clinic for Cardiovascular Surgery, University of Cologne, Joseph-
  Stelzmann-Strasse 9, 5000 Cologne 41, F.R.G.
  Co-authors: H. Nigbur, J. Kalotai, A. Schmitz-Koehler

DeBakey, M.E.
  Department of Surgery, Baylor College of Medicine, 1200 Moursund Ave,
  Houston, TX 77030, U.S.A.
  Co-author: G.M. Lawrie

De Leval, M.R.
  The Hospital for Sick Children, Great Ormond Street, London WC1N 3JH,
  United Kingdom

De Vivie, E.R.
  Department of Thoracic and Cardiovascular Surgery, University of
  Goettingen, Robert-Koch-Strasse 40, 3400 Goettingen, F.R.G.
  Co-authors: H. Hartung, K. Hellberg, K. Neuhaus, W. Ruschewski, U.
  Tebbe

Effert, S.
  Department of Internal Medicine I, RWTH Aachen, Pauwelstrasse 1, 5000
  Aachen, F.R.G.
  Co-author: M. Sigmund

Erbel, R.
  Medical Clinic II, Johannes Gutenberg University, Langenbeckstrasse 1,
  6500 Mainz 1, F.R.G.
  Co-authors: T. Pop, K.J. Henrichs, K. von Olshausen, T. Meinertz, H.J.
  Rupprecht, R. Zahn, C. Steuernagel, F. Beck, J. Meyer

Evans-Bell, G.T.
  University of California, Room 312, Moffitt Hospital, School of Medicine,
  San Francisco, CA 94143, U.S.A.
  Co-authors: M.M. Scheinmann & the Executive Committee of the
  Percutaneous Cardiac mapping and Ablation Registry

Fisher, J D.
Cardiology Division, Montefiore Hospital and Medical Center, Moses
Division, Albert Einstein College of Medicine, 111 East 210th Street, Bronx,
NY 10467, U.S.A.

Fontaine, G.
Hospital Jean-Rostand, Centre of Cardiac Stimulation and Rythmology,
39–41 rue Jean le Galleu, 94200 Ivry-sur-Seine, France
Co-authors: R. Frank, J.L. Tonet, G. Farenq, Y. Grosgogeat

Gallagher, J.J.
Diagnostic Cardiology and Hemodynamics-Adult, The Sanger Clinic, P.A.,
1960 Randolph Road, Charlotte, NC 28207, U.S.A.
Co-authors: J.G. Selle, W.C. Sealy, J.M. Fedor, R.H. Svenson, S.H.
Zimmern

Hacker, R.W.
Cardiovascular Clinic, Salzburger Leite 1, 8740 Bad Neustadt/Saale, F.R.G.
Co-author: M. Torka

Hannekum, A.
Clinic for Cardiovascular Surgery, University of Cologne, Joseph-
Stelzmann-Strasse 9, 5000 Cologne 41, F.R.G.
Co-authors: G. Arnold, V. Hombach, A. Kux, B. Herse

Heger, J.
Krannert Institute of Cardiology, Department of Medicine, Indiana
University School of Medicine, 1100 West Michigan Street, Indianapolis, IN
46223, U.S.A.
Co-authors: E.N. Prystowsky, W.M. Miles, D.P. Zipes

Hilgenberg, A.
Cardiovascular Surgical Unit, Warren II, Massachusetts General Hospital,
Boston, MA 02114, U.S.A.
Co-author: W.M. Daggett

Hilger, H.H.
Medical Clinic III, Department of Cardiology, University of Cologne,
Joseph-Stelzmann-Strasse 9, 5000 Cologne 41, F.R.G.

Hombach, V.
Medical Clinic III, Department of Cardiology, University of Cologne,
Joseph-Stelzmann-Strasse 9, 5000 Cologne 41, F.R.G.
Co-authors: H.W. Hoepp, F.M. McDonald, M. Fuchs, A. Hannekum, A.
Heinen, A. Osterspey, T. Eggeling, H. Hirche, H.H. Hilger

Hugenholtz, P.G.
Thorax Center, Erasmus University Rotterdam, P.O. Box 1738, 3000 DR
Rotterdam, The Netherlands
Co-authors: P.W. Serruys, P.J. de Feyter, M. van den Brand, H.J.
Suryapranata, M. Haalebos, E. Bos

Huegel, W.
Clinic for Cardiovascular Surgery, University of Cologne, Joseph-
Stelzmann-Strasse 9, 5000 Cologne 41, F.R.G.
Co-authors: A. Hannekum, T. Peuster, V. Hombach

Klein, H.H.
Department of Cardiology, University of Goettingen, Robert-Koch-Strasse
40, 3400 Goettingen, F.R.G.
Co-author: H. Kreuzer

Klepetko, W.
Second Surgical Department, University of Vienna, Spitalgasse 23, 1090
Vienna, Austria
Co-author: E.W. Wolner

Lee, G.
Western Heart Institute, St. Mary's Hospital and Medical Center, 450
Stanyon Street, San Francisco, CA 94117, U.S.A.
Co-authors: M.C. Chan, R.M. Ikeda, D.T. Mason

Leimgruber, P.P.
Department of Medicine, Emory University School of Medicine, 1364
Clifton Road N.E., Atlanta, GA 30322, U.S.A.
Co-author: A.R. Gruentzig

Leonhard, J.
Thoracic & Cardiovascular Surgery, Suite 318, South Center, Medical
Building, West 105 Eighth Avenue, Spokane, WA 99204, U.S.A.

Lichtlen, P.R.
Division of Cardiology, Department of Medicine, Hannover Medical
School, Karl-Wiechert-Allee 9, 3000 Hannover 61, F.R.G.

Meyer, J.
Medical Clinic II, Johannes-Gutenberg University, Langenbeckstrasse 1,
6500 Mainz, F.R.G.
Co-authors: J. Erbel, H.J. Schmitz, T. Pop, K. v. Olshausen, B. Henkel,
H.J. Rupprecht, H. Kopp, S. Effert

Mirowski, M.
Coronary Care Unit, Sinai Hospital of Baltimore, The Johns Hopkins
University, Baltimore, MD 21215, U.S.A.
Co-authors: E.P. Veltri, M.M. Mower, P.R. Reid, J.M. Juanteguy

Mohl, W.
Department of Surgery, General City Hospital, Spitalgasse 23, 1000 Vienna,
Austria
Co-author: E. Wolner

Nathan, A.W.
Department of Cardiology, St. Bartholomew Hospital, West Smithfield,
London EC1A 7BE, United Kingdom

Oelert, H.
Clinic for Thoracic and Cardiovascular Surgery, Johannes-Gutenberg
University, Langenbeckstrasse 1, 6500 Mainz, F.R.G.

Peters, P.E.
Institute of Clinical Radiology, Wilhelms University of Westphalia, Albert-
Schweitzer-Strasse 33, 4400 Muenster, F.R.G.
Co-authors: V. Fiedler, J. Sciuk, A.R. Fischedick, H. Vetter

Prystowsky, E.N.
Indiana University School of Medicine, Dept. of Medicine, 1100 West
Michigan Street, Indianapolis, IN 46223, U.S.A.
Co-authors: J.R. Windle, W.M. Miles, R.F. Gilmour, B.T. Skale, D.P.
Zipes

Radley-Smith, R.C.
Thoracic and Cardiac Surgical Unit, Harefield Hospital, Harefield,
Uxbridge, Middlesex UB9 6JH, United Kingdom
Co-author: M.H. Yacoub

Rashkind, W.J.
Cardiovascular Laboratories, The Children's Hospital of Philadelphia, One
Children's Center, 34th Street and Civic Center Bvd, Philadelphia, PA
19104, U.S.A.

Roth, F.J.
Department of Radiology, Aggertal Clinic, 5250 Engelskirchen, F.R.G.
Co-authors: P. Berliner, W. Krings, I. Schmidtke, B. Koppers, B. Gruen

Rupprath, G.
Department of Pediatric Cardiology, University of Goettingen, Waldweg
33, 3400 Goettingen, F.R.G.
Co-author: K.L. Neuhaus

Schroeder, R.
Department of Cardiology and Pneumology, Steglitz Clinic, Free University
of Berlin, Hindenburgdamm 30, 1000 Berlin, F.R.G.

Schwarz, F.
Internal Medicine Clinic III, Department of Cardiology, University of
Heidelberg, Bergheimerstrasse 58, 6900 Heidelberg 1, F.R.G.
Co-authors: H.C. Mehmel, G. Schueler, M. Hofmann, J. Manthey, W.
Kuebler

Sievert, H.
Center of Internal Medicine, Department of Cardiology, University Clinic,
Theodor-Stern-Kai 7, 6000 Frankfurt/Mainz 70, F.R.G.
Co-authors: W.D. Bussmann, M. Kaltenbach

Steinbach, K.
Medical Department III (Cardiology), Wilhelminen Hospital, Laudongasse
20, 1080 Vienna, Austria
Co-author: G. Joskowicz

Tauchert, M.
Medical Clinic I, Municipal Hospital, Leverkusen, Dhuennberg 60, 5090
Leverkusen, F.R.G.
Co-authors: A. Gaczkowski, H. Borberg, K. Oette, W. Stoffel

Van de Loo, J.C.W.
Department of Internal Medicine, Wilhelms University of Westphalia,
Albert Schweitzer-Strasse 33, 4400 Münster, F.R.G.

Von Essen, R.
Stiftsklinikum Augustinum, Stiftsbogen 74, 8000 München 70, F.R.G.
Co-authors: R. Uebis, B. Bertram, S. Effert, B. Vondenbusch, J. Silny, G. Rau

Winter, U.J.
Medical Clinic III, Department of Cardiology, University of Cologne, Joseph-Stelzmann-Strasse 9, 5000 Cologne 41, F.R.G.
Co-authors: D.W. Behrenbeck, M. Hoeher, Th. Brill, H. Ebeling, H.J. Hirche, H.H. Hilger

Wirtzfeld, A.
Medical Clinic I, 'Rechts der Isar', Munich Technical University, Ismaningerstrasse 22, 8000 Munich 80, F.R.G.
Co-authors: G. Schmidt, K. Stangl

# Table of contents

# I. Congenital malformations

# Balloon catheter procedures in congenital heart disease

W.J. RASHKIND

## Introduction

Cardiac catheterization has only achieved widespread use in man in the last thirty years. The first attempt on a human subject was described in 1833, by J.F. Dieffenbach. From animal experimentation he learned that the introduction of foreign bodies into the large vessels and the heart 'was tolerated in a wonderful way'. He added that it was known that the external surface of the heart possessed a certain degree of insensibility to mechanical stimuli and that 'this was the case to a certain extent with its interior walls'. Based on the theory that cholera sufferers accumulated blood in the heart, thus emptying the periphery and overloading the heart; Dieffenbach attempted his first human cardiac catheterization in an effort to remove this 'extra blood'. 'In an almost dying patient, I opened . . . the brachial artery in its upper third. As not a drop of blood flowed, I introduced, as I had planned, an elastic catheter into the vessel approximately as far as the heart. No blood appeared through the catheter. The heart became clearer and more rapid, and I now withdrew the catheter . . . It is greatly to be regretted that this operation of interest for all physiology was performed on a man who was so near to death and who shortly afterwards was seized by convulsions and rendered up his soul.' His pioneering in human cardiac catheterization should not be downgraded because his theories were misguided [1].

Although his studies were the first, there is serious doubt as to whether he actually reached the heart. The same criticism applies to the studies of Bleich-roeder, Unger, and Loeb, who published descriptions of experiments performed in 1922 on animals and humans using catheterization techniques. Unger and Loeb catheterized Bleichroeder and reached the axillary vein and the inferior vena cava. During one such attempt, Bleichroeder complained of a stabbing pain in his chest, suggesting that the heart *may* have been reached [2]. None of these earlier studies should in any way detract credit for priority, courage, and significance from Forssmann's studies on himself, reported in 1929 as 'Catheterization of the Right Heart', for he clearly was the first to *document* catheterization of the right

4

heart in humans [3]. Cournand and his colleagues Richards, Ranges, and Riley, in a series of papers in the early 1940's put cardiac catheterization on the map. Cournand's studies with Baldwin and Himmelstein culminated in their volume, *Cardiac Catheterization in Congenital Heart Disease* [4]. The method soon achieved widespread use for physiologic studies in man and for making precise anatomical and physiologic analyses of congenital heart defects.

**Therapeutic use of cardiac catheters**

Rubeo-Alvarez and Limon-Lason (1950) described a cardiac catheter method to treat pulmonic stenosis. No subsequent reports have ever been published by them [5]. In 1966, we reported a method for balloon atrioseptostomy, a technique that has had wide and continued application since that time [6]. Subsequently, several procedures have been developed to expand the role of balloon tipped cardiac catheters as therapeutic instruments.

*Balloon atrioseptostomy*

Infants with certain congenital cardiac defects require the presence of an atrial septal defect to survive. The first balloon atrial septostomy was performed at The Children's Hospital of Philadelphia in 1965. This report summarizes the 15 year experience with balloon atrioseptostomy in over 300 children with certain congenital heart lesions at that institution.

A special balloon-tipped catheter is used for the procedure. Initially, a double-lumen catheter was used to assist in localization of the balloon in the left atrium. However, the widespread availability of biplane fluoroscopy, has obviated the need for a second lumen. The current equipment, therefore, is a single-lumen balloon-tipped catheter, generally 4.5 F to 6 F, which can be introduced via a 6 F sheath. Cardiac catheterization is performed in the usual manner to achieve a complete diagnosis. After the diagnosis has been established, the balloon-tipped catheter is passed via the sheath into the inferior vena cava, to the right atrium, across the foramen ovale into the left atrium. The balloon is slowly dilated with dilute radio-opaque material. If the balloon happens to be in a pulmonary vein, slow dilatation will result in the balloon being extruded to lie free in the left atrial chamber. Once certain that the catheter tip is in the left atrium, the balloon is inflated to a volume of approximately 2 ml, or to a diameter of approximately 15 mm. At this point, the catheter is vigorously jerked through the atrial septum into the right atrium, being careful not to wedge it into the inferior cava. It is allowed to float free in the right atrial chamber while the balloon is deflated.

From May 1965 through April 1980, 307 patients have been treated by the balloon atrioseptostomy technique at The Children's Hospital of Philadelphia.

This report describes the follow-up data on the first 300 of these patients. The most frequent lesion for which this method was used was d-Transposition of the Great Arteries. There were 186 patients (62%) whose primary diagnosis was transposition. Seventy-four (40%) had isolated d-TGA (included in this group were patients with hemodynamically insignificant ventricular septal defect or patent ductus, and patients with mild pulmonic stenosis with peak left ventricular to pulmonary artery systolic gradient of under 35 mm Hg), thirty (16%) had ventricular septal defects, and 14 (7%) had ventricular septal defect and pulmonic stenosis. In addition, 30 (10%) had d-TGA associated with extremely complex additional cardiovascular anomalies. On the remaining patients, the distribution by lesions was as follows: pulmonary atresia with intact ventricular septum, 32 patients (11%); total anomalous pulmonary venous return, 31 patients (10%); tricuspid atresia, 28 patients (10%); left ventricular hypoplasia complexes, 16 patients (5%); and there were 5 patients (2%) with a variety of other congenital cardiac defects.

In the following description of the results of the use of this technique, the term effective palliation rate is defined as the rate of survival from the first admission to the present time or to *elective* surgical correction. In the group of transposition patients classified as isolated, and in the group with ventricular septal defect, 86% were discharged improved from their first admission, and 72% had effective palliation. (The long term results of corrective surgery for these patients is beyond the scope of this report.) The presence of hemodynamically significant patent ductus arteriosus, with or without a coexisting ventricular septal defect, was generally lethal. In the nontransposition group of patients, the best effective palliation rate was obtained in tricuspid atresia. Eighty percent of those patients were long term survivors: all had additional treatment consisting of some type of aortic-pulmonary shunting. Three of that group died from left ventricular failure ten years or more after initial palliation. In those patients with pulmonary atresia and intact ventricular septum, and in those with total anomalous pulmonary venous return, the effective palliation rate was approximately 60%. Many patients were successfully palliated for long enough periods of time to facilitate total surgical correction.

Generally, the atrial septum is paper thin and balloon atrioseptostomy may be performed easily. Occasionally, the atrial septum is too thick to permit production of an adequate atrial defect with a balloon catheter. Park [7] has reported excellent results in such patients with a retractable blade catheter. We have employed his technique on a few patients with satisfactory results. The largest group of patients for whom balloon atrioseptostomy will continue to be used is transposition of the great arteries. We have made some interesting ancillary observations about transposition in the past 15 years. There has been a striking change in the clinical profile of the infant presenting to us with transposition. In the first five years of septostomy, only half of the patients appeared in the first week of life. In the last five years, almost *all* have appeared in the first week of life. Indeed, whereas only 13% arrived on the first day of life in the first five years, now nearly 70% are seen within the first 24 hours of life. We have also noticed a striking change in the occurrence of sub-pulmonic stenosis. In the first five years, less than 30% of the patients developed this complication. This has increased to an incidence of 62% in the most recent five year period. In the last five years, 70% of the infants ballooned within the first 24 hours of life acquired pulmonic stenosis, many within the first few months after septostomy. Fortunately, our management of these patients currently is facilitated by the fact that Mustard's operation can be performed successfully in early infancy. Another observation of interest about transposition was made in our laboratory by Dennis Wood. If one makes a short axial cut across the heart in the normal infant, the cavity of the anterior right ventricle has the shape of a banana, and the cavity of the postorior left ventricle has the shape of a grapefruit. In transposition, the situation is reversed, and the anterior right ventricle has the shape of the grapefruit and the posterior left ventricle, the shape of a banana. This is well demonstrated on a short axis two-dimensional echocardiogram. The grapefruit-banana shape relationship is sustained after Mustard's operation and provides an interesting comment on the biological adaptability of human tissue. Moreover, it offers encouragement regarding the ability of the modified right ventricle to function as a systemic ventricle for a long period of time.

As alternative approach to venous switching for infants with transposition of the great arteries, is arterial switching. If this can be performed successfully in early infancy, the problems described above may be obviated. In calendar year 1984, Dr. William Norwood performed arterial switching in eighteen infants at The Children's Hospital of Philadelphia, without mortality. Fifteen of them were less than two weeks of age, and eleven of the fifteen were younger than one week of age. Eight of the patients had hemodynamically significant ventricular septal defects which were closed at the time of surgery. The current management sequence at this institution is immediate diagnosis by echocardiography, palliation by balloon atrioseptostomy, clinical medical stabilization with or without the use of prostaglandins for eight to twenty-four hours, followed by the arterial switch operation.

Balloon atrioseptostomy has proved its worth in the palliation of many infants with life-threatening cardiac lesions. The technique has been successfully employed, worldwide. The major benefit has been to change the infant mortality rate in transposition of the great arteries from 90% death rate to nearly 90% survival rate.

*Balloon valvoplasty and angioplasty*

The principal current usage for these procedures in pediatrics is for dilation of pulmonic valve stenosis, re-coarctation of the aorta, and peripheral pulmonary artery stenosis. In addition, there have been recent reports of successful aortic valvoplasty [8], dilation of unoperated coarctation of the aorta [9], dilation of certain types of venous obstruction [10], and dilation of mitral stenosis [11].

*Pulmonic stenosis*
Kan et al [12] reported the experimental basis for balloon valvoplasty for pulmonary valve stenosis. They also reported [13, 14] early clinical trials, with very encouraging results. Other groups have performed the procedure, and have described favorable results. In a recent survey, over 300 pulmonic stenosis dilatation procedures were reviewed. Early analysis of this data confirms the safety and efficacy of this technique.

*Coarctation of the aorta*
Sos et al [15] suggested application of the balloon angioplasty technique to the discreet type of coarctation of the aorta, and tested it on postmortem specimens. Lock et al extended Sos' work to excised Ao coarctation from 6 children who underwent resections and reanastomosis. Dilatation was attempted within 2 hrs of resection using a Gruntzig polyvinyl chloride catheter [16]. Encouraged by their data on specimens, they created an animal model of coarctation, and were successful in dilatating these in vivo [17]. They and several other authors have found the method to be most helpful in patients with recurrent coarctation of the aorta. Lock suggests high inflation pressures are necessary, using a balloon with a maximum diameter up to 1.5 times the diameter of the aorta proximal to the coarctation.

*Peripheral pulmonic stenosis and hypoplastic pulmonary arteries*
Lock and associates have described the experimental approach to this problem. They created an animal model in the newborn lamb, and achieved good results in

*Table 1.*

| Lesion | # | Complications |
|---|---|---|
| Pulmonic stenosis | 300 | 1 death |
| Coarctation of aorta, recurrent | 120 | 3 deaths |
| | | 3 cerebro-vascular accidents |
| Coarctation of aorta, unoperated | 60 | 4 deaths |
| | | 1 cerebro-vascular accident |
| Peripheral pulmonic stenosis | 150 | 2 deaths |
| Aortic stenosis | 45 | ? aortic insufficiency |

dilating branch stenoses [18]. They have also reported early clinical trials [19] with satisfactory initial results. In addition, they have had some intriguing success in dilating hypoplastic pulmonary arteries. Some of the vessels they have succeeded in dilating are beyong the hilum of the lung, and, thus, inaccessible by surgery. This offers some hope to children who currently are labeled as inoperable.

## *Children's Hospital of Philadelphia experience*

Thirty-three procedures have been performed on thirty patients. There were fifteen patients with pulmonic stenosis; the only failures were in very small infants in whom access to the pulmonary artery was not possible with the current equipment. Six patients with recurrence of coarctation were all treated successfully. In addition, four patients with previously untreated coarctation were dilated in the operating room. The dilating catheter was introduced via a pursestring incision in the thoracic descending aorta. Inflation of the balloon was achieved under direct inspection and palpation. All four procedures were successful. Two attempts at dilating stenotic right ventricle to pulmonary artery valve conduits resulted in relief of obstruction, but increased conduit valve insufficiency. Two patients with post-Mustard caval obstruction (one superior vena cava and one inferior vena cava) had successful relief of these narrowings. The superior vena cava obstruction was complete, but a track could be made with a guidewire, over which the dilating catheter was passed. Sufficient dilation was achieved to abolish the pressure gradient, and to permit transvenous pacemaker implantation. Two of three patients with peripheral pulmonic stenosis were treated successfully. A single patient with a narrowed Blalock-Taussig shunt failed to respond to this therapy.

## Summary

Cardiac catheterization has proved its value as a major tool in the diagnosis of congenital cardiac defects. The advent of non-invasive imaging of various sorts has altered the role of diagnostic catheterization. Within the past two decades balloon tipped cardiac catheters of various types have been used to provide therapy for many lesions. Improvements in design and methods will expand the use of therapeutic catheterization. It is inevitable that better results will be obtained for those defects currently being treated that way, and that the method will be applied to other conditions.

# References

1. Dieffenbach JF (1832) Physiologisch-Chirurgisch Beobachtigen die Cholera-Kranken. Cholera Arch 1: 86–105
2. Bleichroeder F, Unger E, Loeb W (1912) Intraarterielle Therapie. Klin Wochenschr 49: 1502
3. Forssman WTO (1929) Die Sondierung des rechten Herzens. Klin Wochenschr 8: 2085–2087
4. Cournand A, Baldwin JS, Himmelstein A (1949) Cardiac Catheterization in Congenital Heart Disease. New York: The Commonwealth Fund
5. Rubeo-Alvarez V, Limon-Lason R (1950) Treatment of Pulmonary Valvular Stenosis and Tricuspid Stenosis with a Modified Cardiac Catheter. Proc First National Conference on Cardiovascular Disease, Washington, D.C.
6. Rashkind WJ, Miller WW (1966) Creation of an atrial septal defect without thoracotomy. JAMA 196: 991–992
7. Park SC et al (1978) Clinical use of blade atrial septostomy. Circulation 58: 600–606
8. Lababidi Z, Jiunn-Ren W, Walls JT (1983) Percutaneous balloon aortic valvuloplasty: Results in 23 patients. Am J Cardiol 53: 194–197
9. Cooper RS, Ritter SB, Golinko RJ (1984) Balloon dilatation angioplasty: nonsurgical management of coarctation of the aorta. Circulation 70: 903–907
10. Lock JE et al (1984) Dilation angioplasty of congenital or operative narrowings of venous channels. Circulation 70: 457–464
11. Inoue K et al (1984) Clinical application of transvenous mitral commissurotomy by a new balloon catheter. J Thorac Cardiovasc Surg 87: 394–402
12. Kan JS, Anderson JH, White RI Jr (Oct. 1982) Experimental basis for balloon valvuloplasty of congenital pulmonary valvular stenosis. Proc Sect Cardiol Amer Acad Ped, New York, p. 101A
13. Kan JS, White RI Jr, Mitchell SE, Gardner TJ (1982) Percutaneous balloon valvuloplasty: A new method for treating congenital pulmonary valve stenosis. New England J Med 307: 540
14. Kan JS, White RI, Mitchell SE, Gardner TJ (1983) Transluminal balloon valvuloplasty for the treatment of congenital pulmonary valve stenosis. J Am Coll Cardiol 2: 588
15. Sos T, Sniderman KW, Rettek-Sos B, Strupp A, Alonso DR (1979) Percutaneous transluminal dilatation of coarctation of thoracic aorta post mortem. Lancet 2: 970
16. Lock JE, Castaneda-Zuniga WR, Bass JF, Fcker JE, Amplatz K, Anderson RW (1982) Balloon dilatation of excised aortic coarctation. Radiology 143: 689
17. Lock JE, Niemi T, Burke BA, Einzig S, Castaneda-Zuniga WR (1982) Transcutaneous angioplasty of experimental aortic coarctation. Circulation 66: 1280
18. Lock JE, Neimi BA, Einzig S, Amplatz K, Burke B, Bass JL (1981) Transvenous Angioplasty of Experimental Branch Pulmonary Artery Stenosis in Newborn Lambs. Circulation 64, No. 5, 886–893
19. Lock JE, Castaneda-Zuniga WF, Fuhrman BP, Bass JL (1983) Balloon Dilation angioplasty of hypoplastic and stenotic pulmonary arteries. J Am Coll Cardiol 2: 588
20. Stanger P, Personal Communication

# Balloon angioplasty in congenital heart disease

G. RUPPRATH and K.L. NEUHAUS

## Introduction

Successful transluminal recanalisation of arteriosclerotic obstructions using large dilating catheters was reported in 1964 by Dotter and Judkins [1]. The method was extended by Grüntzig to transluminal dilation by a double-lumen catheter with a non-elastic balloon [2, 3]. In congenital cardiac malformations there have been recent reports of angioplasty for coarctation [8–15] and recoarctation [18], peripheral pulmonary arterial stenosis [20–22], pulmonary venous obstruction [23–25], superior vena cava [26, 27, 29] or baffle obstruction [28] and stenosis of a Blalock-Taussig-shunt [30–32]. Balloon dilatation technique has also been applied in patients with pulmonary [33–37, 40] and aortic valve stenosis [38–41].

## Coarctation of the aorta

Dilation of coarctation was attempted by Sos in 1979 in a postmortem specimen on a newborn with coarctation and hypoplastic left heart syndrome [4]. Experimental studies by Lock in 1982 [5] demonstrated the feasibility of balloon dilation in excised segments of coarctations. With a Grüntzig balloon catheter he achieved in vitro a significant increase of the diameter of the stenotic aorta at pressures up to 8 athmospheres. Intimal, medial and transmedial tears were observed without rupture of the aortic wall. In experimental studies on an animal model with surgically created aortic coarctation, dilation was successfully performed [6, 7]. By stretching the narrow segment, intimal and medial tears occurred without early or late aneurysm formation despite medial thinning of the aorta in two lambs [6]. The best hemodynamic results were achieved with balloons twice to three times the diameter of the coarctation. In Table 1 results and complications of balloon angioplasty (BA) in coarctation are reviewed. In 20 of the patients dilation was performed within the first year of life (Table 2), the risk appears to be higher in this age group than in childhood or adolescence. One death reported by

Finley [9] occurred when the catheter was exchanged without the use of a wire causing perforation of the aortic wall within the dilated segment at the site of the ductus origin. The 7-year old patient reported by Kan [18] died 6 hours after an uncomplicated angioplasty probably by a vagal event. One infant died following resection after an unsuccessfull dilation of a coarctation and banding of the pulmonary artery for complex heart disease [8], and another infant in the series by Suarez De Lezo [11] of unknown reasons. It is not mentioned whether a post-mortem study had been performed.

*Table 1.* Summary of the already published experience with balloon angioplasty in coarctation and recoarctation; 16 out of 60 patients had evidence of restenosis at follow-up. Grad = systolic gradient. Results of balloon angioplasty in coarctation.

| Study and year | No. of pts | Age | Previous surgery | Early good (pts) | Complications (pts) | Restenosis (Grad >20 mmHg) |
|---|---|---|---|---|---|---|
| Singer [15] (1982) | 1 | 7 w | 1 | 1 | 0 | 0 |
| Sperling [8] (1983) | 2 | 3 w–1 yr | 0 | 2 | 0 | 1 |
| Lock [10] (1983) | 8 | 1 w–22 yr | 5 | 4 | 1 death | 5 |
| Finley [9] (1983) | 4 | 2 w–3 mo | 1 | 3 | 1 death | 3 |
| Suarez [11] (1984) | 6 | 2 w–7 w | 0 | 4 | 1 death | 1 |
| Lababidi [12] (1984) | 27 | 1 w–27 yr | 7 | 24 | 0 | 5 |
| Cooper [14] (1984) | 5 | 1 yr–17 yr | 0 | 5 | 0 | 0 |
| Kan [18] (1983) | 7 | 10 mo–17 yr | 7 | 6 | 1 death | 1 |
| Total | 60 | | 21 | 49 | 4 (±) | 16 |

*Table 2.* The reported incidence of restenosis (see Table 1) is higher in infancy than in childhood. Early results of balloon dilation seem to be better in recoarctation than in native stenosis. Results of balloon angioplasty (BA) in coarctation.

| | | Total no. | Restenosis No. (%) | Early death BA related | Early death Unknown reason |
|---|---|---|---|---|---|
| Infants | Primary dilation | 17 | 12 (71%) | 1 | 2 |
| | Previous surgery | 3 | 1 (33%) | 0 | 0 |
| Children/Adults | Primary dilation | 22 | 3 (14%) | 0 | 0 |
| | Previous surgery | 18 | 1 ( 6%) | 0 | 1 |

*Results*

The reported early results were satisfactory (Table 1) especially in older children and in patients with restenosis (Table 2). Recoarctation was observed in the majority of infants with a higher risk than older patients. Success depends on the type of coarctation and the presence of additional malformations. Especially long segment coarctations and forms with a tubular hypoplasia are less suitable for angioplasty. Perhaps the different results are related to different types of obstructions.

Recently Pellegrino and coworkers have analysed in an anatomopathological study 42 specimens of coarctation with respect to a possible treatment by operation or dilation. They concluded, that only 22 of 42 coarctations would have been suitable for a transluminal angioplasty.

*Conclusion*

Angioplasty of coarctation in children older than 1 year and in patients with recoarctation appears to be an alternative method to operation. In infant coarctation early results are unsatisfactory and dilation should only be performed as a palliative procedure in the presence of a favourable anatomy and a high operative risk. It should be kept in mind that angioplasty works by producing a disruption of the intima and parts of the media. The larger the balloon, the better the gradient relief but the higher the chances of complete vascular disruption [16]. Formation of a pseudoaneurysm following BA war recently reported [17]. It is well known, that years after patch aortoplasty for coarctation aneurysms may develop [53]. Due to the unknown and potentially fatal late complications we would not recommend witespread use of balloon angioplasty. Further investigations and follow-up data over a longer period are required.

**Peripheral pulmonary arterial stenosis**

Peripheral pulmonary stenosis may occure as a congenital (single or multiple) or aquired lesion, frequently following an aorto-pulmonary shunt operation. Surgical treatment is difficult and often ineffective or impossible. Lock [19] described the feasability of dilating stenotic pulmonary arteries in an experimental animal model. He observed an average reduction of the gradient of 79% and an increase in vessel diameter of 63%. The clinical results were not as favourable as the experimental ones. Lock [19] reported successful dilation of peripheral pulmonary stenosis in 5 of 7 patients and Rocchini [21] in 5 of 13 patients with a satisfactory relief of the obstruction. In 4 patients the stenosis was not dilatable and in the case of 4 additional children it could not be performed. He reported one nonfatal perforation of the pulmonary artery. The balloon size was 3 to 4 times the diameter of the stenosis and the filling pressure of 4–6 athmospheres was maintained for 30 seconds.

Recently the morphologic changes of dilated pulmonary arteries were described in detail by Edwards [22]. Intimal and medial tears were present in all 7 cases extending in 5 of them through the adventitia. The adventitia remained intact. The transmedial tear resulted in a gap that represented up to 25% of the wall circumference being responsible for the increase of the internal diameter. The intimal and medial tears had healed by the deposits of collagen and elastic fibers.

*Conclusion*

Balloon angioplasty of peripheral pulmonary arterial stenosis offers an alternative method of treatment in patients in whom traditional operative management is usually unsuccessful. Perforation of the pulmonary artery may occure especially when the inflated balloon ruptures. Dilation should be performed only with operative stand by. More experience and follow-up data are needed in order to define the advantages and limitations of this procedure.

**Pulmonary venous obstruction**

Results of medical or surgical treatment of pulmonary venous stenosis are poor. BA has been attempted so far in 7 patients [23–26]. Relief of obstruction was only transient and all patients died later on. These limited data suggest BA is not an effective treatment for this lesion.

**Superior vena cava or baffle obstruction**

The reports concerning the use of BA in superior vena cava obstruction indicated initial hemodynamic and symptomatic improvement [26, 27, 29]. The patient reported by Rocchini [26, 27] exhibited restenosis later on and died 14 hours after BA during the insertion of a venous catheter. At autopsy there was no evidence of perforation or hemorrhage. Lock [29] recently described early good results in 5 patients with caval obstruction following repair of transposition of the great arteries. The patient with mid-cavity baffle obstruction treated by Waldman [28] exhibited restenosis later on. Whether dilation will be an important alternative to surgical repair in this entity remains to be seen.

14

## Stenotic Blalock-Taussig shunts

Unsatisfactory results following BA for stenotic Blalock-Taussig shunts have been reported by Fellows and coworkers [30]. In 7 dilating procedures there was no success in 3 cases, unknown success in further 3 and an early good result in only 1 patient. They observed partial dissection of the right pulmonary artery in 1 patient perhaps induced by the guidewire. Recently, Fischer performed BA in 1 patient with incorrectable heart malformation with good relief of the obstruction.

We have limited experience with 4 dilations of a stenotic Blalock-Taussig shunt in 3 patients aged 10 to 14 years [31]. Two of them had dextrocardia with complex incorrectable cyanotic heart disease. In the first patient a 4.3 F steerable Grüntzig coronary dilation catheter* with a 4.2 mm balloon was passed over a 0.014" guidewire* across the stenotic segment. The balloon diameter was 2.5 times the diameter of the stenosis. 4 dilations with a pressure of 6 atmospheres were performed each time for 1 minute without complications. Oxygen saturation increased from 80% to 84% and the continous murmur from 1/6 to 3/6 grade. 10 months later the patient is still in a better clinical condition than before BA.

In 2 additional patients catheterization was performed percutaneously from the right femorals vein. The ascending aorta was reached over the outlet foramen of a single ventricle or through the VSD. A long guide sheath* with a Judkins curvature for the right or left coronary artery facilitated the passage of the Grüntzig dilation catheter into the left or right Blalock-Taussig anastomosis. The dilation catheter was advanced through the stenotic segment over a 0.014" guidewire with a long flexible tip. These thin wires allow the passage through severely stenotic regions and are nearly atraumatic. In one of the children oxygen saturation increased from 73% to 80% whereas in the other child the saturation remained unchanged at 80%. There was still a 50% stenosis at the anastomotic site.

## Conclusion

In patients with cyanotic heart disease being dependent upon the function of a Blalock-Taussig shunt stenosis at the anastomotic site may be dilatable. Early results are satisfactory but follow-up data remain discordant. The use of coronary dilation catheters and guidewires facilitates the passage across the stenosis [31]. The ideal size of the balloon, either 2–3 times the diameter of the stenosis [20] or 2 mm larger than the vessel [32] remains to be determined.

* Schneider Medintag, Zürich

**Valvar pulmonary stenosis**

The first successful balloon valvuloplasty (BVP) of a stenotic pulmonary valve was reported by Kan 1982 [33]. Table 3 summarizes the experience with BVP in this lesion. There have been no serious complications so far.

*Technique of valvuloplasty*

The diameter of the pulmonary valve annulus is determined by 2d-echo and right ventricular angiography. The ideal balloon size is still in question, a diameter equal to the annulus [36, 37], 1 mm larger [36] or smaller [35, 40] is recommended. We have used diameters equal to or 1 mm smaller than the valve ring. Over a previously advanced guidewire which is left in place in the left pulmonary artery the balloon catheter is passed across the stenotic valve and rapidly inflated and deflated with pressures of 3 to 5 atmospheres. Under continous fluoroscopic monotoring the waist of the balloon produced by the narrow valve should disappear and the balloon should be kept within the valve annulus. A balloon length of 3 cm is sufficient, a larger one leads to longer inflation-deflation times. A significant infundibular stenosis may cause balloon fixation and retraction of the balloon into the right ventricle during systole thereby producing avulsive forces to the cusps [40]. The relief of valvar pulmonary stenosis by BVP can occur from commissural splitting, cusptearing and avulsion of a cusp [40]. In our limited experience we have not observed any complications during or following this procedure (Table 3).

*Table 3*. In 68 patients reported in the literature an average pressure gradient of 85 mmHg between right ventricle and pulmonary artery was reduced to approximately 31 mmHg by balloon valvuloplasty.
Results of balloon pulmonary valvuloplasty (BVP).

| Study and year | No. of pts | Age (years) | PSG Pre BVP mmHg | Post BVP mmHg | Follow up No. of pts | PSG mmHg |
|---|---|---|---|---|---|---|
| Kan [33] (1982) | (1) | 8 | 48 | 14 | (1) | 20 |
| Kan [36] (1984) | 18 | 0.5–56 | 68 ± 27 | 23 ± 8 | 9 | 22 ± 5 |
| Pepine [34]1 (1982) | 1 | 59 | 140 | 32 | 1 | 38 |
| Lababidi [35] (1983) | (18) | 0.9–19 | 81 ± 31 | 23 ± 11 | – | – |
| Walls, Lababidi et al [40] (1984) | 33 | 0.9–19 | 85 ± 35 | 27 ± 15 | 11 | 23 ± 12 |
| Rocchini [26] (1984) | 13 | 0.5–9 | 83 ± 21 | 43 ± 12 | 7 | 29 ± 10 |
| Our series (1985) | 3 | 0.2–50 | 102 ± 43 | 48 ± 10 | 1 | 25 |
| Total | 68 | | 85 | 31 | 29 | |

**Critical pulmonary valve stenosis**

BVP in critical pulmonary valve stenosis has not been described previously. SEMB 1979 reported an attempt to treat a valvular pulmonary stenosis in a 2-day-old newborn withdrawing a $CO_2$-filled 5 F Berman angiocardiographic balloon catheter from the main pulmonary artery into the right ventricle. The infant was in cardiac failure due to massive tricuspid insufficiency and had a transvalvular gradient of 20 mmHg prior to balloon valvulotomy; the gradient fell to 6 mmHg and the child's condition improved rapidly.

We have successfully performed BVP on a 2-month-old infant with critical pulmonary valve stenosis, intact ventricular septum hypoplastic right ventricle, tricuspid insufficiency, right-to-left shunt on atrial level and persistent ductus arteriosus (Figure 1). At the age of 6 weeks a first attempt to dilate the stenotic pulmonary valve failed. A 0.014′ guidewire was passed into the main pulmonary artery but the Grüntzig coronary dilation catheter could not be advanced over the guidewire. At a second attempt 2 weeks later the pressure in the right ventricle had increased from 120 to 160 mmHg (left ventricle pressure 85 mmHg) and we could now advance a 0.014′ wire into the right pulmonary artery and subsequently pass a 4.3 F Grüntzig dilation catheter with a 3.7 mm balloon diameter across the stenotic valve. Pulmonary valve annulus was 5 mm in diamter. 6 dilations, each one lasting 30 seconds with pressures up to 8 atmospheres were performed without any complications or evidence of premature beats. Subsequently the previous catheter was replaced by a 4.3 F Grüntzig catheter with a 4.2 mm balloon diameter and a balloon length of 2 cm. During valvuloplasty pulmonary perfusion was maintained by the patent ductus. E-type prostaglandins were not required.

The pressure gradient decreased from 140 to 60 mmHg, systemic oxygen saturation increased from 56% to 74% and the child's condition improved markedly. During the following days the continuous murmur of the ductus disappeared without deterioration of the clinical status. Dopplerechocardiographic investigation disclosed no flow through the ductus.

From this limited experience we presume that BVP may become an alternative method of treatment to operation. Coles [52] has recently reviewed the risk of different operative procedures in 36 infants with critical pulmonary stenosis. Overall operative mortality within the first month of life was 42%. Perioperative administration of $PGE_1$ resulted in a significant improvement of early survival. According to these observations we would recommend $PGE_1$ therapy if necessary pre, during and post BVP. If the pulmonary blood flow does not improve following BVP $PGE_1$ infusion should be continued until a systemic-pulmonary shunt is accomplished.

17

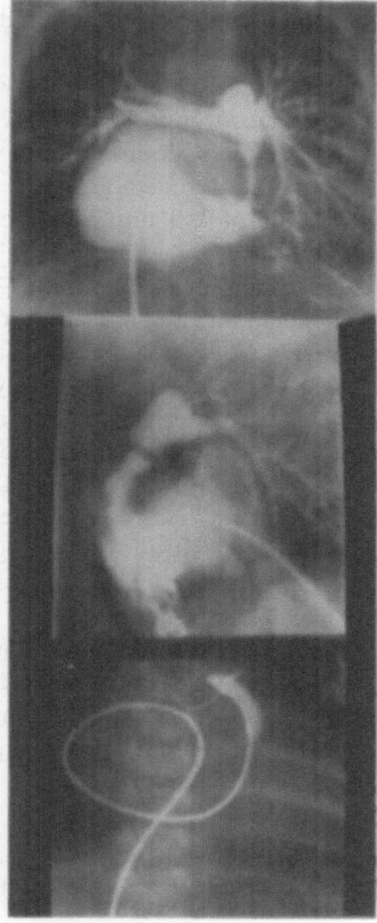

*Figure 1.* Right ventricular angiogram in a 30° sitting-up position in a 2-month-old infant with severe valvar pulmonary stenosis, hypoplastic right ventricle and tricuspid insufficiency (A and B). Dilating of the pulmonary valve with 4.2 mm balloon (C) resulted in a decrease of the pressure gradient from 140 to 60 mmHg.

## Aortic valve stenosis

Lababidi and coworkers reported 1984 successful BVP in aortic valve stenosis in 23 children and adolescents aged 2–19 years, the number of patients increased in the meantime up to 27 [40]. The peak systolic gradient decreased from 108 ± 40 to 32 ± 16 mmHg following BVP. They observed no serious complications; mild aortic incompetence developed in 7 and moderate in 1 patient. In 10 patients a previous mild aortic regurgitation remained unchanged [40]. Hemodynamic follow-up in 14 patients revealed an average residual gradient of $37 \pm 29$ mmHg [40].

BVP in critical aortic stenosis was attempted recently by Waller [39] on a 2-day-old infant. The gradient decreased from 70 to 40 mmHg without improvement of the clinical condition. During BVP the balloon ruptured without evidence of an aortic damage. The child was operated some hours later and died after 2 days.

We reported recently early results of BVP during infancy [41]. In the meantime we have performed BVP on 4 infants and 3 adolescents (Table 4) with good early results (Table 5). Recatheterization in the 4 infants 4 to 7 month later revealed nearly the same residual gradient in 2 and a significant restenosis in the remaining 2 infants (patient No. 2 and 3; Table 5). On patient No. 2 a commissurotomy was performed at the age of 2 weeks. The child improved only slightly and remained in severe cardiac insufficiency. A recatheterization at the age of 8 weeks revealed significant restenosis (Table 5). We performed BVP despite the previous operation and the gradient decreased from 75 to 28 mmHg. This child had poor left ventricular function due to endocardial fibrosis (Table 4) but her condition improved in the weeks following BVP. Restudy at the age of 9 months showed significant restenosis with normal left ventricular function. After a second BVP the gradient decreased only from 80 to 60 mmHg.

In the second patient with significant restenosis following BVP the balloon diameter had been 3 mm smaller than the aortic annulus and this may have been responsible for the residual gradient. Despite this, the clinical condition had been improved by the first BVP and the repeated BVP at the age of 7 months reduced the gradient from 70 to 40 mmHg.

*Table 4.* Clinical data of the infants and adolescents having had balloon valvuloplasty for aortic valve stenosis (AS). AVA = aortic valve annulus diameter; CoA = coarctation of the aorta; PDA = persistent ductus arteriosus.

| Pt | Age (weeks) | Weight (kg) | Diagnosis | Associated lesions |
|---|---|---|---|---|
| 1 | 4 | 2.6 | Valvular AS Narrow AVA | Mitral hypoplasia, preductal CoA PDA with R-L-shunt, pulmonary hypertension |
| 2 | 8 | 3.6 | Valvular AS Narrow AVA | Endocardial fibrosis, mitral hypoplasia PDA with R-L-shunt, pulmonary hypertension |
| 3 | 6 | 4.0 | Valvular AS | – |
| 4 | 1 (years) | 3.0 | Valvular AS | PDA |
| 5 | 13 | 48 | Valvular AS | – |
| 6 | 17 | 65 | Valvular AS Narrow AVA | – |
| 7 | 17 | 72 | Valvular AS | – |

Table 5. Clinical and hemodynamic data before and after balloon aortic valvuloplasty. AVA = aortic valve annulus diameter; BD = balloon diameter (inflated); LV = left ventricle.

| Pt | AVA (mm) | BD (mm) | Before valvuloplasty | | | After valvuloplasty | | | Follow up (6±1 months) | | | After 2nd valvuloplasty | | | | |
|---|---|---|---|---|---|---|---|---|---|---|---|---|---|---|---|---|
| | | | LV mmHg | PSG mmHg | CI L/min/m² | LV mmHg | PSG mmHg | CI L/min/m² | LV mmHg | PSG mmHg | CI L/min/m² | BD mm | AVA mm | LV mmHg | PSG mmHg | CI L/min/m² |
| 1 | 5 | 4.2 | 140 | 75 | 0.6 | 145 | 35 | 0.9 | 130 | 40 | 1.5 | – | 7 | – | – | – |
| 2 | 5 | 4.2 | 140 | 70 | 0.7 | 128 | 28 | 1 | 160 | 80 | 2.2 | 8 | 8 | 150 | 60 | 3.2 |
| 3 | 7 | 4.2 | 125 | 75 | 0.8 | 90 | 40 | 1.1 | 190 | 75 | 4.7* | 8 | 8 | 150 | 30 | 6.5* |
| 4 | 7 | 8 | 155 | 80 | 1.2 | 115 | 30 | 1.8 | 135 | 40 | 2.1 | | 9 | | | – |
| 5 | 22 | 18 | 250 | 120 | 4.6* | 200 | 60 | 4.9* | | | | | | | | |
| 6 | 20 | 18 | 245 | 140 | 6.8* | 205 | 65 | 7.3* | | | | | | | | |
| 7 | 21 | 18 | 200 | 80 | 4.7* | 150 | 35 | 5* | | | | | | | | |

* determined by thermodilution.

Mild aortic incompetence was observed in 1 patient on whom an 8 mm balloon diameter was used at an aortic annulus diameter of 7 mm, determined by 2d-echo and 8 mm by angiography. This patient exhibited the best relief of obstruction (Figure 2).

*Technique of balloon valvuloplasty*

Percutaneous left and right heart catheterization was performed through the right or left groin. Cardiac output was measured by the Fick principle or by thermodilution. If the foramen ovale was patent a left ventricular angiogram was performed and the pressure monitored before, during and after BVP. A 5 F multipurpose catheter with 1 endhole and 2 sideholes was introduced percutaneously over a 0.014' inch guidewire, aortic pressure recorded and an aortography performed. The extremely soft flexible tip of this guidewire facilitated the crossing of the stenotic valve. Leaving the guidewire in the left ventricle the catheter was replaced by a 4.3 F Grüntzig coronary dilation catheter* with a balloon length of 2 cm and an inflated balloon diameter of 4.2 mm (patient No. 1–3). A 5 F 8 mm balloon catheter* was used in patient No. 4. The dilation catheter was passed into the left ventricle over the 0.014" guidewire. Crossing of the stenotic valve should not be attempted without the use of this guidewire which remains in the balloon catheter during BVP, the soft flexible end overlapping the tip of the catheter about 1–2 cm. An Y-connector* at the proximal end of the catheter allows pressure monitoring and perfusion of the catheterlumen without withdrawing the guidewire. The balloon was placed across the valve and several times inflated up to 6–8 athmospheres. Attention was paid to the disappearing of the hourglass shape of the balloon produced by the stenotic valve. There were no complications during or following BVP. Some premature beats occurred in 13 of a total of 19 dilations. The balloon catheter was then replaced by the former multipurpose catheter, pressure in the left ventricle and aorta was again recorded and a second aortography performed. All patients remained fully heparinized during the following 2 days. In 2 patients femoral artery pulses were slightly deminished for some days without the need of surgical intervention. The results are delineated in Figure 2 and in Table 5.

*Comment*

In critical aortic stenosis in infancy medical treatment is almost invariably ineffective. Operative mortality is higher than in older children (Table 6). The operative

---

* Schneider Medintag, Zürich

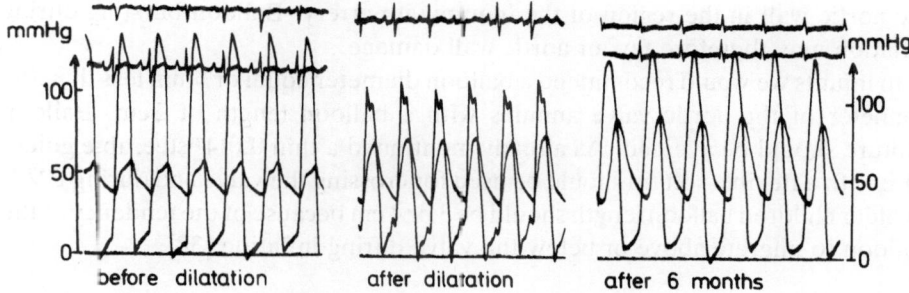

*Figure 2.* Simultaneous pressure recordings of the left ventricle and aorta before and after balloon valvuloplasty in a 13-day-old infant (patient No. 4). Peak systolic gradient decreased from 80 to 30 mmHg and was 40 mmHg at a restudy.

risk is about 32% and depends on the age and associated lesions [43–50]. Closed commissurotomy was proposed by Trinkler 1975 [42].

In 4 infants he dilated a stenotic valve with a vascular dilator introduced from the apex of the left ventricle. The effect on the valve is comparable with the BVP.

We have not observed any complications following BVP. Waller [39] reported a transversal intimal and medial aortic wall tear resulting from a rupture of a dilating balloon during BVP on a 2-day-old infant. The patient died two days after commissurotomy which was performed some hours following BVP. The aortic wall tear occurred in the ascending aorta at the level of the innominate artery. Waller could demonstrate in further studies on unfixed aortic specimens that balloon rupture with inflated balloon diameter similar or oversized to the aorta resulted in aortic damage [40]. In most patients with aortic valve stenosis the diameter of the ascending aorta is larger than the valve annulus which should result in balloon diameters smaller than the ascending aorta. The inflation pressure should not exceed the recommended maximal value. Long balloons (over 2 cm) tend to migrate in the ascending aorta during BVP and may stretch

*Table 6.* Operative mortality was about 32% in 140 infants with critical aortic valve stenosis.

| Study and year | No. of pts | Age | Mortality No. (%) |
|---|---|---|---|
| Lakier [43] (1974) | 7 | 1 w–3 w | 5 (71%) |
| Keane [44] (1975) | 28 | 1 w–6 mo | 8 (28%) |
| Kugler [45] (1979) | 39 | 1 w–1 yr | 13 33% |
| Bühlmeyer [46] (1979) | 18 | 1 w–6 mo | 4 (22%) |
| Edmunds [47] (1980) | 14 | 1 w–4 w | 7 (50%) |
| Rupprath [48] (1982) | 15 | 1 w–1 yr | 3 (20%) |
| Huhta [49] (1984) | 8 | 1 w–7 mo | 4 (50%) |
| Messina [50] (1984) | 11 | 1 w–4 w | 1 ( 9%) |
| Total | 140 | | 45 (32%) |

the aortic wall in the region of the innominate artery. Balloon bursting during inflation may therefore favour aortic wall damage.

In infants we would recommend a balloon diameter equal or 1 mm less than the diameter of the aortic valve annulus with a balloon length of 2 cm. Balloon rupture should be avoided. As already mentioned a thin 0.014″ steerable guidewire with a flexible soft tip should be used for crossing the valve and during BVP. In older children balloon length should be 3 or 4 cm because of the tendency of the balloon to migrate above or below the valve during inflation [38].

## Summary

In our opinion BVP is the method of choice in critical valvar aortic stenosis in infancy and should be considered in critical pulmonary valve stenosis, too. Aortic and pulmonary valve stenosis in childhood can also be successfully treated. BVP should not be applied on patients with calcified aortic valves, pressure gradients less than 50 mmHg or with moderate aortic incompetence. Peripheral pulmonary arterial stenosis seems to be amenable to dilation as well. At present we do not recommend a witespread use of BA for coarctation or recoarctation in children despite satisfactory early results. We are not sure about the incidence of late complications. Operative procedures have a very low risk in this lesion. In the same way BA may be applied for stenotic Blalock-Taussig shunts or vena cava obstruction. Late results are lacking. Presently BA can not be recommended in coarctation in infancy and in pulmonary venous obstruction.

Balloon angio- and valvuloplasty is a new therapeutic approach with good early results. Very few complications have been reported. As in all new procedures the duration of benefit and the incidence of late complications has yet to be established.

## References

1. Dotter CT. Judkins MP (1964) Transluminal treatment of arteriosclerotic obstruction. Description of a new technic and a preliminary report of its application. Circulation 30: 654–670
2. Grüntzig A, Hopff H (1974) Perkutane Rekanalisation chronischer arterieller Verschlüsse mit einem neuen Dilatationskatheter. Modifikation der Dotter-Technik. Dtsch Med Wochenschr 99: 2502
3. Grüntzig A, Senning A, Siegenthaler WE (1979) Nonoperative dilatation of coronary-artery stenosis. Percutaneous transluminal coronary angioplasty. N Engl J Med 301: 61–68
4. Sos T, Sniderman KW, Rettek-Sos B et al (1979) Percutaneous transluminal dilatation of coarctation of thoracic aorta post mortem. Lancet 2: 970–971
5. Lock JE, Castaneda-Zuniga WR, Bass JL, Foker JE, Amplatz K, Anderson RW (1982) Balloon dilatation of excised aortic coarctations. Radiology 143: 689–691
6. Lock JE, Niemi T, Burke BA, Einzig St, Castaneda-Zuniga WR (1982) Transcutaneous angioplasty of experimental aortic coarctation. Circulation 66: 1280–1285

7.  Castaneda-Zuniga WR, Lock JE, Vlodarer Z et al (1982) Transluminal dilatation of coarctation of the abdominal aorta. Radiology 143: 693–697
8.  Sperling DR, Dorsey TJ, Rowen M, Gazzaniga AB (1983) Percutaneous transluminal angioplasty of congenital coarctation of the aorta. Am J Cardiol 51: 562–564
9.  Finley JP, Beaulieu RG, Nanton MA, Roy DL (1983) Balloon catheter dilatation of coarctation of the aorta in young infants. Br Heart J 50: 411–415
10. Lock JE, Bass JL, Amplatz K et al (1983) Balloon dilatation angioplasty of coarctation in infants and children. Circulation 68: 109–116
11. Suarez de Lezo J, Fernandez R, Sancho M, Concha M, Arizon J, Franco M, Alemany F, Barcones F, Lopez-Rubio F, Valles F (1984) Percutaneous transluminal angioplasty for aortic isthmic coarctation in infancy. Am J Cardiol 54: 1147–1149
12. Lababidi ZA, Daskalopoulos DA, Stoeckle jr H (1984) Transluminal balloon coarctation angioplasty: experience with 27 patients. Am J Cardiol 54: 1288–1291
13. Lababidi ZA, Madigan N, Wu JR, Murphy TJ (1984) Balloon coarctation angioplasty in an adult. Am J Cardiol 53: 350–351
14. Cooper RS, Ritter SB, Golinko RJ (1984) Balloon dilatation angioplasty: nonsurgical management of coarctation of the aorta. Circulation 70: 903–907
15. Singer MI, Rowen M, Dorsey TJ (1982) Transluminal aortic balloon angioplasty for coarctation of the aorta in the newborn. Am Heart J 103: 131–132
16. Lock JE (1984) Now that we can dilate, should we? Am J Cardiol 54: 1360
17. Pellegrino A, Derverall PB, Anderson RH, Smith A, Wilkinson JL, Russo P, Girod DA, Tynan M (1985) Aortic coarctation in the first three months of life. An anatomopathological study with respect to treatment. J Thorac Cardiovasc Surg 89: 121–127
18. Kan JS, White RI, Mitchell SE et al (1983) Treatment of restenosis of coarctation by percutaneous transluminal angioplasty. Circulation 68: 1087–1094
19. Lock JE, Niemi T, Einzig St, Amplatz K, Burke B, Bass JL (1981) Transvenous angioplasty of experimental branch pulmonary artery stenos s in newborn lambs. Circulation 64: 886–892
20. Lock JE, Castaneda-Zuniga WR, Fuhrman BP, Bass JL (1983) Balloon dilatation angioplasty of hypoplastic and stenotic pulmonary arteries. Circulation 67: 962–967
21. Rocchini AP, Kveselis D, Dick MacD, Crowley D, Snider R, Rosenthal A (1984) Use of balloon angioplasty to treat peripheral pulmonary stenosis. Am J Cardiol 54: 1069–1073
22. Edwarcs BS, Lucas RV, Lock JE, Edwards JE (1985) Morphologic changes in the pulmonary arteries after percutaneous balloon angioplasty for pulmonary arterial stenosis. Circulation 71: 195–201
23. Massumi A, Woods L, Mullins ChE, Nasser WK, Hall RJ (1981) Pulmonary venous dilatation in pulmonary veno-occlusive disease. Am J Cardiol 48: 585–589
24. Driscoll DJ, Hesslein PS, Mullins CE (1982) Congenital Stenosis of Individual Pulmonary Veins: Clinical spectrum and unsuccessful treatment by transvenous balloon dilatation. Am J Cardiol 49: 1767–1772
25. Lock JE, Fuhrman BP, Castaneda-Zuniga WR, Bass JL (1982) Dilatation angioplasty (DA) of congen tal cardiac defects: preliminary results. Circulation 66, Supp. II–360
26. Rocchini AP, Kveselis D (1984) The use of balloon angioplasty in the pediatric patient. Pediatr Clin North Am 31: 1293–1305
27. Rocchini AP, Cho KJ, Byrum C, Heidelberger K (1982) Transluminal angioplasty of superior vena cava obstruction in an 15-month-old child. Chest 82: 506–508
28. Waldman JD, Waldman J, Jones MC (1983) Failure of balloon dilatation in mid-cavity obstruction of the systemic venous atrium after the Mustard operation. Ped Cardiol 4: 151–154
29. Lock JE, Fuhrman BP, Rashkind WJ et al (1984) Dilatation angioplasty of postoperative 'caval' obstructions: Preliminary results. (abstract). J Am Coll Cardiol 3: 532
30. Fellows KE jr(1984) Therapeutic catheter procedures in congenital heart disease: Current status and future prospects. Cardiovasc Intervent Radiol 7: 170–177

24

31. Neuhaus KL, Rupprath G, Hellberg K, Kühn R, Tebbe M (1985) Valvuloplastie und periphere Angioplastie mit Koronardilatationskathetern. Dtsch Med Wschr 118: 703–708
32. Fischer DR, Park SC, Neches WH et al (1985) Successful dilatation of a stenotic Blalock-Taussig anastomosis by percutaneous transluminal balloon angioplasty. Am J Cardiol 55: 861–862
33. Kan JS, White RI, Mitchell SE, Gardner TJ (1982) Percutaneous balloon valvuloplasty: a new method for treating congenital pulmonary-valve stenosis. N Engl J Med 370: 540–542
34. Pepine CJ, Gessner IH, Feldmann RL (1982) Percutaneous balloon valvuloplasty for pulmonic valve stenosis in the adult. Am J Cardiol 50: 1442–1445
35. Lababidi ZA, Wu JR (1983) Percutaneous balloon pulmonary valvuloplasty. Am J Cardiol 52: 560–562
36. Kan JS, White jr. RI, Mitchell SE, Anderson JH, Gardner TJ (1984) Percutaneous transluminal balloon valvuloplasty for pulmonary valve stenosis. Circulation 69: 554–560
37. Rocchini AP, Cho KJ, Byrum L et al (1984) Percutaneous balloon valvuloplasty for treatment of congenital pulmonary valve stenosis in children. JACC 3: 1127–1135
38. Lababidi ZA, Wu JR, Walls JT (1984) Percutaneous balloon aortic valvuloplasty: results in 23 patients. Am J Cardiol 53: 194–197
39. Waller BF, Girod DA, Dillon JC (1984) Transverse aortic wall tears in infants after balloon angioplasty for aortic valve stenosis: relation of aortic wall to diameter of inflated angioplasty balloon and aortic lumen in seven necropsy cases. JACC 4: 1235–1241
40. Walls JT, Lababidi ZA, Curtis JJ, Silver D (1984) Assessment of percutaneous balloon pulmonary and aortic valvuloplasty. J Thorac Cardiovasc Surg 88: 352–356
41. Rupprath G, Neuhaus KL (June 1985) Percutaneous balloon valvuloplasty for aortic valve stenosis in infancy. Am J Cardiol, in press
42. Trinkle JK, Norton JB, Richardson JD, Grover FL, Noonan AJ (1975) Closed aortic valvotomy and simultaneous correction of associated anomalies in infants. J Thorac Cardiovasc Surg 69: 758–762
43. Lakier JB, Lewis AB, Heymann MA, Stanger P. Hoffman JIE, Rudolph AM (1974) Isolated aortic stenosis in the neonate. Natural history and hemodynamic considerations. Circulation 50: 801–808
44. Keane JF, Bernhard WF, Nadas AS (1975) Aortic stenosis surgery in infancy. Circulation 52: 1138–1143
45. Kugler JD, Campbell E, Vargo TA, McNamara DG, Hallman GL, Cooley DA (1979) Results of aortic valvotomy in infants with isolated aortic valvular stenosis. J Thorac Cardiovasc Surg 78: 553–557
46. Bühlmeyer K, Simon B, Mocellin R, Sauer U (1979) Clinical angiocardiographic and functional studies in the assessment of critical valvular aortic studies. In: Paediatric Cardiology, Vol. 2, edited by Godman MJ, Marquis RM, Churchill Livingstone, Edinburgh, London, New York
47. Edmunds LH Jr, Wagner HR, Heymann MA (1980) Aortic valvulotomy in neonates. Circulation 61: 421–427
48. Rupprath G, Vogt J, Wesselhoeft H, de Vivie ER, Beuren AJ (1982) Früh- und Spätergebnisse nach Kommissurotomie kritischer Säuglingsaortenstenosen. Herz/Kreisl 11: 623–624
49. Huhta JC, Latson LA, Gutgesell HP, Cooley DA, Kearney DL (1984) Echocardiography in the diagnosis and management of symptomatic aortic valve stenosis in infants. Circulation 70: 438–444
50. Messina LM, Turley K, Stanger P. Hoffman JIE, Ebert PA (1984) Successful aortic valvotomy for severe congenital valvular aortic stenosis in the newborn. J Thorac Cardiovasc Surg 88: 92–96
51. Semb BKH, Tjönneland S, Stake G, Aabyholm G (1979) 'Balloon valvulotomy' of congenital pulmonary valve stenosis with tricuspid valve insufficiency. Cardiovasc Radiol 2: 239–241
52. Coles JG, Freedom RM, Olley PM, Coceani F, Williams WG, Trusler GA (1984) Surgical management of critical pulmonary stenosis in the neonate. Ann Thorac Surg 38: 458–465
53. Bergdahl L, Ljungqvist A (1980) Long-term results after repair of coarctation of the aorta by patch grafting. J Thorac Cardiovasc Surg 80: 177–181

# Closure of left-to-right shunts by catheter techniques

H. SIEVERT, W.-D. BUSSMANN, and M. KALTENBACH

During the last two decades a number of catheter techniques for the closure of left-to-right shunts have been developed. Most of these techniques are still under investigation, but some are now applicable as an alternative to surgery.

## Atrial septal defect

In 1974 King and Mills [4] used double umbrellas (Fig. 1) to occlude experimentally created septal defects in dogs. Two years later, they were able to use this technique in a seventeen year old girl [5] and in 1984 they reported excellent longterm results in five patients without any complications [8]. Rashkind reported adequate closure of atrial septal defect by a single-disc, hooked prothesis in thirteen out of 20 patients [14].

## Ventricular septal defect

Some experimental work concerning the closure of a ventricular septal defect has been done by Mills et al as early as 1971 [9]. Using a disc-shaped balloon on a double lumen catheter, it was possible to occlude temporarily an experimentally produced ventricular septal defect.

## Arterio-venous fistulae

Steel coils (Fig. 2) introduced by a catheter have been used by Gianturco [3] to occlude renal arteries. Wallace [20] et al applied this technique to arterio-venous fistulae. It is also possible to occlude coronary artery fistulae, as was recently shown by a Russian group.

The closure of arteries by detachable balloons is a common technique. Re-

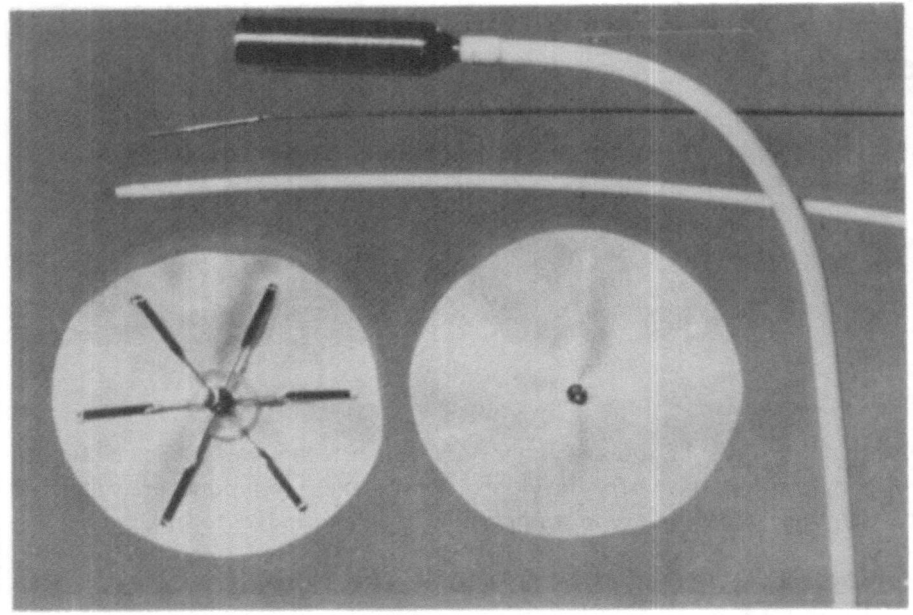

*Figure 1.* Atrial umbrella device developed by Mills and King (1976). It is introduced in a capsule at the tip of a catheter. A snap device locks the umbrellas across the atrial septal defect.

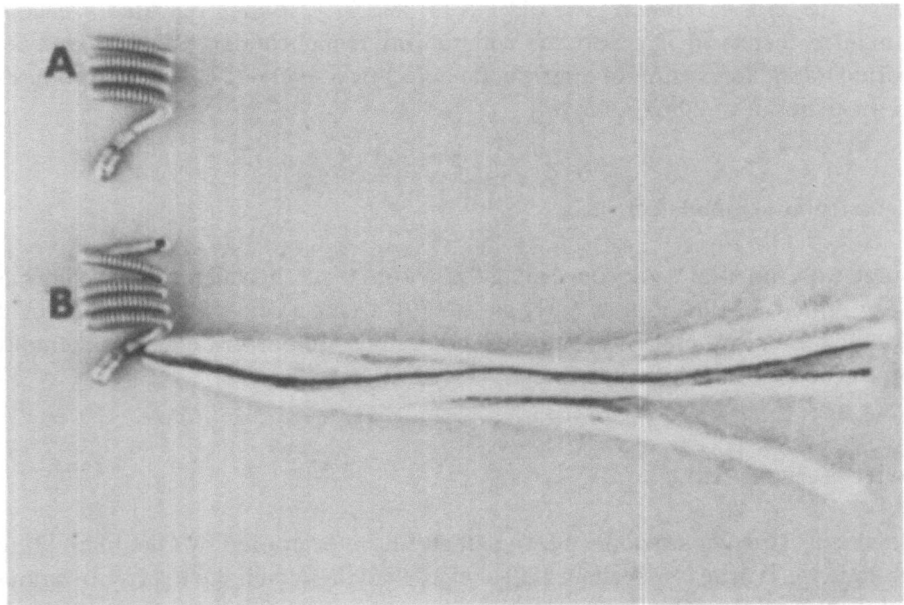

*Figure 2.* Steel coil (A) with attached woolen strands (B) for the occlusion of larger arteries or arterio-venous fistulae (Gianturco et al 1975).

cently Reidy [17] reported a case of coronary to bronchial anastomosis, successfully occluded by such a balloon. This device was also used to occlude a Blalock-Taussig shunt [16].

## Persistent ductus arteriosus

More than eighteen years ago, Porstmann [11] described the closure of a patent ductus in a seventeen-year old boy. He used a plug made of polyvinyl alcohol (Ivalon), that was introduced transfemorally. Because it seems to be applicable as a routine therapy, at least in adult patients, we will describe this technique in detail later.

The closure of a patent ductus by an umbrella (Fig. 3) has been developed by

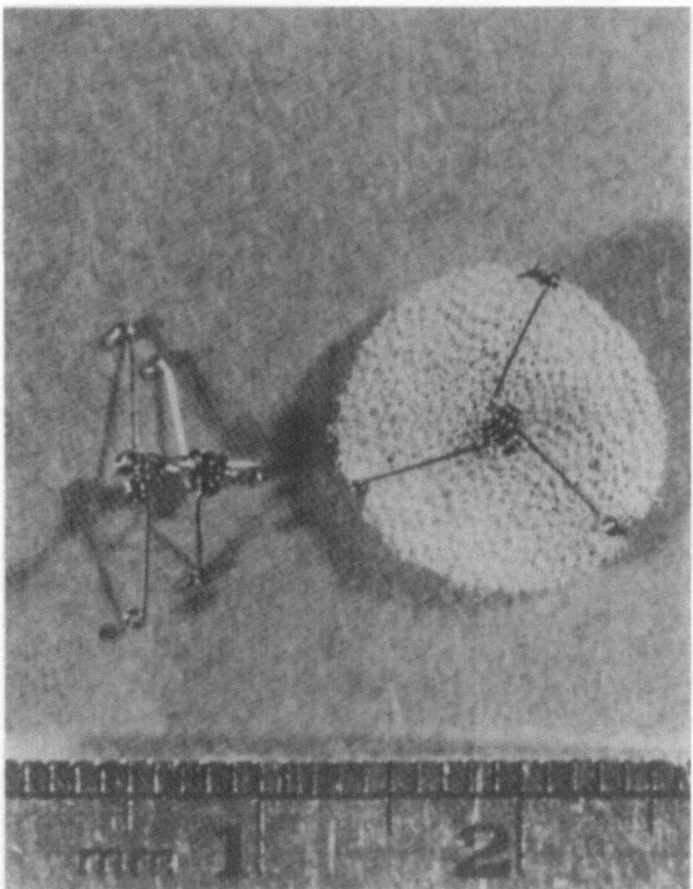

*Figure 3.* Double-disc prosthesis for patent ductus arteriosus. Left: steel frame in profile. Right: frontal view of the same prosthesis covered by foam disc (Rashkind 1983).

Rashkind [14] in 1979. This technique has the advantage to be applicable in small infants. A great problem has been the risk of embolisation of the prosthesis. Bash et al [1] attempted a ductus closure with a double-umbrella occluder device in thirty-four patients. Embolisation into the pulmonary artery (seven patients) and aorta (one patient) occurred in twenty-three percent. But with growing experience it may be possible – as shown by Rashkind [15] – to avoid this complication.

## Plug closure of patent ductus

Most of the described catheter techniques are still under investigation or applicable only in very rare disorders. The closure of a patent ductus by an Ivalon plug has achieved clinical significance. Meanwhile it has been performed in several hundred patients [2, 6, 10, 12, 13, 18, 19]. Favorable results have been reported with a high success rate of up to ninety-six percent, a low complication rate, and no mortality at all. Nevertheless this technique did not replace surgery. Besides the Charité in East Berlin, where it was developed by Porstmann, it is routinely used only in two clinics in Japan [6, 18, 19].

## Method

Prior to the closing procedure detailed information about the size and shape of the ductus have to be obtained. Therefore an aortogram in lateral view is performed (Fig. 4) during a first diagnostic catheterisation. After this the patient usually leaves the hospital to come back some weeks later for the ductus closure.

According to the size and the shape of the ductus an Ivalon (polyvinyl alcohol) plug is prepared (Fig. 5a, b). For stabilization it contains an inner steel wire frame.

This plug has to be moved into position along an arterial transductal venous track wire (Fig. 6). Due to this approach it is possible to remove the plug via the venous side, if it is too small to occlude the ductus. The track-wire is introduced through a preshaped arterial catheter into the pulmonary artery. From the femoral vein a 10 F-cathether is introduced. Inside of this venous catheter there is a double folded snare wire which can be opened in the pulmonary artery. Capturing of the track wire with the snare wire takes about five to ten minutes. (Fig. 7). An arterial transductal venous loop is established by withdrawing the snare wire together with the trapped track wire from the venous side. Then the arterial catheter is replaced by a tubular applicator with a diameter according to the size of the plug. Usually the introduction of the applicator causes no problems. Only a few patients have been described in the literature in whom surgical reconstruction has been necessary [10]. In those patients with a comparably small femoral artery, the applicator may be introduced after exposure of the vessel.

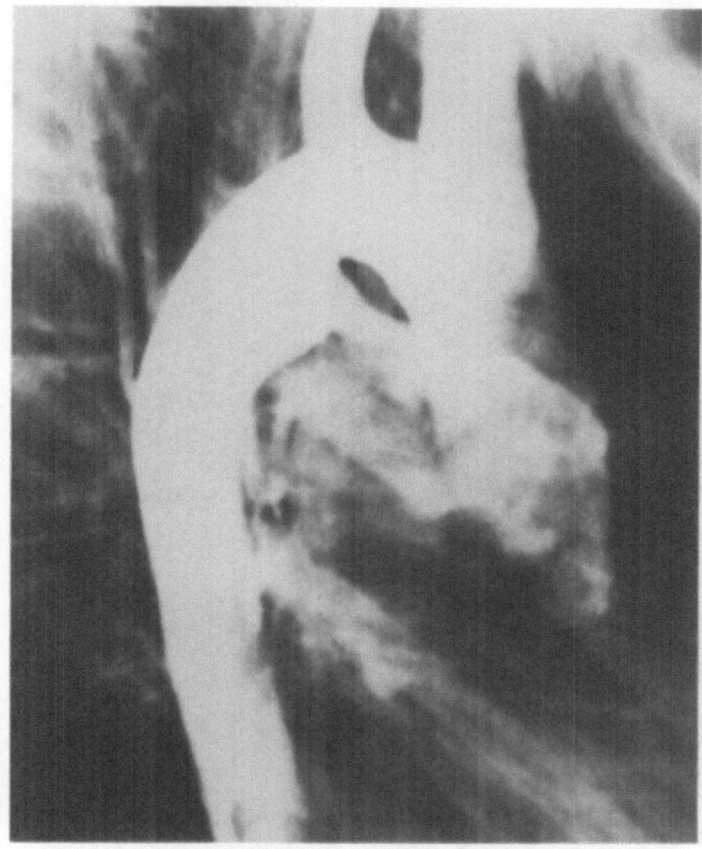

*Figure 4.* Aortogram in the lateral view showing a typical conically shaped ductus with a diameter of 7 mm.

The plug, threaded over the track wire, is introduced through the applicator by a strong pushing-cannula and advanced into the ductus by a pushing catheter, that is also threaded over the track wire. When a gentle pulling from the arterial side confirms wedging of the plug in the ductus, the track wire is withdrawn via the venous side. The plug remains in position due to the friction in the conical duct. The whole procedure takes one or two hours. Hemostasis at the puncture site is achieved by manual compression. Usually the patient is discharged from hospital three to five days after the procedure.

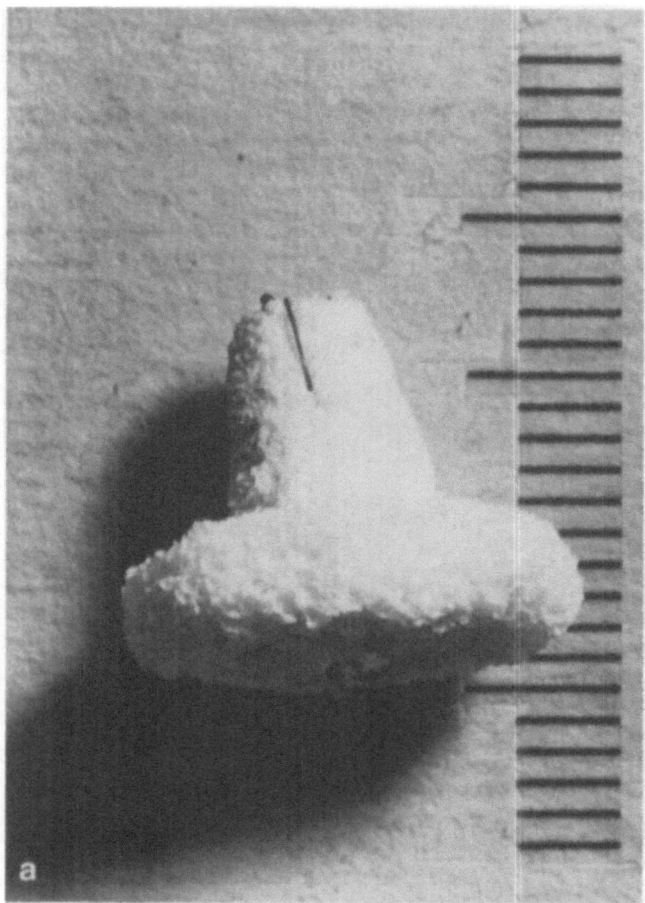

*Figure 5*. Plug made of polyvinyl alcohol (a) for ductus closure. For stabilisation it contains an inner steel wire frame (b) (Porstmann, Wierny 1981).


## Results

From June 1983 to April 1985 transfemoral plug closure of a patent ductus arteriosus was attempted in twelve patients, the youngest was a fifteen-year-old boy, the oldest a fifty-three-year-old woman (Table 1). The pressure in the pulmonary artery ranged from 15/5 to 55/25 mmHg, the diameter of the ductus from 2 mm to 9 mm, the left-to-right shunt from sixteen to ninety percent. Eleven patients had puncture, in one patient a cutdown of the femoral artery was necessary to introduce the applicator. All patients have been followed for a period of two to twenty-one months. Complete closure of the ductus was docu-

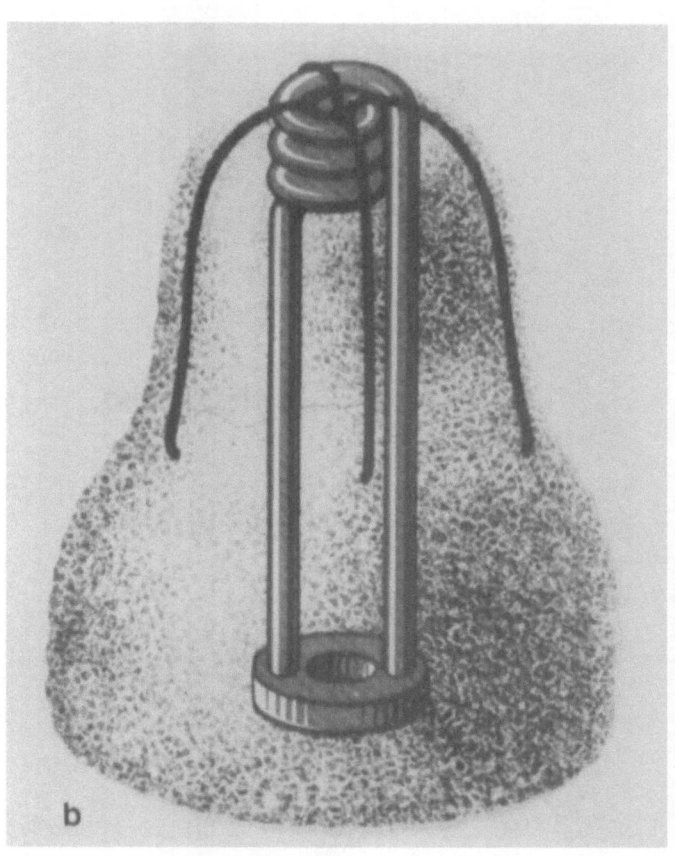

b

RESULTS:

| patient | sex | age | L-R Shunt % | PA- pressure mm Hg | diameter of PDA mm | of fem. art. mm | complications / remarks | follow-up months |
|---|---|---|---|---|---|---|---|---|
| S. H. | ♀ | 17 | 21 | 20/12, $\overline{15}$ | 3.0 | 8.0 | ∅ | 21 |
| H. K. | ♀ | 43 | 66 | 35/18, $\overline{25}$ | 5.0 | 8.5 | ∅ | 21 |
| E. S. | ♀ | 53 | 90 | 35/20, $\overline{25}$ | 9.0 | 9.5 | ∅/arteriotomy | 17 |
| M. Y. | ♂ | 15 | 33 | 20/11, $\overline{14}$ | 3.5 | 11.5 | ∅ | 17 |
| M. G. | ♀ | 25 | 33 | 23/10, $\overline{14}$ | 3.5 | 8.5 | ∅ | 17 |
| G. S. | ♂ | 27 | 33 | 55/25, $\overline{35}$ | 5.0 | 10.0 | ∅ | 17 |
| A. D. | ♀ | 17 | 32 | 26/19, $\overline{22}$ | 4.0 | 8.0 | ∅ | 14 |
| M. S. | ♀ | 25 | 20 | 22/13, $\overline{26}$ | 2.0 | 6.0 | ∅ | 11 |
| E. L. | ♂ | 46 | 36 | 30/13, $\overline{22}$ | 6.0 | 11.5 | late dislocation | 7 |
| T. R. | ♀ | 18 | 16 | 18/ 6, $\overline{8}$ | 4.5 | 9.5 | ∅ | 5 |
| H. M. | ♀ | 17 | 25 | 15/5, $\overline{8}$ | 4.0 | 9.0 | ∅ | 4 |
| H. K. | ♀ | 16 | 21 | 25/ 6, $\overline{15}$ | 5.0 | 9.0 | ∅ | 2 |

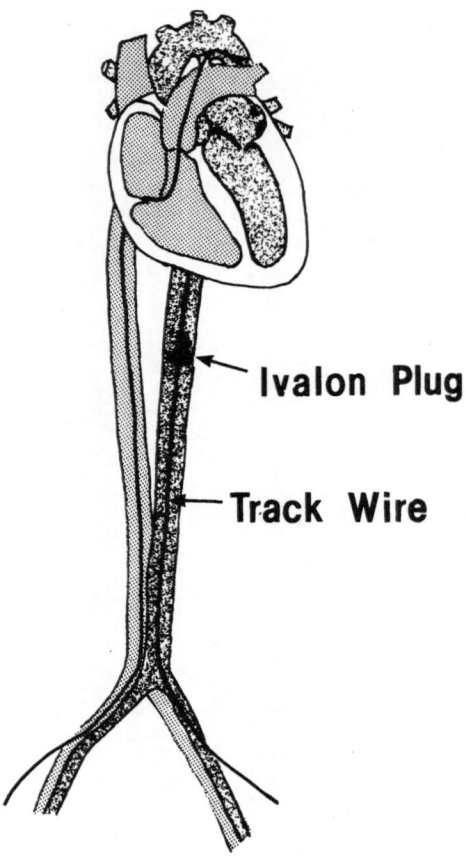

*Figure 6.* Transfemoral closure of persistent ductus arteriosus. The plug is moved into position along an arterial-transductal-venous track wire.

mented by phonocardiography and dye dilution curves (Fig. 8a, b). Those patients with elevated pressure in the pulmonary artery and clinical symptoms reported dramatic improvement within a few days. This happened also in the case of the 53-year-old woman. Pulmonary congestion and heart size decreased considerably within three days after ductus closure (Fig. 9a, b).

In one of our patients the Ivalon plug dislodged seven weeks after PDA-closure and embolized into a side branch of the left pulmonary artery. The patient experienced short-lasting pain and fever for some days. No further symptoms occurred. In the meantime the transfemoral closure has been performed successfully without complications.

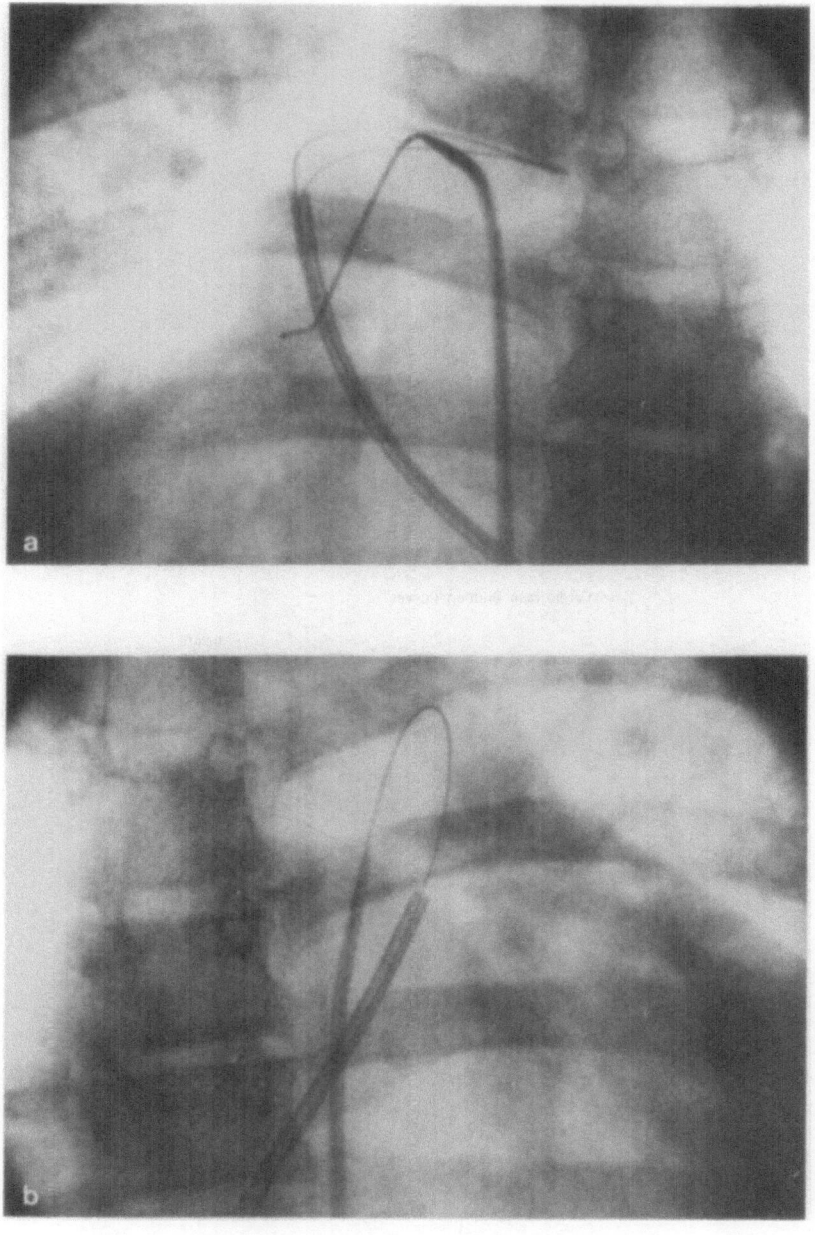

*Figure 7.* Capturing of the track wire with the snare wire within the pulmonary artery (a). To establish the arterial-transductal venous loop, the track wire is pulled out to the venous side.

34

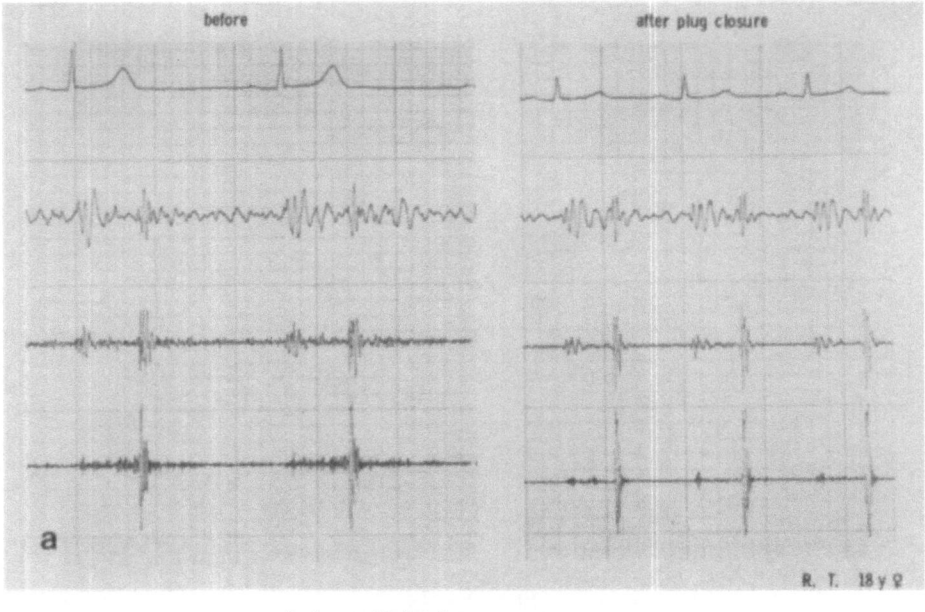

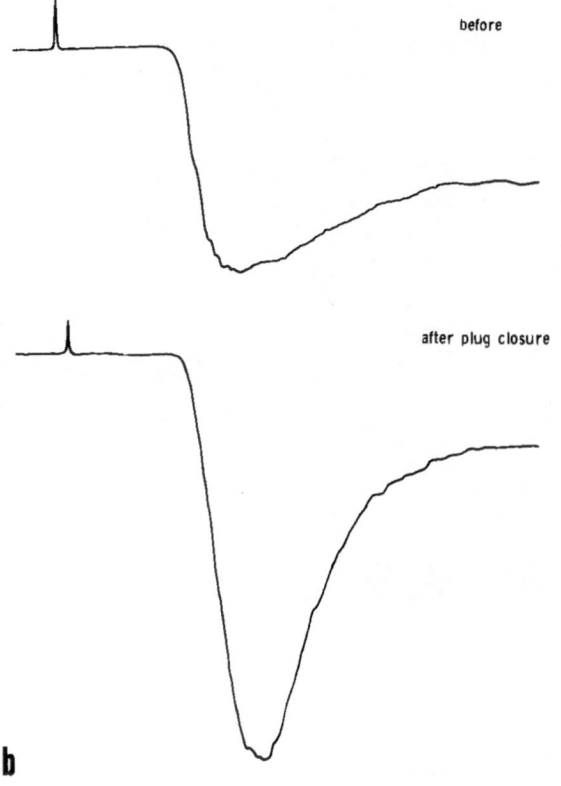

Cardiogreen Dilution Curves

before

after plug closure

Sa. E. 44 y ♀

*Figure 8.* Phonocardiography (a) and dye-dilution curves (b) before and after plug closure of PDA.

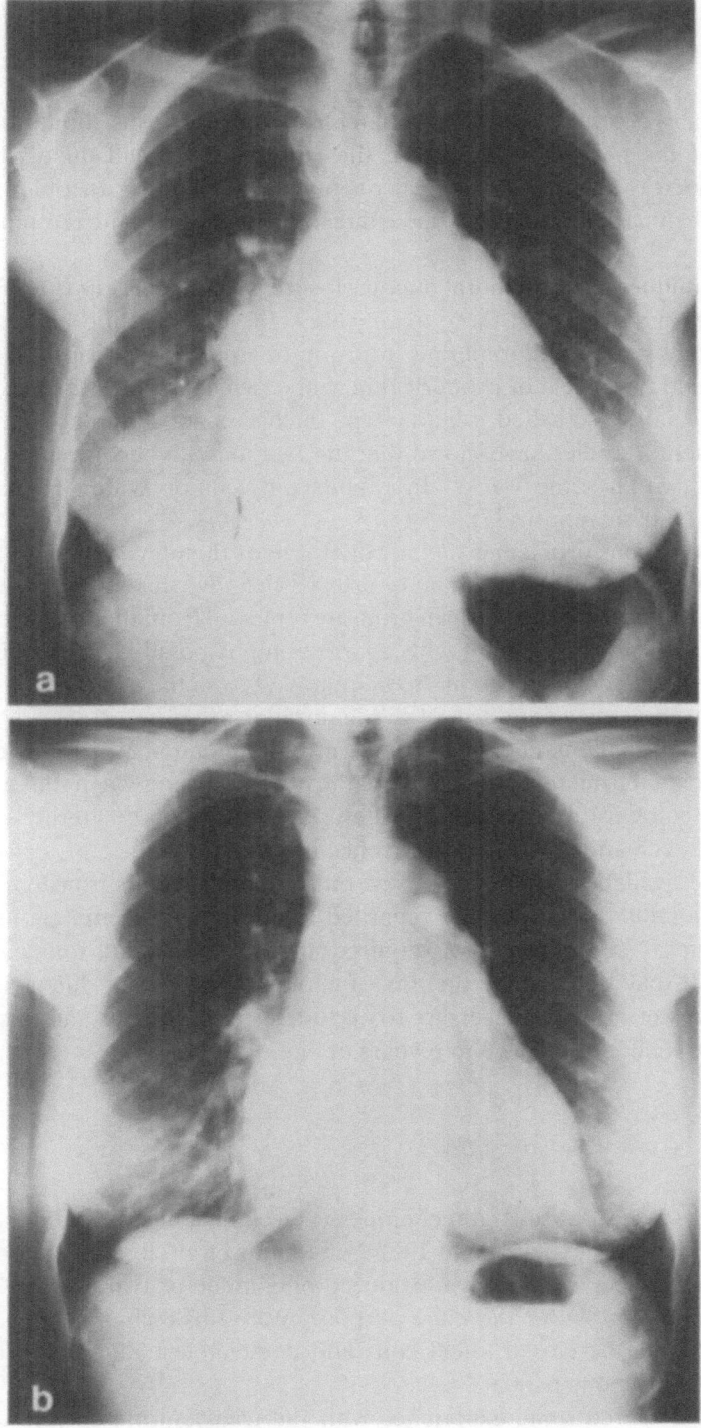

*Figure 9.* Enlarged heart and severe pulmonary congestion on the day before ductus closure (a); considerably improved 3 days later (b).

## Discussion

It is generally accepted that a large patent ductus arteriosus should be closed. Because of the risk of ductitis, even the closure of a small ductus is usually recommended. Mortality of surgical ductus closure is low. In older patients, however, technical problems may arise due to calcification of the infundibulum of the ductus.

The technique of transfemoral ductus closure without surgery is applicable to patients beyond the age of three to six years. In younger children the femoral artery usually is too small to permit insertion of a plug of appropriate size. The ductus should be conical or cylindrical in shape, which is the case in most of the patients. Usually a so called 'window-type ductus' is not suitable.

Experimental studies have shown that the Ivalon foam becomes infiltrated by tissue cells within some weeks. In rabbits only minor Ivalon residues were detectable after six months [7].

The most serious problem is an improper size of the plug. When a plug is too small, it may slip into the pulmonary artery. Usually, this happens during the procedure. In that case the plug can be easily removed from the track wire via the venous side. A second attempt with a larger plug is possible. If the plug is too large to wedge in the ductus, it has to be removed from the aorta with a Fogarty-catheter. In this case a cut down of the femoral artery is necessary.

In one of our patients the plug slipped into the pulmonary artery two months after closure of the ductus. Dislocation of the plug after removal of the catheters is a very rare complication. It was never described before in the literature. On the other hand even after surgery a recurrence is not unknown.

From the available experience in several hundred patients transfemoral plug closure of a patent ductus can be regarded as a relatively secure catheter technique. General anesthesia is not required and hospitalisation for one week is sufficient. It may become the therapy of choice in the patent ductus in adults. Further investigations are necessary to occlude oversize ductus and to adapt the technique to children below 3 to 6 years of age.

## Summary

In the last two decades several techniques to occlude congenital shunts without surgery have been developed. In 1967 Porstmann et al closed a patent ductus arteriosus with a transfemorally introduced plug made of Ivalon. In 1977 Rashkind used an umbrella for the same purpose. With this technique also an atrial septal defect can be closed. Steel coils and detachable balloons are useful to occlude arteriovenous fistulae.

We have acquired some experience with the transfemoral closure of patent ductus arteriosus by a plug. Prior to the closure it is necessary to get detailed information about the size and shape of the ductus. Therefore an aortography in the lateral view is performed as a first diagnostic step. Then a plug of Ivalon (polyvinyl alcohol) is made according to the size of the ductus. In a second intervention an arterio-transductal venous loop – using a long track wire – is established. Threaded over the track wire, the plug is advanced into the ductus by a pushing catheter.

During the last two years we attempted a transfemoral closure of a persistent ductus arteriosus in twelve patients. The youngest was a fifteen-year-old boy, the oldest a 53-year-old woman. The pressure in the pulmonary artery ranged from 15/5 to 55/25 mmHg, the diameter of the ductus from 2 mm up to 9 mm. In all patients transfemoral plug closure of the ductus was possible. The patients were followed-up for a period of two to twenty-one months. Patients with complaints and increased heart size became symptom-free and heart volume decreased considerably. In one patient, however, the plug dislocated seven weeks after the procedure into a side branch of the pulmonary artery, without serious consequences. A second transfemoral closure was performed successfully in this patient.

A high success rate, a low complication rate and no mortality for the use of this technique has been reported in the literature. Transfemoral closure of a persistent ductus arteriosus is a catheter technique, that can replace surgery in most of the patients.

## References

1. Bash SE, Mullins CE (1984) Insertion of patent ductus arteriosus occluder by transvenous approach: A new technique. Circulation 70 (Suppl II): 285
2. Bussmann W-D, Sievert H, Kaltenbach M (1984) Transfemoraler Verschluß des Ductus arteriosus persistens. Dtsch Med Wschr 109: 1322
3. Gianturco C, Anderson JH, Wallace S (1975) Mechanical devices for arterial occlusion. Am J Roentgenol 124: 428
4. King TD, Mills NL (1974) Nonoperative closure of atrial septal defects. Surgery 75, 383
5. King TD, Thompson SL, Steiner C, Mills NL (1976) Secundum atrial septal defect. JAMA 235, 2506
6. Kitamura S, Sato K, Naito Y, Shimizu Y, Fujino M, Oyama C, Nakano S, Kawashima Y (1976) Plug closure of patent ductus arteriosus by transfemoral catheter method. Chest 70, 631
7. Mai J, Hackensellner HA, Porstmann W (1967) Zur Reaktion der Gefäßwand auf die intravasale Applikation von Ivalon. Frankfurter Zeitschrift für Pathologie 77, 252
8. Mills N, King T, Joyce D (1984) Transvenous closure of ASD's with a double umbrella device – 7–year minimum follow-up. Circulation 70, Supple II, 317
9. Mills NL, Vargish T, Kleinman LH, Bloomfield DA, Reed GE (1971) Balloon closure of ventricular septal defect. Circulation 43/44, Supple I, 111
10. Porstmann W, Wierny L (1981) Percutaneous transfemoral closure of the patent ductus arteriosus – an alternative to surgery. Semin Roentenol 16, 95
11. Porstmann W, Wierny L, Warnke H (1967) Der Verschluß des Ductus arteriosus persistens ohne Thorakotomie. Thoraxchirurgie 15, 199

12. Porstmann W, Wierny L, Warnke H (1968) Der Verschluß des Ductus arteriosus persistens ohne Thorakotomie (2. Mitteilung). Fortschr Röntgenstr 109, 133
13. Porstmann W, Wierny L, Warnke H, Gerstberger G, Romaniuk A (1971) Catheter closure of patent ductus arteriosus. Radiol Clin N Amer 9, 203
14. Rashkind WJ (1983) Transcatheter treatment of congenital heart disease. Circulation 67, 711
15. Rashkind WK, personal communication
16. Reidy JF, Baker E, Tynan M (1983) Transcatheter occlusion of a Blalock-Taussig shunt with a detachable balloon in a child. Br Heart J 50, 101
17. Reidy JF, Sowton E, Ross DN (1983) Transcatheter occlusion of coronary to bronchial anastomosis by detachable balloon combined with coronary angioplasty at same procedure. Br Heart J 49, 284
18. Sato K, Fuijino M, Kozuka T, Naito Y, Kitamura S, Nakano S, Ohyama C, Kawashima Y (1975) Transfemoral plug closure of patent ductus arteriosus. Experience in 61 consecutive cases treated without thoracotomy. Circulation 51, 337
19. Takamiya M, Tadokoro M, Okada Y (1973) Nonsurgical closure of PDA. Report of 23 cases. J Jap Ass thorac Surg 21, 196
20. Wallace S, Gianturco C, Anderson JH, Goldstein HM, Davis LJ, Bree RL (1976) Therapeutic vascular occlusion utilizing steel coil technique: clinical applications. Am J Roentgenol 127, 381

# Atrial inversion in TGA according to Mustard or Senning

H. OELERT

Transposition of the great arteries (TGA) was considered a lethal disease until Senning, in 1958, for the first time successfully transposed the atrial inflow in order to match the malformation of the ventricular outflow [27].

The technique he used was considered quite complex at the time and there was a high mortality with that procedure which was also caused by immature methods of extracorporeal circulation and lack of understanding of the perioperative course. In 1964, Mustard described his simpler atrial baffle procedure for redirection of the venous return which has become 'standard' in the ensuing years [19]. In both large and small series the Mustard operation could be applied with a mortality risk of 5 to 10% for TGA and intact ventricular septum [4, 20, 31]. Serious late complications and deaths, however, were numerous and resulted from atrial dysrhythmias [15, 32, 33] right ventricular dysfunction [12, 13, 14] and systemic and/or pulmonary venous obstruction [2, 3, 12, 13, 17, 31, 35].

Consequently, they lead to a variety of modifications of the Mustard procedure [23, 25, 31, 33, 34] and, at the same time accounted for a revival of the Senning approach [21, 24]. Together with progress in myocardial preservation and bypass techniques, operative mortalities and complication rates could be significantly reduced almost everywhere with either method [20, 22, 23, 35].

Most interests nowadays concentrate on non-lethal postoperative complications, and although many hemodynamic and electrophysical studies have been performed, no clear-cut conclusions on the superiority of the Mustard or Senning variety of atrial inversion have been drawn. It therefore seems appropriate to review our total experience in surgery of TGA, and to compare it with the techniques and results of others. This report is, however, restricted to inflow correction of TGA with intact ventricular septum to avoid the variability introduced by the presence and repair of other defects.

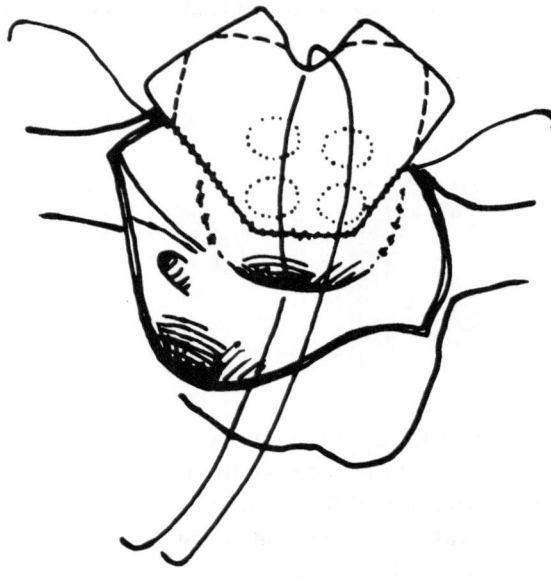

*Figure 1.* Brom's modification of the Mustard operation using a trousers shape intraatrial baffle [23].

## Methods

In January, 1974, we started operating on children with TGA using a technique closely related to the procedure of Mustard. In principle (Fig. 1) this method consisted of implantation of a tortuous baffle in the modification of Brom's trousers shape [23]. Because of an early and high (28%) incidence of systemic and/or pulmonary venous obstruction we were urged to modify our method repeatedly during the following years [20]. The changes applied not only to the surgical procedure but also to the material and design of the intraatrial baffle. Presently, the heart is opened by an oblique atrial incision which extends into the right upper pulmonary vein, the superior and inferior rim of the atrial septum are excised, and a standard size triangular patch is inserted (Fig. 2) so as to redirect the venous return. By taking most of the space of the atrial cavities, a large straight caval tunnel is created. Reconstruction of the pulmonary venous atrium is performed through a direct or indirect atrial wall plasty.

The baffle within the atrium (Fig. 3) is constructed from a Gore-Tex prosthesies. This material, in which patch fibrosis is less extensive and consequently less constructive than in pericardium or Dacron, allows the implantation of a dimensionally small patch which in addition has the curvature of a vascular graft and is therefore unlikely prone to distortion. Its teardrop configuration takes advantage of the anatomical larger diameter of the left atrium in the horizontal

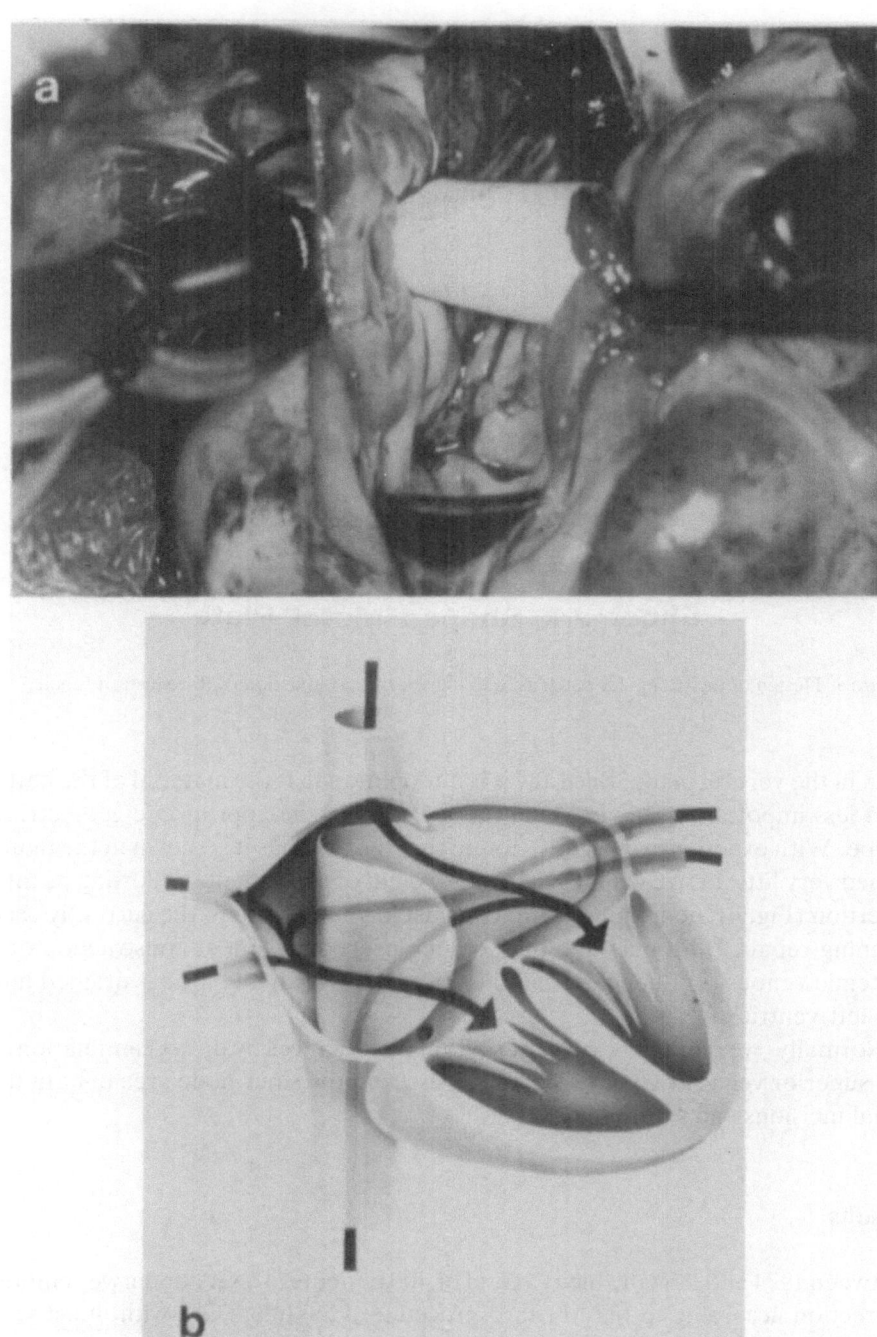

*Figure 2.* Insertion of the new designed triangular patch from a Gore-Tex prosthesis. It allows the creation of a straight caval tunnel within the atria: a) intraoperative view, b) diagramatic view.

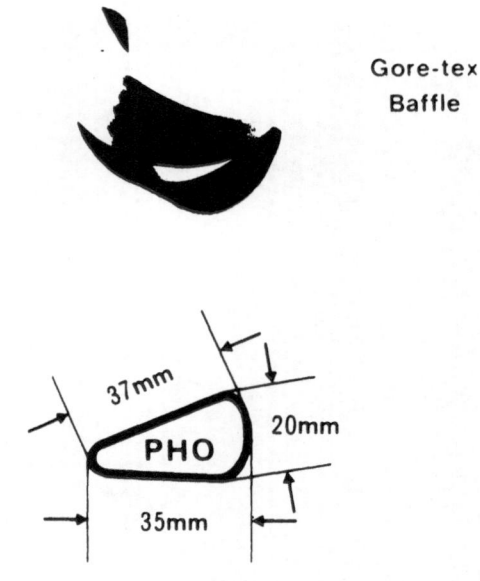

Gore-tex
Baffle

**Shoemark Shaped Metal Plate**

*Figure 3.* Design of the triangular patch used in our recent modification of the Mustard repair.

than in the vertical plane. Basically it is our opinion that the material of the baffle is of less importance as long as the baffle itself has the appropriate geometrical shape. With experience it was also found that the patch as it is shown in the figure varied very little in size with regard to the weight of the patient. Following its final insertion (Fig. 4), no major differences exist in comparison to the currently used Senning repair. Both ours and the Senning procedure aim at construction of a systemic venous confluence within the atria from which all blood is drained into the left ventricle.

Normally, we attempt to prevent rhythm disturbances by direct cannulation of the superior vena cava and by staying away from the sinus node area in both the atrial incisions and suture lines.

**Results**

Between 1974 and 1984 (Table 1) a total of 400 patients of TGA underwent inflow correction according to the Mustard procedure. 260 had TGA with intact ventricular septum or an insignificant ventricular septal defect (VSD) and 140 had TGA with associated anomalies, such as large VSD, left ventricular outflow obstruction, and/or pulmonary vascular disease. The overall early mortality

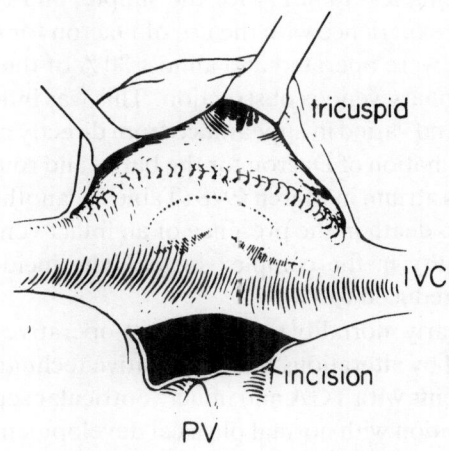

*Figure 4.* Diagramatic view of the currently used Senning operation.

TRANSPOSITION OF THE GREAT ARTERIES

Total Experience

(1974 - 1984)

| Anatomical Type | No.of cases | (% ) | early deaths | (%) |
|---|---|---|---|---|
| intact  VS | 260 | (65%) | 2 | ( 1%) |
| large   VSD | 49 | (12%) | 7 | (14 %) |
| LVOTO | 39 | (10%) | 4 | (10 %) |
| VSD, LVOTO | 41 | (10%) | 2 | ( 5 %) |
| VSD, PVD | 11 | ( 3%) | 2 | (18 %) |
| total | 400 | (100%) | 17 | ( 4 %) |

VS(D)  =  Ventricular Septal (Defect)

LVOTO  =  Left Ventricular Outflow Tract Obstruction

PVD    =  Pulmonary Vascular Disease

*Table 1.* Total experience with the Mustard operation, 1974–1984.

amounted to 4.3% being less than 1% for the simple, and 11% for the complex varieties. Early in our experience with the use of Dacron for the intraatrial baffle (Table 2) 138 patients were operated and almost 30% of the survivors sustained systemic and/or pulmonary venous obstruction. This was independent of the age at primary operation and varied in appearance from directly postoperative up to 5 years later. Since elimination of Dacron for the baffle and routine enlargement of the pulmonary venous atrium in March 1978 (Table 3), another 262 patients have been operated with no death in the presence of an intact ventricular septum and an 8.5% early mortality in the complex forms. The incidence of late inflow obstruction could be reduced to 1%.

According to this, early mortality as well as post-operative complications were significantly improved by alterations in the operative techniques. With regard to the late results of patients with TGA and intact ventricular septum, 95% are in an excellent clinical condition with normal physical development. Sinus rhythm was recorded in 80% of the survivors and junctional rhythm in another 18%. Two patients suffered from sick sinus syndrome but could be controlled by antiarrythmic drugs.

TRANSPOSITION OF THE GREAT ARTERIES

early experience (1974 - 3/1978)

| | No.of cases | Incidence of inflow obstruction | |
|---|---|---|---|
| | | n | (%) |
| simple TGA | 92 (2) | | |
| complex TGA | 46 (7) | 39 | (28%) |
| Total | 138 (9) | | |

Table 2. Early experience using a Dacron baffle, 1974–3/1978.

TRANSPOSITION OF THE GREAT ARTERIES

recent experience (3/1978 - 1984)

| | No. of cases | Incidence of inflow obstruction | |
|---|---|---|---|
| | | n | % |
| simple TGA | 168 (-) | | |
| complex TGA | 94 (8) | 3 | (1 %) |
| TOTAL | 262 (8) | | |

Table 3. Recent experience using a Gore-Tex triangular patch, 3/1978–1984.

## Discussion

Following introduction of the original Mustard operation, the mortality of children with TGA has been substantially reduced and was considered acceptable in most centers. However, numerous early and late complications of the inflow obstruction and rhythm disturbances rendered the procedure far from being curative. When early in the experience pericardium was used for the baffle, it soon became obvious that some degree of cicatricial adherence occurred which could result in hindrance of the venous inflow [5, 18, 31, 32]. This was found predominantly in infants because, with a small initial orifice constructed in small atria, a given degree of shrinkage more severely compromised the flow in the smaller patient as compared to the larger child.

During the following years varying degrees of obstruction to the venous return were identified. Because this was attributed to constriction of baffles constructed from pericardium [5, 37], Dacron was proposed as an appropriate substitute [31], at least in the infant. However, rather than decreasing the incidence of late fibrosis by substituting Dacron for pericardium, pulmonary as well as systemic venous obstruction was markedly increased [1, 6, 12, 31]. During reoperation, thickened neointima and buildup of fibrotic tissue were demonstrated all along the synthetic material adjacent to the venous blood stream.

When other centers similarly experienced [1, 6, 18, 26, 31] an increased incidence of late complication, it became obvious that despite the relatively low immediate surgical mortality and the symptomatic improvement of the survivors there was a need for a better operation. At this time, in 1977, the Senning operation was rediscovered by Brom [24] and those surgeons who did join this renewed method in order to improve results, developed a personal modification of the Mustard repair [34]. From then on, utilizing both methods, the operative risk was minimal and early as well as late inflow obstruction has become rare even in the newborne infant [22, 30, 32].

Starting in 1978, we still continue to use Gore-Tex for the intraatrial baffle. We thereby take advantage not only of its athrombogenic character but also of its natural curvature which offers creation of a new patch design. With this method of repair (Table 3), only three newborns developed late pulmonary venous obstruction, probably because of their initially small atria.

In parallel, the popularity of the Senning procedure has grown in different centers, largely due to reports of others that have concluded that baffle material in principle should be avoided. Including minor but important modifications by Brom [24] and others [21], the Senning procedure has been successfully applied particularly in infants [21, 22, 23, 36]. The presumption that the living tissue can be expected to grow and to conform to the blood flow within is most attractive. More and more surgeons have turned to the Senning operation not only because the incidence of reoperation previously has been high in their patients [7], but also because of the major advantage which lies in the potential of growth and contraction of the new atria [5, 21]. Since introduction of this method, the incidence of venous obstruction has been exceedingly rare [22, 23]. As in the Mustard operation damage to the sinus node and its artery through incisions and suture lines are carefully avoided [22, 23]. A comperative series from the Munich heart center [8] demonstrated sinus rhythm in 80% of the patients following the Senning operation, and in 91% of the patients after the Mustard repair. Parenzan published postoperative sinus rhythm in all of his 35 patients [22], and in a series of Martin et al [17a], 86% of patients resumed sinus rhythm within a mean interval of 15 months after the Senning operation. Sinus rhythm following the modified Mustard repair has been reported in a range from 76 to 96% [1, 22, 25, 33, 34]. According to the atrial myocardium at risk in both operations no different incidence of such arrythmias consisting of sick sinus syndrome, sinus bradycardia, junctional rhythm or a wandering pacemaker has been found nor can it be expected to exist [17b]. Rarely have dysrhythmias caused important hemodynamic alterations after correction of simple TGA.

Having reduced early mortality rate as well as the major complications of inflow obstruction and rhythm disturbances, several areas of concern have remained during the late postoperative course. These include functional adequacy of the newly created atria, long term competence of the tricuspid valve in a high-pressure ventricle, and the ability of the right ventricle to sustain the necessary systemic cardiac output.

Residual shunts at the atrial level are generally small and of minor concern [32, 37]. They have occurred regardless of the operative method and suggest that some technical improvement still can be made. While most of the intraatrial space is used to construct the systemic venous confluence, patch enlargement of the pulmonary venous atrium in Mustard operation was advised to secure an unobstructed blood flow also through this channel. However, increase in the pulmonary venous atrial reservoir may decrease the effectiveness of atrial contraction and thus depress cardia output. Particularly in infants under the age of one year we therefore recommend a direct atrial wall plasty, which makes the procedure even more similar to the Senning repair.

Tricuspid insufficiency has been infrequently encountered in patients with an essentially intact ventricular septum [2, 9]. While some authors suggest that the final result must still be awaited, others have drawn an analogy between TGA after the Mustard operation and naturally corrected TGA in which incompetence of the left sided tricuspid valve is a common occurrence in the long term.

However, because of the high incidence of abnormalities of the valve, naturally corrected TGA is not a valid model for the prediction of tricuspid valve function in surgically corrected TGA. The hitherto rare incidence of tricuspid regurgitation suggest that this valve may well sustain systemic pressure load following inflow correction of TGA with intact ventricular septum [2, 30, 33, 37].

Finally, a distinct worry has been the occurrence of a diminished right ventricular contractility in some children, with or without tricuspid valve incompetence some months or years later after the operation [12, 13, 32]. Although it was mainly seen in patients who already had preoperative depression of right ventricular function [14] and who suffered from associated lesions such as VSD and/or left ventricular outflow obstruction which per se may alter ventricular function, Graham et al [11] have described similar observations in the simple post-Mustard patient. It must, however, be argued, that these results were obtained from earlier series or from patients in whom surgical correction had been unduely delayed because of young age.

Myocardial injury may occur at operation or even in the early postoperative days [11], but it has also been suspected that the right ventricle in TGA is more susceptible to hypoxia than the left ventricle in a normal heart [13, 32].

Since all efforts have been made not to postpone surgery in symptomatic infants and to protect the myocardium during the operation by limiting the period of ischemia using hypothermic cardioplegic arrest, the incidence of impaired right ventricular function has become vary rare [10]. Recatherisation data from our laboratory and from others indicate that in patients with isolated TGA and preoperative unimpaired right ventricular function the contractility of the right ventricle remains unaltered following the correctly performed Mustard operation [16]. To the contrary, tricuspid incompetence and severe depression of right ventricular function was found in a substantial number of patients when inflow correction was performed in complex TGA [12, 14, 17]. It is suspected that in these cases some instances of myocardial damage are related to episodes of dysrhythmias, because they often occur together in the same child. It remains to be seen if fundamental physiologic and structural differences eventually will provide more information on the right ventricular behaviour as a systemic ventricle in TGA.


## Summary

In summary the modified Mustard procedure has come very close to the Senning repair. Both operations restore the normal circulatory pattern, but leave the anatomy unaltered.

From the point of operative techniques, some foreign material is required in the Mustard operation, while in the Senning procedure the patient's own atrial tissue is exclusively used. While the Mustard operation is easier to perform because of its standardised techniques, the advantages of the Senning repair are primarily related to the increased potential of growth.

The operative mortality of both procedures is low. In a series from several centers it was shown to be 1.4% for the Mustard operation and 1.3% for the Senning operation [30]. Amongst surgical complications, caval as well as pulmonary obstruction could be eliminated in the Senning procedure [22, 23] and have been reported with diminishing incidence in the modified Mustard repair [20, 25,

32, 34]. It may continue to be a problem in the small heart of the neonate, but recent investigations have demonstrated adequate growth following both operations, the condition being that wide pathways have been achieved during primary insertion of the baffle [32, 33]. Similarly, because of technical modifications, the current incidence of serious arrythmias after the Mustard and Senning operation is low [1, 22, 25, 29, 33, 34]. Tricuspid incompetence may exist isolated or secondary to poor right ventricular function. However, because of the high incidence of abnormalities of the valve, naturally corrected TGA is not a valid model for the prediction of tricuspid valve function in surgically corrected TGA. The hitherto rare incidence of tricuspid regurgitation suggest that this valve may well sustain systemic pressure load following inflow correction of TGA with intact ventricular septum [2, 30, 33, 37].

Finally, a distinct worry has been the occurrence of a diminished right ventricular contractility in some children, with or without tricuspid valve incompetence some months or years after the operation [12, 13, 32]. Although it was mainly seen in patients who already had preoperative depression of right ventricular function [14] and who suffered from associated lesions such as VSD and/or left ventricular outflow obstruction which per se alter ventricular function, Graham et al [11] have described similar observations in the simple post Mustard patient. It must, however, be argued, that these results were obtained from earlier series or from patients in whom surgical correction had been unduely delayed because of young age.

Myocardial injury may occur at operation or even in the early postoperative days [11], but it has also been suscepted that the right ventricle in TGA is more suspectible to hypoxia than the left ventricle in a normal heart [13, 32].

However, it has not longer been seen in patients with simple TGA during the last years, so that this problem following intraatrial repair may have antedated it in earlier series [1, 2, 9, 10, 12, 32]. Hemodynamic studies indicate that the right ventricle in patients who underwent surgery in the first year of life and with improved methods of myocardial protection, continues to function well. Additionally, long term results have shown that the majority of survivors can lead a normal life [22, 28, 30]. It would therefore appear that both the Mustard and the Senning operation, the choice depending on the surgeon's experience and preference, continue to be recommended for children with TGA and intact ventricular septum.

## References

1. Arciniegas E, Farooki ZQ, Hakimi M et al (1981) Results of the Mustard operation for d-transposition of the great arteries. J Thorac Cardiovasc Surg 81: 580
2. Balderman SC, Athanasuleas AB, Anagnostopoulos CE (1974) The atrial baffle operation for transposition of the great arteries. A review of 591 reported cases. Ann Thorac Surg 17: 114–121

3. Berman MA, Barask PS, Hellenbrand WE et al (1976) Late development of severe pulmonary venous obstruction following the Mustard operation. Circulation 56 (Suppl. 2): 91–94
4. Champsaur GL, Sokol DM, Trusler GA, Mustard UT (1973) Repair of transposition of the great arteries in 123 pediatric patients. Early and long term results. Circulation 47: 1032–1041
5. Cobanoglu A, Abbruzzese PA, Freimanis J et al (1984) Pericardial baffle complications following the Mustard operation. J Thorac Cardiovasc Surg 87: 371–378
6. Driscol DD, Nibill MR, Vargo TA et al (1977) Late development of pulmonary venous obstruction following Mustard operation using a Dacron baffle. Circulation 55: 484–488
7. Egloff LP, Freed MD, Dick M et al (1978) Early and late results with the Mustard operation in infancy. Ann Thorac Surg 26: 474–484
8. Feder E, Meisner H, Bühlmeyer K et al (1980) Operative Treatment of TGA: Comparison of Senning's and Mustard's operation in patients under 2 years. Thorac cardiovasc Surgeon 28: 7–12
9. Flemming WH (1979) Why switch? J Thorac Cardiovasc Surg 78: 1–2
10. Godman MJ, Friedli B, Pasternac A et al (1976) Hemodynamic studies in children four to ten years after the Mustard operation for transposition of the Great Arteries. Circulation 53: 532–538
11. Graham TP, Aturood GF, Boucek JR et al (1975) Abnormalities of right ventricular function following Mustard's operation for transposition of the great arteries. Circulation 52: 678–684
12. Hagler D.J., Ritter DG, Mair DD et al (1978) Clinical, Angiographic, and Hemodynamic Assessment of Late Results After Mustard operation. Circulation 57: 1214–1220
13. Hagler DJ, Ritter DG, Mair DD et al (1979) Right and left ventricular function after the Mustard procedure in transposition of the great arteries. Am J Cardiol 44: 276–283
14. Jarmakani JMM, Canent RV jr (1974) Preoperative and postoperative right ventricular function in children with transposition of great vessels. Circulation 50 Sup II: II, 39: II–45
15. Lewis AB, Lindesmith GG, Takashashi et al (1977) Cardiac rhythm following the Mustard procedure for transposition of the great vessels. J Thorac Cardiovasc Surg 73: 919–926
16. Luhmer I, Weber L, Wuttke S, Oelert H, Kallfelz HC (1981) Zur Funktion des rechten Ventrikels bei Transposition der Großen Arterien nach Vorhofumkehr (Mustard). Herz 6: 352–355
17. Mair DD, Danielson G, Wallace RB, McGoon DC (1974) Long term follow up of Mustard operation survivors. Circulation 50, Suppl. 2: 46–53
17a. Martin TC, Smith L, Hernandez A, Weldon CS (1983) Dysthythmias following the Senning operation for dextro-transposition of the great arteries. J Thorac Cardiovasc Surg 85: 928–932
17b. Marquez-Montez J, O'Connor F, Burgos R et al (1983) Comparative electrophysiological evaluation of atrial activation and sinoatrial node function following Senning and Mustard procedures: An experimental study. Am Thor Surg 36: 692–699
18. Mohri H, Barnes RW, Rittenhouse EA et al (1970) Fate of autologous pericardium and Dacron falzic used as substitutes for total atrial septum in growing animals. J Thorac Cardiovasc Surg 59: 501–511
19. Mustard WT (1964) Successful two-stage correction of transposition of the great vessels. Surgery 55: 469–472
20. Oelert H, Borst HG (1977) Atrial inversion for transposition of the great arteries using an intraatrial Dacron baffle. Surgical technique and results in: Modern cardiac Surgery, D.B. Longmore ed., Londen, Medical Technical Press
21. Otero Coto E, Norwood WJ, Lang P, Castaneda AR (1979) Modified Senning operation for treatment of transposition of the great arteries. J Thorac Cardiovasc Surg 78: 721–729
22. Parenzan L, Locatelli G, Alfieri O et al (1978) The Senning operation for transposition of the great arteries. J Thorac Cardiovasc Surg 76: 305–311
23. Quageneur JM, Brom AG (1978) The trousers-shaped Baffle for use the Mustard operation. Ann Thorac Surg 25: 240–242
24. Quageneur JM, Rohmer J, Brom AG, Tinkelenberg J (1977) Revival of the Senning operation in the treatment of transposition of the great arteries. Thorax 32: 517–524
25. Replogle RL, Lin CY (1972) Surgical correction of transposition of the great vessels. A technical

suggestion. J Thorac Cardiovasc 63: 196–198

26. Reul GJ, Cooley DA, Sanidorfd FM, Hallman GL (1974) Complications following the contaused Dacron baffle in correction of transposition of the great arteries. Surgery 76: 946–954

27. Senning Å (1959) Surgical correction of transposition of the great vessels. Surgery 45: 966–980

28. Schmitz JP, Taylor JFN, Graham GR, Stark J. Late Results of Mustard operation for transposition of the great arteries. Proc 7th Europ Congress Cardiology, p. 291

29. Southall DP, Keeton BR, Leangage R et al (1980) Cardiac rhythm and conduction before and after Mustard's operation for complete transposition of the great arteries. Br Heart J 43: 21–30

30. Stark J (1983) Evaluation of inflour-type repairs for transposition of the great arteries. Ped Cardiol 4, Suppl. 1: 159–164

31. Stark J, Silove ED, Taylor JFN, Graham GR (1974) Obstruction to systemic venous return following the Mustard operation for transposition of the great arteries. J Thorac Cardiovasc Surg 68: 742–749

32. Trusler GA, Williams WG, Izukawa T, Olley PM (1980) Current results with the Mustard operation in isolated transposition of the great arteries. J Thorac Cardiovasc Surg 80: 381–389

33. Turley K, Ebert PA (1978) Total correction of transposition of the great arteries. Conduction disturbances in infants younger than three month of age. J Thorac Cardiovasc Surg 76: 312–320

34. Ullal RR, Anderson RH, Lincoln C (1979) Mustard's operation modified to avoid dysthythmias and pulmonary and systemic venous obstruction. J Thorac Cardiovasc Surg 78: 431–439

35. Venables AW, Edis B, Clarke CP (1974) Vena caval obstruction complicating the Mustard operation for complete transposition of the great arteries. Eur J Cardiol 1: 401

36. Weldon CS, Hartmann AF Jr, Kelly JP (1983) Current management of transposition of the great arteries: Immediate septostomy, occasional prostaglandin infusion, and early Senning operations. Ann Thorac Surg 36: 10–18

37. Zavarella C, Subramanian S (1978) Review: Surgery for transposition of the great arteries in the first year of life. Ann Surg 187: 143–150

# Switch-over procedure in transposition of the great arteries

R.C. RADLEY-SMITH and MAGDI H. YACOUB

## Summary

Between 1975 and 1985, 110 children underwent anatomic correction of transposition of the great arteries at Harefield Hospital. Forty five patients aged between 3 weeks and 26 years had complex lesions and underwent a primary correction. Sixty five had intact septum. Of these, 38 patients aged 4.5–24 months had a 2-stage procedure with preliminary banding to prepare the left ventricle. Seventeen neonates and 10 children with dynamic subpulmonary stenosis underwent primary correction. There were 14 (31%) early deaths in the complex group and 8 (10%) in the simple group. Coronary artery transfer was accomplished safely in all patients and was not a factor in early death. One patient at restudy has occlusion of his left coronary artery. Three methods have been used for reconstruction of the pulmonary arteries. Four patients have gradients of more than 40 mm Hg across the right ventricular outflow tract and one has required reoperation. Two patients have mild, non progressive aortic regurgitation. Left ventricular function assessed by echocardiography and catheterisation in 56 is normal in all but one patient. Anatomic correction of transposition of the great arteries gives encouraging medium term results.

It is now 10 years since Jatene [1] performed the first successful anatomic correction of transposition of the great arteries (TGA) in a baby with an additional large ventricular septal defect (VSD). This technique has now largely been accepted as the treatment of choice for TGA with VSD, but controversy still exists as to its place in the treatment of the majority of patients with TGA – those with intact septum.

Since our first successful anatomic correction at Harefield Hospital, also in 1975, we have analysed our experience and identified several potential or actual problems and attempted to provide some answers.

These problems include:
1. The initial high mortality (learning curve).
2. Transfer of the different anatomic types of coronary artery without torsion,

tension, or kinking.

3. The ability of the left ventricle to take over the systemic load.
4. Its ability to function normally long-term.
5. Bridging the gap between the proximal and distal pulmonary artery.
6. The ability of all the anastomotic sites; coronary, aortic and pulmonary, to grow normally.
7. The ability of the new aortic valve and sinuses of Valsalva to function normally without progressive dilatation or regurgitation.

**Patients and methods**

Between October 1975 and April 1985, 110 patients have undergone anatomic correction of TGA at Harefield Hospital. Forty-five patients had complex TGA with a high left ventricular pressure. Additional lesions included a large VSD in 41, persistent ductus arteriosus (PDA) in 3 and an aorto-pulmonary window in 1. Their ages were between 3 weeks and 16 years.

Sixty-five patients had an intact interventricular septum – simple TGA. Thirty-eight patients aged 4.5–24 months underwent a 2-stage procedure with pulmonary artery banding ± a shunt as a first stage to prepare the left ventricle. The age at banding varied from 1 day to 13 months and the interval between banding and correction 2–11 months.

Since May 1982, 17 patients presenting at Harefield in the neonatal period have undergone primary correction, aged 3–42 days, weighing 1.5–4.5 kg. These babies are now operated upon as emergencies on echocardiographic diagnosis alone and in the last 6 patients without even a balloon septostomy.

Ten patients aged 3.5–48 months with simple TGA, had dynamic subpulmonary obstruction maintaining a high left ventricular (LV) pressure, also underwent primary correction. The outflow tract gradient disappeared completely after operation without any resection of the subvalve region.

Fifty-six out of 59 patients who have been followed up for more than 12 months since operation, have undergone routine re-investigation, at least once by cardiac catheterisation and angiography. Twelve patients had an early restudy and 53 patients had a late restudy 1–4.6 (mean 2.0) years after operation. Twelve patients have undergone more than 1 restudy.

**Early and late mortality**

Fourteen patients (31%) with complex TGA died within 30 days of operation. Seven of these had advanced pulmonary vascular disease. Other contributory factors were an abnormal positioned or undiagnosed VSD in 2 and a poorly developed left ventricle in 1.

In patients with simple TGA there were 4 deaths (10%) in patients undergoing banding as a first stage procedure. Two of these deaths were thought to be preventable. There were 8 deaths (10%) at correction, four in the group undergoing the second stage correction, 2 in the neonatal group and 2 in patients with subpulmonary stenosis. Left ventricular failure due to an inadequately prepared LV was thought to be responsible for death in 4 patients. One patient aged 24 months had severe pulmonary vascular disease. Eleven deaths occurred between 1975 and 1978 – a period that we consider was our learning curve for this operation. Since 1979, there have been 11 further deaths in 89 patients.

With a follow up of 1–103 months, there have been 2 late deaths in the complex group due to progressive pulmonary vascular disease 18 months after operation in 1 and a cerebrovascular accident 3.5 years after operation in another. One patient with simple TGA died 6 months after operation from pneumonia. There have been no unexplained sudden deaths.

## Coronary transfer

Because anatomic correction of TGA involves transfer of the coronary ostia from the aorta to the pulmonary artery (new aorta), it is essential to be familiar with the different modes of origin, course and early branching of the coronary arteries in this condition. Despite the existance of many variations of coronary anatomy, the great majority of patients have one of 3 types: designated Types A, D and E [2] (Fig. 1), in order of frequency of presentation. Type E is present only in patients with side by side great arteries. Types B and C are very rare. Variants of the basic anatomic types also occur, but rarely (Table 1). The type of coronary anatomy can usually be diagnosed preoperatively from the angiogram.

With attention to detail, contrary to some opinions, we believe that all types of

Table 1. Coronary anatomy.

| Type | Simple [65] | | Death | Complex [45] | | Death |
|---|---|---|---|---|---|---|
| A | 42 | 66% | 3 | 30 | 69% | 1 |
| Variant | 1 | | | 1 | | |
| B | 1 | 1% | | – | 4% | |
| Variant | | | 1 | 2 | | 2 |
| C | 2 | 3% | 1 | 2 | 4% | 1 |
| D | 11 | 22% | | 3 | 7% | 1 |
| Variant | 3 | | 3 | – | | |
| E | 3 | 8% | | 3 | 16% | |
| Variant | | | | 4 | | 2 |

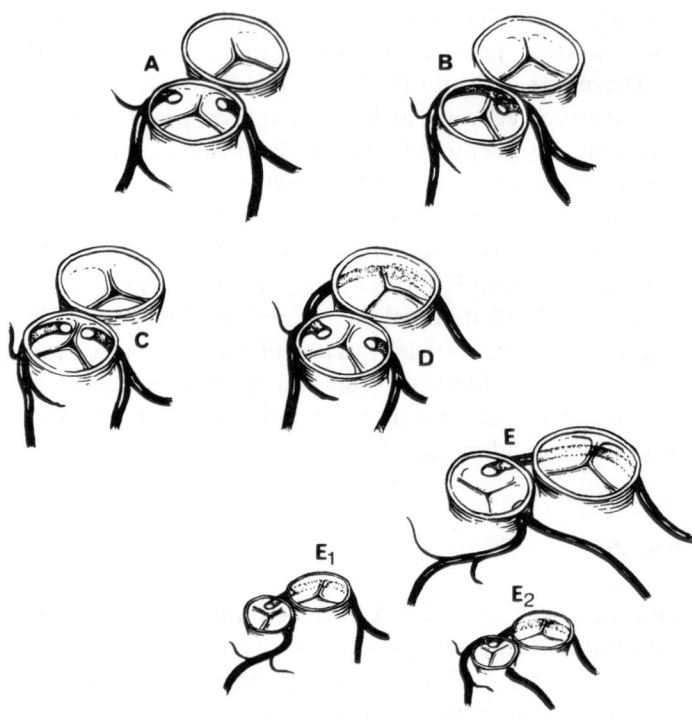

*Figure 1.* The origin and modes of branching of the coronary arteries.

coronary anatomy can be transferred. The technique used should avoid tension, torsion or kinking of the main coronary arteries and avoid injury to the proximal branches and allow for growth of the origin of the coronary arteries from the aorta. To achieve these objectives the following principles should be observed:

1. The angle of rotation of the coronary ostia in the horizontal plane should not be more than 90 degrees.
2. The level of coronary anastomosis should correspond to the site of origin from the anterior vessel in the frontal plane. As the aortic valve and sinuses in TGA are higher than that of the pulmonary valve, it is usually necessary to anastomose the coronary ostia at a point above the level of the pulmonary artery (new aortic) sinuses.
3. The special relationship between the mobilised aortic discs surrounding the coronary ostia and the proximal coronary artery should be maintained as any rotation of the discs during anastomosis may produce torsion of the proximal coronary artery.
4. Kinking or injury of early branches should be avoided. This can be achieved by identifying the early branches and performing minimal mobilisation.

5. Apposition between the proximal coronary artery and the aortic wall for a distance of more than a few milimetres should be avoided, as future distension of the aorta during exercise may result in stretching of the coronary artery and sudden myocardial ischaemia, as is known to happen in abnormal origin of the left coronary artery from the anterior sinus [3].

The technique commonly used for most patients who have Type A, D or E involves direct transfer with a generous disc of aortic wall and to allow for growth of the ostia (Fig. 2). During transfer, care should be taken not to distort the components of the new aortic valve, because this may result in postoperative aortic regurgitation.

In patients with Type B or C in whom the coronary ostia (or ostium) is facing almost directly forward, rotation of the disc would involve severe torsion of the proximal coronary arteries. For these patients, another technique which requires no rotation of the disc has been devised [2] (Fig. 3). Other methods have been described [4, 5] that re-locate the coronary arteries without transfer or manipulation. These have the disadvantage of creating a recess that may interfere with future coronary flow. In analysing the results in our patients (Table 1), the coronary artery anatomy was not a factor in early mortality except perhaps in patients with Type B (single orifice) anatomy. However, 2 of these patients also had severe pulmonary vascular disease and 1 had a poorly developed left ventricle.

Postoperative restudy in 56 patients has shown that the ostia have grown in all patients (Fig. 4). One patient had proximal occlusion of the left coronary artery with consequent reduction in left ventricular ejection fraction. This occlusion probably occurred early in the postoperative period which was protracted and stormy.

**Ability of the left ventricle to take over the load of the circulation after correction**

After birth, the left ventricle develops normally in patients with TGA and additional lesions, such as a large VSD, PDA or subpulmonary stenosis which maintains a high peak systolic pressure in the left ventricle, which is therefore capable of taking over the load of circulation.

In patients with simple TGA – who constitute the majority, the normal drop in pulmonary vascular resistance after birth results in progressive fall in the left ventricular pressure and failure of development of the LV muscle mass. This fall in pressure occurs largely in the first 4 weeks of life [6] but can be variable. The interval between pressure drop and the diminution of LV muscle mass so as to render it incapable of supporting the systemic circulation is not known, but is also probably about 4 weeks. If primary correction is to be undertaken in these patients, it would appear that it should be performed during this period. This approach has become feasible with the better understanding of neonatal physiol-

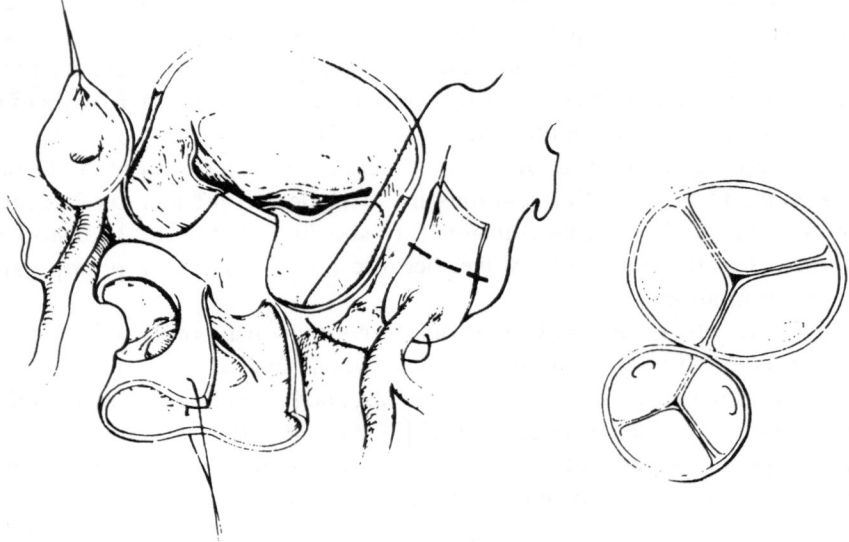

*Figure 2.* Method of transfer for types A, D and E coronary anatomy.

ogy, specialist neonatal care and better myocardial protection. It is now our preferred method of treatment, and has been successfully accomplished in a baby of 32 weeks gestation weighing 1.5 kg.

Early in our experience and for late referrals, we have used a 2-stage technique for correction [7]. The first stage operation consists of banding the pulmonary artery with an additional aortopulmonary shunt in patients with a preoperative low total pulmonary blood flow. The interval between banding and correction depends on the pressures achieved at banding. In patients with a peak LV/RV ratio of more than .8 an interval of 3 months seems adequate to prepare the ventricle. If however, the ratio is less than this, an interval of 6–9 months appears to be necessary. Other helpful guides to the state of the LV have been the Frank vectorcardiogram and a subcostal four chamber view of the ventricles. If the echo shows a normal appearance of the ventricular septum committed to the LV then the ventricle will support the systemic load.

## Late LV function

Most patients following operation have varying degrees of LV failure requiring intensive medical treatment for periods up to 3 months. At late evaluation, 1 year or more after operation, all patients apart from the patient already mentioned with left coronary artery occlusion appear to have a normal LV function. Echo-

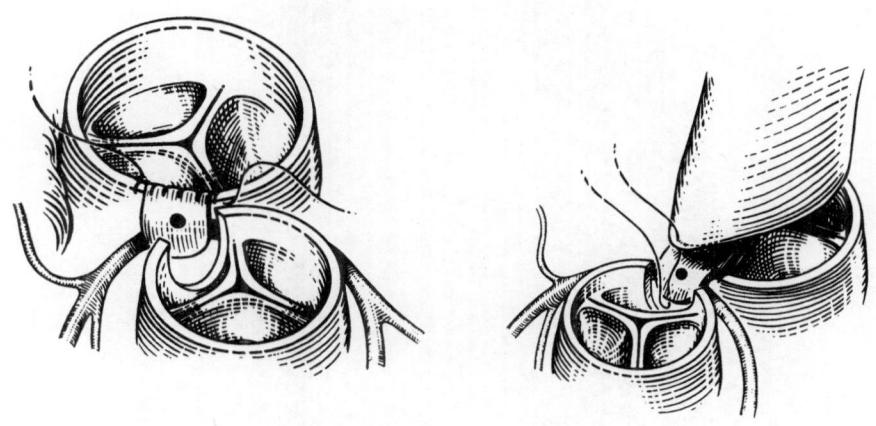

*Figure 3*. Method of transfer of types B and C, with no rotation of the coronary ostium.

cardiographically, the shortening fraction and therefore the ejection fraction are within normal limits. Posterior wall thickness is normal but the septum as in other postoperative states, is flat. At catheterisation, the LV end diastolic pressure and ejection fraction is normal and the ventricles contract with a normal pattern. Assessment of the contractile state using a methoxamine challenge [8] has shown a normal response in 10 out of 12 patients studied. The 2 abnormal results were obtained in a patient studied early postoperatively still in the adaptive phase, and in a patient corrected at the age of 2 years. From this study it would appear that the LV function is better the earlier the patient is corrected.

**Bridging the gap between the proximal pulmonary artery and distal pulmonary artery**

Although direct anastomosis of the pulmonary artery is feasible in a small number of patients – particularly if the great arteries are side by side, in the majority of patients, direct anastomosis results in undue tension and narrowing of the distal pulmonary arteries and compression of the new aortic root. To overcome this difficulty, three techniques have been used (Fig. 5). Early in our experience a variable sized dacron tube was used depending on the age of the patient. Supravalve gradients occurred in the two smallest patients necessitating re-operation, which was successful in 1. A large (2.5 cm diameter) tube of homologous dura mater placed to the left of the aorta was used in 33 patients. Placement to the right aorta results in kinking and supravalve stenosis due to compression. The technique described by Le Compte [9] with mobilisation of the pulmonary arterial bifurcation and branches into the hilum and threading the aortic arch

58

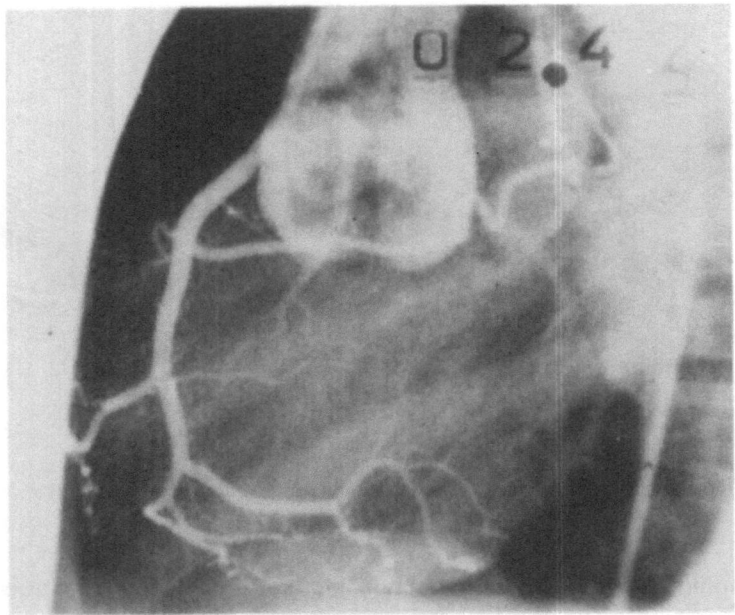

*Figure 4.* Aortogram showing normal growth of the coronary ostia and distribution of the coronaries 18 months after operation.

behind the bifurcation allowing for direct anastomosis of the pulmonary artery has been used in 71 patients. However, gradients of up to 40 mmHg in the right ventricular outflow tract have been recorded at 1 year after operation in some patients in the neonatal group, both by ourselves and the Boston group [10].

## Fate of the new aortic valve and growth of the aortic anastomoses

Although the 2 semilunar valves are similar in thickness and structure at birth, the pulmonary valve undergoes adaptive changes which include thinning of the cusps due to the fall in pulmonary artery pressure. After correction this valve becomes the aortic valve. However, this pulmonary valve developmentally is an aortic valve, with the normal attachment to the subaortic curtain and fibrous skeleton of the heart. Repeat angiography up to 4.6 years after operation has shown mild aortic regurgitation in two patients, one of whom had an extremely large pulmonary valve root preoperatively because of advanced pulmonary vascular disease. In neither patient has the regurgitation or dilatation of the aortic root increased with time either angiographically or echocardiographically with no increase in LV end diastolic volume.

Anatomic correction entails circumferential anastomosis of the aorta at a

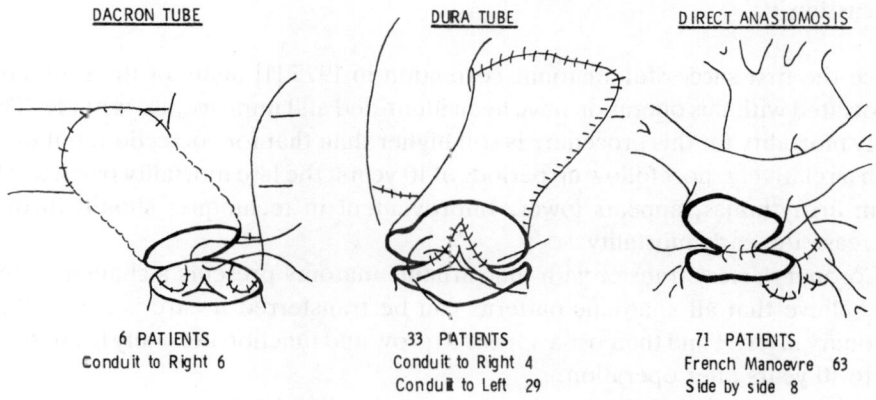

| DACRON TUBE | DURA TUBE | DIRECT ANASTOMOSIS |
| --- | --- | --- |
| 6 PATIENTS | 33 PATIENTS | 71 PATIENTS |
| Conduit to Right 6 | Conduit to Right 4 | French Manoevre 63 |
| | Conduit to Left 29 | Side by side 8 |

*Figure 5.* The three methods used for pulmonary artery reconstruction.

young age and the long term success of this procedure depends on continued growth of the anastomotic site. At repeat cardiac catheterisation the aortic root is measured at the level of the top of the sinuses and above the anastomotic site and the ratio measured. There has been no change in these measurements between early and late reinvestigations and no gradients have been measured on the left side of the heart.

**Pulmonary hypertension**

One patient with a large VSD, banded at 18 months and corrected at 5.5 years, died 18 months after correction. In the simple group, 1 patient died at correction aged 24 months and 1 patient corrected at 17 months has, 1 year after operation, a peak pulmonary artery pressure of 67 mmHg.

**Postoperative cardiac rhythm**

All patients routinely have standard 12-lead electrocardiogram at every visit and Holter monitoring at the time of their restudy catheterisation. All patients are in sinus rhythm without ectopic beats, except 1 who developed complete heart block following a repair of a large septectomy. She has not, with a 7 year follow up, required pacing. There has been no cases of sudden death or life threatening arrhythmias.

60

## Discussion

Since the first successful anatomic correction in 1975 [1] many of the problems associated with this operation have been identified and improvements made. The early mortality for this procedure is still higher than that for correction, but even with a relatively short follow up periods of 10 years, the late mortality particularly from arrhythmias, appears lower. Improvement in techniques should further decrease the early mortality.

Coronary artery transfer with the variable anatomy presents a challenge, but we believe that all anatomic patterns can be transferred if care is taken. The coronary arteries and their ostia appear to grow and function normally for periods up to 10 years after operation.

Although modifications in technique have simplified pulmonary artery reconstruction and the Le Compte [9] technique allows for direct anastomosis without inter-position of foreign material, recent evidence from the neonatal group has led one to believe that other methods of direct anastomosis may have to be developed for this age group.

Concern over the ability of the pulmonary valve to function long term as an aortic valve without progressive regurgitation, as yet appears to be unfounded and the anastomotic sites continue to grow. Progressive pulmonary vascular disease is a feature of TGA both with intact septum and particularly in the presence of VSD. Anatomic correction has not influenced the incidence of this complication which continues to be a problem.

The ability of the left ventricle to take over systemic load immediately after correction is of extreme importance. In the majority of patients with TGA – those with intact interventricular septum, the ventricle is incapable of supporting circulation after the first few weeks of life. If a 2-stage procedure with preparation of the ventricle is to be avoided, these babies will have to undergo correction as a semi-emergency procedure in the first month of life and currently we are operating as early as possible without prior septostomy.

The rationale for performing anatomic correction is to normalise the roles of the ventricles and depends on the assumption that the LV is normal before correction. Therefore, the evaluation of the late LV function is and will continue to be of extreme importance. At present is appears that after an initial period of adaptation the LV appears to function normally for periods up to 10 years.

## References

1. Jatene AD, Fontes VF, Paulista PP, Souza LCB, Neger F, Galantier M, Sousa JEMR (1975) Successful anatomic correction of transposition of the great vessels. A preliminary report. Arq Bras Cardiol 28: 461–464
2. Yacoub MH, Radley-Smith R (1978) Anatomy of the coronary arteries in transposition of the

great arteries and methods for their transfer in anatomical correction. Thorax 33: 418–424
3. Mustafa I, Gula G, Radley-Smith R, Durrer D, Yacoub MH (1981) Anomalous origin of the left coronary artery from the anterior aortic sinus: A potential cause of sudden death. Anatomic characterisation and surgical treatment. Thorac Cardiovasc Surg 82: 297–300
4. Damus PS (1975) Letter to the Editor. Ann Thorac Surg 20: 724
5. Danielson GK, Tabru IF, Mair DD, Fulton RE 1978 Great vessels switch operation without coronary relocation for transposition of the great arteries. Mayo Clin Proc 53: 675–682
6. Tynan M (1972) Transposition of the great arteries. Changes in circulation after birth. Circulation 46: 809–815
7. Yacoub MH, Radley-Smith R, MacLaurin R (1977) Two-stage operation for anatomical correction of transposition of the great arteries with intact interventricular septum. Lancet 1: 1275–1278
8. Borow KM, Arensman FW. Webb C, Radley-Smith R, Yacoub MH (1984) Assessment of left ventricular contractile state following anatomic correction of transposition of the great arteries using afterload challenge. Circulation 69: 106–112
9. Le Compte Y, Zannini L, Hazan E, Jarreau MM, Bex JP, Tran Viet Tin, Neveux JY (1981) Anatomic correction of transposition of the great arteries. A new technique without use of prosthetic conduit. J Thorac Cardiovasc Surg 82: 629–631
10. Hougen TJ, Colan SD, Norwood WI, Sanders SP, Lang P, Jones RA, Castaneda AR (1984) Haemodynamic results of arterial switch operation for transposition of the great arteries, intact ventricular septum (abstract). Circulation 70 (Suppl. II): 11–26

# Operative management of patients with pulmonary atresia and intact ventricular septum

M. DE LEVAL

Accounts of the management of pulmonary atresia with intact ventricular septum (PA:IVS) often constitute a catalogue of early and late failures of surgical treatment. A significant fall in early mortality in most series is attributable to a more reliable and durable augmentation of the pulmonary blood flow before, during and after the operation. Right ventricular hypoplasia is the main cause for the persistent dismal late outlook of this condition. This report reviews the Great Ormond Street experience and summarises our current thoughts on the definitive repair of this condition.

## Clinical material and methods

We first studied 32 specimens of patients who died with PA:IVS during the neonatal period and correlated these anatomic findings with the angiocardiograms of 45 newborns with PA:IVS. This analysis was based on the tripartite concept of the right ventricle dividing the chamber into an inlet, a trabecular and an outlet component. In addition the diameter of the tricuspid valve was utilised as a indicator of right ventricular cavity size.

The second part of the study consisted of a retrospective analysis of the early results of the surgical treatment of 60 neonates with PA:IVS. The third part of the study relates to decision making in the definitive repair of 51 patients.

## Results

Hearts with PA:IVS were classified anatomically and angiographically into three groups. In the first group all three portions of the right ventricular cavity were present and the anomaly consisted of a more or less severe degree of generalised hypoplasia. In the other hearts, besides the smallness of the cavity at least one portion was missing. All cases by definition had a patent tricuspid valve and thus an inlet portion to the ventricle but the trabecular (Group 2) or both trabecular and infundibular (Group 3) portions of the cavity can be so overgrown by hypertrophic myocardium as to be affectively absent. No specimen with a trabecular portion but no infundibular cavity was found. The tricuspid valve diameter was smaller than normal in all hearts. The largest tricuspid valve annulae were in the group in which all components of the ventricular cavity was present and the smallest in those with only an inlet portion to the ventricular cavity. Autopsy and angiographic estimates of tricuspid valve diameter correlate closely, the angiographic figures exceed the autopsy estimate by a factor of approximately 1.43:1. With this appreciation of the variety of ventricular morphology encountered we have reviewed the results of our surgical management of PA:IVS. The main objective of the treatment in the neonatal period is to increase the pulmonary blood flow. This is indispensible to achieve early survival. The quality of the definitive repair is closely related to right ventricular size and function. In the neonate the treatment must therefore increase the pulmonary blood flow and enable the right ventricle to serve the pulmonary circulation whenever possible.

The dramatic fall in early mortality is partly due to the pre- and peri-operative use of prostaglandin which allows the patient to come to surgery less acidotic, better oxygenated with a much better cardiac output.

Surgically the pulmonary blood flow can be increased by opening the right ventricular outflow tract or by the creation of a systemic to pulmonary artery fistula. The opening of the right ventricular outflow tract can be achieved by a closed transventricular or transpulmonary valvotomy, an open valvotomy on cardiopulmonary bypass or inflow occlusion or by combining the open valvotomy on cardiopulmonary bypass with a patch enlargement of the right ventricular outflow tract. Because of the poor results of the procedures performed on cardiopulmonary bypass as well as the transventricular valvotomies we adopted, a few years ago, a policy of doing transpulmonary valvotomies. This appeared to give satisfactory early results. However, the incidence of restenosis of the pulmonary valve was high and we now prefer pulmonary valvectomy under inflow occlusion. The presence of an infundibular component to the right ventricular cavity is of course a pre-requisite for an opening of the right ventricular outflow tract. A variety of shunt procedures have been utilised for these patients. We currently prefer the Blalock-Taussig shunt or the modified Blalock-Taussig shunt consisting of interposing a prosthesis between the subclavian artery and the pulmonary artery.

The neonatal management of PA:IVS based on the right ventricular size and morphology is summarised in Figure 1. In a small number of patients with a tripartite right ventricle of good size the relief of the right ventricular outflow tract obstruction can be sufficient to achieve a normal pulmonary perfusion with normal right ventricular haemodynamics. For these exceptional cases the definitive repair is achieved in infancy. Patients with a three portion right ventricle of a small size or a two portion right ventricle are currently submitted to a shunt

64

## PA:IVS MANAGEMENT IN NEONATES

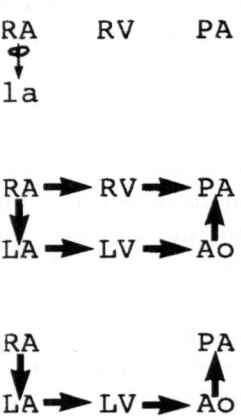

*Figure 1.*

procedure and a relief of the right ventricular outflow tract obstruction. We usually perform the two procedures during the same operating session. Because the relief of the right ventricular outflow tract obstruction via the trans-pulmonary valvotomy has not given us good long term results one could conceive that the two procedures could be done in two stages. The first operation consisting of a systemic to pulmonary artery shunt and the second stage would consist of a relief of the right ventricular outflow tract obstruction on cardiopulmonary bypass. For those right ventricles with an inlet portion only it is of course not possible to open up the right ventricular outflow tract and the pulmonary blood flow will rely on a systemic to pulmonary artery anastomosis. For that particular group of patients in whom the whole systemic venous return has to go into the left atrium through an atrial septal defect a balloon atrial septostomy might be advisable.

By the time definitive repair is undertaken most of these right ventricular cavities are still somewhat hypoplastic. The question then arises as to how small the diminitive right ventricular cavity can be to be usefully and safely incorporated into a surgical repair. We have retrospectively correlated the outcome of these patients with the preoperative right ventricular cavity size assessed by tricuspid valve diameter measurement and with the right ventricular morphology. The repair was considered to be definitive when it was expected to be the final management. The definitive repair was considered as complete when it consisted of a relief of the right ventricular outflow tract obstruction with separation of the pulmonary and systemic circulations by closure of intracardiac and extracardiac shunts (when present). The latter included persistent ductus arteriosus and surgically created systemic to pulmonary artery shunts. The definitive repair was considered as a definitive palliation when the atrial communication and the extracardiac shunts were left open. For these patients the right ventricular cavity was just too small to carry the whole cardiac output and this is why the shunts were left open. A complete separation of the systemic and pulmonary circulations was established using the Fontan procedure in a third group of patients.

The diameter of the tricuspid valve was estimated by measuring the diameter of the annulus as seen in diastolic frames of the anterior/posterior and the lateral right ventricular angiograms that preceeded the definitive repair. The diameter of the catheters was ued as the magnification factor and a table was prepared from the autopsy data of Rowlatt et al (1963) [1] adjusted for angiographic assessment [2] to establish normal ranges of tricuspid valve diameters by weight. All but one of the 29 patients who underwent a complete repair had a tricuspid valve diameter below the mean normal. This exceptional patient had massive tricuspid valve regurgitation. There were ten deaths among these 29 patients. Comparing the tricuspid valve diameter of the patients who died with those who survived it became apparent that the great majority of the survivors had a tricuspid valve diameter larger than the lower 99% confidence limits (CL) of mean normal (3 standard deviations). This was the case for 19 patients, 16 of whom survived (84%). All three patients who died with apparently adequate tricuspid valves were repaired as neonates. Two had free tricuspid valve regurgitation and one had a two portion right ventricle. There were eight deaths among the ten patients whose tricuspid valve diameter was smaller than the lower 99% CL of mean normal. This demarkation line between the survivors and the non-survivors of attempted complete repair was highly significant (p<0.01).

Twenty four of the 29 patients who underwent a complete repair had a three portion right ventricle. Five patients had an absent trabecular component and three died. Retrospectively all five had a tricuspid valve diameter around the lower 99% CL. Haemodynamic data were available for the two survivors and both had high venous pressures and their pulmonary arterial pressure tracing showed an 'a' wave corresponding to forward flow into the pulmonary artery giving atrial contraction.

All 11 patients who underwent a definitive palliation had a tricuspid valve diameter below the lower 99% CL. There were ten survivors all of them with some degree of systemic arterial desaturation and some exercise intolerance.

The theoretical attraction of the definitive palliation was that the right ventricle is used for what it can provide. The remaining pulmonary blood flow coming from the left ventricle via a systemic to pulmonary artery shunt. At first glance this might appear to be a fairly flexible circulation capable of maintaining pulmonary blood flow in the face of an elevated pulmonary vascular resistance that could not be tolerated by a Fontan circulation. However, there are drawbacks. One disadvantage relates to systemic desaturation which tends to increase with exercise. The second one relates to the increased left ventricular workload in a circulation with intra and extracardiac shunts. A Fontan procedure was performed in 11 patients of whom three died. These three patients did not fulfill the Fontan circulation criteria.

## Conclusion

Our data suggests that a three portion right ventricle with tricuspid valve diameter above the lower 99% CL can safely be used to support the pulmonary circulation providing major tricuspid valve regurgitation is not present. Such hearts are capable of producing a normal right ventricular dependent circulation with a systolic 'v' wave in the pulmonary artery and a normal central venous pressure. The above criteria can be fulfilled following palliative surgery but sometimes neonates would qualify for primary definitive repair.

Patients without a trabecular portion of the right ventricular cavity are of particular interest. If their tricuspid valve is within the 99% CL of the mean normal these right ventricles can be incorporated in a complete repair if the pulmonary arterial pressure and the resistance are low and if there is no gradient across the right heart pathway. These right ventricles have a stroke volume which is less than that of the left ventricle and right atrial systole must be able to effectively contribute to pulmonary blood flow (right atrial pulmonary dependent circulation). If the tricuspid valve is too small for complete repair the choice between a definitive palliation or a Fontan procedure must be made. From the point of view of haemodynamic economy the Fontan procedure is more appealing though long term results of this operation are not yet available. We would currently advise a definitive palliation for patients who are not suitable for a complete repair and do not fulfill the Fontan criteria.

## References

1. Rowlatt UF, Fimoldi HJA, Lev M (1963) The quantitative anatomy of the normal child's heart. Pediatr Clin North Am 10: 499
2. Bull C, De Leval MR, Mercanti C, Macartney FJ, Anderson RH (1982) Pulmonary atresia and intact ventricular septum: A revised classification. Circulation 66: 266

# The Fontan procedure in tricuspid atresia and single ventricle

J. BUSQUET, G. FERNANDEZ and F. FONTAN

Since the first successful surgical repair of tricuspid atresia performed in 1968, 125 patients have been operated upon using the Fontan procedure. In addition, this technique has been applied in 26 patients with single ventricle. This report reviews our experience.

## Single ventricle

In this group of cardiac malformation, double inlet univentricular heart, both atrial chambers are connected to only one ventricular chamber of right or left morphology; it may exist a rudimentary sub-arterial ventricular chamber.

*Patients and methods*

Between 1972 and 1984, 26 consecutive patients with double inlet univentricular heart underwent surgical repair. There were 14 male and 12 female patients ranging in age from 3.7 to 28 years with an average age of 14.7 years. Nineteen patients had undergone previous palliative operations (Table 1). All patients had preoperative hemodynamic and angiographic evaluation. Postoperative angiograms and exercise tests were available in 9 patients.

*Operative technique*

The type of repair was the creation of an atrio-pulmonary connection using antibiotically sterilized human aortic homograft valve. Standard methods of cardiopulmonary bypass and myocardial protection were used. Through a right atriotomy, the atrial septal defect was closed. The main pulmonary artery was divided and proximally closed. Since 1979, as advised by Dr. Danielson, a dacron patch was sutured one centimeter above the right atrioventricular valve annulus and the coronary sinus, in order to avoid the atrioventricular node. In all patients a postoperative cardiac output thermodilution catheter was implanted.

*Results*

Hospital mortality occured in seven of the 26 patients (27%). They died from different causes: septicemia in one, cardiac arrhythmia in two, renal failure in one, tracheal bleeding in one and coagulation disorders in two.

There were 4 late deaths (15%), one each from pericardial drainage, cancer of the liver, heart failure and cerebral vascular disease.

Among 17 patients seen 6 months to 12 years postoperatively 95% of them were in good functionnal status (N.Y.H.A. class I or II). Pulmonary artery banding previously performed in 4 patients appeared to be an incremental risk factor: two of these patients died, one in the early post operative period, the other later, 6 years after operation (Table 2). Higher pulmonary arterial resistances, non reliable mean pulmonary arterial pressure and arterial saturation higher than 80% seemed to put this group of patients at risk.

On another hand, impairing effects of long standing systemic pulmonary shunts has been identified on the basis of duration of the shunt, mean age at repair and post operative ventricular function (Table 3). By the light of these findings, repair has to be performed before 10 years of age and no later than 6 years of time after shunt creation.

**Tricuspid atresia**

This study concerns patients in whom there is a situs solitus of the atria and absent right atrioventricular connection, with the main ventricular chamber of left

*Table 1.* Previous palliative surgery, 19 patients.*

| Type | n |
|------|---|
| Blalock Taussig anastomosis | 12 |
| Cavo-pulmonary anastomosis | 5 |
| Pulmonary artery banding | 4 |
| Waterston anastomosis | 1 |
| Blalock Hanlon Procedure | 1 |
| Total | 23 |

* Seven patients without previous surgery.

ventricular type and the outlet chamber of right ventricular type, the latter giving rise to either of the great arteries.

## Patients and methods

Among the 125 cases of tricuspid atresia operated upon since 1968, 59 were male and 66 female patients with a mean age of 9 years 2 months, ranging from 15 months to 36 years. The ventriculo-arterial connection was concordant in 93 patients, discordant in 32. Previous palliative surgery was performed in 91 patients with a total of 117 procedures, mainly systemic-pulmonary artery shunts (Table 4).

Preoperative angiograms were performed in all patients; post operative evaluation concerned 54 patients with angiograms and 30 patients with exercise test.

Table 2. Incremental risk factor pulmonary artery banding, 4 patients.

| V.A. Connexion | Age at | | P.A. resistances U.m2 | P.A. pressure (mean) mmHg | $O_2$ arterial saturation % | Result |
|---|---|---|---|---|---|---|
| | Banding (months) | Repair (years) | | | | |
| Discordant | 4 | 3.7 | 4.2 | 10 | 70 | Good |
| Concordant | 7 | 6.7 | 4.4 | 17 | 63 | Excellent |
| Discordant | 4 | 4 | 3.7 | 6 | 84 | Early p.o. death |
| Concordant | 4 | 10 | 5.5 | 10 | 87 | Late death (6 years) |

Table 3. Impairing effect of long standing arterial systemico-pulmonary shunts.

| Duration of shunt (years) | Mean age at repair (years) | Postoperative ventricular function | | |
|---|---|---|---|---|
| | | E.F. % | E.D.V. ml/m2 | E.S.V. ml/m2 |
| 7 | 10 | 0.59 | 114 | 50 |
| 7 | 10 | 0.45 | 168 | 90 |

Proposals: Repair before 10 years of age in case of arterial systemico pulmonary shunt. Repair no later than 6 years after creation of a shunt.

*Operative technique*

In the cases of ventriculo-arterial discordance, a human aortic homograft valve was implanted as a right atrium-pulmonary artery conduit. Four of these patients had left juxtaposition of the atrial appendages. In 3 of them the homograft was inserted to the right of the aorta; in the fourth patient, it was inserted to the left between the left sided right atrial appendage and the pulmonary artery.

In the cases of ventriculo-arterial concordance, an atrioventricular conduit connection was usually established either with an aortic homograft valve, or with a woven dacron tube between the right atrial appendage and the right ventricular outlet chamber. In some patients a direct posterior atrioventricular anastomosis was made with an anterior dacron or pericardial patch roof. Several additional surgical procedures were performed in some patients (Table 5). Insertion of an aortic valve homograft into the inferior vena cava was made in 11 patients, 6 of them operated upon early in the series, 5 more recently. Partially unroofed

*Table 4.* Previous palliative surgery, 117 operations in 91 patients.

| Systemic-pulmonary artery shunts | | | Others | | |
| --- | --- | --- | --- | --- | --- |
| Type | No | % | Type | No | % |
| Blalock-Taussig | 59 | 69 | Glenn | 19 | 61 |
| Waterston | 21 | 24 | Blalock-Hanlon | 1 | 3 |
| Dacron aorto-pulmonary | 5 | 6 | P.A. Banding | 7 | 23 |
| Potts | 1 | 1.2 | P.E.R.O.T.* | 2 | 6 |
| | | | Rashkind | 1 | 3 |
| | | | A.S.D. enlargement | 1 | 3 |
| Total | 86 | | | 31 | |

* Palliative enlargement of right ventricular outflow tract.

*Table 5.* Additional surgical procedures.

| Type | No. pts |
| --- | --- |
| Inferior vena cava valvulation | 11 |
| Glenn anastomosis | 4 |
| Pulmonary valve commissurotomy | 3 |
| Removal of pulmonary artery banding | 2 |
| Pulmonary artery ring enlargement | 1 |
| Mitral valve replacement | 1 |
| Mitral valvuloplasty | 1 |
| Closure of partially unroofed coronary sinus | 1 |
| Left atrial translocation of coronary sinus | 3 |

coronary sinus was closed once and left atrial translocation of coronary sinus was performed in 3 recent patients in order to facilitate venous coronary drainage into a low pressure cardiac chamber. During surgical repair, closure of the atrial septal defect has to be performed rigorously in order to avoid any residual shunt because of increased right postoperative pressure, taking care to respect the whole Eustachian valve. In cases of ventriculo-arterial discordance, the identification of a restrictive ventricular septal defect is important in order to perform adequate enlargement during surgical repair. Two D echocardiography is able to appreciate the reduced size of the defect and TM echocardiography shows an early closure of aortic valve. During angiocardiography, left ventricle-right ventricle pressure gradient and direct vision of the defect are of utmost interest. Concerning high located ventricular septal defect, enlargement has to be made on the superior edge of the defect in order to avoid bundle of His. This can be made through an aortotomy or an incision in the ventricular infundibulum.

In case of muscular ventricular septal defect in a lower position, the enlargement has to be made on the inferior edge of the defect.

*Results*

Hospital mortality affected 14 (11%) of the 125 patients who died within 30 days of operation. Table 6 indicates the number of deaths according to the surgical technique. Age at operation is a significant determinant of hospital mortality. In the group of patients with age less than 4 years, there were 6 deaths (43%). In the group more than 4, there were only 8 deaths (7%). Among 55 patients operated upon, more than 4 years old from 1979 to 1985, only one died and there were only 4 deaths in the 100 last patients more than 4 years old. The mode of ventriculo-

*Table 6.* Tricuspid atresia, 125 patients.

| Type | Technique | N | Hosp. | mortal. | |
|------|-----------|---|-------|---------|---|
| | | | | % | CL 70% |
| Condordant RA-PA | Direct | 1 | 0 | 0 | |
| | Homograft | 5 | 3 | 60 | 29–86 |
| Condordant RAV | Homograft | 15 | 0 | 0 | – |
| | Non valved conduit | 59 | 6 | 0 | 4–12 |
| | Direct anastomosis | 12 | 0 | 0 | – |
| Discordant RA-PA | Homograft | 32 | 5 | 16 | 10–28 |
| | Direct | 1 | 0 | 0 | |
| | | 125 | 14 | 11 | 8–15 |

RAV: right atrium ventricle.
PA: pulmonary artery.

*Table 7.* Causes of reoperation or late failure.

- Second ventricular septal defect
- Residual atrial septal defect
  (including partially unroofed coronary sinus)
- Dacron conduit obstruction
- Sternal compression of conduit
- Proteïn loosing enteropathy
- Heart failure
- Mitral incompetence
- Fate of valved conduits
  - Xenograft
  - Homograft
- Restrictive ventricular septal defect

arterial connection did not influence early mortality. There were 10 late deaths (11%) in patients with ventriculo-arterial concordance, 4 deaths (12.5%) in patient with discordance.

The usual causes of reoperation or late failure after surgical repair are shown in Table 7. The different causes of late mortality were sudden death, infection, chylothorax and residual atrial shunt (requiring reoperation) heart failure and caval thrombosis.

**Comments**

Evaluation of functionnal status exercise capacity, catheterization data and echocardiographic studies tend to demonstrate that a homograft valve is a valuable adjunct to the operative technique. Exercise tolerance was tested in 32 patients. The result is a percentage of normal values for age, sex, weight and height. The best results are obtained in the patients with homograft valve. The test is lower in patients with non valved conduit. Morphology of right atrial pressure curve in patients with concordance and atrioventricular homograft valve shows a low c wave compared to systolic pressure in right ventricle attesting competence of the homograft.

Calculation of the shortening fraction of the right atrium demonstrates a postoperative decrease, but the difference is less marked in the group of concordant patients with homograft. The diastolic diameter of the outlet chamber and trabecular chamber is slightly increased after operation with concordant ventriculo arterial connection. Finally echocardiographic studies in patients after Fontan procedure are able to demonstrate the good function of aortic homograft valve.

Concerning the mode of right atrio-pulmonary connection, non valved Dacron conduit presents a risk of late stenosis or thrombosis because of progressive internal fibrous proliferation. Aortic homograft valve prevents regurgitation into the right atrium during contraction of the right ventricular chamber, unloading the right atrial volume. The presence of this valve permits the trabecular chamber to perform as a ventricle capable of growth after repair. Late results are encouraging in spite of unknown future. Patch technique should be used in the younger age group, because it requires less space than a conduit between sternum and heart.

For patients with concordant ventriculo-arterial connection, the use of homograft valve is particularly recommended. Ventricular septal defect is then closed, the ostium infundibuli enlarged and trabecular chamber put in circuit after internal muscular resection. When for anatomical or technical reasons, a homograft cannot be used, the patch technique has to be employed with exclusion of the trabecular chamber from right circulation by closing the infundibular ostium.

## References

1. Fontan F, Choussat A, Brom AG, Chauve A, Deville Cl, Castro-Cels A (1977) Repair of tricuspid atresia – Surgical considerations and results. In: Anderson RH, Shinebourne EA (eds) (1985) Paediatric Cardiology. Churchill Livingstone, 65: 567–580
2. Fontan F, Deville Cl, Quaegebeur J, Ottenkamp J, Sourdille N, Choussat A, Brom GA (1985) Repair of tricuspid atresia in 100 patients. J Thorac Cardiovasc Surg 85–5: 647–660

# II. Acquired heart diseases

# DeBakey-surgitool pyrolite® aortic valve: results of isolated replacement in 345 patients followed up to 13 years after operation*

E. DEBAKEY and G.M. LAWRIE

## Summary

The clinical and hemodynamic outcome of isolated aortic valve replacement with the DeBakey-Surgitool Pyrolite® aortic valve prosthesis was evaluated in 345 consecutive patients operated on between 1968 and 1978 and followed up to 17 years after operation. Their mean age was 47.8 ± 15.8 years. The perioperative mortality rate was 8.1%. Five-year survival probability (Kaplan-Meier) was 74.0%.

Preoperatively, 53.0% of patients were in New York Heart Association (NYHA) Class III-IV, but postoperatively only 9.9% were in Class III-IV. The overall annual rate of thromboembolism was 2.9%, but for patients maintained on Coumadin® it was 1.7%. In this study, aspirin and Persantine® provided no protection against thromboembolism. Other complications were relatively infrequent, and 5 years after operation the probability of freedom from all major complications was 81.8%.

Follow-up catheterization was performed on 27 patients at a mean interval of 57.7 months (range, 3–146 months). Whereas the preoperative aortic valve gradient was 56.1 ± 49.6 mm Hg (range, 0–165 mm Hg), the prosthetic valve gradient was 4.7 ± 10 mm Hg (range, 0–50 mm Hg). There was no measurable gradient in 19 patients. Three patients had strut fracture at the site of attachment of the titanium cage to the annulus. This problem is rare and has been rectified by changes in the construction of the cage. With the exception of these mechanical failures, the results obtained with this prosthesis compare favorably with other mechanical aortic valve prostheses.

* Supported in part by HEW research grant HL-17269, National Heart and Blood Vessel Research and Demonstration Center, Houston, Texas

## Introduction

In 1967, the senior author, working in close collaboration with Mr. Harry Cromie of Surgitool and Mr. Jack Bokros, who at that time was working with Gulf General Atomic Inc., developed prosthetic heart valves designed for replacement of human heart valves. The hollow-ball occluder and orifice ring of the caged ball prosthesis are coated with Pyrolite® carbon. The valve frame and one-piece cage are formed of titanium. The sewing ring consists of a double layer of Dacron® velour attached to the valve base (Fig. 1). This valve was designed for replacement of human aortic or pulmonic heart valves. The Pyrolite® carbon coating was selected for its demonstrated impermeability, high-wear resistance, non-biogradability, and low thrombogenicity [1–3]. It was also shown by *in vitro* studies that there is less disturbed flow around this ball and less back flow during seating of the ball [4]. A low-profile mitral valve prosthesis was developed using the same materials with a disk-type occluder (Fig. 2).

Between 1968 when the DeBakey-Surgitool Pyrolite® aortic valve was first used clinically and 1978, 345 consecutive patients had isolated aortic valve replacement with the DeBakey-Surgitool Pyrolite® aortic valve. These patients were among a larger series of 623 patients who received DeBakey-Surgitool Pyrolite® aortic valves during this period. Of the 623 patients, 143 had mitral valve replacement in addition to aortic valve implantation. Of the 480 patients receiving only an aortic valve at this operation, 74 also had resection of an aneurysm of the ascending aorta and 61 had coronary artery bypass. Because the purpose of this study was to evaluate the characteristics of the aortic valve prosthesis, detailed analysis of the clinical results has been confined to the subgroup of 345 patients who underwent isolated aortic valve replacement.

## Material and method

The mean age of the 345 patients who had isolated aortic valve replacement was $47.8 \pm 15.8$ years, with a range of 3 to 78 years; 273 were male (79.1%) and 72 female (20.9%) patients. The distribution of the patients according to New York Heart Association (NYHA) Class, preoperative medication, extent of cardiomegaly, and clinical manifestations is shown in Tables 1–4. Cardiac catheterization showed predominantly aortic stenosis in 167 patients (48.4%), aortic regurgitation in 134 patients (38.8%), and both conditions in 44 patients (12.8%).

The preoperative aortic valve gradient in 284 of these patients was $56.1 \pm 49.6$ mm Hg with a range of 0 to 165 mm Hg. The mean preoperative aortic valve area calculated for 37 of the patients with aortic stenosis was $0.61 \pm 0.37 \, cm^2$ with a range of 0.24 to $0.84 \, cm^2$. The aortic regurgitation in 62 patients was graded on a 1 to 4 scale as grade 1–2 in 16 patients (25.8%) and as grade 3–4 in 46 patients (74.2%). Twenty-one patients (6.1%) had associated mitral valve disease not

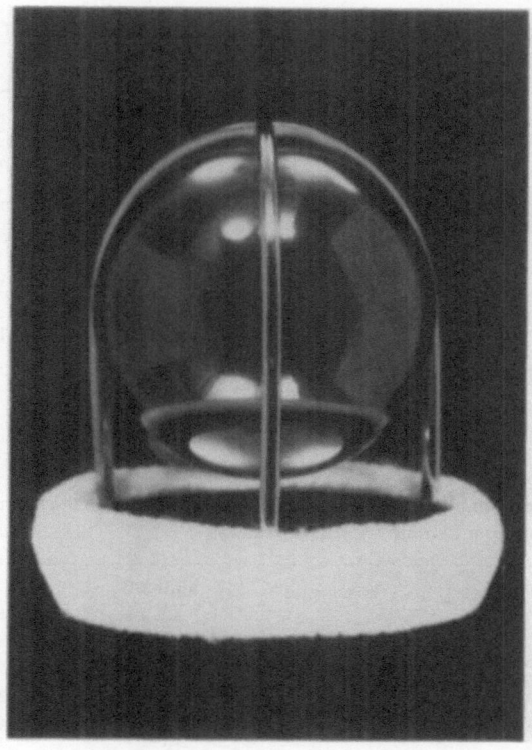

*Figure 1.* Photograph of DeBakey-Surgitool Pyrolite® aortic valve prosthesis.

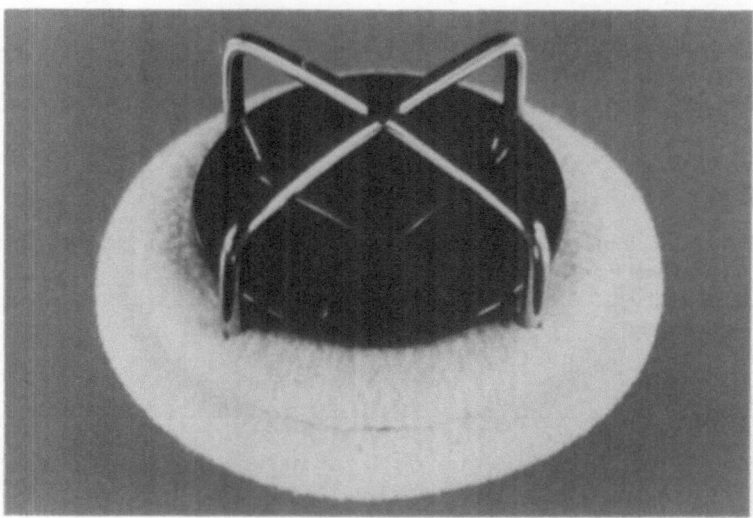

*Figure 2.* Photograph of DeBakey-Surgitool Pyrolite® mitral valve prosthesis.

*Table 1.* Distribution according to New York Heart Association (NYHA) Class of 345 patients having isolated replacement with DeBakey-Surgitool Pyrolite® aortic valves.

| NYHA class | Patients | |
|---|---|---|
| | Number | % |
| I | 29 | 8.3 |
| II | 133 | 38.7 |
| III | 147 | 42.5 |
| IV | 36 | 10.5 |
| Total | 345 | 100.0 |

*Table 2.* Distribution according to preoperative medication of 345 patients having isolated replacement with DeBakey-Surgitool Pyrolite® aortic valves.*

| Preoperative medication | Patients | |
|---|---|---|
| | Number | % |
| Digoxin® | 186 | 53.9 |
| Diuretic | 144 | 41.7 |
| Coumadin® | 18 | 5.2 |
| Aspirin | 4 | 1.2 |
| Persantine® | 6 | 1.7 |
| Other cardiac medication** | 187 | 54.2 |
| None | 55 | 15.9 |

* Many patients were taking more than one drug.
** Includes beta-blockers, antiarrhythmia and antihypertensive agents.

*Table 3.* Distribution according to extent of cardiomegaly in 345 patients having isolated replacement with DeBakey-Surgitool Pyrolite® aortic valves.

| Degree of cardiomegaly | Patients | |
|---|---|---|
| | Number | % |
| None | 78 | 22.6 |
| Mild | 187 | 54.2 |
| Moderate | 49 | 14.2 |
| Massive | 18 | 5.2 |
| Unknown | 13 | 3.8 |

*Table 4.* Results of preoperative resting electrocardiography in 345 patients having isolated replacement with DeBakey-Surgitool Pyrolite® aortic valves.

| Clinical manifestation | Patients | |
|---|---|---|
| | Number | % |
| Sinus rhythm | 134 | 38.8 |
| Atrial fibrillation | 27 | 7.8 |
| Left ventricular hypertrophy | 254 | 73.6 |
| Premature ventricular contraction | 29 | 8.4 |
| Conduction defect | 78 | 22.6 |

requiring prosthetic replacement. Fifteen patients had mitral stenosis, and 5 had mitral regurgitation. Atherosclerotic coronary artery disease was present in 31 patients (9.0%) and aneurysms of the ascending aorta in 6 patients (1.7%). Eleven patients had replacement of a previously inserted aortic valve prosthesis.

The preoperative left ventricular end-diastolic pressure in 271 patients was $14.7 \pm 10.2$ mm Hg (range of 0 to 40 mm Hg). The preoperative cardiac index in 232 patients was $3.06 \pm 1.1$ L/min/m$^2$ (range 0.8–6 L/min/m$^2$).

The surgical technique used during the period of this study consisted in normothermic total cardiopulmonary bypass with myocardial preservation during aortic cross clamping by continuous coronary perfusion with normothermic blood. After excision of the diseased aortic valve, multiple interrupted 2–0 Tycron® everting horizontal mattress sutures were inserted into the annulus. The Pyrolite® carbon ball was removed temporarily from the cage, and the sutures were inserted through the prosthetic valve sewing ring. After the valve was seated and the sutures were tied, the ball was reinserted, and the aortotomy closed. Coronary perfusion was discontinued upon completion of the aortotomy closure. Temporary pacing wires were used in all patients.

*Table 5.* Distribution according to etiology in 345 patients having isolated replacement with DeBakey-Surgitool Pyrolite® aortic valves.

| Etiology | Patients | |
|---|---|---|
| | Number | % |
| Rheumatic | 136 | 39.4 |
| Endocarditis | 11 | 3.2 |
| Degenerative | 174 | 50.4 |
| Congenital | 12 | 3.5 |
| Unknown | 12 | 3.5 |

The perioperative mortality rate (30-day) was 8.1% (28/345), the major cause of death being postoperative left ventricular dysfunction (Table 6). No perioperative death was attributable to the prosthetic valve. In the perioperative period, 18 patients (5.2%) required implantation of a permanent pacemaker system. The medication at discharge is shown in Table 7.

## Results

Late postoperative follow-up was obtained in 97.8% (310/317) of patients at a mean interval of 46.5 ± 40.2 months (range 1 to 204 months). The NYHA functional class at late follow-up was known for 111 of these patients (Table 8).

Late death occurred in 98 patients over this period. Death was definitely not

*Table 6.* Major cause of perioperative death in 28 patients having isolated replacement with DeBakey-Surgitool Pyrolite® aortic valves.

| Cause | Patients | |
|---|---|---|
| | Number | % |
| Left ventricular failure | 7 | 25.0 |
| Myocardial infarction | 4 | 14.3 |
| Arrhythmia | 6 | 21.4 |
| Infection | 2 | 7.1 |
| Renal | 3 | 10.7 |
| Bleeding | 4 | 14.3 |
| Respiratory | 2 | 7.1 |

*Table 7.* Postoperative medication in 345 patients having isolated replacement with DeBakey-Surgitool Pyrolite® aortic valves.*

| Discharge medication | Patients | |
|---|---|---|
| | Number | % |
| Digoxin® | 270 | 85.2 |
| Diuretic | 73 | 23.0 |
| Coumadin® | 135 | 42.6 |
| Aspirin | 86 | 27.1 |
| Persantine® | 66 | 20.8 |
| Other** | 204 | 64.4 |
| None | 3 | 0.9 |

* Many patients were taking more than one drug.
** Includes beta-blockers, antiarrhythmic and antihypertensive agents.

attributable to the prosthetic valve in 64 patients and was sudden in 3 patients. The cause of death could not be determined in 25 patients. Death was due to mechanical failure of the prosthetic valve in 3 patients (0.8%). In one patient, fracture of the base of two struts was identified at reoperation for prosthetic dysfunction, and the patient died in the perioperative period. In 2 other patients, who had been doing well, acute heart failure developed, and at necropsy the Pyrolyte® valve poppets were found lodged at their aortic bifurcations.

The survival data and data relating to freedom from complications obtained from the follow-up studies were analyzed by Kaplan-Meier curves of survival probability and, in the case of the survival data, by Cox multivariate analysis. The Kaplan-Meier estimate of survival curves presented here is given by the equation:

$$P(t) = \prod_{i=1}^{t} (1 - \frac{m_i}{n_i})$$

where $P(t)$ is the probability of survival to time interval $t$, $m_i$ is the number of deaths in the ith interval, and $n_i$ is the number at risk of dying in the ith interval, including those lost to follow-up during the interval i. Each term in this product is the conditional probability of surviving the interval i given survival up to that time. A stepwise nonlinear regression algorithm for the Cox proportional hazards model was used to select variables that significantly affected survival among the patients in the series. Univariate Chi-square statistics, known as Wald statistics, were computed for each variable of interest. The variable with the largest significant Wald Chi-square was entered into the survival model; its coefficient was estimated and incorporated into the likelihood function. The variable was tested for removal by a t test. Adjusted Wald statistics were computed for each variable of interest. The variable with the largest significant Wald Chi-square was entered into the survival model; its coefficient was estimated and incorporated into the likelihood function. The variable was tested for removal by a t test. Adjusted Wald statistics were computed for the remaining variable, adjusted for the variable already in the model. The variable with the largest significant adjusted Wald statistic was added to the model and the coefficients of both

Table 8. Postoperative New York Heart Association (NYHA) Class at late follow-up in 111 patients among 345 patients having isolated replacement with DeBakey-Surgitool Pyrolite® aortic valves.

| Postoperative NYHA class | Patients | |
| --- | --- | --- |
| | Number | % |
| I | 64 | 57.7 |
| II | 36 | 32.4 |
| III | 7 | 6.3 |
| IV | 4 | 3.6 |
| Total | 111 | 100.0 |

variables were jointly estimated. The algorithm continues in this manner either until no Wald statistic is significant or until all variables are removed.

The Cox analysis was performed to determine the influence of the variables shown in Table 8. The most important preoperative predictors of overall survival are shown in Table 9. The most important preoperative predictors of late survival (excluding the perioperative deaths) are shown in Table 10. The data in Tables 9

*Table 9.* Most important preoperative predictors of overall and late survival in 345 patients having isolated replacement with DeBakey-Surgitool Pyrolite® aortic valves.*

| Variable | Chi-square | P | R |
|---|---|---|---|
| Year of operation | 0.19 | 0.6602 | 0.000 |
| Sex | 0.62 | 0.4321 | 0.000 |
| Age | 13.30 | 0.0003 | 0.131 |
| Aortic stenosis | 0.09 | 0.7627 | 0.000 |
| Aortic regurgitation | 1.27 | 0.2602 | 0.000 |
| Aortic, mixed | 1.98 | 0.1591 | 0.000 |
| No mitral lesion | 1.16 | 0.2808 | 0.000 |
| Mitral stenosis | 1.57 | 0.2103 | 0.000 |
| Mitral regurgitation | 0.07 | 0.7953 | 0.000 |
| No tricuspid lesion | 0.24 | 0.6224 | 0.000 |
| Etiology, rheumatic | 0.42 | 0.5171 | 0.000 |
| Etiology, endocarditis | 0.66 | 0.4170 | 0.000 |
| Etiology, degenerative | 0.02 | 0.8830 | 0.000 |
| Etiology, congenital | 2.84 | 0.0917 | − 0.036 |
| Etiology, unknown | 0.87 | 0.3499 | 0.000 |
| Coronary heart disease | 8.10 | 0.0044 | 0.096 |
| Ascending aortic lesion | 0.95 | 0.3293 | 0.000 |
| Previous operation | 0.99 | 0.3201 | 0.000 |
| Previous aortic valve | 0.77 | 0.3814 | 0.000 |
| Previous mitral valve | 0.41 | 0.5211 | 0.000 |
| Previous coronary artery bypass | 0.43 | 0.5136 | 0.000 |
| Other previous operation | 1.98 | 0.1597 | 0.000 |
| NYHA class | 0.31 | 0.5795 | 0.000 |
| Cardiomegaly | 0.05 | 0.8311 | 0.000 |
| Sinus rhythm | 1.22 | 0.2687 | 0.000 |
| Atrial fibrillation | 0.02 | 0.8811 | 0.000 |
| Left ventricular hypertrophy | 1.14 | 0.2864 | 0.000 |
| Premature ventricular contraction | 4.66 | 0.0309 | 0.064 |
| Conduction defect | 0.00 | 0.9951 | 0.000 |
| No preoperative medication | 7.76 | 0.0053 | −0.094 |
| Preoperative Digoxin® | 2.93 | 0.0867 | 0.038 |
| Preoperative diuretic | 7.83 | 0.0052 | 0.094 |
| Preoperative Coumadin® | 0.89 | 0.3465 | 0.000 |
| Preoperative aspirin | 0.15 | 0.7029 | 0.000 |
| Preoperative Persantine® | 0.36 | 0.5481 | 0.000 |
| Preoperative other medication | 4.68 | 0.0304 | 0.064 |
| No coexistent lesions | 0.82 | 0.3654 | 0.000 |
| No discharge medication | 0.71 | 0.4001 | 0.000 |

*Table 9.* Continued.

| Variable | Chi-square | P | R |
|---|---|---|---|
| Discharge Digoxin® | 0.12 | 0.7303 | 0.000 |
| Discharge diuretic | 1.11 | 0.2930 | 0.000 |
| Discharge Coumadin/Warfarin® | 0.12 | 0.7285 | 0.000 |
| Discharge aspirin | 0.02 | 0.8967 | 0.000 |
| Discharge Persantine® | 0.01 | 0.9408 | 0.000 |
| Discharge other medication | 0.00 | 0.9982 | 0.000 |

* Simple unadjusted Chi-square Q statistics for the variables analyzed for their influence on overall and late survival.

and 10 suggest that the perioperative mortality rate in this series was greatly influenced by the year of operation and coexistent cardiac disease at the time of operation. Of interest is the persistent effect of coronary heart disease which, in this subgroup of patients, had not been treated by coronary bypass.

To assess the magnitude of the effect of these preoperative variables, we used the factors shown to be predictive of death to classify the patients into groups of high, medium, and low risk of death. The patients were divided into quartiles according to risk with the medium-risk group containing the two middle quartiles. The results of these analyses indicated that the preoperative variables listed greatly affected the mortality rate (Table II and Figs. 3–5).

The absolute numbers of patients who had late complications are shown in Table 12. In addition, the results of the Kaplan-Meier analyses of probability of freedom from complications are shown in Figures 6 and 7. These curves show the probability of freedom from the listed complication up to 120 months postoperatively. Notable was the 91.4% probability of freedom from thromboembolism for patients 5 years after operation who were maintained on Coumadin® in the postoperative period, an annualized rate of 1.7%.

*Table 10.* Most important preoperative predictors of late survival (excluding perioperative deaths) in 345 patients having isolated replacement with DeBakey-Surgitool Pyrolite® aortic valves.*

| Variable | Beta | Standard error | Chi-square | P | R |
|---|---|---|---|---|---|
| Age | 0.02444322 | 0.00802714 | 9.27 | 0.0023 | 0.086 |
| Cardiomegaly | 0.40277959 | 0.17176327 | 5.50 | 0.0190 | 0.060 |
| Coronary ht. dis. | 0.91241072 | 0.30209435 | 9.12 | 0.0025 | 0.085 |
| Year of operation | 0.63092522 | 0.23008285 | 7.52 | 0.0061 | 0.075 |
| Diuretic | 0.49578661 | 0.21963200 | 5.10 | 0.0240 | 0.056 |

* Final estimates for the Cox model for variable most predictive of overall survival. Note that the presence of preoperative other coexistent lesions was a highly significant predictor of outcome, but for statistical reasons it did not appear in this list of variables.

Also notable is the apparent lack of protection afforded by aspirin and Persantine®. Patients on neither Coumadin® nor an anti-platelet regimen had rates of thromboembolic complications similar to those of patients on aspirin and Persantine® with 5-year annualized rates of 5.5% (aspirin-Persantine®) and 3.4% (no medication). If all patients are considered, regardless of medication status, the overall annual rate was 2.9%.

Of the 63 thromboembolic events noted in Table 12, there were 5 fatal strokes and one fatal coronary embolus (9.5%). Sixteen patients had episodes of cerebral embolism which resulted in permanent neurologic deficits (25.4%). There were 7 transient ischemic attacks, one saddle embolus of the aortic bifurcation, one mesenteric embolus, and one popliteal embolus. The remaining patients experienced cerebral emboli causing deficits which ultimately resolved completely. Serious anticoagulant-related hemorrhage (requiring hospital admission or more than minor treatment) occurred at an annual rate of 1.4%.

When all the valve-related complications listed in Table 12 were considered in

*Table 11.* Final estimates from Cox Model for variables most predictive of late survival having excluded perioperative deaths in 345 patients having isolated replacement with DeBakey-Surgitool Pyrolite® aortic valves.

| Variable | Beta | Standard error | Chi-square | P | R |
|---|---|---|---|---|---|
| Age | 0.02260581 | 0.00959139 | 5.55 | 0.0184 | 0.074 |
| No preoperative medication | − 1.20051720 | 0.52653388 | 5.20 | 0.0226 | − 0.070 |
| Coronary heart disease | 0.78327972 | 0.34902112 | 5.04 | 0.0248 | 0.068 |
| Premature ventricular contraction | 0.71903761 | 0.36279846 | 3.93 | 0.0475 | 0.054 |

*Table 12.* Late complications in 317 survivors up to 200 months among 345 patients having isolated replacement with DeBakey-Surgitool Pyrolite® aortic valves.

| Complication | Patients | |
|---|---|---|
| | Number | % |
| Endocarditis | 11 | 3.4 |
| Valve thrombus | 3 | 0.9 |
| Thromboembolism | 63 | 19.9 |
| Mechanical failure | 3 | 0.9 |
| Perivalvular leak | 10 | 3.2 |
| Hemolysis | 3 | 0.9 |
| Serious Coumadin®-related bleeding | 8 | 2.5 |

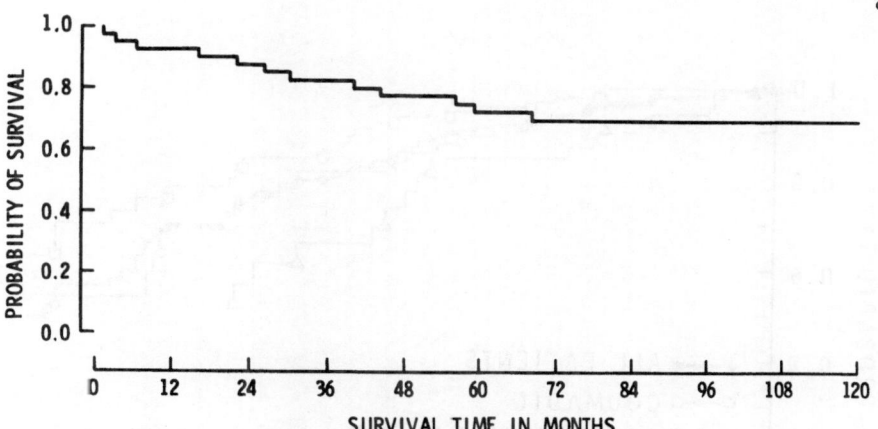

*Figure 3.* Kaplan-Meier curve of survival probability after isolated aortic valve replacement with the DeBakey-Surgitool Pyrolite® prosthesis. (Perioperative mortality rate is excluded).

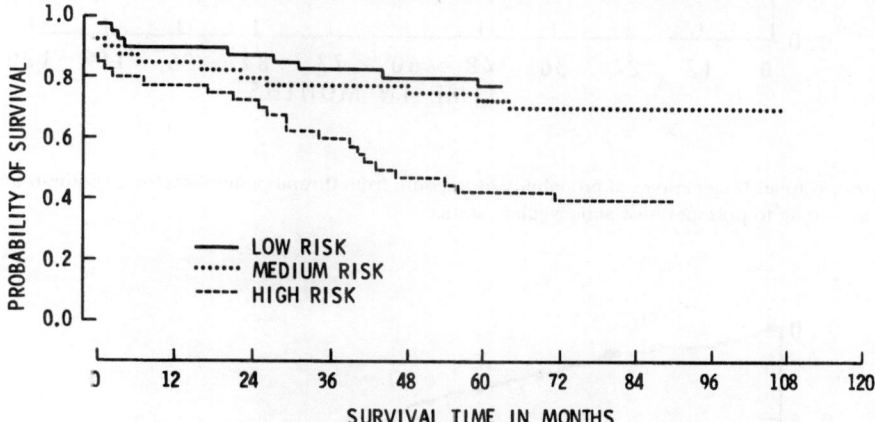

*Figure 4.* Curves of overall survival probability according to preoperative risk categories as defined in the text. These curves include perioperative mortality.

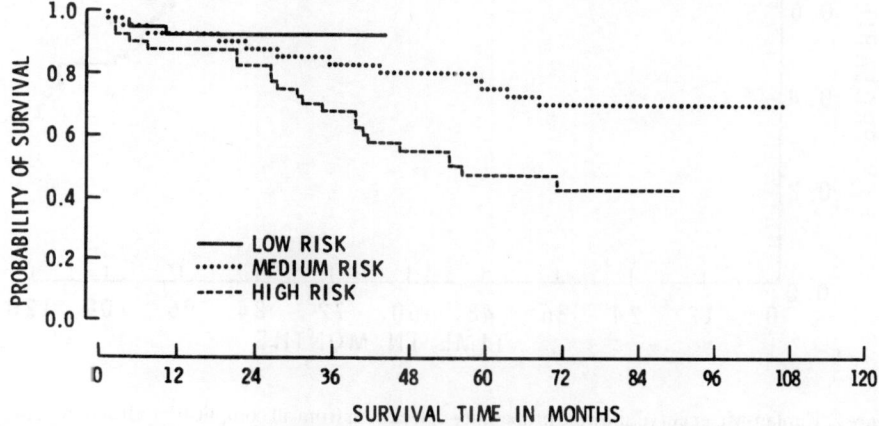

*Figure 5.* Curves of late survival probability as for Figure 2 but excluding perioperative mortality rate.

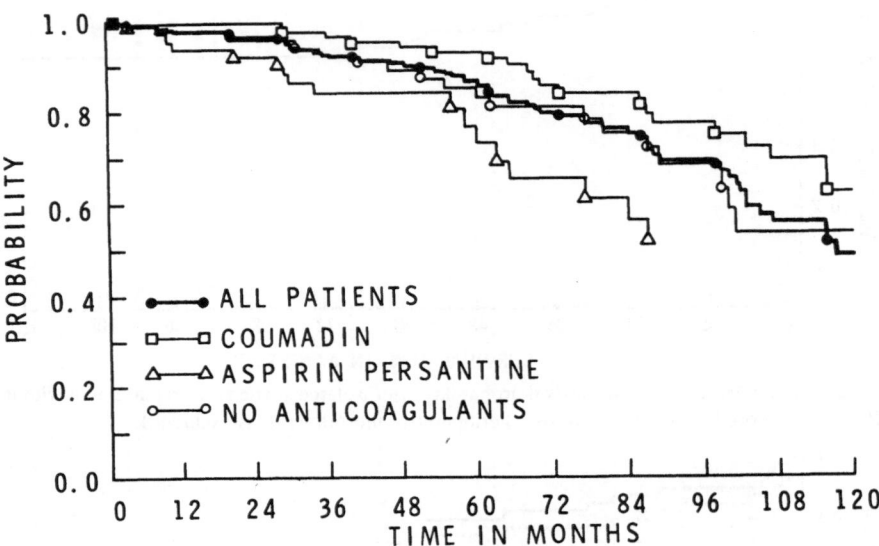

*Figure 6.* Kaplan-Meier curves of probability of freedom from thromboembolism for all patients and also according to postoperative anticoagulant status.

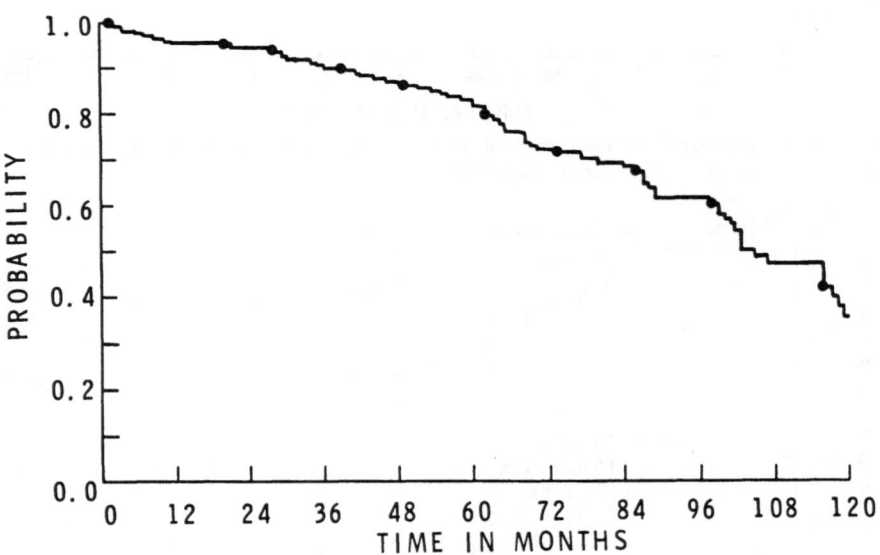

*Figure 7.* Kaplan-Meier curve showing probability of freedom from all complications listed in Table 12 (see text for further details).

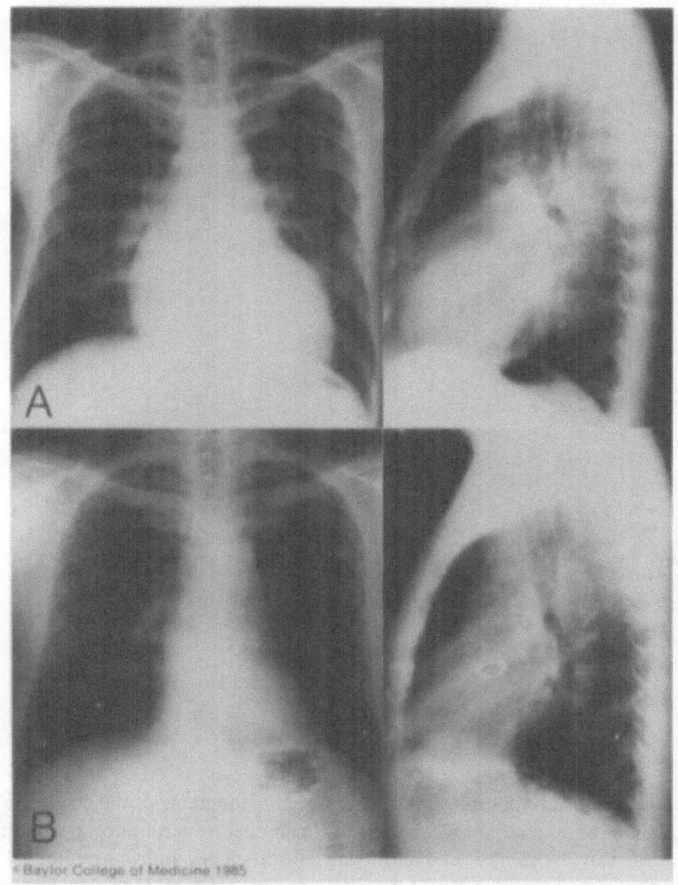

*Figure 8.* A. Preoperative anteroposterior and lateral roentgenograms of chest of 40-year-old white man suffering from severe, calcific aortic stenosis showing moderate cardiac enlargement, left ventricular hypertrophy, and moderate bilateral pulmonary congestion. The stenotic aortic valve was resected and replaced with a DeBakey-Surgitool aortic valve prosthesis. B. Postoperative anteroposterior and lateral roentgenograms of chest made 17 years after operation show restoration of normal cardiac silhouette and pulmonary structure, and valve prosthesis in aortic position.

the Kaplan-Meier analysis, 5 years after operation there was an 81.8% probability of freedom from these complications. This analysis of freedom from valve-complications is therefore more inclusive than the definition of valve failure proposed by Miller and associates [5] in which only complications leading to valve explantation were considered.

Of the overall group of 623 patients who received aortic valve prostheses, 27 underwent follow-up cardiac catheterization at a mean postoperative interval of 57.7 months (range 3 to 146 months). At these studies, the mean postoperative resting aortic gradient was $4.7 \pm 10.7$ mm Hg (range 0 to 50 mm Hg). Nineteen

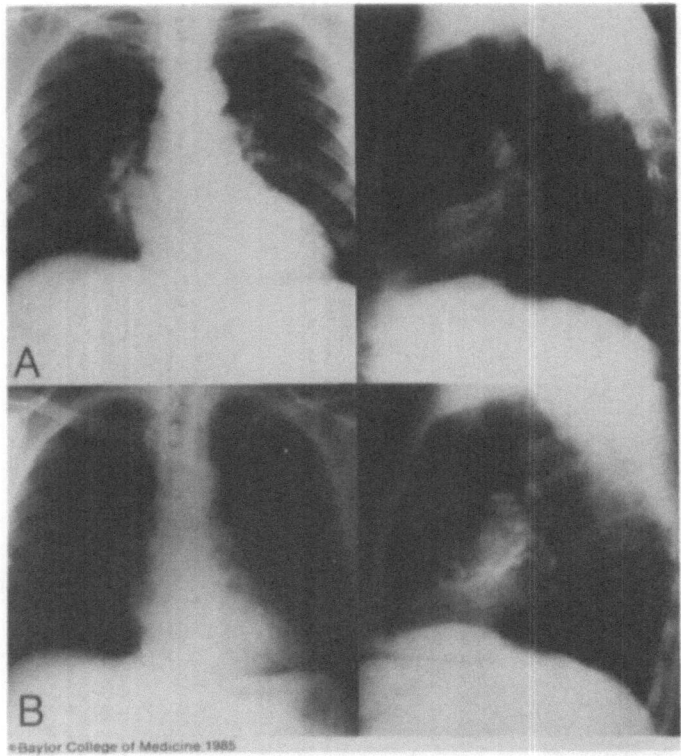

*Figure 9.* A. Preoperative anteroposterior and lateral roentgenograms of the chest of a 57-year-old white man complaining of dyspnea and weakness showing moderate cardiomegaly. Patient was found to have severe aortic valvular stenosis and mitral valve insufficiency and was treated by resection of these valves and replacement with DeBakey-Surgitool aortic valve and DeBakey Disk mitral valve. B. Postoperative anteroposterior and lateral roentgenograms of chest in same patient made 10 years after operation showing relatively normal cardiac size and pulmonary field.

patients had no measurable resting gradient. Only one patient had a gradient of more than 40 mm Hg – a female patient with a small aortic root who had received a number 2A prosthesis and had a gradient of 50 mm Hg.

The long-term clinical and hemodynamic results obtained with this prosthesis compare favorably with the results reported for other aortic valve prostheses and particularly for other ball-in-cage designs, such as the Starr-Edwards 1200/1260 prosthesis and the Smeloff-Cutter prosthesis [6–10]. The improvement in pre-operative functional clinical class observed at late follow-up was striking and correlates well with the excellent hemodynamic data obtained at late follow-up (Figs. 8–10).

It had been hoped that the need for anticoagulation with Coumadin® had been overcome by the use of Pyrolite® in this valve, but as the results indicate,

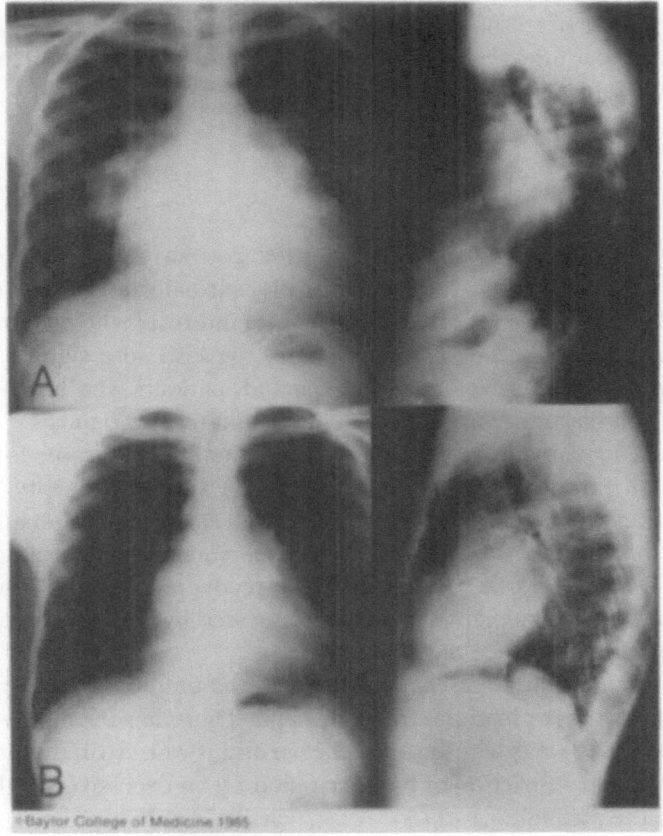

*Figure 10.* A. Preoperative anteroposterior and lateral roentgenograms of chest of 19-year-old white man showing severe cardiomegaly and bilateral pulmonary congestion resulting from severe aortic valvular insufficiency, mitral valvular stenosis and unsufficiency, and tricuspid valvular insufficiency. B. Postoperative anteroposterior and lateral roentgenograms of chest made 13 years after operation show relatively normal cardiac and pulmonary appearances. Patient has remained well.

Coumadin® is required for this prosthesis as it is for all other mechanical prostheses. The patients on Coumadin® had a relatively low annual rate of thromboembolism of 1.7%, and 91.4% were free of thromboembolism 5 years after operation. This compares with a 2.6% annual rate for our own series of patients with Smeloff-Cutter aortic implants on Coumadin® [8] and with results for the Starr-Edwards 1200/1260 prosthesis in which thromboembolism rates have been 3.4% to 6.5% and the embolus-free rate at 5 years was 87% [9]. The rate of serious hemorrhagic complications observed is comparable to those of previous reports for other prostheses. The perioperative mortality rate and the 5-year survival probability of 74% for the DeBakey-Surgitool group is comparable to the Starr-Edwards (77%), Hancock porcine (69%), and Smeloff-Cutter (80%)

prostheses. As has been shown in other series, the duration of operation was an important variable affecting the perioperative mortality rate but not the late survival rate (Tables 10, 11).

## Discussion

The change on our service from normothermic coronary perfusion to moderate systemic hypothermia and cardioplegia for myocardial preservation occurred at the end of the experience reported here. Also of interest is the fact that coronary artery disease not treated by coronary artery bypass had a significant adverse influence on the late survival rate. As expected, patients who had not required preoperative cardiac medication had a better long-term prognosis.

Pyrolitic carbon appears to have many of the qualities desirable for prosthetic valves. It is an extremely durable material of low thrombogenicity. It is highly resistant to fracturing, and our studies [11], as well as those of others [12], showed their exceptional resistance to material loss from abrasion. For example, evaluation of two DeBakey aortic valve prostheses, recovered 48 and 85 months after implantation, showed negligble wear when assessed by scanning electron microscopy and analytical surface profilometry [11].

Similar analysis of the wear-characteristics of the titanium cage of these valves showed minimal loss of material from the cage. There has been only one report [13] of serious cage-wear with this prosthesis, and it was attributed to abnormal ball-motion due to restriction of ball-excursion by an excessively tight fit of the valve within the ascending aorta.

The more serious complication of strut fracture occurred in 3 patients in this series, and 2 other strut fractures were previously reported [14]. This problem has been resolved by redesign of the acute angle at the base of each strut which was the high stress area at which fracture had occurred.

Because of the favorable long-term results obtained with this prosthesis, we believe that in patients requiring aortic valve replacement, the DeBakey-Surgitool Pyrolite® valve in its current modified form will provide a useful addition to available prostheses of a device with documented good long-term clinical and hemodynamic characteristics.

## References

1. Bokros JC (1969) Deposition, structure, and properties of pyrolytic carbon. In: Walker PL Jr (ed) Chemistry and Physics of Carbon, New York: Marcel Dekker, Vol. 5, Chap. 1, pp 1–118
2. Bokros JC, Adkins RJ (1971) Applications of pyrolytic carbon in artificial heart valves: A status report. Proc 4th Buhl Int Conf Materials, Pittsburgh, PA, November 16–18 (1971) Pittsburgh: Carnegie Press, p 243
3. Gott VL (1972) Synthetic materials for valve construction. Adv Cardiol 7: 12–24

4. Wieting DW (1969) Discussion: Sauvage LR et al, *In vivo* testing of prosthetic heart valves and criteria for specimen evaluation. In: Brewer LA III (ed), Prosthetic Heart Valves, Springfield, Illinois: Charles C Thomas, pp 253–255

5. Miller DC, Oyer PE, Stinson EB, Reitz BA, Jamieson SW, Baumgartner WA, Mitchell RS, Shumway NE (1983) Ten to fifteen year reassessment of the performance characteristics of the Starr-Edwards model 6120 mitral valve prosthesis. J Thorac Cardiovasc Surg 85: 1–20

6. Fuster V, Pumphrey CW, McGoon MD, Chesebro JH, Pluth JR, McGoon DC (1982) Systemic thromboembolism in mitral and aortic Starr-Edwards prostheses: A 10-19-year follow-up, Circulation 66 (Suppl 1): I157–I161

7. Oyer PE, Stinson EB, Griepp RB, Shumway NE (1977) Valve replacement with the Starr-Edwards and Hancock prostheses: Comparative analysis of late morbidity and mortality. Ann Surg 186: 301–309

8. Edmunds LH Jr (1982) Thromboembolic complications of current cardiac valvular prostheses. Ann Thorac Surg 34: 96–106

9. Macmanus Q, Grunkemeier GL, Lambert LE, Teply JF, Harlan BJ, Starr A (1980) Year of operation as a risk factor in the late results of valve replacement. J Thorac Cardiovasc Surg 80: 834–841

10. Starr DS, Lawrie GM, Gowell JF, Morris GC Jr (1980) Clinical experience with the Smeloff-Cutter prosthesis: 1– to 12-year follow-up, Ann Thorac Surg 30: 448–454

11. Schoen FJ, Titus JL, Lawrie GM (1982) Durability of pyrolitic carbon-containing heart valve prostheses. J Biomed Mater Res 16: 559–570

12. Shim HS and Schoen FJ (1974) The wear resistance of pure and silicon-alloyed isotropic carbons. Biomater Med Devices Artif Organs 2: 103–118

13. Paton BC, Pine MB (1976) Aortic valve replacement with the DeBakey valve. J. Thorac Cardiovasc Surg 72: 652–656

14. Zumbro GL Jr, Cundey PE Jr, Fishback ME, Galloway RF (1977) Strut fracture in DeBakey valve: Successful reoperation and valve replacement. J Thorac Cardiovasc Surg 74: 469–470

# The Medtronic Hall® valve

I. ALTIERI, E. DEFENDINI, J.M. TORO, H. BANCHS and I. LLADO

The decision of which valve to be used in a certain patient depends on the individual needs of each patient including age, possibility of future pregnancies, anatomic lesion, and the contraindications for the use of anti-coagulation. An aspect which is of crucial importance in the selection is the durability and complications of the valve.

Of the new generation valves, the Medtronic Hall® valve is probably the most durable one at the present time and compares with any of them with fewer complications [1–5]. Due to this, we decided three years ago to use this valve in our patients when no contraindications for anticoagulation exist. It is the purpose of this manuscript to describe our experience with this valve and to compare the results to similar valves in use at the present time.

**Material**

*Description of the valve*

The Medtronic Hall® valve (Fig. 1) is a pivotal disc design which consists of a pyrolytic carbon disc occlucer, a polished titanium housing, and a knitted Teflon fabric sewing ring. There are no welds or introduced bends. The aortic valve disc opens to a full 75° opening angle and the mitral to 70°. The importance of this opening is that it allows for maximum, even flow distribution on both sides of the open disc, reducing the risk of thrombosis and thromboembolic incidence. The elliptical shape housing guide strut provides great strength while reducing resistance to blood flow past its surfaces. Also, oval shapes in the blood stream reduce the potential for thrombus formation more than round shapes projected across the blood stream.

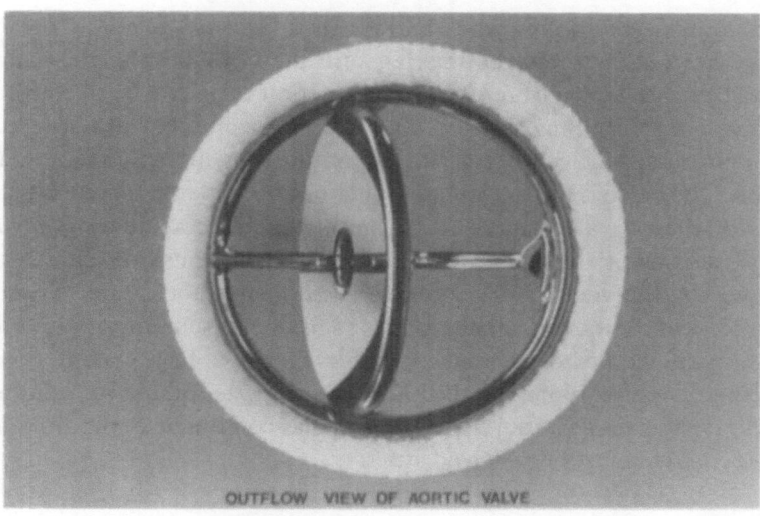

OUTFLOW VIEW OF AORTIC VALVE

*Figure 1.* Outflow view of the aortic Medtronic Hall® valve.

## Patient population

Between December 1981 and December 1984, one hundred and forty seven patients received 157 Medtronic Hall® valves. The mean age of the aortic patients was 47 years and of the mitral 32 years. All had full catheterization including right and left heart catheterization and coronary angiography when needed. The left ventricular function was studied in all. All underwent cardiovascular surgery using standard techniques. None of the patients had coronary disease requiring bypass surgery.

## Mitral valve surgery

Mitral valve surgery was performed through a median sternotomy incision using general hypothermia and crystalloid cardioplegia. When the mitral valve is going to be inserted, the mitral annulus is divided into four equal quadrants by means of four mattress pledgetted blue sutures. The suture is drawn in from the atrial to ventricular side. The obturators are used to determine the correct valve size. The size of the ventricular cavity as well as the size of the annulus is considered in the selection of the mitral prosthesis. An obturator that provides a loose fit in the annulus and can be passed easily into the left ventricle, without impingement on the septum, is selected. The four quadrant sutures are passed through the selected valve sewing ring so that the large orifice is oriented posteriorly with the downward moving portion of the disc posterior, thereby dividing sewing ring into four equal quadrants. Alternating white and green sutures are places in each quadrant. The valve is then lowered making sure there is no entanglement of the sutures. The valve holder is removed and traction is placed by all the sutures. Valve function is tested making sure the ventricular muscle will not restrict the motion of the disc, which may cause improper function, arrhythmias, and thrombosis. Once the valve is in position and functioning properly, all sutures are tied starting with the four quadrant sutures. The valve is tested again *reconfirming* the adequate function. Positioning of the large orifice posteriorly guards against interference by the ventricular septum. Figure 2 shows a patient whose large valve orifice was positioned anteriorly. As seen, there is an intermittent drop of blood pressure without electrocardiographic changes. This patient was taken again to the operating room and the valve housing was rotated so that the large orifice was positioned posteriorly. The patient has continued asymptomatic. This surgical technique must be followed strictly.

*Aortic valve surgery*

The deformed valve is resected leaving only a 2 mm rim of tissue. Any residual calcifications are carefully removed. The largest valve that fits well in the aortic root is selected. Our policy is that if we cannot accommodate a 21 mm valve, a root enlargement is performed using standard techniques, which will include the

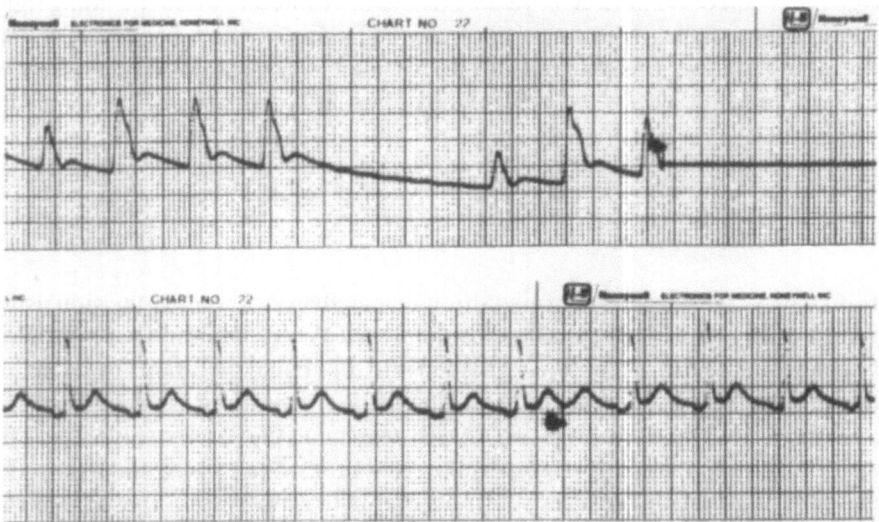

*Figure 2.* Electromechanical dissociation in a patient who had a Medtronic Hall® valve inserted in the mitral position. The large orifice was inserted looking anteriorly producing interference of the disc by the septum. The problem was solved by rotating the valve and orienting the large orifice posteriorly.

aortotomy incision that is extended through the commissure of the noncoronary and left cusp into the septal leaf-let of the mitral valve to enlarge the aortic annulus. Once a valve is selected, it is oriented in the valve holder so that the major orifice is oriented toward the noncoronary cusp area. We start our sutures on the right cusp area followed by the left cusp and finally the noncoronary cusp. The sutures are placed midway high in the sewing ring to prevent encroachment upon the coronary orifices, however, if they are too high they may interfere with free disc motion. Once all sutures are in place, they are made tight and the valve holder is then removed. The valve is seated with the index finger into the aortic root annulus. The valve is tested for adequate function. If any tissue interferes with its motion, such as ventricular or aortic wall calcifications, the interfering tissue is removed and the valve is reoriented. Once adequate function is demonstrated, all the sutures are tied and cut closely to the knots so that they remain below the valve housing. This is important as long suture tails could interfere with free disc motion.

Five patients with Marfan Syndrome had a Medtronic Hall® valve inserted in a Dacron tube graft. This conduit then was sewn to the aortic annulus. The two coronary ostia were then anastomosed successively to the end of a second preclotted Dacron which then is anastomosed to the coronary ostium.

### Sex distribution

Table 1 shows the sex distribution of all patients. Of the 78 aortic valves, 30 were female and 48 male. In the mitral valve 49 were female and 23 were males. One male patient had a tricuspid valve replacement alone.

### Valve size

Table 2 shows the sizes used in the aortic position. As seen in both sexes, the most frequent size used was #21 (when a #21 valve will fit, then aortic root enlarge-

*Table 1.* Sex distribution of all valve replacements.

| Position | Patients | Sex | |
|---|---|---|---|
| | | F | M |
| Aortic | 78 | 30 | 48 |
| Mitral | 72 | 49 | 23 |
| Tricuspid | 1 | – | 1 |
| Total | 151 | | |

ment was done and a #21 valve was then reinserted), followed by #23 and #25. The larger sizes were the least used. We think the use of smaller valve sizes is due to the fact that the aortic root of the Puertorican population, especially females, is smaller than the non-Puertorican population operated on.

Table 3 shows the valve sizes used in the mitral position. The most frequently used valve was #27 followed by #29 and #31.

Table 4 shows the double valve replacements performed. There were 14 patients, eight were males and 6 females, again the most frequent combination was a #21 in the aortic position and a #29 in the mitral position.

Table 5 shows the orifice diameter and orifice area of each size valve in the aortic and mitral position. It is clearly seen that as the size of the valve increases the orifice area also increases.

## Complications

Table 6 shows the total early mortality in our group which is 7.1% and the causes. As seen we haven't had a valve related death, and the two most frequent causes of death have complications due to renal failure in patients operated on with an

*Table 2.* Distribution by sex and size of the aortic valve replacement.

|     | Size | Male | Size | Female | Total |
|-----|------|------|------|--------|-------|
| 1.  | # 21 | 15   | # 21 | 17     | 32    |
| 2.  | # 23 | 12   | # 23 | 7      | 19    |
| 3.  | # 25 | 16   | # 25 | 3      | 19    |
| 4.  | # 27 | 4    | # 27 | 1      | 5     |
| 5.  | # 29 | 1    | # 29 | 0      | 1     |
| 6.  | # 31 | 0    | # 31 | 2      | 2     |
|     |      | 48   |      | 30     | 78    |

# = Size of valve

*Table 3.* Distribution by sex and size of the mitral valve replacements.

|     | Size | Male | Size | Female | Total |
|-----|------|------|------|--------|-------|
| 1.  | # 27 | 4    | # 27 | 23     | 27    |
| 2.  | # 29 | 15   | # 29 | 12     | 27    |
| 3.  | # 31 | 4    | # 31 | 14     | 28    |
|     |      | 23   |      | 49     | 82    |

# = Size of valve

*Table 4.* Double valve replacements, 14 patients. Sex and valve number combinations.

**I. Male = 8 patients**

| Mitral | Aortic |
|--------|--------|
| # 27 | # 21 |
| # 29 | # 23 |
| # 29 | # 23 |
| # 27 | # 23 |
| # 29 | # 25 |
| # 29 | # 21 |
| # 31 | # 27 |
| # 29 | # 25 |

**II. Female = 6 patients**

| Mitral | Aortic |
|--------|--------|
| # 27 | # 23 |
| # 29 | # 25 |
| # 31 | # 21 |
| # 29 | # 21 |
| # 29 | # 21 |
| # 27 | # 21 |

*Table 5.* Comparison between heart valve size, orifice diameter, orifice area of the mitral and aortic Medtronic Hall® valve.

| I. | Mitral valve | Orifice diameter (mm) | Orifice area |
|----|--------------|------------------------|--------------|
| 1. | # 23 | 18 | 2.54 cm² |
| 2. | # 25 | 20 | 3.14 |
| 3. | # 27 | 22 | 3.80 |
| 4. | # 29 | 24 | 4.52 |
| 5. | # 31 | 24 | 4.52 |
| 6. | # 33 | 24 | 4.52 |

| II. | Aortic valve | Orifice diameter (mm) | Orifice area |
|-----|--------------|------------------------|--------------|
| 1. | # 20 | 16 | 2.01 cm² |
| 2. | # 21 | 16 | 2.01 |
| 3. | # 23 | 18 | 2.54 |
| 4. | # 25 | 20 | 3.14 |
| 5. | # 27 | 22 | 3.80 |
| 6. | # 29 | 24 | 4.52 |

elevated B.U.N., severe bleeding during surgery, and sepsis in patients operated on with bacterial endocarditis. It is important to notice that we haven't had any problems with clinically significant hemolysis or any severe embolic episodes. We have had only two cases of transient embolic episodes. No perivalvular leaks have been detected.

Table 7 shows the detail analysis of the patients who had an early death. Also shown are three patients who had late death (1.9%) due to congestive heart failure (all of three had an ejection fraction of less then 30% before surgery) and one who had a reoperation due to the development of a pseudo-aneurysm after aortic root enlargement.

*Table 6.* Early complications producing death in patients with Medtronic Hall® valve replacements.

| | | |
|---|---|---|
| 1. | Valve related deaths | = 0% |
| 2. | Deaths from other causes | = 3.1% |
| | a. Myocardial failure | = 0% |
| | b. Myocardial infarction | = 0.6% |
| | c. Sudden death | = 0% |
| | d. Tamponade | = 6% |
| | e. Sepsis | = 1.9% |
| | f. Pulmonary embolus | = 0% |
| | g. Hemolysis | = 0% |
| 3. | Others: | |
| | Renal failure | |
| | Bleeding | = 4% |
| | Technical problems | |
| | Total mortality | = 7.1% |

*Table 7.* Detail analysis of all the deaths.

| Early death | Late death |
|---|---|
| 1. Cardiac Tamponade | 1. Congestive heart failure (3 patients). |
| 2. Patient operated with Bacterial Endocarditis. Died in sepsis. | 2. Operation for a pseudo aneurysm. |
| 3. Perforation of the left ventricular wall during surgery. | |
| 4. Acute myocardial infarction post-operatively. Patient had minimal coronary disease prior to surgery and was not considered for coronary bypass. | |
| 5. One recognized dislocation of the aortic annulus by a stab wound. | |
| 6. Acute renal failure superimposed in chronic renal disease (2 patients). | |
| 7. Severe bleeding during surgery (2 patients). | |
| 8. Brain ischemia. | |

*Postoperative disc entrapment*

As discussed previously, it is very important to orient the large orifice posteriorly and inferiorly to improve the left ventricular hemodynamics because the flow will be directed toward the apex and not to the septum or free wall. Also, this is done to avoid interference of the septum with the disc. Harvine [6] and associates have reported ten patients with disc entrapment, and as causes they mention:
1. Disc entrapment against the ventricular wall (Bjork-Shiley valve)
2. Disc entrapment by overhanging suture (Medtronic Hall® valve)
3. One disc failed to open (St. Jude valve)
Table 8 shows the mechanism of postoperative disc entrapment.

*Follow-up*

Most of our patients have been followed for two to three years at a special anticoagulation clinic. They are followed with monthly prothrombin time and serial echocardiograms and parameters to detect clinically important hemolysis. We have not experienced any valvular malfunction, thrombosis, or clinically important hemolysis. Only two episodes of transient embolism occurred without neurologic deficits. All of our patients have been in NYHA Class I or II post-operatively.

*Postoperative hemodynamics*

In the aortic and mitral position, several investigators have studied the hemo-dynamic changes produced by several valves. Table 9 shows the comparative

*Table 8.* Mechanism of postoperative disc entrapment.

| I. Mitral valve |
|---|
| a.  Interference by the septum |
| b.  Interference by overhanging suture |
| c.  Inhibition by overhanging tissue |
| d.  Oversizing |

| II. Aortic valve |
|---|
| a.  Disc attached to aortic wall |
| b.  Overhanging suture |
| c.  Disc interference, due to hematoma, between graft and aortic valve |
| d.  Oversizing |

hemodynamics between four of the most frequently used tilting disc valves in the aortic position (St. Jude, Bjork-Shiley, Medtronic Hall®, and Lillehi Kaster [7–12] and Table 10 shows the hemodynamics of the mitral Medtronic Hall® valve. The most frequent valve size used in our group in the aortic position was a #23 and #25, and basically the St. Jude and Medtronic Hall® give similar hemodynamic results, although the smaller St. Jude will give smaller gradients. The same has been found in the mitral position. Horstkotte [13] calculated the effective·valve orifice in the mitral position (#29 size valve) and found to be $3.1 \pm 0.8 \, cm^2$ in the St. Jude; $2.2 \pm 0.5 \, cm^2$ in the Bjork-Shiley, and $1.9 \pm 0.5 \, cm$ in the Medtronic Hall®. Forman [12] reported the hemodynamic parameters in the Lillehei Kaster valve. He showed valves which compared with the other valves.

*Table 9.* Comparative hemodynamics in the aortic position between St. Jude, Bjork-Shiley, Medtronic Hall® valve and Lillehei-Kaster.

| Prostheses | Valve size | | | | | | | |
| | #21 | | #23 | | #25 | | #27 | |
| | AP | EOA | AP | EOA | AP | EOA | AP | EOA |
|---|---|---|---|---|---|---|---|---|
| St. Jude | 5.2 | 2.7 | 3.2 | 3.6 | 3.4 | 3.0 | 2.5 | – |
| Bjork-Shiley | 22 | 1.30 | 14 | 1.7 | 9 | 2.20 | 11 | 2.40 |
| Medtronic Hall® | 12.5 | 1.56 | 9.2 | 2.17 | 3.8 | 2.11 | 2.5 | 2.25 |
| Lillehei-Kaster | 45 | 0.80 | 28 | 1.10 | 22 | 1.30 | 15 | 1.90 |

AP = Trans Valvular Pressure Gradient (MMHG).
EOA = Effective Orifice Area.
References:
1. Chaux A. 2 – Ref. 7
2. Allessandro D. – Ref. 8
3. Medtronic Blood Systems – Ref. 9
4. Bjork-Shiley — Ref. 10
5. Pyle RB – Ref. 11

*Table 10.* Hemodynamics of the Medtronic Hall® valve in the mitral position.

| Valve | E.O.A. | AP (Rest) |
|---|---|---|
| #27 | 3.03 | 6.0 |
| #29 | 2.86 | 2.7 |
| #31 | 3.35 | 2.0 |

AP = Transvalvular Pressure Gradient.
EOA = Effective Orifice Area.
Ref: Medtronic Blood Systems data.

There is little hemodynamic data available on the Omniscience valves. In our opinion of the mechanical valves on the market, the Medtronic Hall® has the potential of producing the least complications.

## Discussion

The decision which valve to be used in a patient depends on many factors, especially the durability and late complications of the prosthesis. Of the new generation of valves, emphasis has been given to the St. Jude and the Medtronic Hall® valve. In our selection of which valve to use, several factors influenced our decision. We wanted a pyrolytic carbon disc due to proven performance of the material, a titanium housing, employing elliptical component shapes which decrease blood flow resistance and increase durability. Oval cross-sectional shapes in the blood stream tend to reduce the risk of thrombus formation. By analyzing the most commonly used mechanical valves (St. Jude, Bjork-Shiley, Lillehei Kaster, Medtronic Hall®), we were concerned regarding the use of two leaflets in the St. Jude valve. We believe this may provide more mechanical chances of failure and the valve hinge mechanism may increase the chance of thrombus formation impairing leaflet mobility [15]. The Bjork-Shiley valve [16] has been shown to be less resistant than both. Due to all of these factors, we selected the use of the Medtronic Hall® valve, which is a durable valve and satisfied our criteria of an improved prosthetic replacement.

At the beginning, our biggest problem was that we were not satisfied where to position the large orifice of the valve in the mitral position. After studying the hemodynamic changes seen in the operating room by positioning the valve in different positions, we decided that it is crucial to orient the large orifice of the valve posteriorly. This will avoid disc interference by the septum and hemodynamically will direct the blood flow to the apex of the ventricle, which will avoid blood turbulence occurring when the flow is directed to the septum or free wall. After using this technique, we have not experienced surgical problems during implantation. As seen in our data, our early surgical mortality was related to surgical technical problems and by operating on high risk patients. Regarding late mortality, three of the patients died of congestive heart failure. These patients were ones with severe left ventricular dysfunction preoperatively. Another died post-operatively after surgery for a pseudoaneurysm developed after aortic root enlargement.

Related to aortic valve replacement we have been impressed by the performance of the small size aortic prosthesis used in our patients. The Puertorican patients have a rather small aortic root. This had required us to perform five aortic root enlargements to be able to introduce a size #21 valve.

Our general complications during follow-up have been minimal. We have not had any valve related deaths nor clinically significant hemolysis. Probably a very important aspect of this low complication rate is that we follow all our patients monthly in a special anticoagulation clinic.

Hemodynamically, as seen in Tables 9 and 10, the St. Jude and Medtronic Hall® valves are similar although the effective orifice area of the St. Jude valves is bigger in the smaller valves, but we agree with Yoganathan [14] who studied the St. Jude hemodynamically in vitro. He said that 'he cannot indicate at the present time whether the in vitro characteristics of reduced shear stress and turbulance will translate to increased valve durability or lessened thromboembolism'.

In conclusion, our experience with the Medtronic Hall® valve has been excellent. We think that this valve compares to any at present regarding effective hemodynamics, extended functional durability, and freedom from thromboembolic complications. We believe it to be superior to the other pivotal valves being used at the present time.

## References

1. Hauge SN, Semb B, Abdal Noor MSC, Hall KV (1983) A 5-Year Experience with the Medtronic Hall® Disc Valve Prosthesis Circulation 68, II: 169–174
2. Starek PJK, Murray GF, Keagy BA, Wilcox BR (1963) Clinical Experience With the Hall Pivoting Disc Valve Thoracic Cardiovascular Surgeon 31/11: 66–68 New York: George Thieme Verlag Stuttgart
3. Beaudet RL, Poirier NC, Guerraty AJ, Doyle D Fifty-Four Month Experience With an Improved Tilting Disk Valve (Medtronic Hall®) Thoracic Cardiovascular Surgeon 31/11: 89–93, New York: George Thieme Verlag Stuttgart
4. Semb B, Hauge SN, Hall KV Intraoperative and Postoperative Hemodynamic Studies in Patients Undergoing Aortic Valve Replacement With the Hall-Kaster Cardiac Disc Prosthesis 27: 92–97, 1979, New York: George Thieme Verlag Stuttgart
5. Hall KV An Improved Pivotal Disc Type Prosthetic Heart Valve Oslo City Hospital, 29: 3–21, 1979
6. Jarvinen A, Virtanen K, Peltolak³, Magmies T, Ketonen P, KKo. Manni A Postoperative Disc Entrapment Following Cardiac Valve Replacement – Report of Ten Cases Thoracic Cardiovascular Surgeon, 32: 152–156, 1984, New York: George Thieme Verlag Stuttgart
7. Chaux A, Gray RJ, Matloff JM, Feldman H, Sustaita H An appreciation of the New St. Jude Valvular Prosthesis Journal of Thoracic Cardiovascular Surgery, 81: 202–211, 1981
8. D'Alessandro LC, St. Jude Medical Prosthesis: Clinical Results, St. Jude Medical Inc., Second Symposium, March 11–14, 1981, San Diego, California
9. Medtronic Blood Systems, Three-Year Clinical Evaluation of the Hall-Kaster Prosthetic Valve, 1980
10. Bjork VO, Holmgren A, Ovenfors CP Olinc Clinical and Hemodynamic Results of Aortic Valve Replacement With the Bjork-Shiley Tilting Disc Valve Prosthesis Scandinavian Journal of Thoracic Cardiovascular Surgery 5: 177–191, 1971
11. Pyle RB, Mayer JE, Lindsay WG, Jorgensen CR, Wang Y, Wicoloff DM Hemodynamic Evaluation of Lillehei-Kaster and Starr-Edwards Prosthesis Ann Thorac Surg 76: 336–343, 1978
12. Forman E, Gersh B, Fraser R, Beck W Hemodynamic Assessment of Lillehei-Kaster Tilting Disc Aortic and Mitral Prostheses Journal of Thoracic Cardiovascular Surgery 75: 595–598, 1978
13. Horstkotte K, Haerten K, Herzer JA, Seipel L, Bircks W, Loogen F Preliminary Results in Mitral Valve Replacement With the St. Jude Medical Prosthesis: Comparison With the Bjork-Shiley

Valve Circulation, 64, II: 203–209, 1981

14. Yogahathan AP, Woo YR, Williams FP In Vitro Hydrodynamic Characteristics of the St. Jude Bileaflet Prosthesis Advances in Cardiac Valves, De Bakey Med., New York Medical Books, 1982

15. Bradley LM, Derry LW, Watson DC Failure of St. Jude Medical Mitral Prosthesis Diagnosed by Two-Dimensional Echocardiography Am J Cardiol 57: 1385, 1984

16. Tull R Complications of Convexo-Concave Heart Valve Devices and Diagnostic Letter 12: 8, 1985

# Experience with the St. Jude medical heart valve prosthesis

H. DALICHAU, H. NIGBUR, J. KALOTAI and A. SCHMITZ-KÖHLER

## I. Introduction

During the past 25 years, numerous different technical conceptions for the development of a suitable artificial heart valve have been followed, only a few of which led to clinical applicability. Among those prostheses which reached the stage of clinical testing, only a small number have proved to be reliable for a certain space of time. The so-called Bileaflet-Valves steadily have been gaining ground upon the Caged-Ball-Valves (e.g. the Starr-Edwards- and the Smeloff-Cutter-Valve) as well as the Tilting-Disc-Prostheses (e.g. Björk-Shiley-, Omni-science-, Lillehei-Kaster-Prosthesis) over the last few years.

One of the Bileaflet-Valves is the St. Jude Medical Heart Valve Prosthesis*, that gained increasing acceptance world-wide since being introduced into clinical usage in 1977. The Duromedics Heart Valve Prosthesis**, available since 1982, is the other representative. They are both based on a valve-design from the mid-sixties from Kalke and Lillehei [3].

According to our most recent knowledge, approximately 70.000 St. Jude Valves and about 2.000 Duromedics Prostheses have been implanted in man up to now.

Our own practical experience is limited to the St. Jude Medical Prosthesis (SJM), which has been used at the Clinic for Cardiovascular Surgery at the University of Cologne since its introduction into German hospitals in 1978.

Up to December 1984 a total of 811 patients underwent heart-valve replacement with the SJM-prosthesis. Initially the SJM was reserved for what we considered our problem-patients, e.g. those with a very small aortic valve annulus. When however subsequent haemodynamic studies on this group of patients showed the clear superiority of the SJM-valve in comparison to its pre-

---

* St. Jude Medical, Inc., St. Paul.
** Hemex Scientific, Inc., Austin.

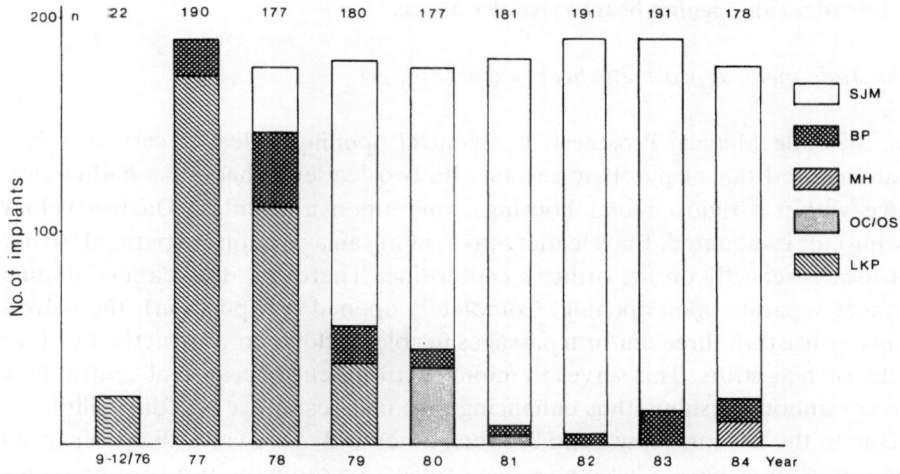

*Figure 1.* Ar ificial heart valve replacement at the University Hospital Cologne from September 1976 to Decembe⁻ 1984. The Lillehei Kaster Valve was preferred until 1978, since then the SJM became the valve of firs⁻ choice.

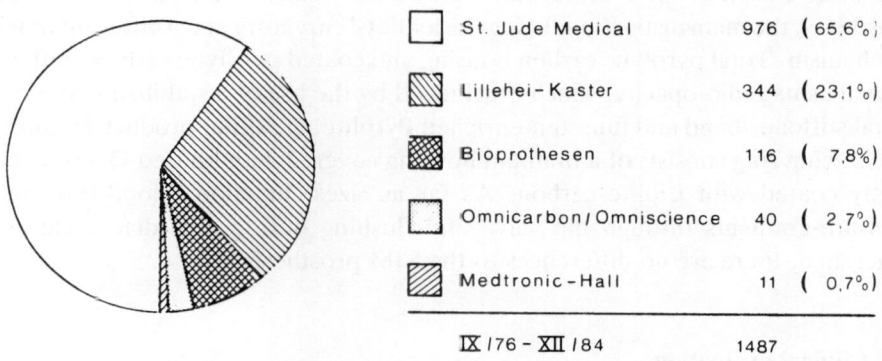

| | | |
|---|---|---|
| St. Jude Medical | 976 | ( 65,6 %) |
| Lillehei-Kaster | 344 | ( 23,1 %) |
| Bioprothesen | 116 | ( 7,8%) |
| Omnicarbon/Omniscience | 40 | ( 2,7 %) |
| Medtronic-Hall | 11 | ( 0,7 %) |
| IX /76 – XII /84 | 1487 | |

*Figure 2.* D stribution of 1.487 heart valve prostheses which have been implanted from September 1976 to December 1984.

decessors this bileaflet prosthesis became the valve of first choice in our hands and has been increasingly used ever since (Fig. 1). A total of 976 SJM-valves have been implanted from May 1978 until December 1984 (Fig. 2).

## II. Bileaflet full-opening heart valve prosthesis

### 1. St. Jude medical prosthetic heart valve (Fig. A)

The St. Jude Medical Prosthesis is a central opening, bileaflet cardiac valve, manufactured out of pyrolytic carbon. Its two leaflets, shaped as half-circles, move within a rigid circular housing, whereupon a seamless Dacron velour sewing cuff is mounted. Each leaflet moves along an axis adjusted parallel to, but not located exactly on the orifice's center-line. Therefore, the leaflets' mating surfaces separate upon opening. Completely opened (85° position), the valve's orifice consists of three uniform passages for blood-flow, un-obstructed by other parts, such as struts. This serves to minimize turbulence because of central flow and continuous flushing, thus enhancing thrombo-resistance and durability.

Due to the advantageous ratio between inner and outer valve-diameter, even small prostheses have a large effective orifice. Accordingly, pressure-gradients across the valve are very low [2, 9, 10].

### 2. The duromedics bileaflet heart valve (Fig. B)

The basic design of the Duromedics Valve differs only little from the St. Jude prosthesis, the main distinctions being the leaflets' curvature and a different hinge mechanism. Total pyrolytic carbon housing and coated pyrolytic carbon leaflets, as well as its radio-opacity, which is achieved by the use of a stabilizing Stellite-metal stiffener-band and tungsten-enriched Pyrolite, are other product-features. The sewing ring consists of a titanium housing covered with knitted Dacron and partly coated with Biolite carbon. As far as sizes, function, blood-flow and pressure-gradients through the valve and flushing during a cardiac cycle are concerned, there are no differences to the SJM prosthesis [4].

## III. Clinical evaluation

### 1. The St. Jude medical prosthetic heart valve

In the summer of 1984 Lillehei [8] reported on a multicenter long-term study, based on the evaluation of 584 cases with isolated aortic (330) or mitral valve (254) replacement with a follow-up of 4.5 to 6.5 years after operation. Seven American and ten European centers, one of them being the Clinic for Cardio-vascular Surgery at the University of Cologne, contributed to the study.

All patients with isolated heart valve replacement, operated upon before December 31st, 1979, have been included without any form of selection.

The probability of a 5-year-survival for patients with isolated aortic or mitral

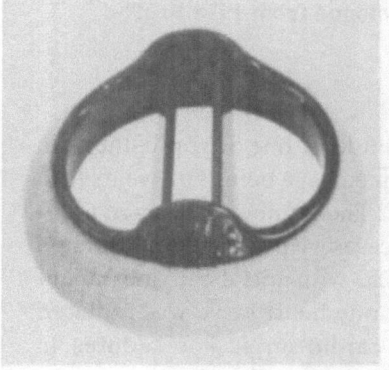

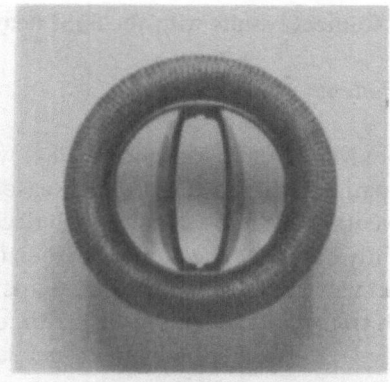

*Figure A.*                                    *Figure B.*

valve replacement was 85.1% and 86.9% respectively, the mean follow-up being 4.1 years and early mortality being excluded (3.6% after aortic valve replacement, 9.5% after mitral valve replacement). The majority of deaths was not valve-related. With patients after aortic valve replacement, the valve-related late mortality was 2.1% and only 1.0% after mitral valve replacement. 65% of all patients remained totally free of complications postoperatively. The incidence of thromboembolism being 0.97% per patient year for the replaced aortic valve and 1.98% for the mitral valve, the embolus-free rate after 5 years amounts to 95.9% ± 2.4% for patients with SJM in aortic position and to 89.4% ± 5.4% for mitral valve replacement. Up to the present, no other mechanical heart valve prosthesis has had such a low embolus-rate. Furthermore, no case was observed, where valve-malfunction could be held responsible for a patient's death or necessitated re-operation.

## 2. *The duromedics bileaflet valve*

For the Duromedics valve, which was introduced into clinical usage considerably later, no comparable long-term evaluations can be referred to. According to the manufacturers, the longest postoperative interval up to May 1985 was 37 months and the mean follow-up for 1.744 patients not yet higher than 9.55 months. The similarity of both artificial heart valves as to design and function however suggests, that long-term results will be similar to the SJM.

Prospective randomized studies still have to be published. Taking into account some preliminary reports, already available today, the SJM valve, however, seems to be slightly superior to the Duromedics prosthesis, as regards the thrombo-embolus-free rate [1].

# IV. Clinical results with the SJM heart valve in Cologne from 1978 to 1984

## 1. Patients

From May 1978 to December 1984, we implanted at least one SJM prosthesis in 811 patients with cardiac valve disease (Fig. 3), the mean age being 50.9 years (1 to 76 years) with a peak in the sixth decade (39.6%). The number of women (409) slightly exceeded the number of men (402). In 521 cases we performed an isolated heart valve replacement: 268 patients with aortic, 252 with mitral and one patient with tricuspid valve disease. 122 times more than one heart valve was replaced (Fig. 4). 180 additional patients needed associated cardio-surgical procedures, in most cases because of concomitant coronary heart disease (Fig. 5).

## 2. Early mortality

Early mortality of our patients with an isolated singular heart valve replacement came up to 4.2%, with a significant difference, however, between aortic (2.2%) and mitral valve replacement (6.3%). The highest rate of early death was found among patients with combined procedures. Further analysis revealed a distinct correlation between the high early-mortality-risk and the degree of the pre-existing left ventricular malfunction. Concomitant coronary heart disease as well as pulmonary or renal insufficiency proved to be particularly responsible for higher risk of early mortality. No death, however, has been caused by a valve-related complication (Fig. 6).

## 3. Long-term results

In 1984, the Clinic for Cardiovascular Surgery at the University of Cologne contributed to Lillehei's [8] multi-center, long-term study of patients after iso-

Patients :  $\boxed{811}$

Age :  1-76 years (m = 50.9)

Sex :  409 female, 402 male

Implants :  $\boxed{976}$

*Figure 3.* Patient age and sex distribution.

| | n | ✝ |
|---|---|---|
| Singular HVR | 521 | 22 ( 4,2 % ) |
| Multiple HVR | 122 | 14 ( 11,5 % ) |
| HVR + ass. surgery | 168 | 25 ( 14,9 % ) |
| incl. Redos | 811 | 61 ( 7,5 % ) |

*Figure 4.* Heart valve replacement (HVR) with the SJM from May 1978 to December 1984 in 811 patients. Number of operations and hospital mortality.

ASSOCIATED SURGERY IN 168 PATIENTS
WITH SJMVP IMPLANTATION (N = 179)

| | |
|---|---|
| CABG | 64 |
| VAR (± CABG) | 5 |
| AORTA ASC.REPLACEMENT | 5 |
| LVOTE, MYOTOMY ETC. | 28 |
| MITRAL RECONSTRUCTION | 22 |
| TRICUSPID RECONSTRUCTION | 13 |
| OTHERS | 42 |

*Figure 5.* Associated procedures in addition to heart valve replacement with the SJM in 168 patients (CABG = coronary artery bypass grafting, LVOTE = left ventricular outflow tract enlargement, VAR = ventricular aneurysma resection).

lated heart valve replacement with SJM. We extended this follow-up to patients operated upon until the end of 1980. Out of 242 patients from May 1978 until December 1980, 21 died within 30 days after the operation (8.7%). Three survivors were lost to follow-up due to the return to their home countries (Fig. 7). The remaining total of 218 patients comprises 122 [26] with aortic, 61 [9] with mitral and 35 [7] with more than one heart valve replacement, the numbers in parenthesis indicating associated cardiac procedures.

Mean follow-up time was 56.4 months. 4.7 years respectively and varied from 48 to 78 months (12.291 patient months for the whole group) with no significant variations in the subsets (Fig. 8). During the time of follow-up 26 patients out of

## CAUSES OF EARLY DEATH  (N = 61)

| | |
|---|---:|
| LCO | 33 |
| MYOCARDIAL INFARCT | 6 |
| VENTRICULAR TACHYCARDIA | 4 |
| RENAL INSUFFICIENCY | 5 |
| PNEUMONIE | 2 |
| NEUROLOGIC PROBLEMS | 3 |
| SEPTICEMIA | 3 |
| HEMMORRHAGE | 4 |
| LATE TAMPONADE | 1 |

*Figure 6.* Causes of early death in 61 patients (LCO = low cardiac output).

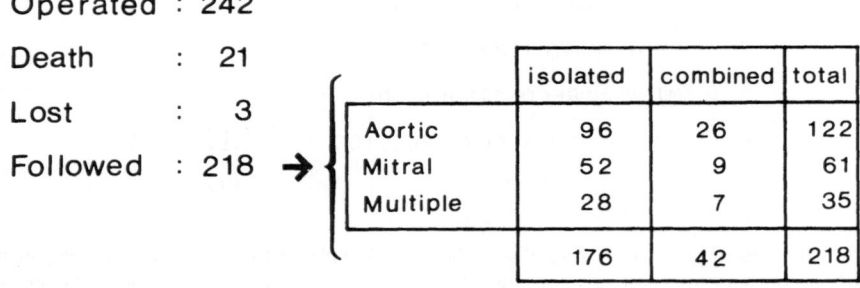

Operated : 242
Death : 21
Lost : 3
Followed : 218 →

| | isolated | combined | total |
|---|---:|---:|---:|
| Aortic | 96 | 26 | 122 |
| Mitral | 52 | 9 | 61 |
| Multiple | 28 | 7 | 35 |
| | 176 | 42 | 218 |

*Figure 7.* Long term follow-up study after SJM implantation. Patient cohort followed and distribution of operative procedures.

218 died (11.9%): 14 after aortic, 6 after mitral and one after tricuspid as well as 5 after multiple heart valve replacement. Thus, the calculated probability for a 4-year-survival is 88.5%, 90.2% and 85.7% for patients after aortic-, mitral- and multiple heart valve replacement, respectively (Fig. 9). In no case was death caused by mechanical valve malfunction, up to today. The majority of patients studied who died were lost because of progressive cardiac failure. The following deaths were associated directly or indirectly with valve-malfunction: 3 patients died from cerebral bleeding due to excessive anticoagulation, 3 from undiagnosed

113

| | |
|---|---|
| Patients at follow-up | : 218 |
| Time of follow-up | : 48-78 months |
| Mean time of follow-up | : 56,4 months |
| Total time at risk | : 12.291 months |

*Figure 8.* Long term follow-up study of patients operated between May 1978 and December 1980.

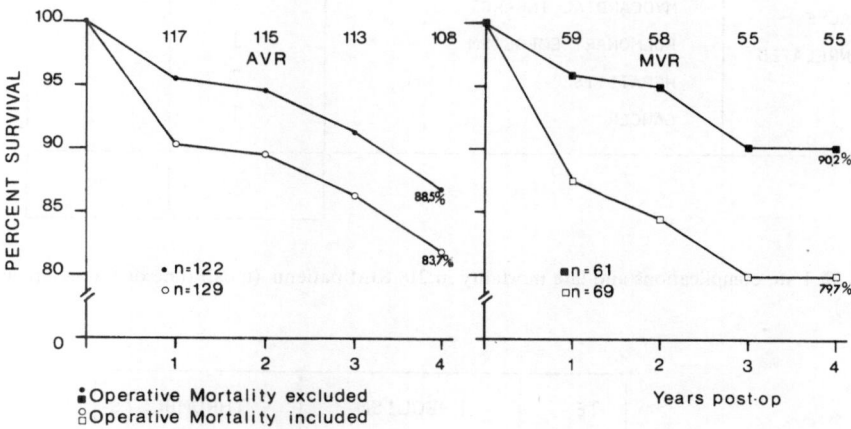

*Figure 9.* Actuarial survival curves for patients with aortic (AVR) or mitral (MVR) valve replacement using SJM.

progressive valvular thrombosis, 2 after cerebral embolism and one other in the course of septicaemia due to bacterial endocarditis (Fig. 10).

We saw a total of 9 patients with thrombo-embolic complications (Fig. 11): 3 cases of complete thrombotic valve obstruction and 6 of cerebral embolism. In all cases, valve thrombosis could not be recognized in time to rescue the patient. 2 patients out of 6 died after cerebral embolism, whereas the other 4 survived with slowly receding neurological symptoms. Thus, the incidence of thrombo-embolic complications for a total time at risk of 12.291 months could be calculated with 0.88% per patient year for aortic-, 1.03% for mitral patients and 0.62% for patients after multiple valve replacement (Fig. 12).

Compared to the thrombo-embolic rates of other artificial heart valves previously used in our clinic, these results suggest a particularly low risk of thrombo-embolism after SJM heart valve replacement with subsequent permanent anti-coagulation.

|  |  | N | + |
|---|---|---|---|
| VALVE - RELATED | MALFUNCTION | - | - |
|  | BACTERIAL ENDOCARDITIS | 2 | 1 |
|  | LEAKAGE | 1 | - |
|  | THROMBOSIS | 3 | 3 |
|  | EMBOLISM | 6 | 2 |
|  | HEMORRHAGE | 20 | 3 |
| VALVE - UNRELATED | CONGESTIVE HEART FAILURE | 13 | 13 |
|  | MYOCARDIAL INFARCT | 2 | 2 |
|  | PULMONARY EMBOLISM | 1 | 1 |
|  | HEPATITIS | 7 | - |
|  | CANCER | 1 | 1 |
|  |  | 56 | 26 |

*Figure 10.* Late complications and late mortality in 218 SJM patients (mean time of follow-up 56,4 months).

|  | TE | EMBOLISM | THROMBOSIS |
|---|---|---|---|
| AORTIC | 5 | 3  (+ 1) | 2  (+ 2) |
| MITRAL | 3 | 2 | 1  (+ 1) |
| MULTIPLE | 1 | 1  (+ 1) | - |
|  | 9 | 6  (+ 2) | 3  (+ 3) |

*Figure 11.* Thromboembolic late complications (TE) in SJM patients.

On the other hand, the rate of haemorrhage due to excessive anticoagulation was comparatively high: 20 patients developed extended bleeding with 3 cases of lethal cerebral or spinal haemorrhage (Fig. 10).

|  | Aortic | Mitral | Multiple | Total |
|---|---|---|---|---|
| Patients at risk | 122 | 61 | 35 | 218 |
| Time at risk (months) | 6.856 | 3.495 | 1.939 | 12.290 |
| No. of TE | 5 (⊥3) | 3 (⊥1) | 1 (⊥1) | 9 (⊥5) |
| TE / pat. year (%) | 0.88 | 1.03 | 0.62 | 0.88 |

*Figure 12.* Thromboembolic risk for patients with aortic, mitral and multiple SJM implants (TE = thromboembolism).

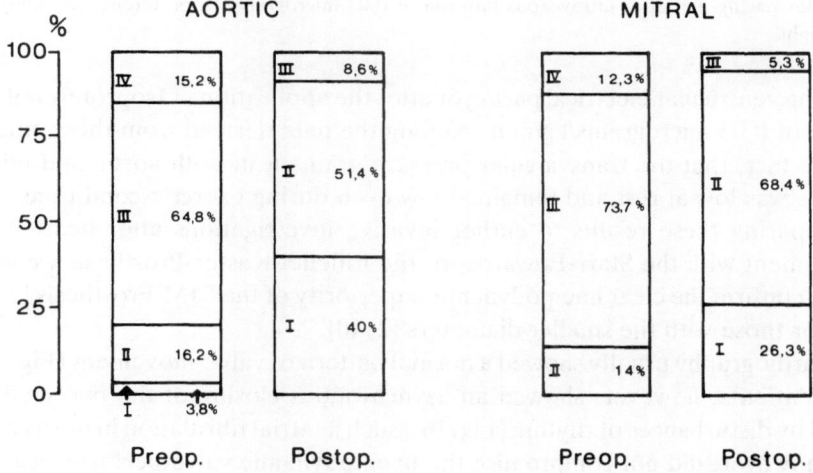

*Figure 13.* Clinical improvement according to NYHAC 48 to 78 months after aortic and mitral valve replacement using SJM.

## 4. Clinical and haemodynamic studies

The majority of patients after heart valve replacement improved clinically resulting in a rise of at least one grade in the New York Heart Association's functional classification – with aortic patients having a significant advantage over mitral patients (Fig. 13). These results proved to be in accordance with our haemodynamic studies of 112 patients (79 aortic- and 33 mitral valves), followed-up from 2 to 48 months after heart valve replacement, the mean time being 8.1 months (Fig. 14).

The haemodynamic performance of the prosthesis was determined at rest as well

| Position | Nr. of pat. | Condition | Δ P (mm Hg) | ΔP mean |
|----------|-------------|-----------|-------------|---------|
| Aortic | 73 | Rest | 0 - 20 | 3,8 ± 1,2 |
| | 19 | Pacing | 0 - 14 | 3,1 ± 0,9 |
| | 18 | Isoproterenol | 0 - 42 | 13,8 ± 4,8 |
| Mitral | 39 | Rest | 0 - 4 | 0,8 ± 0,3 |
| | 9 | Pacing | 0 - 4 | 3,0 ± 0,8 |
| | 12 | Isoproterenol | 0 - 5 | 2,4 ± 0,5 |

Time of study   2 - 48 months p. op  (mean 8,1 mo.)

Total time of follow - up 907 months

*Figure 14.* Results of hemodynamic reinvestigations in 73 aortic and 39 mitral patients at rest, with ventricular pacing and after intravenous infusion of 0,03 micrograms Isoproterenol per kilogram bodyweight.

as during ventricular electrical pacing or after the application of Isoproterenol in a dosage of 0.03 micrograms/kg/min. Among the data derived from these studies was the fact, that the transvalvular pressure-gradient in both aortic and mitral patients was low at rest and remained low even during exercise-conditions.

Comparing these results to earlier invasive investigations after heart valve replacement with the Starr-Edwards- or the Lillehei-Kaster-Prosthesis we were able to confirm the clear haemodynamic superiority of the SJM-Prosthesis [2, 7], even for those with the smaller diameters [2, 10].

Echocardiography usually showed a normal pattern of valve-movement (Fig. 15). Some patients, however, showed an asynchronous closing of the two leaflets, caused by disturbances of rhythm (Fig. 16), such as atrial fibrillation in most cases. This, however, did not compromise the haemodynamic valve-performance and disappeared in all cases on return to regular sinus rhythm after cardioversion [5]. On high speed cinefilm studies, normal bileaflet movement could be confirmed at rest as well as during exercise or during high-frequency electrical ventricular pacing (Fig. 17).

## 5. Conclusions

A cardiac surgeon's choice for a suitable artificial heart valve substitute will always be influenced by his previous clinical experience and – to no lesser extent – by his personal philosophy. This may be the reason why new artificial heart valves meet with various degrees of acceptance.

On the other hand, it has to be emphasized, that the clinical introduction of a new heart valve prosthesis – its evident improvements apart – may lead to unforeseen complications. The premature destruction of the Starr-Edward's cloth-covered

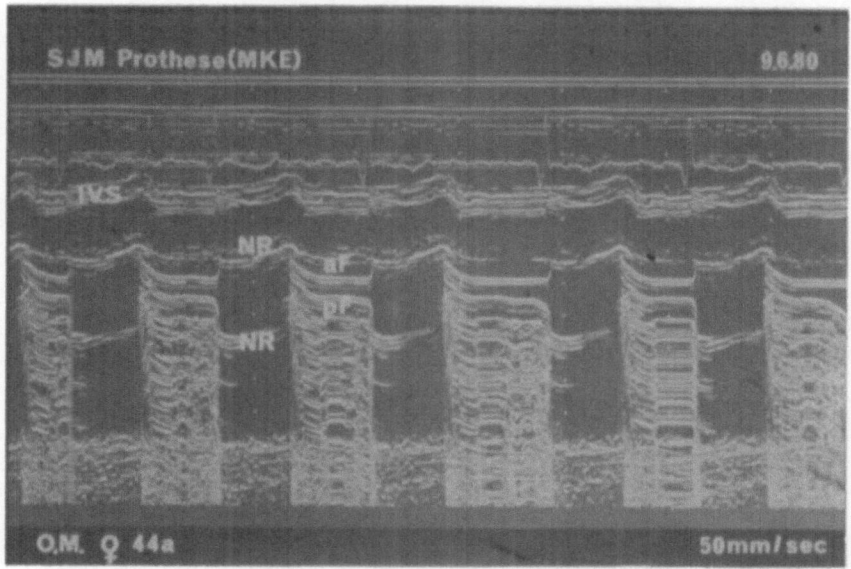

*Figure 15.* Echocardiogram of a normally functioning SJM in mitral position, aF = anterior leaflet, pF = posterior leaflet, NR = suture ring, IVS = interventricular septum.

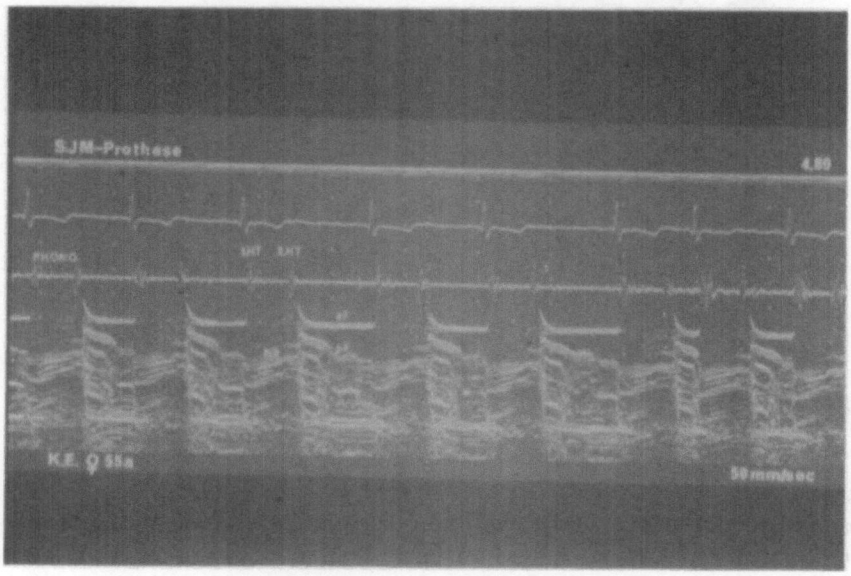

*Figure 16.* Asynchronous leaflet closure of a SJM in mitral position caused by ventricular arrhythmia due to atrial fibrillation.

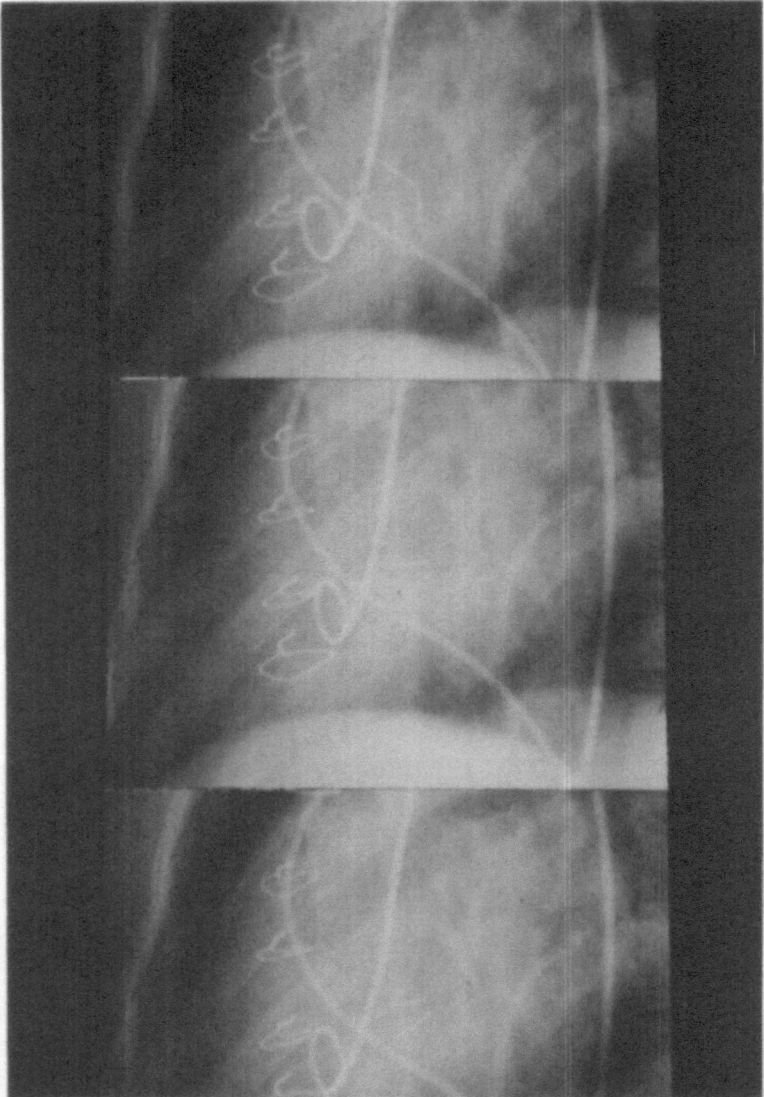

*Figure 17.* Normal opening and closure of a SJM at high speed cinefilm study.

cage with subsequent valve-failure may serve as an example.

The introduction of the SJM-valve into our clinic in 1978 was facilitated by the fact, that for problempatients better haemodynamic results could be attained with the SJM-valve than with others previously implanted. Evidence for this may be the significant decrease of cases where the aortic annulus had to be enlarged, in order to accomodate a larger prosthesis (Fig. 18).

| PROSTHESIS | AORTIC VALVE IMPLANTS | LVOTE |
|------------|----------------------|-------|
| LKP | 179 | 20 (11,2 %) |
| SJMVP | 532 | 10 ( 1,9 %) |

COLOGNE 1976 - 1984

*Figure 18.* Incidence of left ventricular outflow tract enlargement (LVOTE) in patients with a small aortic annulus with regard to the implanted prosthesis (LKP = Lillehei-Kaster Prosthesis).

Patients with SJM in aortic position appeared to have much lower pressure-gradients across the prosthesis than patients after valve replacement with a Lillehei-Kaster-Valve of comparable size.

After 6.5 years of experience with the SJM-Valve-Prothesis, it seemed appropriate to evaluate whether its haemodynamic advantages have any effect on the survival-time, on the number of complications and on the risk of mechanical malfunction and thrombo-embolism.

Our results are in agreement with the above-mentioned multi-center long-term study [2, 8], and they seem to justify our view of the SJM being the most advanced type of mechanical heart valve prosthesis at the present time. It is regrettable that since the autumn of 1984 the manufacturers are unable to provide a sufficient supply of valves for centers outside of the USA – even for those involved in the valve's first clinical tests.

This provides an opportunity for the other bileaflet valve prosthesis available (Duromedics), to furnish proof of its equality.

## Acknowledgement

The authors wish to express their appreciation to Priv.- Doz. Dr. W. Jansen from the Medical Clinic III (Dep. of Cardiology) at the University Hospital of Cologne for providing Figures 15, 16, and 17 and to Dr. J. Lynch for his assistance preparing the manuscript.

## References

1. Abbate M (1985) Comparative clinical evaluation of S.J.M. and Duromedics Valves: 3 years experience. International Symposium on Cardiac Surgery. Roma, May 13–15, Abstracts p 37
2. Dalichau H, Hehrlein FW, Lübbing H, Scheld HH (1981) Early clinical follow-up of 400 patients with the St. Jude Medical Heart Valve Prosthesis, a joint study of two, cardiovascular departments in West Germany. Proc Second Internation Symposium on the St. Jude Valve. San Diego, March 11–14, pp 38–52

3. Duromedics Report, Update 17, May 1985
4. Hemex Symposium on Duromedics Bileaflet Valve, Vail/Colorado, January 23–27, 1985, Abstracts
5. Jansen W, Niehues B, Hombach V, Schlütter A, Lie T, Behrenbeck DW, Hilger HH (1980) Echokardiographische Kriterien der 'St. Jude-Medical-Prothese' in Mitralposition. Herz/Kreisl 12: 309–316
6. Kalke BR, Lillehei WC, Kaster RL (1969) Evaluation of a double-leaflet prosthetic heart valve of a new design for clinical use. In: Charles C. Thomas, Springfield: Prosthetic Heart Valves. Brewer III LA (ed), pp 285–302
7. Lillehei CW (1982) Worldwide Experience with the St. Jude Medical Valve Prosthesis: Clinical and Hemodynamic Results. Contemporary Surgery Vol 20 Nr 1: 17–37
8. Lillehei CW (1984) St. Jude Medical Prosthetic Heart Valve – Results from a five-year multicenter experience. IXth European Congr Cardiol. Düsseldorf, July 8–12
9. Trieb G, Faßbender D, Schuster P, Mannebach H, Schmidt H, Ohlmeier H, Gleichmann U (1982) Hemodynamics of the St. Jude Medical Aortic Prosthesis in Comparison to the Björk-Shiley and Lillehei-Kaster-Prostheses. Z Kardiol 71: 830–838
10. Wortham DC, Tri TB, Bowen ThE (1981) Hemodynamic evaluation of the St. Jude Medical valve prosthesis in the small aortic anulus. J thorac cardiovasc Surg 81: 615–620

# Surgery for bacterial endocarditis and prosthetic valve endocarditis

W. HUEGEL, A. HANNEKUM, T. PEUSTER and V. HOMBACH

## Introduction

In spite of the introduction of effective antimicrobial therapy, the incidence of bacterial endocarditis has not been diminished. To the contrary: the number of publications regarding this disease increased over the last years [1–5]. In our patients we also found an increasing incidence of infective endocarditis (Fig. 1).

However, clinical symptoms and course of that disease have changed. The leading cause of death in those patients is no longer sepsis but congestive heart failure. Therefore early surgical intervention is preferable to procrastination in the management of severe heart failure due to infective endocarditis. Patients with persistent symptoms or relapse of infection on medical therapy and with hemodynamic stability may particularly benefit from surgical sanitation.

A major and special problem remains prosthetic valve endocarditis. This group of patients is rarely responsive to medical therapy [6, 7].

## Patients

Out of 1265 patients with prosthetic valve replacement from 1977 through April 1985 the leading indication for surgical intervention was infective endocarditis in 50 cases. 43 patients suffered from primary or native endocarditis (group 1). 7 patients had undergone reoperation due to early prosthetic valve endocarditis (group 2). The age ranged from 14 to 69 years with a mean of 36,8 years. 33 were male, 17 female. The most common localization was the aortic valve (29 patients). 12 patients had an infection of the mitral valve, 8 of aortic and mitral valve. One young woman suffered from infective endocarditis of the tricuspid valve caused by an embolized intraveneous catheter.

Figure 2 shows the functional classes of heart failure according to the New York Heart Association criteria present at the time of operation.

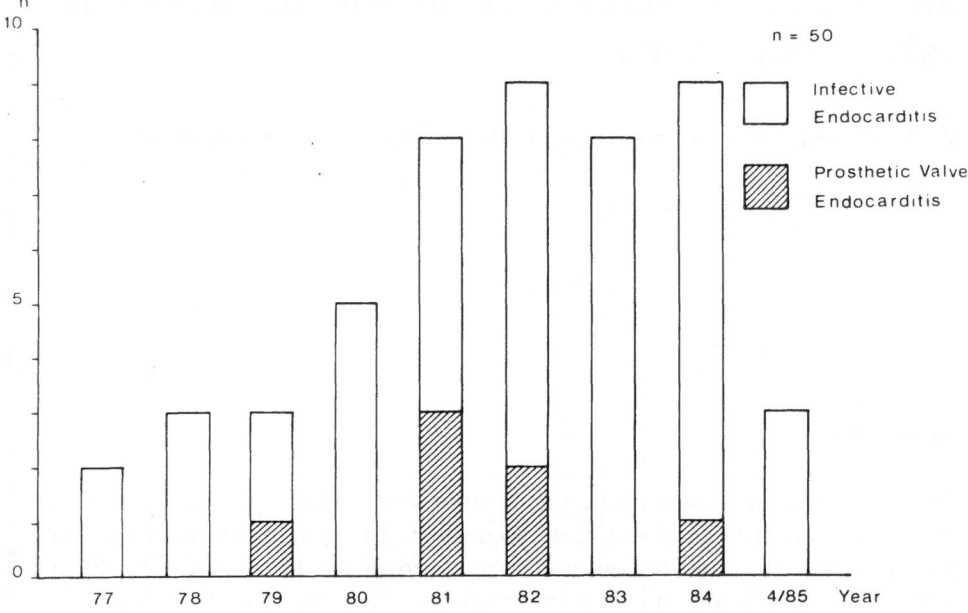

*Figure 1.* Distribution of 50 patients undergoing valve procedures for infective endocarditis and prosthetic valve endocarditis from 1977 to April 1985.

### Microbial etiology

Active infection was proved by cultures of blood or excised valves. The predominant microorganism in native endocarditis was viridans streptococcus, whereas the most common causative organism of prosthetic valve endocarditis was staphylococcus aureus or staphylococcus epidermidis (Fig. 3). In 18 cases blood cultures were negative, probably due to response to effective antibiotic therapy.

### Indications for surgery

The most important factor in determining the timing of surgical intervention is the hemodynamic status. Our approach to the management of infective endocarditis is as follows (Fig. 3): patients in functional class II or III according to NYHA are treated medically. In responsive cases cardiac valve replacement may be carried out later on if necessary. If there is no response within several days cardiac valve replacement is mandatory.

Severe cardiac failure requires urgent cardiac valve replacement. Especially a sudden onset of severe aortic insufficiency is an absolute indication for surgery.

| PATIENTS | GROUP 1 | PRIMARY ENDOCARDITIS | | EARLY MORTALITY | % | CAUSE OF DEATH |
|---|---|---|---|---|---|---|
| N = 50 | 43 | NYHA II - III | 8 | - | | |
| (4 - 69 YEARS) | | III | 32 | 1 | 9,3 | PERS. SEPSIS |
| (MEAN 36.8) | | IV | 3 | 3 | | LCO |
| MALE: 33 | | | | | | |
| FEMALE: 17 | | | | | | |
| | GROUP 2 | PROSTHETIC VALVE ENDOCARDITIS | | | | |
| | 7 | NYHA III | 5 | 1 | | PERS. SEPSIS |
| | | IV | 2 | 2 | 42,9 | LCO |

COLOGNE 1977 - 4/85

*Figure 2.* Functional classification present at the time of operation and results: LCO = low cardiac output syndrom.

| ORGANISM | NATIVE E. | PROSTHETIC VALVE E. |
|---|---|---|
| STREPT.VIRIDANS | 13 | 1 |
| STAPH.AUREUS | 3 | 3 |
| STAPH.EPIDERMIS | | 2 |
| OTHER GRAM-POS.COCCI | 4 | |
| PSEUDOMONAS | 2 | |
| GRAM-NEG.BACILLI | 4 | |
| CULTURE NEG. | 17 | 1 |
| TOTAL | 43 | 7 |

*Figure 3.* Mycrobial etiology of native endocarditis and prosthetic valve endocarditis; E = endocarditis.

An attempt to stabilize the hemodynamic situation by medical therapy usually results in death from cardiac failure.

Large and mobile vegetations on the valves with multiple emboli may be a further indication for early operation. Table 1 shows a synopsis of the absolute and relative indications for surgical intervention.

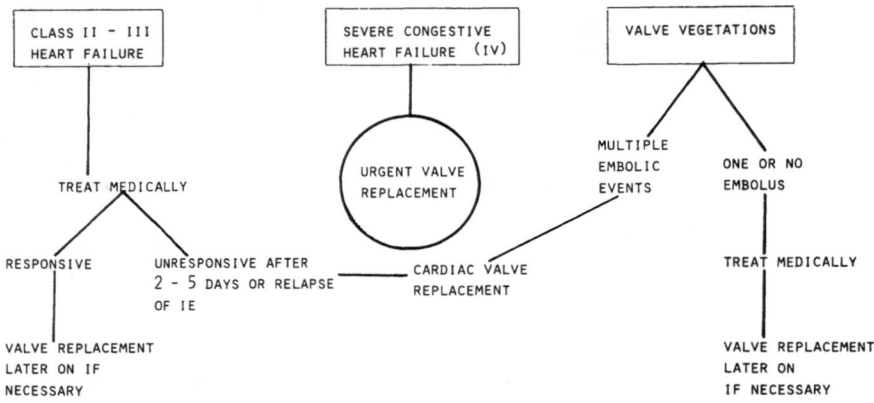

*Figure 4.* Diagram of our approach to management of patients with infective endocarditis (= IE).

## Surgical aspects

Technical advances in surgical management have considerably improved the outcome of patients with infective endocarditis. In the majority of our patients (about 60%) with localization of the infection at the valvular tissue a conventional surgical approach can be employed. After debridement of the infected tissue and an intensive local desinfection the valve can be replaced in the usual technique.

However, in 40% of our patients we observed severe extensive annulus myocardial abscesses with predominant location at the aortic annulus. In these instances a more radical surgical procedure can be necessary [2, 3, 9]. It is very important to remove all infected tissues and to excavate abscess cavities. Resulting defects of cardiac structures have to be reconstructed with patch material. Small annulus abscess cavities can be closed directly. Larger abscesses should be

*Table 1.* Absolute and relative indications for surgery.

| Absolute: | Severe congestive |
| | Heart failure (valve related) |
| | Persistent signs of IE, |
| | Despite antibiotic therapy |
| | Multiple embolic events |
| | Prosthetic valve dysfunction |
| | Fungal etiology |
| Relative: | Congestive heart failure class III |
| | Valve vegetations with no or one embolus |
| | Paravalvular leak |
| | First relapse after medical therapy |

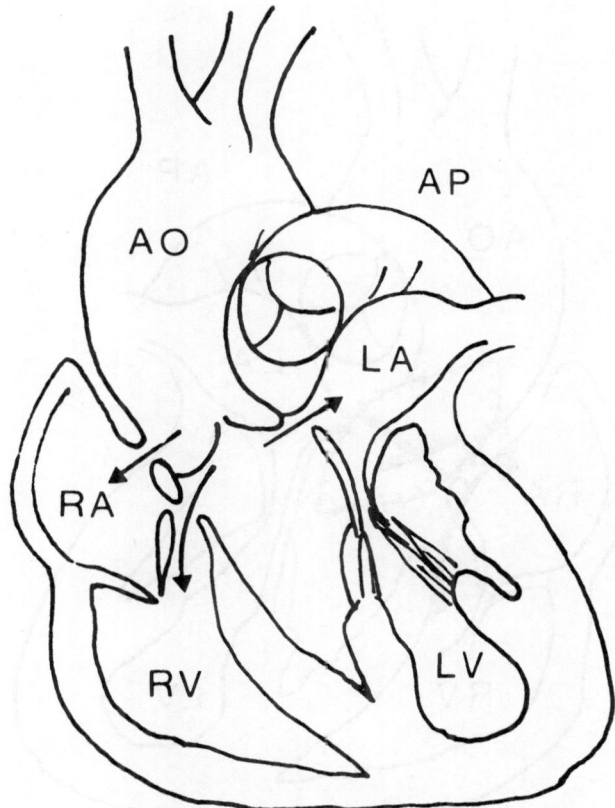

*Figure 5.* Abscess formation in the aortic root with penetration into the right atrium (RA), right ventricle (RV) and left atrium (LA); dehiscence of aortico-mitral curtain.

excavated. According to Hetzer [5] the remaining cavities between inserted patches and abscess wall are filled with a suspension of fibrin glue and antibiotics. All patients with annulus distruction treated in this way survived without any relapse of infection.

One case may demonstrate this procedure (Figs. 5 and 6): A 20 year old man suffered from bacterial endocarditis caused by viridans streptococcus. His hemodynamic status was compensated. Two weeks after onset of medical therapy severe congestive heart failure required urgent operation. Intraoperatively a distruction of the aortic root was found with penetrations into the right atrium and the right ventricle. The subaortic curtain was destroyed. The septal leaflets of the tricuspid and mitral valve were separated from the valve annulus. The surgical procedure was similar to the approach of correcting an av-canal. The ventricular and atrial septum was reconstructed with a common fabric patch. The abscess cavities in the subaortic curtain and the aortic root were excavated and closed

126

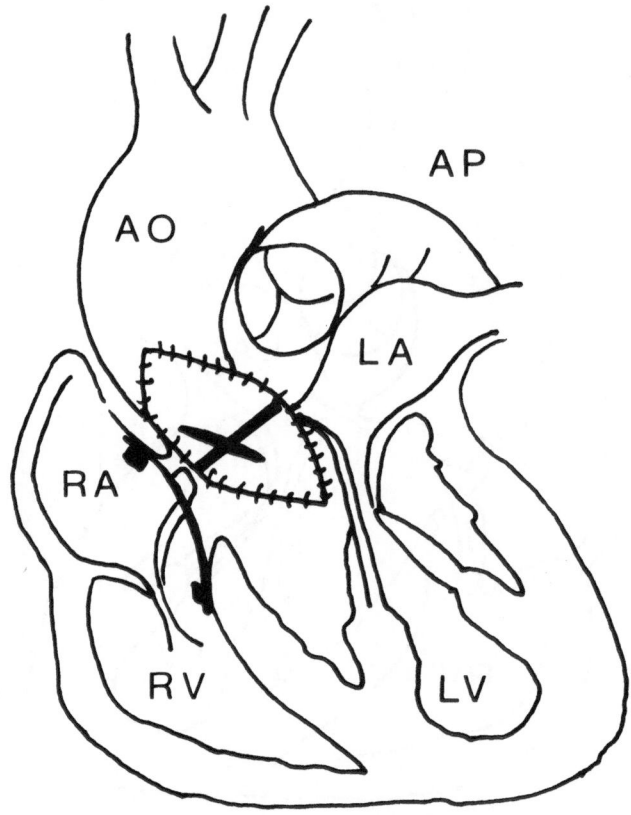

*Figure 6.* Reconstruction of the ventricular and atrial septum with fixation of the septal tricuspid leaflet; reconstruction of the subaortic curtain, fixation of the mitral septal leaflet and implantation of aortic valve prosthesis.

with a second patch. Finally the septal leaflets of mitral and tricuspid valve were fixed to the patches. The remaining cavities were filled with fibrin glue and antibiotics. The outcome was quite well. The patient was discharged from hospital two weeks later on. After antibiotic therapy for 6 months he is now – two years after operation – free of relapse of infection.

**Results**

In patients with native infective endocarditis, surgical therapy can be carried out with early mortality as low as 9.3% (Fig. 2). These results include aortic-, mitral-, tricuspid- and double valve replacements and are comparable to patients with elective non infective valve replacements.

In contrast, the mortality rate of prosthetic valve endocarditis remains with 42.9% very high.

All surviving patients are free from recurrent infection without any late death. The follow-up period ranged from three months to 7 years with a mean of 3.4 years.

## Discussion

Surgical therapy is increasingly playing an important role in the management of infective endocarditis. In patients with severe congestive heart failure early surgical intervention is preferable to procrastination. There is little to be gained by delaying surgery in order to stabilize the hemodynamic situation.

In patients with infective endocarditis, surgical intervention can be carried out with low hospital mortality of less than 10%, comparable to that with elective cardiac valve replacement. There was no late mortality in our material. These findings correspond to the lower range of results published by other groups [1, 3, 4, 5].

Especially the rate of early death is related both to an optimal timing of surgery and to the surgical technique itself. Careful debridement and local desinfection of the infected area are very important. Larger abscess cavities should be closed with a fabric patch. In case of extensive destruction of the aortic root alternative methods can be employed as suggested by Danielson [8], Reitz [9] or Lau [10]. We try to avoid remaining cavities within the lumen of the left ventricular outflow tract. On the other hand the implantation of biological material [6] bears a higher risk of persistent infection. Therefore, in case of circular dehiscence of the aortic annulus we prefer the implantation of an artifical valve bearing conduit with reimplantation of the coronary ostia according to Frantz [11].

A major remaining problem is the prosthetic valve endocarditis. The early mortality is higher than 40%. In our opinion and according to other publications [6, 7, 10] these poor results are not due to surgical problems but to the type of causing microbial organisms and their medical therapy. This problem remains to be solved.

## References

1. Nelson RJ, Harley DP, French WJ, Bayer AS (1984) Favorable ten-year experience with valve procedures for active infective endocarditis. J Thorac Cardiovasc Surg 87: 493–502
2. Prager RL, Maples MD, Hammon JW, Friesinger GC, Bender HW (1981) Early operative intervention in aortic bacterial endocarditis. Ann Thorac Surg 32: 347–350
3. Wilson WR, Geraci JE (1983) Cardiac valve replacement in patients with active infective endocarditis. Herz 8: 332–343
4. Borst HG, Hetzer R, and Deyerling W (1982) Surgery for Active Infective Endocarditis. Thorac

Cardiovasc Surg 30: 345–349

5. Hetzer R, Deyerling W, Oelert H, Borst HG (1985) Operative Procedures in Infective Valve Anulus Destruction. Thorac Cardiovasc Surg 33: 60

6. Baumgartner WA, Miller DC, Reitz BA, Oyer PE, Jamieson SW, Stinson EB, Shumway NE (1983) Surgical treatment of prosthetic valve endocarditis. Ann Thorac Surg 35: 87–104

7. Gnann JW, Dismukes WE (1983) Prosthetic valve endocarditis: an overview. Herz 8: 320–331

8. Danielson GK, Titus JL, DuShane JW (1974) Successful treatment of aortic valve endocarditis and aortic root abscesses by insertion of prosthetic valve in ascending aorta and placement of bypass grafts to coronary arteries. J Thorac Cardiovasc Surg 67: 443–449

9. Reitz BA, Stinson EB, Watson DC, Baumgartner WA, Jamieson SW (1981) Translocation of the aortic valve for prosthetic valve endocarditis. J Thorac Cardiovasc Surg 81: 212–218

10. Lau JKH, Robles A, Cherian A, Ross DN (1984) Surgical treatment of prosthetic endocarditis. J Thorac Cardiovasc Surg 87: 712–716

11. Frantz PT, Murray GF, Wilcox BR (1980) Surgical Management of Left Ventricular-aortic Discontinuity Complicating Bacterial Endocarditis. Ann Thorac Surg 29: 1

# Transient mechanical support of the failing heart

E.R. DE VIVIE, H. HARTUNG, K. HELLBERG, K. NEUHAUS,
W. RUSCHEWSKI and U. TEBBE

## Summary

Mechanical aids for the failing heart are necessary in patients with postoperative low-output syndrome (LOS) following cardiac surgery and in cardiologic patients with impending cardiogenic shock due to unstable angina pectoris and acute myocardial infarction (MJ). The IABP is routinely used either in the ICU, the catheter laboratory or in the operation room. Its hemodynamic effects improve the myocardial energy imbalance by a reduction in systolic and an increase in diastolic arterial pressure. The device generally produces a 10% to 20% increase in cardiac output (CO) and at the same time enhances the coronary blood flow (CBF). Nowadays the balloon-catheter is usually inserted transcutanously via femoral artery into the thoracic aorta. From 1975 to 1984, 138 patients (pts) of 6022 pts undergoing open heart surgery at the University of Goettingen required IABP. Another group of 28 pts with cardiogenic shock following acute myocardial infarction without cardiac surgery needed IABP-treatment. Only 28,5% (n = 8) could be weaned from IABP, and 5 pts were discharged from the hospital. Our experience show the coronary artery disease group of IABP patients to be increasing, whereas the intra- and postoperative groups are decreasing, probably as a result of better intraoperative myocardial protection by cardioplegia.

Partial venoarterial bypass (VABP) in combination with IABP is hemodynamically more effective than IABP and can be used in more severe LOS and in presence of right heart failure. Our own experimental results indicate, that VABP of only 35% of cardiac output (CO) combined with IABP can be an effective method to support the failing heart. A bypass of 48% of CO decreased significantly $dp/dt_{max}$ (30%) and calculated myocardial oxygen requirement (E.g. according to Bretschneider, 16%). A simple system is the combination of VAPB cannulating the axillary artery and IABP.

## Introduction

Mechanical aids for the failing heart are necessary in patients with postoperative low-output syndrome (LOS) following cardiac surgery and in cardiologic patients with impending cardiogenic shock due to unstable angina pectoris and or acute myocardial infarction (MJ) [5, 6, 17, 24, 31]. Since Kontrowitz and Kantrowitz [19] introduced the concept of counterpulsation by phase-shift-diastolic augmentation a wide spectrum of circulatory assist devices have been developed [1, 2, 10, 11, 12, 19, 20, 21, 25, 27, 29, 30, 32, 35]:

1.   Circulatory assist by external cardiac massage system,
2.1. Cardiopulmonary bypass (CPB) with continous blood flow and
2.2. membrane oxygenator (ECMO),
2.3. venoarterial bypass (VABP),
2.4. veno-venous bypass (VVBP),
2.5. Combination with counterpulsation,
3.   Counterpulsation,
3.1. external counterpulsation (ECP),
3.2. intraaortic balloon counterpulsation (IABP),
3.3. pulsatile assist device (PAD),
4.   left ventricular assist devices (LVAD).

Out of these the intraaortic balloon pumping (IABP) has become the most common form of mechanical circulatory assistance, and is routinely used either in the intensive care unit (ICU), the catheter laboratory or in the operation room [3, 13, 14, 15, 16, 22, 23, 31, 34].
However, to function poperly, the IABP requires a reasonable amount of remaining left ventricular function. Thus, the need for a device that can support the failing circulation even more effectively remained. The left ventricular assist device (LVAD) was devised to fill this need (Fig. 1), [1, 2, 10, 28].
   It is the purpose of this paper to discuss the circulatory assist with different methods of counterpulsation and the combination of venous-arterial bypass (VABP) together with IABP.

## History

The concept of counterpulsation, as the basis of intraaortic balloon pulsation (IABP), was first described by Harken [18] in 1958. During the systole blood was removed via femoral artery and the same blood was rapidly reinfused during the diastole in reverse direction to improve the coronary blood flow. The hemodynamic effects of counterpulsation pursue the goal to break the vicious cycle that entraps patients in cardiogenic shock, including deterioration of myocardial

# TRANSIENT CIRCULATORY ASSIST DEVICES

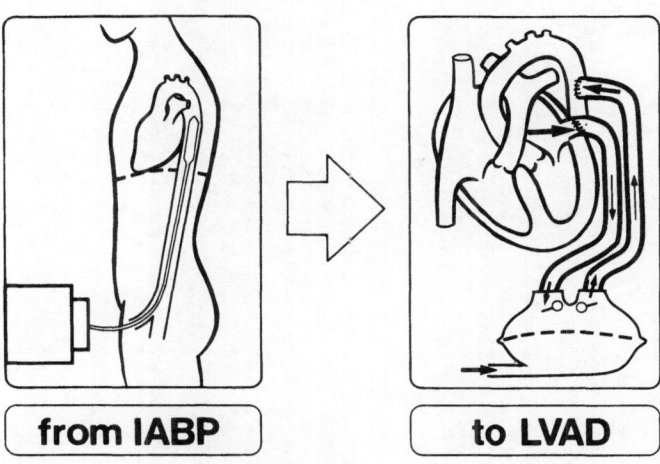

*Figure 1.* Two of the most important transient circulatory assist devices in the mechanical treatment of the failing heart, the intra-aortic balloon counterpulsation (IABP) and the left ventricular assist device (LVAD).

blood flow and organ perfusion on the one hand and increased hypoxemic myocardial failure on the other hand.

The myocardial oxygen demand and supply is a delicate balance, factors affecting myocardial oxygen *demand* are heart rate, myocardial contractility and left ventricular wall tension, and oxygen *supply* are coronary blood flow, coronary resistance and diastolic blood pressure [4]. The well known hemodynamic effects of IABP – reduction of systolic aortic and left ventricular enddiastolic pressure (LVEDP) and diastolic augmentation improve the myocardial energy imbalance (Fig. 2). It has been widely demonstrated both in laboratory and clinically that IABP generally produces a 10 to 20% increase in cardiac output and at the same time an increase in coronary blood flow (CBF) [3]. The tension time index (TTI) is representative of oxygen consumption during systole and the diastolic tension time index (DTTI) correlates with oxygen supply [3, 9]. A summary of the metabolic effects of IABP is shown in Table 1. It is estimated by reports and used balloon-catheters that more than 5000 patients have been treated by IABP [25]. The mean survival rate of 54% depends on the patient selection and is ranging from 13 to 70%. The frequency of IABP treatment in open heart surgery decreased markedly from 16% in 1977 to 4% in 1982 ranging from 1,1 to 6,8%, probably as a result of better intraoperative myocardial protection by cardioplegia.

132

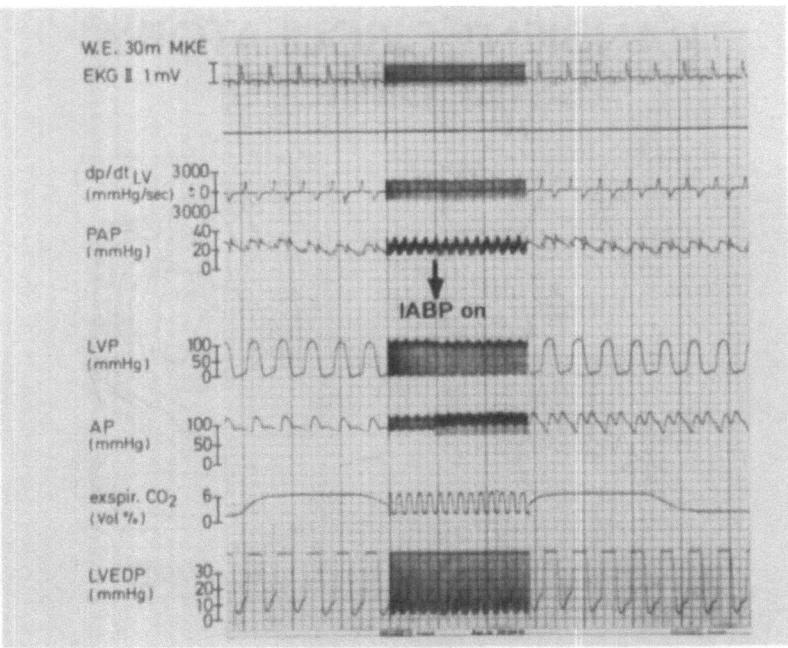

*Figure 2.* Registration in a 30 years old man after mitral valve replacement (MKE). Note the typical effects of IABP with increasing diastolic aortic pressure (AP), and decreasing systolic aortic and left ventricular enddiastolic pressure (LVED) in addition with reduction of systolic left ventricular pressure (LVP). MKE = mitral valve replacement, EKG = electrocardiogram, dp/dt$_{LV}$ = rise in left ventricular pressure, PAP = pulmonary arterial pressure, exspir. $CO_2$ = exspiratory carbon dioxide.

# METABOLIC EFFECTS OF IABP

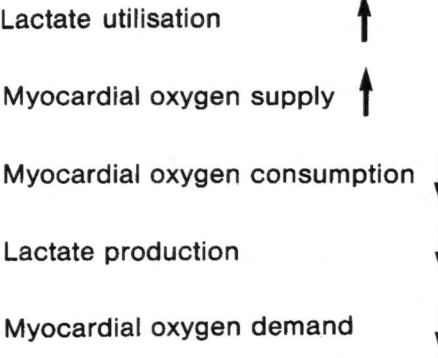

Lactate utilisation

Myocardial oxygen supply

Myocardial oxygen consumption

Lactate production

Myocardial oxygen demand

**Patient material**

From 1975 to 1985 169 patients were treated with the IABP either in our Institution and in the Department of Cardiology at the University of Goettingen (Table 2).

The average age of the patients was 53,5 years – range from 4 to 75 years –. There were 107 male and 62 female patients. Out of these 13 were children aged between 4 and 16 years (mean age 9). The volume of the pediatric balloons ranged from 9 to 23 cc, a 9 cc single chamber balloon size Nr. 7 F was used in 6 cases. The site of insertion was: femoral artery [1], iliacal artery [10] and aorta ascendens [2]. In these cases a postoperative low-output syndrome (LOS) was seen after repair of different congenital complex heart malformations. The patients undergoing IABP were devided into three groups (Table 3):

A. IABP was used intra- and/or postoperatively in 74 patients after open-heart-surgery. During the 10 year time period 5300 patients had corrective open-heart-operations. All patients in this group had low cardiac output, the need for inotropic drugs, or rhythm disturbances. 73% (n = 54) could be hemo-dynamically stabilized, 58,1% (n = 43) were longterm survivors. The duration of mechanical assistance was 36 hours on average (from 4 to 50 hours).

## IABP - PATIENT MATERIAL

| | | |
|---|---|---|
| Patients | | 169 |
| Age (average) | | 53,5 (range 4-75) |
| Sex | male | 107 |
| | female | 62 |
| | | |
| Pediatric patients (out of 169 pts) | | 13 |
| Age (average) | | 9 (range 4-16) |
| Balloon volume | | 9 - 23 cc |
| Site of insertion | | |
| art. femoralis | | 1 |
| art. iliaca | | 10 |
| aorta ascendens | | 2 |

Clinic THG
1985

B. In this group 64 patients had preoperative balloon support and cardiac surgery. The IABP treatment was started in the ICU or in the catheter laboratory, all patients had either crescendo angina refractory to medical therapy, impending infarction, or cardiogenic shock prior to cardiac catheterisation. The patients had to be pumped on average of 6 hours prior to cardiac surgery (from 1 to 15 hours), and the postoperative treatment maintained on average of 67 hours (from 6 to 96 hours). 84,4% (n = 54) in this group could be weaned from IABP, but only 43,7% (n = 28) were longterm survivors. In comparison to the surgical group the longterm results are statistically different to the medical group A.

C. In this group of 28 patients with refractory heart failure and/or cardiogenic shock state due to diffuse coronary heart disease, ventricular aneurysm or acute myocardial infarction with bad condition for cardiac surgery the IABP was used in combination with maximal pharmalogical support. The results have been disappointing, only 28,5% (n = 8) could be temporarily stabilized, and 17,5% (n = 5) were discharged from the hospital. Some of these patients would have been candidates for cardiac transplantation.

Another 3 patients with cardiogenic shock due to septicemia were assisted with IABP, no patient survived.

## INTRA-AORTIC BALLOON PUMPING (IABP)
### GOETTINGEN 1975 - 1985

| Cardiogenic shock and/or postop. LOS | Patients (n) | Hemodynamically stabilized | % | Longterm survivors | % |
|---|---|---|---|---|---|
| A. Open-heart-surgery | 74 | 54 | 73 | 43 | 58,1 |
| B. Preoperative balloon support and cardiac surgery | 64 | 54 | 84,4 | 28 | 43,7 |
| | 138 | 108 | 78,3 | 71 | 51,4 |
| C. Balloon support without cardiac surgery | 28 | 8 | 28,5 | 5 | 17,8 |
| Others (septic shock) | 3 | 1 | | 0 | |

Clinic THG
1985

A special group of patients resulted out of the category A and B (Table 4). Fifty-eight patients developed low-cardiac output after coronary bypass surgery and/or aneurysmectomy, 40 patients could not be disconnected from heartlung-bypass. Out of 38 hemodynamically stabilized patients, 34 (85%) were longterm survivors. Eighteen patients of this group has LOS postoperatively after 4 to 24 hours refractory to medical treatment. Thus IABP was indicated. Fourteen patients could be weaned from the assist device after 12 to 78 hours, 4 patients died. Alltogether 75% out of this special group were longterm survivors. Even a significant decrease of cardiac arrhythmias was noticed due to the improvement of myocardial energy balance, which resulted from the hemodynamic effects of IABP. These beneficial results permits the conclusions that most of the myocardial damage was reversible and the indication for IABP was early enough.

Figure 3 demonstrates the significant preoperative hemodynamic improvement of the left ventricular function in 26 patients with cardiogenic shock after 60 minutes. The enddiastolic volume index (EDVI) and the endsystolic volume index (ESVI) decreased and the ejection fraction (EF) increased from $28 \pm 5\%$ to $38 \pm 7\%$.

Usually the balloon is inserted into the thoracic aorta via femoral artery. Nowadays the application of the balloon-catheter has become much easier by using the guide-wire technique. The percutaneous intra-aortic-balloon can be inserted within a few minutes in more than 90% of the cases (Fig. 4). It was reported by the Massachusetts General Hospital in Boston that the application of

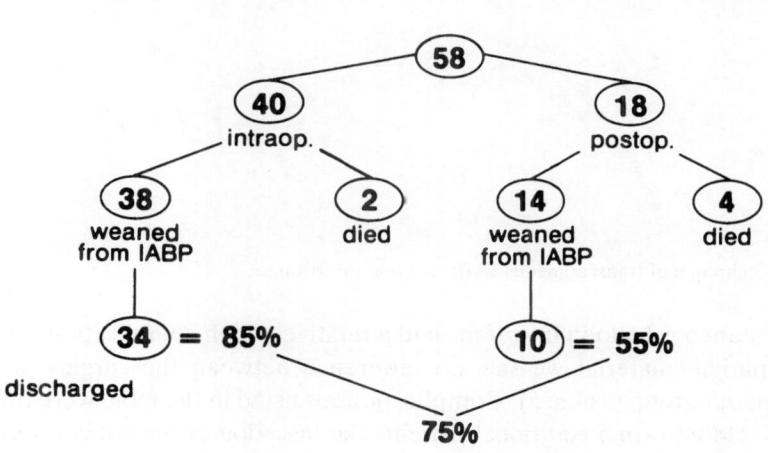

**IABP IN PATIENTS
FOLLOWING CORONARY BYPASS
SURGERY AND/OR ANEURYSMECTOMY**
n = 58

136

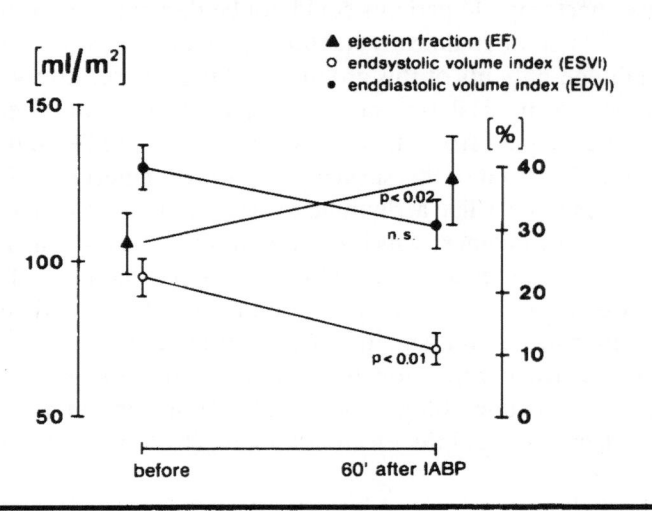

$[ml/m^2]$

▲ ejection fraction (EF)
○ endsystolic volume index (ESVI)
● enddiastolic volume index (EDVI)

150

$[\%]$

40

30

p < 0.02
n.s.

100

20

10

p < 0.01

50

0

before          60' after IABP

* cardiogenic shock - 9 patients
impending cardiog. shock with unstable angina - 17 patients

*Figure 3.* The left ventricular function in 9 patients with cardiogenic shock and 17 patients with unstable angina before and 60 min. after IABP. EF = ejection fraction, ESVI = endsystolic volume index, EDVI = enddiastolic volume index.

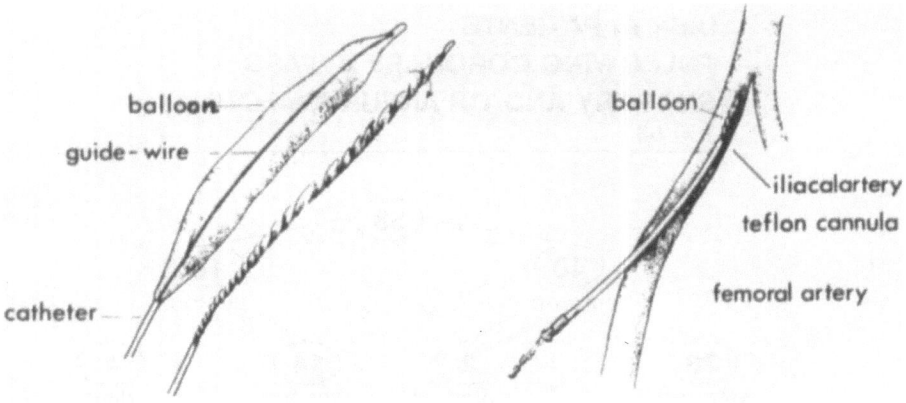

balloon
guide-wire
catheter

balloon
iliacalartery
teflon cannula
femoral artery

*Figure 4.* Technique of transcutaneous IABP balloon insertion.

100 percutaneous balloon insertions had a relatively high complication rate [26]. In our patient material we saw no difference between the surgical and the percutaneous group (Table 5). Complications as listed in the table were revealed in 10,6% (18/169). In 5 additional patients the insertion of the balloon failed.

## Indications for IABP

The indications for the use of intra-aortic balloon counterpulsation covers a wide spectrum, from angina pectoris up to the prelude of a heart-transplantation (Fig. 5). The criterion for the application of IABP with cardiological and surgical heart patients overlap each other in the preoperative diagnostic phase by means of coronary angiography and also during the induction of anaesthesia with high risk patients, this includes patients with so called main-stem stenosis. The postoperative low-output syndrome appears to be seldom due to the improved myocardial protection during cardiac arrest. Today IABP is mainly used in patients showing critical coronary heart disease, and when urgent treatment of an acute myocardial infarction is necessary, that means the indication has changed from surgical to cardiologic patients.

The advantages of IABP for cardiac support are summarized:
1. Easy insertion and removal
2. Easy and safe operation and control
3. Requires little manpower
4. Effective hemodynamics

## BALLOON RELATED COMPLICATIONS

|  | surgical n = 96 | percutaneous n = 73 |
|---|---|---|
| Ischemia of the leg | 2 | 1 |
| Peripheral embolism | 3 | 1 |
| Bleeding | 2 | 3 |
| Infection | 2 | 2 |
| Retrograd aortic dissection | 1 | 0 |
| Balloon rupture | 0 | 0 |
| Vascular injury | 0 | 1 |
|  | 10 | 8 |
| Inability of balloon placement | 3 | 2 |

## COMPLICATION RATE IN IABP: 10,6% (18/169)

Clinic THG
1985

138

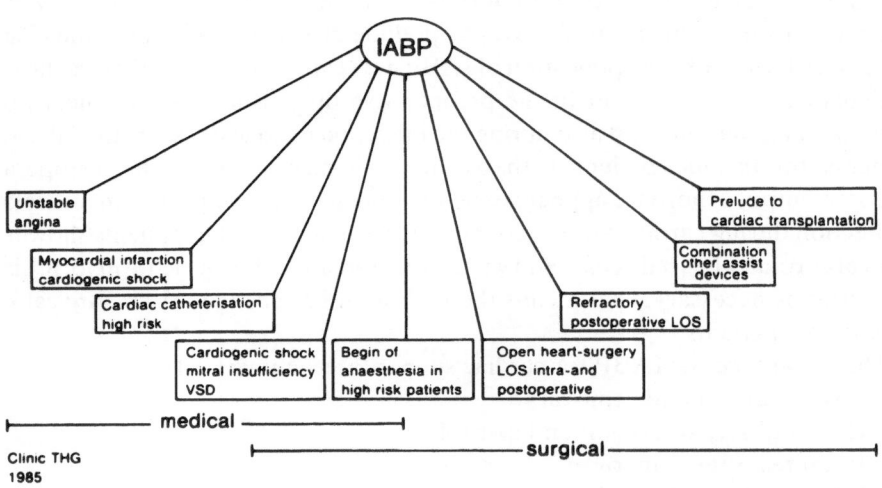

## INDICATIONS FOR IABP

*Figure 5.* The wide spectrum of indications for IABP in cardiological and surgical heart patients.

5. Portable console
6. Reasonable cost
7. Acceptable complication rate
8. No need for anticoatulation
9. Possible for prolonged use (days)
10. Bedside application
11. Production of pulsatile flow during cardiopulmonary bypass (PAD)

### Pulsatile assist device (PAD)

The pulsatile assist device (PAD) covers the principles of IABP, it is employed externally in the cardiopulmonary bypass (Fig. 6). The PAD is a flexible, valveless polyurethan balloon contained within a plastic chamber, which is connected to an IABP console. The system is inserted in the arterial line of the extracorporeal circulation. When cardiopulmonary bypass begins PAD is pulsed synchronously with the ECG in diastole to create pulsatile flow. During ventricular fibrillation an internal trigger is used. While weaning the patient from bypass, the PAD is again utilized as a counterpulsator.

In a series of experiments the PAD was applied during cardiopulmonary bypass, this showed a 10% reduction of the systolic aortic pressure, a 90% enhancement of the diastolic pressure and 62% the cardiac output. An increased hemolysis could not be determined [6, 7]. With a constant perfusion pressure,

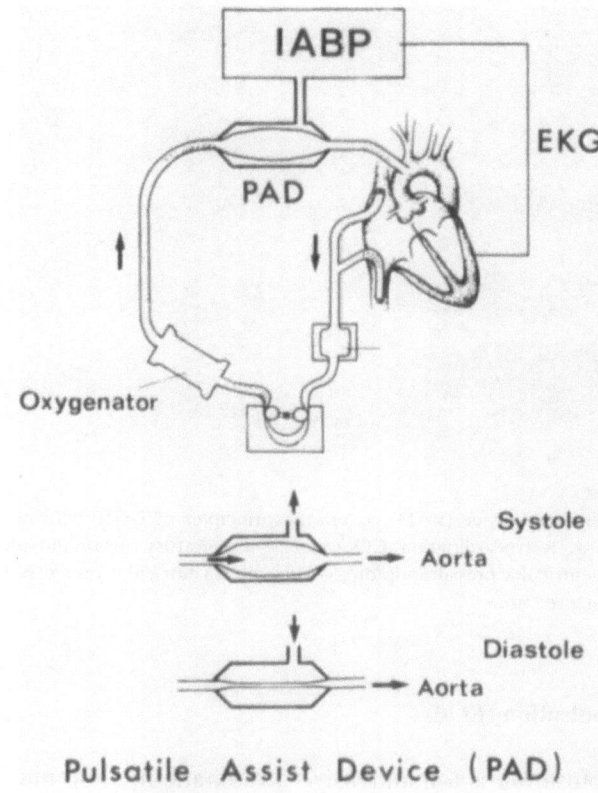

Pulsatile Assist Device (PAD)

*Figure 6.* The principle of the pulsatile assist device (PAD) in combination with the intraaortic balloon pumping (IABP). EKG = electrocardiogram, PAD = pulsatile assist device, IABP = intraaortic balloon pumping.

pulse amplitudes between 40 and 60 mmHg could be achieved. Bregman [7], who introduced this method, has reported more than 3000 clinical applications. An increased blood flow of more than 20% through the bypass-vein could be obtained after coronary artery surgery. The amount of perioperative myocardial infarction and postoperative low-output syndrome could be clearly reduced, using the PAD as an additional method to the application of the extracorporeal circulation. The PAD can be triggered synchronously in the systolic phase as well as counterpulsated in the diastolic phase. This system can only be used in combination with cardiopulmonary bypass. As a result of the long perfusion times a higher blood traumatization is caused in comparison with the use of IABP.

The typical hemodynamic effects during PAD-counterpulsation could be seen in patients after cardiac surgery before discontinuing ECC, as shown in (Fig. 7).

140

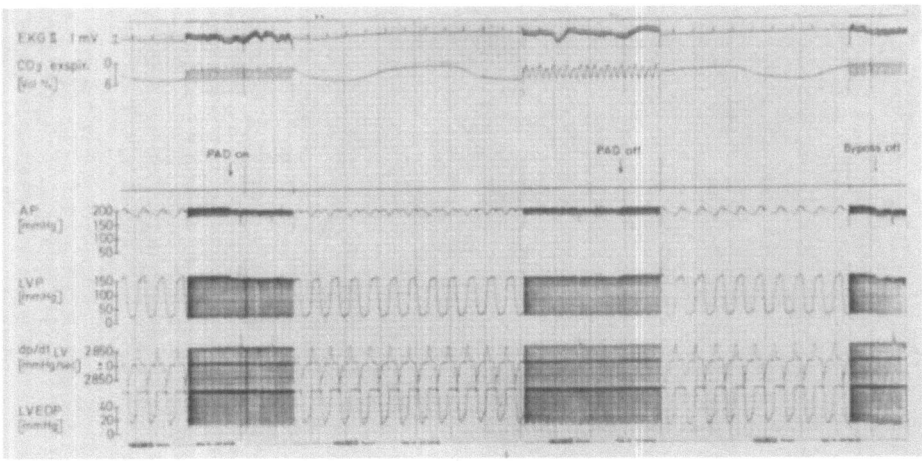

*Figure 7.* The pulsatile assist device (PAD) covers the principles of IABP with its typical hemo-dynamic effects. EKG = electrocardiogram, $CO_2$ exspir. = exspiratory carbon dioxide, AP = aortic pressure, LVP = left ventricular pressure, dp/dt$_{LV}$ = rise in left ventricular pressure, LVEDP = left ventricular enddiastolic pressure.

**External counterpulsation (ECP)**

External counterpulsation is a noninvasive atraumatic method and the indications for the application are the same as those for IABP (Fig. 8). The lower part of the patients body is placed into an occlusive water bag, a pulsatile pressure is then applied. Arterial as well as venous counterpulsation is produced, triggered by the patients ECG ([29, 35]. Our experimental results and also our completed examinations of patients with coronary heart disease have demonstrated better hemodynamic efficiency. Figure 9 shows an original registration in a patient with chronical coronary heart disease (CHD) and angina pectoris (AP).

Experimental examinations have shown the comparison between the control group (plain column) and the counterpulsated group (crossed column) of patients (Fig. 10). The calculated effective left (ELVW) and right ventricular work load (ERVW) results in a minor increase of the myocardial oxygen consumption ($MVO_2$), on the other hand the coronary blood flow (Vcor) is significantly enhanced by diastolic augmentation, consequently the dp/dt$_{max}$ of the right and left ventricles is increased. In case of patients with severe coronary artery disease the augmentation of the diastolic aortic pressure led to an increased coronary bloow flow, from 79 to 92 ml/min $\times$ 100 g. The cardiac work index (CWI) increased, the stoke volume (SV) rose to 5,9% and the cardiac output (CO) up to 8,6%, simultaneously the myocardial oxygen supply increased to 25,4%. Although ECP could not be routinely clinically established because of the technical

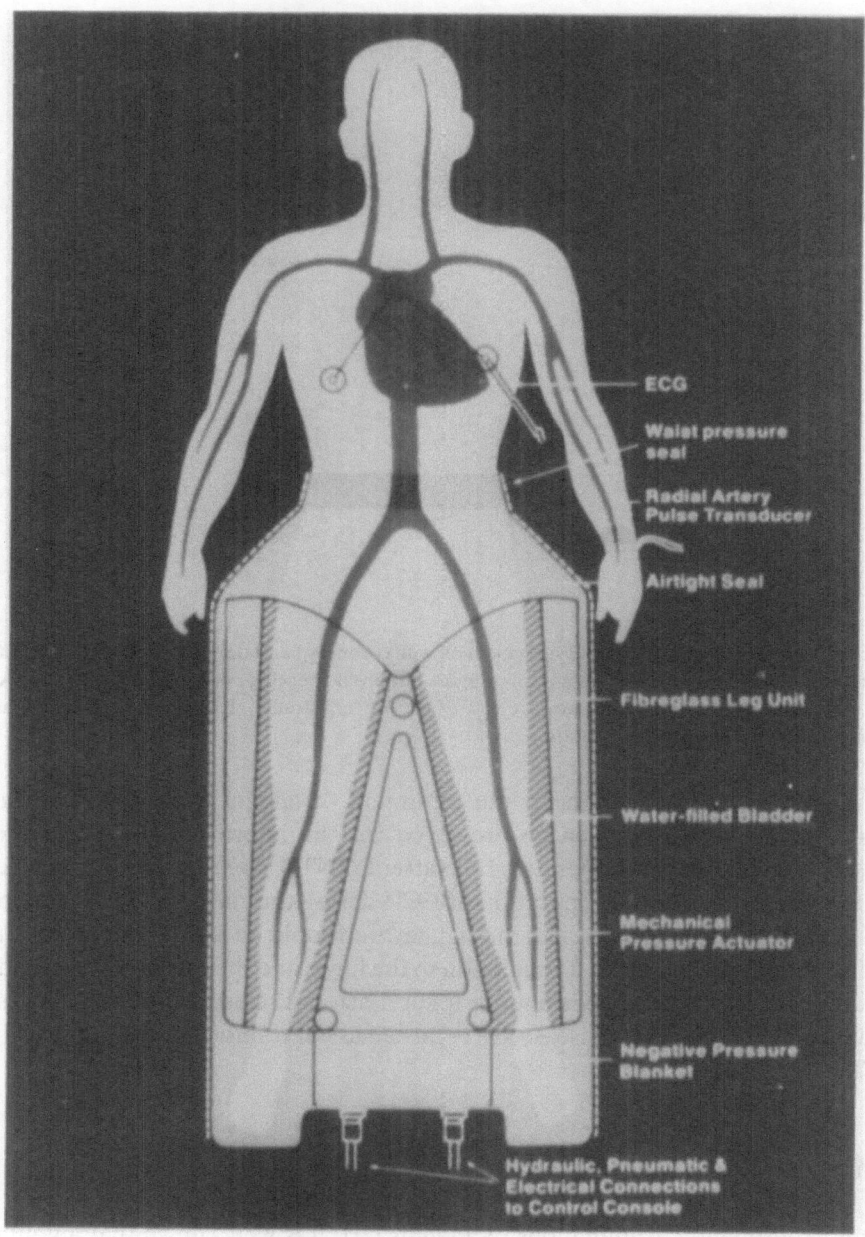

*Figure 8*. The complete scheme of external counterpulsation (ECP) and its clinical use.

142

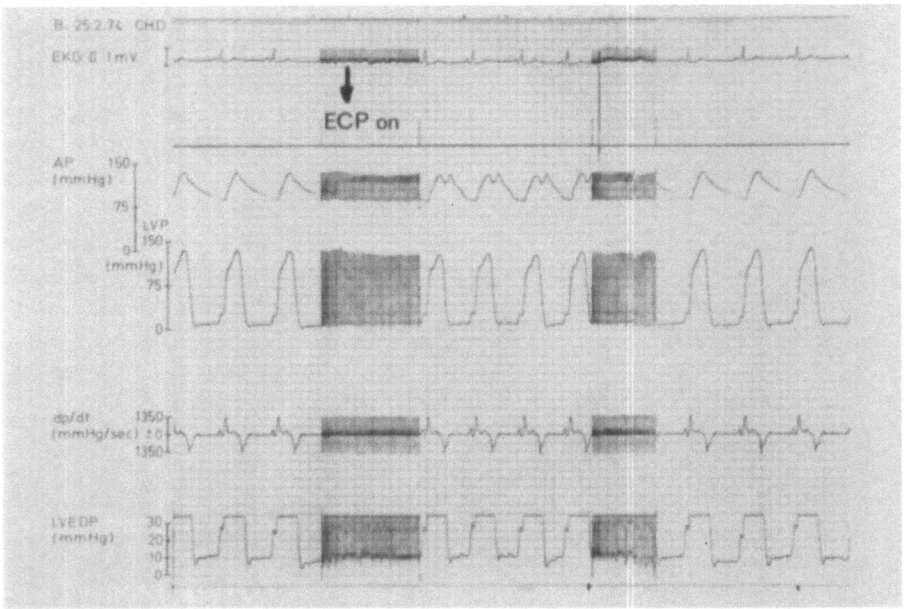

*Figure 9.* Original registration in a 47 years old man with coronary heart disease (CHD). Starting ECP the typical hemodynamic effects of diastolic augmentation, decreasing systolic aortic pressure (AP) and left ventricular enddiastolic pressure (LVEDP) are registrated. EKG = electrocardiogram, dp/dt = rise in left ventricular pressure.

requirements, the indication for the treatment of angina pectoris and diffuse coronary artery sclerosis can be preserved for the improvement of collateral vessels. Patients with postoperative LOS after FONTAN procedure (FP) can be a seldom indication for the application of ECP. Using this method in a 12 year old boy after FP the venous return to the right atrium could be 3–4 mm increased and at the same time an improved circulation to the lungs and the cardiac output could be attained. Abvanced pelvic and peripheral arterial sclerosis, aortic aneurysm and thromboembolic vein disease are regarded as contraindications for the use of ECP.

## Left heart bypass

After experimental examinations by Dennis [11], it is well known that a volume load reduction of 90% decreased the myocardial consumption to 30% and with a 50% reduction the oxygen consumption was reduced to only 20%. In 1976 Litwark [24] introduced a left heart bypass system with a roller pump, with which a 90% volume reduction could be achieved through centrally placed cannulas. This system was clinically tested in 18 patients, a 38% survival rate was the result,

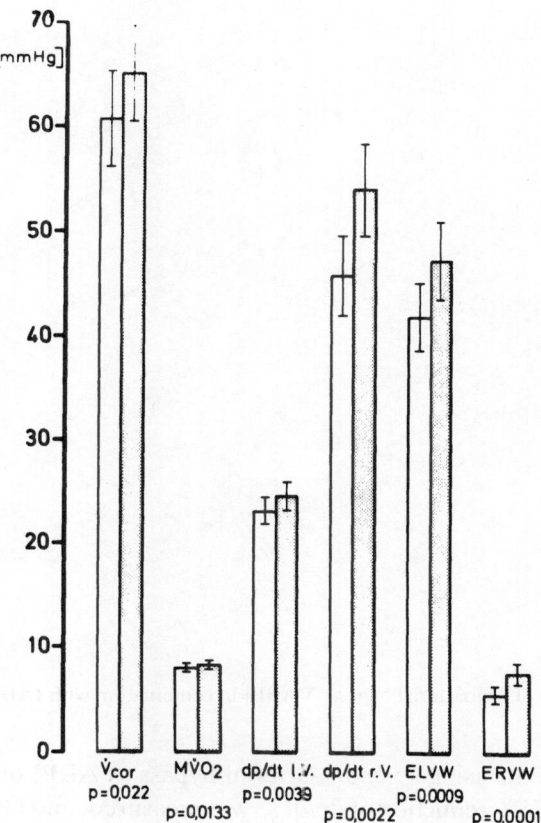

*Figure 10.* Relation of coronary blood flow (Vcor), myocardial oxygen consumption (MVO₂), rise in left ventricular pressure (dp/dt LV), rise in right ventricular pressure (dp/dt RV, effectiv left (ELVW) and right ventricular work load (ERVW) before (plain column) and 15 minutes after ECP (crossed column). Vcor = coronary blood flow, MVO₂ = myocardial oxygen consumption, dp/dt LV = rise in left ventricular pressure, dp/dt RV = rise in right ventricular pressure, ELVW = left ventricular work load, ERVW = right ventricular work load.

this of course was disappointing. Further developments led consequently to the left ventricular assist device (LVAD).

## Partial venous-arterial bypass (VABP) in combination with IABP

The combination of a partial venous-arterial bypass (VABP) [33] and IABP reduced the pressure and the volume in the left and right heart (Fig. 11). No invasive procedure is necessary when peripheal transcutaneous cannulation of the iliac veins is made for removal of venous blood and central cannulation of the ascending aorta via the axillary artery for the arterial recirculation.

144

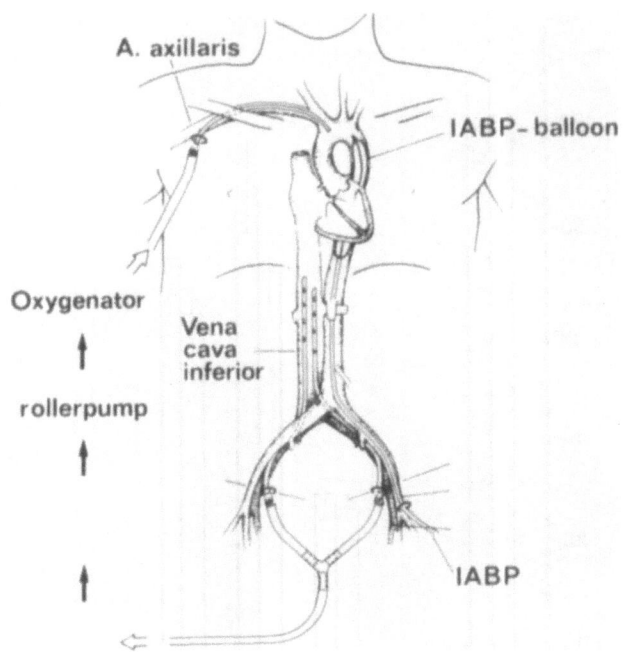

*Figure 11*. The principle of venoarterial bypass (VABP) in combination with IABP.

Animal experiments using a venous-arterial bypass (VABP) of only 10% and IABP a significant 25% reduction of $dp/dt_{max}$ was measured, and further improvement was achieved with 30% and 50% shunt volume (Fig. 12). Regarding to the left ventricular oxygen consumption calculated by the Bretschneider [8] parameter the combination of a VABP with IABP resulted in a 10% reduction. A 50% bypass led to a decreased systolic aortic pressure of 18%, the left ventricular $dp/dt_{max}$ was 25% and the calculated left ventricular oxygen consumption was 22% reduced. The original registration shows the measured parameters in animal experiments (Fig. 13). The combination of a partial VABP with IABP increase the hemodynamic stroke work indexes. This system can be applied to patients

*Figure 12*. Maximal rise in left ventricular pressure ($dp/dt_{max}$ LV) during VABP shunting 10%, 30% and 50% of the cardiac output (crossed column) and during VABP + IABP (stripted column). control = control group (K 1, K 2, K 3), VAB = venousarterial bypass, VAB + IABP = venousarterial bypass + intraaortic balloon pumping.

*Figure 13*. Original registration of veno-arterial continuous flow bypass (VABP) shunting 50% of the cardiac output in combination with intraaortic balloon pumping (IABP). EKG = electrocardiogram, RAP = right atrial pressure, PAP = pulmonary artery pressure, AP = aortic pressure, LVP = left ventricular pressure, $dp/dt_{LV}$ = rise in left ventricular pressure, LVEDP = left ventricular end-diastolic pressure.

145

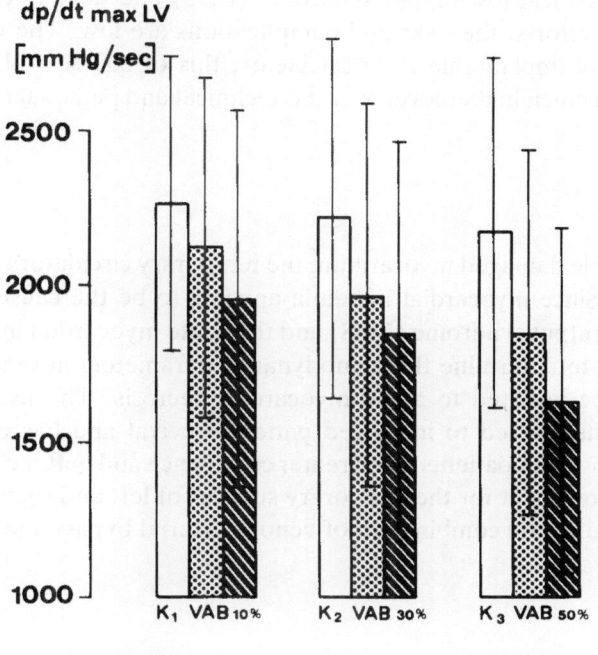

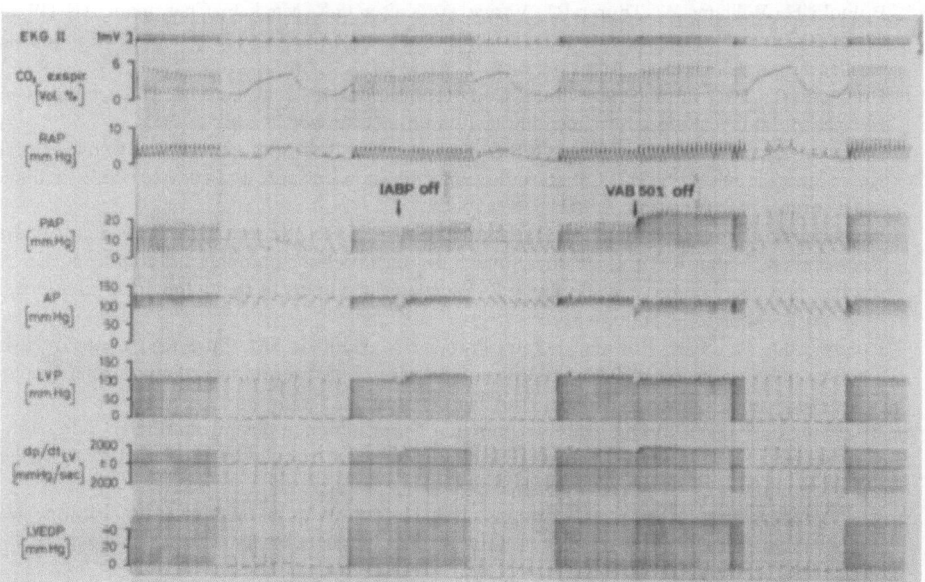

suffering from critical low-output syndrome (LOS) and does not require very much technical efforts, the risks and complications are low. The next step is a partial or a total implantable Artifical Heart, this of course will increase the dimensions to a much higher level of costs, technical and personal requirements.

## Conclusion

For the reversible damaged myocardium the temporary circulatory assist devices are indicated. Since myocardial ischemia appears to be the cause of the post-operative low-output syndrome (LOS) and the acute myocardial infarction (MI) it is postulated to determine the hemodynamic parameters in time if adequate therapy is to be initiated to avoid myocardial necrosis. The use of IABP in selected patients has led to improved patient survival and has enabled us to operate upon high risk patients with greater confidence and better clinical results. A further improvement for the temporary support of left and right heart failure can be achieved by the combination of venous-arterial bypass and IABP.

## References

1. Bernhard WF, La Farge CG, Bernhorst WJ (1973) Development of a left ventricle-to-aorta assist device. Final Progress Report to Division of Technological Applications, National Heart and Lung Institute, U.S. National Institutes of Health. PH 43-67-1116-6, pp 1–130
2. Bernstein EF, De Laria GA, Johansen KH, Shuman RL, Stasz P, Reich S (1975) Twenty-four hour left ventricular bypass with a centrifugal blood pump. Ann Surg 181, 412–417
3. Bolooki H, Williams W, Thurer RJ, Vargas A, Kaiser GA, Mack F, Charamani AR (1976) Clinically and hemodynamic criteria for use of the intra-aortic balloon pump in patients requiring cardiac surgery. J Thorac Cardiovasc Surg 72, 756
4. Bregman D (1981) Intraaortic Balloon Counterpulsation. In: Ionescu M (ed) Techniques in Extracorporal Circulation. Second Edition. London: Butterworths, pp 516–600
5. Bregman D, Parodi EN, Haubert SJ, Szarnicki R, Edie RN, Spotnitz HM, Bowman FO Jr, Reemtsma K, Malm JR (1977) Counterpulsation with a new pulsatile assist device (PAD) in open heart surgery. Med Instrum 11, 292
6. Bregman D, Parodi EH, Haubert SJ, Szarnicki R, Edie RN, Spotnitz HM, Bowman FO Jr, Reemtsma K, Malm JR (1977) Unidirectional intra-aortic balloon pumping and counterpulsation during open heart surgery. In: Bregman D, Mechanical support of the failing heart and lungs. New York: Appleton-Century-Crofts
7. Bregman D, Bailin M, Bowman FO Jr, Parodi EN, Haubert SM, Edie RN, Spotnitz HM, Reemtsma K, Malm JR (1977) A pulsatile assist device (PAD) for improved myocardial protection during cardiopulmonary bypass. Ann Thorac Surg 24, 574
8. Bretschneider HJ (1972) Die hämodynamischen Determinanten des myokardialen Sauerstoffverbrauches. In: Dengler HJ (Hrsg): Die therapeutische Anwendung β-sympathikolytischer Stoffe. Schattauer, Stuttgart-New York, S. 45
9. Buckly MJ, Craver JM, Gold HK, Mundth ED, Daggett WM, Austen WG (1973) Intraaortic balloon pump assist for cardiogenic shock after cardiopulmonary bypass. Circulation Suppl III 47, 48, 90–94

10. De Bakey ME (1971) Left ventricular bypass pump for cardiac assistance: Clinical experience. Am J Cardiol 27, 3

11. Dennis C, Hall DP, Moreno JR, Senning A (1962) Reduction of the oxygen utilization of the heart by left bypass. Circ Res 10, 298

12. Derks C, Jaspar N, Francquen de Ph, Vanderhoeft P (1976) Extracorporeal oxygenation with various experimental venoarterial bypass during prolonged apnea. Thorac Cardiovasc Surg 71, 666–672

13. Disler PB, Scott Miliar RN, Obel IWP (1978) Prolonged circulatory support with the intra-aortic balloon pump after myocardial infarction. Thorax 33, 504

14. Feola M, Wiener L, Walinsky P, Kasparian H, Duca P, Gottlieb R, Brest A, Templeton J (1977) Improved survival after coronary bypass surgery in patients with poor left ventricular function: role of intra-aortic balloon counterpulsation. Amer J Cardiol 39, 1021

15. Gold HK, Leinbach RC, Buckley MJ, Mundth ED, Daggett WM, Austen WG (1976) Refractory angina pectoris: follow-up after intra-aortic balloon pumping and surgery. Circulation 54 (Suppl III), 41

16. Gunstersen J, Goldmann BS, Scully HS, Hukkell VF, Adelman AG (1976) Evolving indications for preoperative intra-aortic balloon pump assistance. Ann Thorac Surg 22, 535

17. Harken DE (1976) Editorial: Circulatory assist devices. Med Instrum 10, 215

18. Harken DE, Lefemine AA (1960) Myocardial and circulatory assistance by synchronized counterpulsation. Dig 15. Annual Conf Eng Med

19. Kantrowitz A, Kantrowitz A (1953) Experimental augmentation of coronary flow by retardation of arterial pressure pulse. Surgery 34, 628

20. Kolff WJ, Akutsu T, Dreyer B, Norton H (1959) Artificial heart in the chest and use of polyurethane for making hearts, valves and aortas. Trans Am Soc, Artif Intern Organs 5, 298

21. Kolff WJ and Lawson J (1975) Status of the artificial heart and cardiac assist devices in the United States. Transactions of the American Society for Artificial Internal Organs 21, 160

22. Kreuzer H, Blanke H, Rentrop P, de Vivie ER, Hellberg K (1977) IACP and ECP in pump failure during acute myocardial infarction. In: The first 24 hours in myocardial infarction. Edited by: Kaindly F, Pachinger O, Probst P (eds), p 174, Verlag Gerhard Witzstrock

23. Lefemine AA, Kosowsky B, Madoff I, Black H, Lewis M (1977) Results and complications of intra-aortic balloon pumping in surgical and medical patients. Amer J Cardiol 40, 416

24. Litwak RS, Koffsky RM, Jurado RA, Lukban SB, Ortiz AF, Jr, Fischer AP, Sherman JJ, Silvay G, Lajam FA (1976) Use of a left heart assist device after intracardiac surgery: Technique and clinical experience. Ann Thorac Surg 21, 191

25. Leinbach RC, Goldstein J, Gold HK, Moses JW, Collings MB, Subramanian V (1982) Percutaneous wire-guided balloon pumping. Am J Cardiol 49, 1707–1710

26. Martin RS, Moncure AC, Buckley MJ, Austen WC, Akins C, Leinbach RC (1983) Complications of percutaneous intra-aortic balloon insertion. J Thorac Cardiovasc Surg 85, 186–190

27. Moulopoulos SD, Topaz S, Kolff WL (1962) Diastolic balloon pumping (with carbon dioxide) in aorta: Mechanical assistance to failing circulation. Am Heart J 63, 669

28. Schenk WG, Jr, Delin NA, Camp FA, McDonald KE, Pollack L, Gage A, Chardack WM (1964) Assisted circulation: an experimental evaluation of counterpulsation and left ventricular bypass. Arch Surg 88, 327

29. Soroff HS, Clautier CT, Birtwell WC, Begley LA, Messer JV (1974) External counterpulsation. Management of cardiogenic shock after myocardial infarction. J Amer Med Ass 229, 1441–1450

30. Unger F (1977) Konstruktion und tierexperimentelle Befunde mit einer neuen Form eines künstlichen Herzens: das Ellipsoidherz. Wien Klin Wochenschr. 89 (Suppl 76) 3

31. de Vivie RE, Kettler D, Hellberg K, Klaess G. Kontokollias J, Sonntag H (1974) Prevention of heart failure during arterial hypoxemia by means of intraaortic balloon pumping. Resuscitation 3, 214–248

32. de Vivie RE, Hellberg K (1977) Clinical results of intraaortic balloon pumping in selected groups

of patients. In: Assisted Circulation, Ed F. Unger pp 40–46, Berlin, Heidelberg, New York: Springer-Verlag

33. Wakabayashi A, Nakamura Y, Murphy KJ, Kubo T, Charney KJ, Connolly JE (1973) Controlled veno-arterial bypass without oxygenation in the treatment of cardiogenic shock. Trans Am Suc Artif Intern Organs 19, 511

34. Wolner E (1979) Indications for intraaortic balloon pumping. In: Assisted Circulation, Ed F. Unger pp 47–55, Berlin, Heidelberg, New York: Springer Verlag

35. Wright PW (1975) External counterpulsation for cardiogenic shock following cardiopulmonary bypass surgery. Amer Heart J 90, 231

36. Zwart HH, Kralios AC, Eastood N, Kolff WF (1972) Effects of partial and complete unloading of the failing left ventricle by transarterial left heart bypass. J Thorac Cardiovasc Surg 63, 865

# Implantable artificial heart devices

W. KLEPETKO and E. WOLNER

Mechanical support of a failing heart is a matter of great interest, since the number of patients dying from cardiac insufficiency is large. To estimate the number of patients, whom might be helped by mechanical circulatory support, first of all it is necessary to identify the groups of possible candidates for such an intervention.

Commonly there are three populations:

1. Patients who cannot be weaned off cardiopulmonary bypass, despite successful operative procedure. The incidence of this event is estimated in about 0,1 to 1,0% of open heart operations. However, this collective of patients is by far the largest, and the only chance for these patients lies in a mechanical support of the heart.

2. Patients suffering from end-stage intractable cardiac failure. Although today this group is favourably treated by heart transplantation, there are still patients with contra-indications to this therapy.

3. The cardiogenic shock-myocardial infarction group, mainly arising in the cardiac care unit. In these patients, mechanical support can be life saving until further recovery or until a donor heart can be found for ultimate heart transplantation.

Two ways of application of a mechanical circulatory assist device arise from these indications:

a. temporary support until myocardial recovery, or until a donor heart is available for cardiac transplantation, and
b. ultimate solution, as total artificial heart.

From the theoretical point of view the demand for mechanical support is large, and stands in clear contrast to the small number of clinical applications up to now. This surprising difference between theoretical demand and practical use is even more striking, when we consider the 30 years of scientific research on this topic and the great amount of financial as well as human energy spent on the evaluation of a practicable device. The specific emphasis of this lecture is therefore not only on giving a concise outline of mechanical cardiac support, but also on discussing the problems, which partly are still unsolved and therefore hinder from a broader application.

**Methods of cardiac assistance**

Unloading of a failing heart can be achieved by four different principles [1]:

1. Systems for volume relief: i.e. CPBP = Cardiopulmonary bypass with the heart lung machine.
2. Systems for pressure relief: i.e. IABP = Intra aortic balloon pump.
3. Combined system: VAD = Ventricular assist devices.
4. TAH = Total artificial heart.

The use of CPBP is temporary limited by high blood traumatisation. IABP does not achieve sufficient circulatory support below a certain level of cardiac performance, which limitates its application in moderate cardiac insufficiency. In case of severe medicamental untractable cardiac failure only the application of VAD or TAH devices are promising approaches (Fig. 1).

The need for mechanical support can result either from isolated right heart or left heart failure. Accordingly, the application of a VAD system on the left side (LVAD) or on the right heart side (RVAD) is necessary. As additional support an IABP can be applied.

In cases of biventricular failure, two VAD systems on both heart sides can be applied temporary (BVAD), or the human heart can be replaced by a TAH, either as a temporary bridge to cardiac transplantation, or as an ultimate solution if counterindications for heart transplantation exist.

**Indications**

The specifications of haemodynamic criterias for mechanical support has been a controversial subject. A VAD implantation performed too early can imply possible harm to the patient, whereas performed too late, can involve irretrievable damage to the heart, that otherwise might have had the chance for recovery.

Pierce, Norman, and Pennington [2] have set up clear indications for left and right heart assistance, especially in postbypass patients. They consider left heart

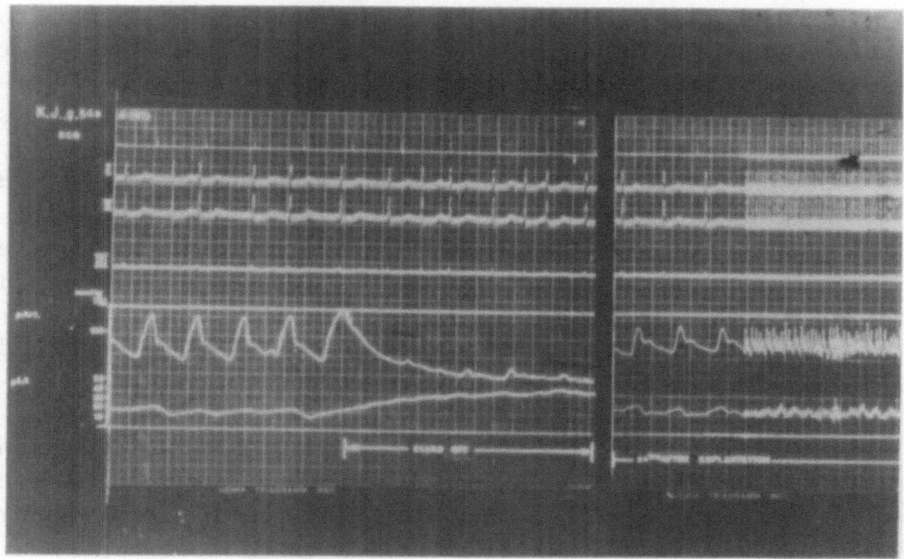

*Figure 1.* Hemodynamic registation of human LVAD application. Switching off the pump results in rapid decrease of arterial pressure (pArt) and increase of left atrial pressure (pLA). 24 hours after LVAD explantation, the patient presents in a stable clinical situation.

assistance to be indicated in cases of left atrial pressure $>25$ mm Hg, arterial pressure $<90$ mm Hg and cardiac index $<1,8$ l/min/m².

Right heart assistance is considered to be indicated in case of cardiac index below 1,8 l/min/m² and the inability to volume load the left ventricle despite a right atrial pressure $>20$ mm Hg. All these parameters presume that conventional therapy with inotropic and vasodilatory drugs, cardiac pacing, and application of IABP have failed to support myocardial function. An additional demand is the satisfactory surgical repair of the underlying cardiac disease.

## Comparison of pulsatile and nonpulsatile pumps

From the technical aspect we distinguish between two main principles of blood pumps: pulsatile and nonpulsatile ones.

By far, the majority of clinically applied systems are pulsatile pumps, whereas the nonpulsatile systems have not yet reached this widespread use. Partly this is due to a backlog in technical evolution when compared with pulsatile systems, but may be this will change with increasing scientific research in the field of nonpulsatile blood pumps.

Possible advantages of nonpulsatile systems are of great promise.
No artificial valves are needed for direction of blood flow, problems with the

blood sac membrane are avoided, no dead space and flow stop in the cannulas occurs. Blood supply to coronary arteries is maintained during the whole cardiac cycle and the system is therefore independent from heart frequency. In comparison with pulsatile systems, a higher volume output can be achieved, as well as complete pressure and volume decompression of both ventricles.

Several disadvantages stand in opposite to this: The pump flow is directed proportional to the number of rotations and indirect to peripheral resistance. Blood flow measurements are therefore necessary and high positive and negative pressures arise at stenoses or occlusions. Areas of high temperature, so called hot spots, can be found within the pump.

A special problem of nonpulsatile blood pumps lies in the dangerous effect of complete unloading of the ventricle with consequent decreasing left atrial pressure to zero. Collapse of the lung vessels can be the deleterious consequence.

However, the physiological and biological questions in regard to longterm nonpulsatile blood flow are, despite the investigations of Bernstein and Nose and our own experiences, not yet answered. Own investigations as well as other studies have found no negative effect on myocardial energy metabolism. Rather we could observe a significant reduction of transmural myocardial blood flow combined with a significant decrease in oxygen consumption during complete decompression of the left ventricle [3]. Further investigations will show, in how far this decrease in oxygen consumption corresponds to an actual reduction of oxygen demand.

## Pulsatile blood pumps

The design of pulsatile blood pumps is based on a blood chamber with variable volume content. By means of compression of this chamber, the blood is sqeezed out. Unidirectional blood flow is achieved by one inlet and one outlet one-way valve. The pump action is generated either by a pusher plate or hydraulic activated diaphragm. Accordingly, it is possible to distinct between electrically and hydraulically driven devices.

The use of pneumatic blood pumps implies the need for large diameter percutaneous lines for transmission of airpulses, generated by an external pneumatic unit. The size of the extracorporeal driving units has been continuously reduced in the last years, now reaching that of a small suitcase [4]. For use in TAH systems it can be installed into a wheelchair offering the patient improved mobility.

The entrance site of the percutaneous lines into the body remains a permanent zone of disturbance to the skin, effecting epidermal down growth and sinus tract formation along the tubes, with the subsequent risk of infection.

The hazard of eventual invasive sepsis originating at the percutaneous tube site, and the tethering effect of a large external driving unit points out the possible advantages of an electrical driving system [5]. For transmission of electrical energy only small percutaneous wires are necessary. The implantation of a subcutaneous battery offers complete independence from an external energy source to the patient. Several systems of energy transmission through intakt skin are now under development. These devices are mainly based on the principle of inductance [6] and include two transformers, an extracorporeal one as an external recharging unit, and a fully subcutaneously implanted one. Further research is also done in the field of nuclear fuel sources.

One significant problem remains in the development of a completely intracorporeable pulsatile blood pump: the need for variable compensation of volume [7]. With the blood pump in a full condition, there is little residual volume between pump housing and the back surface of the diaphragm. At the end of pump ejection, however, the residual volume behind the diaphragm must be increased by the stroke volume that has left the pump. Otherwise the driving unit would have to provide a partial vacuum, a work which would far exceed the work required to pump blood against systemic vascular resistance. This demands the use of an aditional compliance chamber, supplying air or a suitable fluid whenever the pump ejects blood.

The problems combined with the goal of fully implantable VAD systems actuated several working groups to use paracorporeal VAD systems in postcardiotomy patients. In that case the pump usually lies on the patients chest with cannulas passing the thoracic wall. As an advantage, no additional intrathoracic space for the implantation of the device is needed. On the other hand the risk for infection is clearly enlarged and the system as a whole makes the patient fully immobilized.

Another important fact is the technique of cannulation. The need for cannulas of large diameter with good hemodynamic properties clearly stands opposite to the damage of myocardial tissue, which increases with the size of the cannula. Furthermore kinking and twisting of the tubes must be avoided as well as angulation between the inflow cannula and the heart wall. Usually the outflow cannula is sewed onto the thoracic aorta by means of a dacron graft. The most favoured site is the ascending aorta, seldom the descending thoracic or abdominal aorta is used.

Inflow cannulas are usually placed through the apex of the heart into the left ventricle, or through the appendix into the left atrium. Sometimes the cannula is introduced through the left atrium and the mitral valve into the left ventricle. The rationale of this cannulation technique is to avoid damage of the contractile myocardium of the left ventricle, combined with the better inflow condition of the high pressure zone.

Besides the risk of infection, there are several other problems occuring with the contact of artificial surfaces with the human blood. The risk of thromboembolism has been lowered by the use of anticoagulants and the development of biocompatible materials which minimize the interactions between artificial and natural materials. Since several years, a polymer of polyurethane named Cardiothane has provided the best results [8]. With the same considerations bioprosthetic valves have been used in some devices. However, these valves show far lower mechanical stress tolerance than artificial valves. The design of the pump is also of great influence, since especially all regions of recirculation, of blood stagnation, and all kinds of edges are risk factors for thromboembolism.

A new approach towards the ideal of an antithrombogenic surface in artificial heart devices has been started at our institution two years ago. The goal of it is to cover the artificial surface with human endothelial cells [9]. First results have demonstrated the possibility of in vitro cultivation of human endothelial cells on different kinds of synthetic materials commonly used for artificial hearts.

Another special problem lies in the flex life of the blood sac, which often is the ultimate limit to the duration of pumping. Although in vitro tests have exceeded several years, this situation is not comparable with the situation in vivo, where deposition of calcium oxalat at the membrane leads to reduction of flexibility and life. Since this experience was gained in calves, it is not yet clear, whether this is only a special problem in the growing organism, or has also any meaning in adults.

**Nonpulsatile blood pumps**

Besides the pulsatile form of circulation support, nonpulsatile blood pumps have been investigated for 15 years. The most simple system is that of the roller pump, as used for CPBP.

Kletschka [10] has developed a non implantable pump based on the vortex principle, which is under production by the Biomedicus company. One outstanding feature of this device is the lack of need for anticoagulation.

The pump is commercially available, which brought along a great number of experimental and clinical applications.

Another implantable nonpulsatile pump, based on the impeller principle was developed by Bernstein [11] and produced by the Medtronic company. The pump head has a blood compartment, containing an impeller fabricated from pyrolytic carbon. The housing is made of epoxy and internal coated with Avcothane, thus all surfaces are composed of thromboresistant material. Nevertheless, the major limitations to chronic use of this system are seal leakage and accumulation of an amorphous material at the shaft and seal area under the impeller. The device was therefore produced and sold only for a short time.

In Vienna [12] we are at present developing an implantable vaneless centrifugal pump (Fig. 2), based on the friction principle. The size of the latest prototype could be reduced to 80 mm in diameter and only 40 mm in axial length, including the electric driven motor. This type has 2 lamellas made of stainless steel. The lammellas are strapped together by 6 bolts placed 0,2 mm apart and are laser welded. The housing of the hydraulic part was made of vacuum molded polyurethane sheet. For improvement of biocompatibility, future lammelas will be

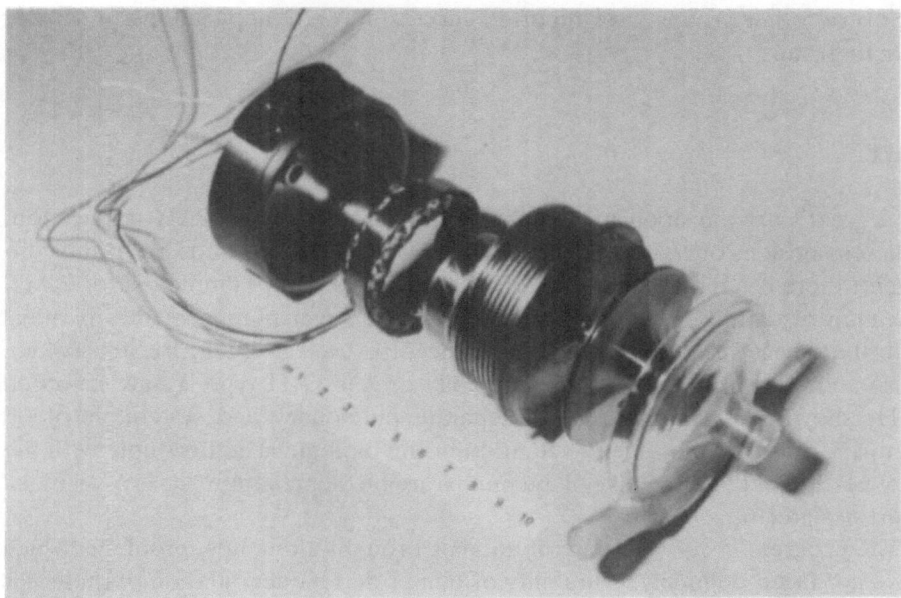

*Figure 2.* Implantable centrifugal pump.

covered with a biocompatible coating. Cooling of the pump is performed with water to keep the pump below body temperature, thus preventing thrombo-embolism formation.

## Clinical results

The largest series of clinical VAD applications have been reported by Pierce [13], Pennington [14], and Bernhard [15]. From 1980 to 1985, Pierce and Donachy at Hershey have applied their device in 21 patients with the result of 11 weaned off patients and 9 discharged patients. 15 of these patients received left heart bypass, 2 right heart bypass and 4 biventricular assistance, none of whom could be weaned off.

Pennington's group at St. Louis university has used the same device in 34 postcardiotomy patients. In 23 a LVAD was applied, in 7 RVAD combined with IABP on the left heart side was performed, and 4 patients needed biventricular assistance. All of the patients could be weaned off cardiopulmonary bypass. Circulatory support was maintained between 3 hours and 18 days. 10 patients could be weaned off the device and 7 were longtime survivors. Bernard's group at Boston has applied their device in 22 postcardiotomy patients, of whom 9 could be returned to the intensive care unit. Four patients survived one month and three patients several years.

Several other groups have reported successful VAD applications in smaller patient groups.

## TAH

In a great part the upon made considerations are true of TAH application. Whereas designs of VAD systems of the single working groups are rather different, there is a remarkable similarity in the blood pumps employed for TAH. The majority consists of two separated pneumatic driven pumps, mainly identical with the devices used for VAD. This concept is used in Utah, Berlin, Tokyo, Brno and Vienna (Fig. 3). The electrically driven TAH type is only favoured at Hershey/Pennsylvannia. Use of separate pulmonary and systematic blood pumps, orthotopic placement, retention of the biologic atria to couple with the inlet portion of the respective blood pumps are further common ideas of artificial heart design [16].

The progress in survival time of animals brought along new problems which were not faced originally. Durability of pumps and biodegradation of materials are the main factors, which became more important. Another problems lies in the use of calves for experimental implantation. At implantation the calf usually is about 3 months of age, with about 90 kg body weight. Daily weight gain of about 0,6 kg results in a body weight of about 210 kg after 200 days of survival. This presents the problem of a growing recipient with a non growing pump. Nevertheless, the calf is the animal of choice of almost all researching groups except of Dr. Atsumi's group in Tokyo, who continues to use goats [17].

A special problem of TAH is pannus formation at the junction of the inflow sewing cuff and the inlet valve. It leads to inflow obstruction with consequently reduced cardiac output. Pannus formation has been observed in most instances combined with bacterial or fungal infection, occasionally the pannus was found to be sterile.

To summarize this paper, there are several problems already solved and others still remaining unsolved. Already solved items are the specification of indications, the control unit, the implantation technique of TAH and some questions of the pump like hemolysis and pump performance, whereas the driving unit, danger of infection, implantation technique of VAD, and concerning the pump, questions of biocompatibility, thromboembolism, and durability remain still unsolved mainpoints.

It remains to be expected, that the continuing scientific research will steadily increase the number of solved problems and thus the application of improved devices will bring along improved clinical results. As a final approach fully implantable systems are considered to combine adaequate hemodynamic performance with satisfactory quality of life.

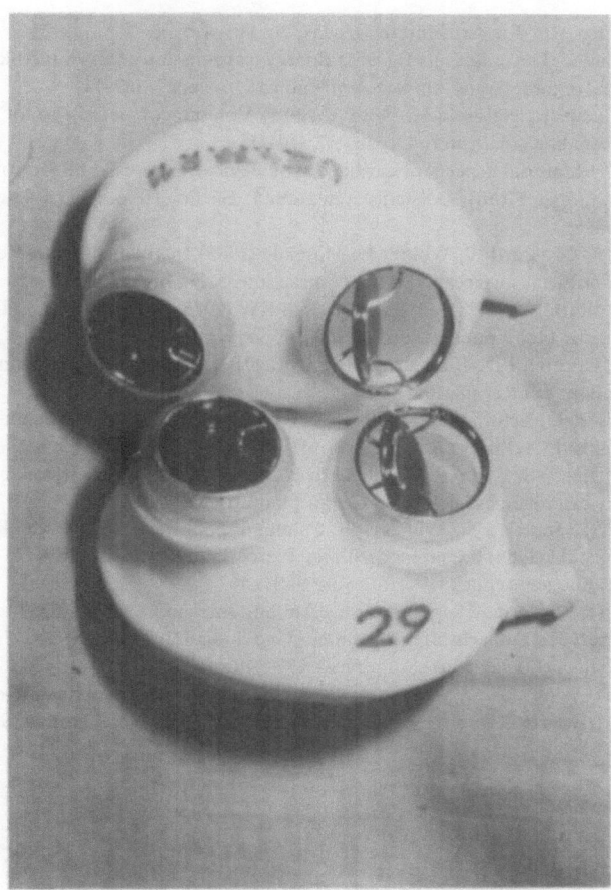

*Figure 3.* Ellipsoid heart.

## References

1. Wolner E, Thoma H, Deutsch M, Eckersberger F, Fasching W, Losert U, Stellwag U, Stöhr F, Unger H, Weisskirchner R, Polzer K (1979) Das Forschungsprojekt Künstliches Herz an der II. Chirurgischen Universitätsklinik Wien. Wien klin Wschr 91: 74–81
2. Pennock JL, Pierce WS, Wisman CB, Bull AP, Waldhausen JA (1983) Survival and complications following ventricular assist pumping for cardiogenic shock. Ann Surg 198: 469–478
3. Losert U, Glogar D, Mayr H, Mohl W, Ogris E, Stöhr H, Wolner E (1982) Regional myocardial blood flow during nonpulsatile left ventricular bypass in calves. Trans Am Soc Artif Intern Organs 28: 86–92
4. Hennig E (1984) The artificial heart program in Berlin – Technical aspects. In: Unger F (ed) Assisted Circulation 2. Berlin, Heidelberg, New York, Tokyo: Springer 229–253
5. Ozawa K, Snow J, Sukalac R, Takatani S, Kitagawa M, Valdes F, Harsaki H, Hillegass D, Castle C, Jacobs G, Kiraly R, Nose Y (1980) Totally implantable left ventricular assist device for human

application. Trans Am Soc Artif Intern Organs, 26: 461–465

6. Sherman C, Clay W, Dasse K, Daly B (1981) Energy transmission across intact skin for powering artificial internal organs. Trans Am Soc Artif Intern Organs 27, 137–141

7. Whalen RL, Snow JL, Harasaki H, Nose Y (1981) Volume compensation for pulsatile blood pumps. Trans Am Soc Artif Intern Organs 27, 110–115

8. Nyilasi E (1979) Material aspects of cardiac assist devices. The case history of Avcothane 51 Elastomer. In: Unger F (ed) Assisted Circulation 1, Berlin, Heidelberg, New York, Tokyo: Springer, 483–496

9. Fasol R, Zilla P, Groscurth P, Wolner E, Moser R (1985) In vitro cultivation of human endothelial cells on artificial surfaces; ASAIO Transactions 31, in press

10. Kletschka HD, Rafferty EH, Olsen DA, Clausen EW (1975) Artificial Heart. Development of efficient atraumatic blood pump; Minn Med 58, 756

11. Bernstein EF, Dorman FD, Blackshear PL, Scott DR (1970) An efficient compact pump for assisted circulation. Surgery 68, 105

12. Thoma H, Losert U, Schwanda G, Stöhr H, Wolner E (1985) Development of implantable centrifugal pumps; ISAO in press

13. Pennock JL, Pierce WS, Bull AP, Waldhausen JA (1983) Use of the ventricular assist pump for postcardiotomy cardiogenic shock. Heart Transplantation 3, 26–29

14. Pennington DG, Samuels LD, Williams G, Palmer D, Schwartz MT, Codd JE, Merjavy JP, Lagunoff D, Joist JH (1985) Experience with the Pierce-Donachy assist device in postcardiotomy patients with cardiogenic shock; World J Surg 9, 37–46

15. Bernhard WF (1980) Cardiac Support. Trans Am Soc Intern Organs 26, 625

16. Pierce WS, Myers JL, Donachy JH, Rosenberg G, Landis DL, Prophet GA, Snyder AJ (1981) Approaches to the artificial heart. Surgery 90, 137–148

17. Atsumi K (1984) Ventricular assistance – Development and clinical application of a new device. In: Unger F (ed) Assisted Circulation 2. Berlin, Heidelberg, New York, Tokyo: Springer, 100–114

# Current status of cardiac and cardiopulmonary transplantation

J.C. BALDWIN and N.E. SHUMWAY

## Summary

Cardiac transplantation has emerged as a standard mode of clinical therapy for end-stage heart failure. Since clinical application began in 1967, there has been continual improvement in donor management, surgical techniques, post-operative management, and the diagnosis and treatment of rejection. More than 350 cardiac transplant operations have been performed in our institution, and one-year survival currently exceeds 80%. Current immunosuppressive techniques involve the use of cyclosporine, and experience with this agent and its adverse side effects has prompted institution of low-dose cyclosporine regimens. Principal complications of cardiac transplantation include infection, rejection, malignancy related to immunosuppression, and graft atherosclerosis. During the past four years, clinical cardiopulmonary transplantation has emerged as a therapeutic alternative for patients with end-stage pulmonary vascular disease. Problems of donor identification and management, post-operative pulmonary failure due to rejection and infection, and long-term obstructive pulmonary changes are being addressed in both the clinical and laboratory efforts.

## History

The history of the development of cardiac transplantation as a viable therapeutic alternative spans the course of this century and reflects the development of cardiovascular surgery in general, as well as other fields, such as immunology, oncology, and infectious disease. The first reported cardiac transplant, performed in a canine cervical heterotopic model, appeared in the journal *American Medicine* in 1905 [1]. Alexis Carrel reported this successful transplant, in which the heart was noted to beat for approximately two hours. No less important to the overall development of this field than the transplant itself was Carrel's pioneering contribution in the area of vascular surgical technique. There were gradual refinements in related surgical techniques over the next forty years; and Demikhov, working in the Soviet Union during the 1950's, was the first to demonstrate the ability of a heterotopically-transplanted canine heart to sustain the circulation independently [2]. The development of safe cardiopulmonary bypass techniques, through the work of Gibbon and others, transformed the possibilities for cardiac transplantation as it did the possibilities for other forms of cardiovascular surgery [3]. The first series of successful orthotopic cardiac transplantations were reported by Lower and Shumway in 1960 [4]. In this work, they described a technique which involved reliable cardiopulmonary bypass, topical hypothermic preservation of the cardiac graft, and excision and reimplantation of the heart at the mid-atrial level. The methods used in this study served as the cornerstone for subsequent developments in cardiac transplantation, both in the laboratory and in the clinical sphere.

In December 1967, Barnard performed the first human orthotopic cardiac allograft operation in South Africa [5]. Although this patient did not achieve long-term survival, the performance of this operation led to a dramatic increase in worldwide interest in clinical application of cardiac transplantation. More than 100 cardiac transplant operations were performed throughout the world during 1968, but clinical results were generally dismal. In the following years, the decline in interest in clinical application was equally dramatic.

Based on a long laboratory experience, a program in clinical cardiac transplantation was started at the Stanford University Medical Center in January of 1968. This program has continued on an uninterrupted basis since that time, with progressive improvement in survival and rehabilitation.

**Recipient selection**

Recipients for cardiac transplantation are chosen from the group of patients with end-stage congestive heart failure, in the New York Heart Association Class IV for symptoms. Currently, we apply an upper age limit of 60 years, and there is no lower age limit. Pediatric applications of this technique are the subject of continuing investigation, and certain entities, such as familial-cardiomyopathy and hypoplastic left heart syndrome may prove to be successfully treatable with cardiac transplantation.

Patients should have no other life threatening systemic illness, such as malignancy or collagen vascular disease. Although many patients with end-stage congestive heart failure will have reversible degrees of prerenal azotemia and hepatic congestion, irreversible degrees of renal failure and hepatic failure are generally considered to be contraindications to cardiac transplantation. In addition, patients with recent pulmonary infarctions are not transplanted because of the possibilities of bleeding and infection in the area of pulmonary infarction. Insulin-requiring diabetes mellitus is a relative contraindication, because of the likelihood of exacerbation of the condition with post-operative steroid therapy.

Elevated pulmonary vascular resistance also represents a relative contraindication. We currently limit cardiac transplantation to patients with pulmonary vascular resistance less than 5–6 Wood units. Certain extenuating factors, such as reversibility of elevated pulmonary vascular resistance with vasodilator therapy, availability of on-site donors, and availability of donors with body mass greater than that of the potential recipient, may be considered in cases of borderline ranges of pulmonary hypertension. It may also be that selective pharmacologic maneuvers and temporary right ventricular assist/afterload reduction devices may facilitate successful cardiac transplantation in patients with higher ranges of pulmonary vascular resistance.

## Donor selection

Cardiac donors are selected from among brain dead patients less than 35 years of age. This upper age limit is chosen in the hope of avoiding occult atherosclerotic and other diseases. Potential donors should have no history of cardiac disease and should have no active infection. In general, appropriate donors for cardiac transplantation can be weaned to little or no vasopressor support, with appropriate volume replacement and pharmocologic management of diabetes insipidus.

Since 1977, the majority of cardiac transplant operations performed in our institution have employed distant graft procurement. This program of distant graft procurement has facilitated the personal needs of donors' families and physicians, who prefer that the body not be moved; has increased our ability to work cooperatively with other organ procurement teams, during this period of increasing interest in transplantation; and has generally increased the size of the donor pool. Although laboratory experience at our institution and elsewhere has suggested the possibility of longer ischemic times, we currently limit total graft ischemia to four hours.

## Donor-recipient matching

When a prospective donor for cardiac transplantation becomes available, the cardiac allograft is matched with an appropriate recipient. Given the continuing shortage of donors and the exigencies of timing in organ procurement, immunologic matching in clinical transplantation is usually rudimentary. Donor recipient matching is carried out on the basis of ABO blood group compatibility and size matching. The donor body mass should not be more than 20% smaller than that of the recipient. Cytotoxic antibody screening, using recipient serum and random donor lymphocytes, is carried out in all prospective recipients. In cases where this screening indicates positive cross matches or in cases where previous surgeries/blood transfusions or pregnancies pertain, lymphocytes cross matching is performed prior to transplantation.

A limited retrospective analysis of HLA compatibility in our patients showed no identifiable correlation between degree of HLA incompatibility and incidence or severity of rejection [6]. Incompatibility at the HLA A2 locus between donor and recipient was previously thought to correlate with incidence of coronary artery disease, but more recent retrospective analyses have failed to support this correlation.

**Technique**

Despite emphasis in the literature on immunologic aspects and postoperative care, surgical technique is of paramount importance in the success of cardiac transplantation. The donor operation is carried out without cardiopulmonary bypass. A standard median sternotomy incision is emloyed, and the heart and great vessels are carefully inspected for evidence of occult coronary artery disease, valvular disease, trauma, or congenital anomaly. The donor procurement operation represents the last opportunity for hemodynamic and anatomic assessment. The venae cavae and great vessels are dissected out in the usual fashion. Inflow occlusion is achieved by ligation of the superior vena cava and inferior vena cava, and the heart is allowed to beat for several cycles to empty. The aorta is cross-clamped near the take-off of the innominate artery, and cold potassium cardioplegic solution is administered via the aortic root. Immediately after commencement of instillation of cardioplegic solution, the superior vena cava and right superior pulmonary vein are incised to obviate the possibility of distention of either the right or left side of the heart. Concomitantly with administration of potassium cardioplegic solution via the aortic root, topical cooling is carried out using normal saline at 4 degrees Celsius. The most common causes of graft dysfunction related to organ procurement are distention and inadequate cooling.

The recipient operation is carried out in a fashion which does not differ significantly from that first described by Lower and Shumway in 1960. A standard median sternotomy incision is employed, and cannulation of the aorta is carried out near the take-off of the innominate artery. Cannulation of the superior and inferior venae cavae is carried out laterally, to maximize the amount of residual right atrial cuff. Snares are placed around the cavae to exclude air. Cardiopulmonary bypass is instituted, and systemic cooling is commenced. The heart is excised after placement of the aortic cross-clamp, beginning with incision of the right atrium along the atrio-ventricular groove, through the coronary sinus, and through the atrial septum to empty the left side of the heart of blood. The aorta and pulmonary artery are then transsected at the immediate supravalvular level, and the excision of the heart is completed, by incision of the left atrium just posterior to the left atrial appendage.

The implantation of the graft is carried out, commencing with the left atrium, in the area of the recipient left superior pulmonary vein and the donor left atrial appendage. The left atrial anastomosis is carried out using a continuous poly-propylene technique. Graft preservation is achieved by application of topical cold saline. In addition, after completion of the left atrial anastomosis, a second line containing cold saline is placed into the tip of the left atrial appendage. Placement of this line at this point in the operation enhances endomyocardial cooling, and excludes air from the left side of the graft during the remainder of the operation.

The right atrial anastomosis is commenced in the area of the midseptum and carried out in a continuous fashion, using a polypropylene suture. Systemic warming is begun at the time of commencement of the aortic anastomosis, which is carried out in an end-to-end fashion, using continuous polypropylene.

The aortic cross-clamp is removed, and spontaneous defibrillation usually occurs. It is quite possible to perform the pulmonary arterial anastomosis with the aortic cross-clamp removed and the heart beating. This provides for reduction of the total ischemic time.

Patients are ordinarily maintained on vasopressor support with isoproterenol for 4–5 days post-operatively, based on clinical observation of graft dysfunction when pressor support is weaned earlier and presumed intramyocardial edema and decreased high-energy phosphate stores. Early extubation and ambulation are emphasized.

## Immunosuppression and diagnosis and treatment of rejection

Current immunosuppression technique is based around the fungal metabolite cyclosporine. We have employed cyclosporine immunosuppression since December 1980, and its use has been associated with considerable improvement in survival. However, observation of several significant adverse side effects, including renal failure, hepatic toxicity, hypertension, hirsuitism, and malignancy, has prompted recent institution of a low-dose cyclosporine protocol. This protocol, depicted in Table 1, involves a two-pronged study with one group receiving maintenance steroid therapy, and the other group receiving maintenance therapy with cyclosporine and azathioprine alone.

It is distinctly unusual to observe cardiac rejection before the seventh post-operative day. Accordingly, endomyocardial biopsy is ordinarily performed on the seventh post-operative day using the Caves bioptome. This technique is now well-established and involved percutaneous insertion of the bioptome under local anesthesia, using Seldinger technique. The bioptome is advanced under fluo-rescopic control into the right ventricle and then apposed against the inter-ventricular septum. Multiple biopsies are taken, and the importance of multiple biopsies has recently been emphasized, because of the heterogeneity of histologic involvement with rejection on cyclosporine immunosuppression.

Biopsies are ordinarily carried out on a weekly basis, unless rejection intervenes. When rejection with myocyte necrosis does occur, current therapy involves intravenous methylprednisolone, which is administered as a single bolus of 1,000 mg on a daily basis for 3 days. Histologic resolution can ordinarily be expected to occur within 4 days, and repeat endomyocardial biopsy is carried out on the fourth day. When rejection persists, a second course of three days of intravenous methylprednisolone is administered. When rejection is particularly severe and clinically significant, or when rejection occurs on a third consecutive biopsy, intravenous methylprednisolone therapy is combined with intramuscular rabbit antithymocyte globuline therapy. This latter therapy is also administered for three days, unless T cell rosette counts fall below the 15% level. When rejection is fulminant and life threatening or when it is persistent and clinically significant despite maximal medical therapy, consideration for retransplantation must be made.

**Complications**

The range of causes of death indicated in Table 2 depicts the variety of complications that may occur after cardiac transplantation. Infection and rejection remain the principal complications and causes of death after cardiac transplantation.

The range of infections which may occur after cardiac transplantation is broad, both in terms of types of organisms involved and in terms of sites of involvement. Vigilance for the protean manifestations of infection in the immunosuppressed host is the key to successful care for these patients. However, it should be noted that although cyclosporine immunosuppression has not reduced the incidence of infection in a statistically significant fashion, it has been observed by most investigators that the response of patients to infection is less morbid and that their response to appropriate antimicrobial therapy is more reliable and prompt than

*Table 1.* Current immunosuppression regimens.

| Protocol 1 | |
| --- | --- |
| I. | Cyclosporine – 18 mg/kg orally as a pre-operative loading dose and 9–10 mg/kg/day post-operatively (target level 200–300 ng/ml). |
| II. | Azathioprine – 2 mg/kg/day as maintenance |
| III. | Intravenous equine antithymocyte globulin – 10 mg/kg/day for 7 days (depending on T cell rosette counts) |
| IV. | Prednisone – 0.2 mg/kg/day as maintenance |

| Protocol 2 |
| --- |
| Same as Protocol 1 except for absence of maintenance prednisone therapy. |

that seen among patients treated with conventional immunosuppression.

Similarly with rejection, cyclosporine immunosuppression has not statistically significantly reduced the incidence of the complication. However, it has been generally observed that rejection occurring in cyclosporine-treated patients has been a less morbid and fulminant process which is generally amenable to pulse steroid therapy. These observations with respect to infection and rejection among cyclosporine patients are undoubtedly pivotal factors in the improvement and survival which has obtained.

Graft atherosclerosis is a persistent and disturbing complication after cardiac transplantation. It is noteworthy that more than one-third of patients will have angiographically-identifiable atherosclerotic lesions present when catheterized three years after transplantation. Furthermore, it appears that the incidence of graft atherosclerosis is no longer among patients who underwent transplantation for cardiomyopathy as their initial diagnosis than it is for those patients who underwent transplantation for coronary artery disease. The atherosclerosis which occurs in these grafts is typically a diffuse process, which involves the distal vessels and is therefore not amenable to coronary artery bypass grafting.

In the denervated heart, the onset of graft atherosclerosis is ordinarily and insidious phenomenon, presenting with the gradual onset of congestive heart failure or sudden death. When angiographically identified lesions are severe or particularly threatening in their anatomy, it is important to consider the possibility of retransplantation. In our series, we have performed 18 retransplant operations for graft atherosclerosis.

Malignancy is many times more common among transplant patients than among the general population, and lymphomas of the large-cell immunoblastic type have been observed frequently among cardiac transplant patients [7]. A particularly high incidence of lymphomas occurring in the initial group of cyclosporine-treated cardiac transplant patients prompted an empiric reduction in

*Table 2.* Causes of death among cardiac transplant patients (N = 307, 177 deaths).

| | |
|---|---|
| Infection | 93 |
| Rejection | 30 |
| Graft atherosclerosis | 18 |
| Malignancy | 12 |
| Pulmonary hypertension | 7 |
| Cerebrovascular accident | 3 |
| Pulmonary embolism | 2 |
| Cerebral edema | 1 |
| Myopathy | 1 |
| Suicide | 1 |
| Acute graft failure | 2 |
| Hepatic failure | 1 |
| Sudden death, unknown etiology | 6 |

overall degree of immunosuppression, with elimination of prophylactic rabbit antithymocyte globulin, and adjustment of cyclosporine dosages according to serum levels. Since these adjustments, the incidence of lymphoma has been markedly reduced, and no instances of lymphoma have occurred in the last 100 cardiac transplant patients. A recent retrospective analysis of quantitative measures of immunosuppression among cardiac transplant patients developing lymphoma suggested that the occurrence of lymphoma was related to the overall degree of immunosuppression, with mean cyclosporine levels during the first three months after transplantation and mean cyclosporine levels during T cell suppression showing greatest statistical significance [7].

### Results

Since the inception of the cardiac transplant program at Stanford University in January of 1968, more than 360 cardiac transplant operations have been carried out in 338 patients. There has been steady improvement in survival, and current one-year survival exceeds 80%. Actuarial survival comparing the results of cardiac transplantation with cyclosporine immunosuppression with survival among prospective recipients for whom no donor is found demonstrates the dramatic efficacy of this form of therapy in terms of survival. The mean survival among patients for whom no donor is found is three months, while 84% of cyclosporine-treated patients are alive at one year. It is expected that 55–60% of patients treated with cyclosporine will experience five-year survival.

Since cardiac transplantation is performed in a relatively young group of patients with disease limited to the cardiac axis and its direct ramifications, rehabilitation is similarly gratifying. Among one-year survivors, rehabilitation, as defined by ability to return to school or work, exceeds 80%.

### Cardiopulmonary transplantation

Patients with end-stage pulmonary vascular disease, from any etiology, frequently represent difficult challenges for medical therapy. Similarly, cardiac transplantation alone cannot suffice. Therefore, there has been a long-standing interest in combined heart and lung transplantation [8, 9]. Early laboratory efforts, particularly in the canine model, were frustrated by post-operative pulmonary insufficiency. However, with continued laboratory effort, the advent of cyclosporine and its associated improved survival in cardiac transplantation, and improved results with cardiopulmonary transplantation in primates, a clinical cardiopulmonary transplantation was begun in our institution in 1981 [10, 11].

A wide variety of patients with end-stage pulmonary vascular disease could be considered as potential candidates for cardiopulmonary transplantation. Our early clinical experience has been limited to patients with primary pulmonary hypertension and Eisenmenger's Syndrome. Among other potential indications are chronic obstructive pulmonary disease with cor pulmonale, cystic fibrosis, interstitial pulmonary diseases, and long-standing left ventricular dysfunction, due to coronary artery disease, cardiomyopathy, or valvular disease.

The rate limiting factor in clinical cardiopulmonary transplantation at present is the availability of donors. The basic criteria for donor selection are similar to those employed in cardiac transplantation. However, stringent criteria must be applied with respect to the lungs. We require that PO2 be in excess of 100 mm mercury on 40% inspired oxygen, that peak inspiratory pressures be less than 30–35 mm, and that the chest radiograph be normal. Because of the well-known predisposition toward atelectasis, infection, and neurogenic pulmonary edema in the brain dead, intubated patient, it is important to identify a prospective organ donor early on and to move quickly with organ procurement. Furthermore, maintenance of the cardiopulmonary donor prior to organ procurement requires meticulous attention to treatment of diabetes insipidus, relatively strict fluid restriction, and manipulation of peripheral vascular resistance with alpha vasopressor agents when required.

The recipient operation has been described in detail, and several points deserve special mention [12]. The safe removal of the recipient native organs is achieved by sequential excision of the heart, as in cardiac transplantation, the left lung, and the right lung. Particular attention must be paid to preservation of both phrenic nerves on their pedicles, the vagi, and the recurrent laryngeal nerve. In addition, it is essential to obtain meticulous hemostatis in the bronchial circulation, particularly among patients with Eisenmenger's Syndrome, as these vessels are particularly large and friable and are subjected to systemic arterial pressure at the conclusion of cardiopulmonary bypass.

Post-operative management after heart and lung transplantation is particularly challenging. Current post-operative immunosuppression involves the use of azathioprine and cyclosporine. Steroid therapy is ordinarily deferred for two weeks, to permit early tracheal healing. The early post-operative phase in the clinical sphere, as in the laboratory, has been characterized by difficulties with pulmonary insufficiency, associated with the interrelated problems of pulmonary edema with surgical interruption of the lymphatics, denervation, infection, 'reimplantation response', and rejection. Strict fluid restriction and assiduous attention to the possibility of infection versus rejection are the keys to successful post-operative pulmonary management.

Surveillance for rejection after cardiopulmonary transplantation is identical to that employed in cardiac transplantation. However, it should be noted that cases of isolated pulmonary rejection have occurred, and, in the absence of other explanations for radiographic abnormalities, the possibility for pulmonary rejection must be entertained when the clinical findings suggest it. In such instances, open lung biopsy may be required to confirm the diagnosis.

## Results

We have performed 26 combined heart and lung transplant operations in 25 patients as of April 1985. Fifteen of the 25 patients are surviving at intervals of one month to fifty months after operation. Actuarial survival in this small sample appears comparable with that seen in cardiac transplantation at present.

Long-term complications have been observed in this group. In a study of 17 long-term survivors, 7 were found to develop obstructive pulmonary disease. In 5 patients in whom adequate biopsy tissue was available, a histologic pattern of obliterative bronchiolitis was noted, and it has been posited that the development of these changes may represent a chronic rejection phenomenon. Graft atherosclerosis has also been observed, and one patient succumbed 18 months after operation from anterior myocardial infarction.

## References

1. Carrel A, Guthrie CC (1905) The transplantation of veins and organs. Amer Med 10: 1101–1102
2. Demikhov VP (1962) Experimental transplantation of vital organs. Basil Haigh, translator, New York: Consultants Bureau, p 126
3. Gibbon JH (1954) Application of a mechanical heart and lung apparatus to cardiac surgery. Minn Med 37: 171
4. Lower RR and Shumway NE (1960) Studies on orthotopic transplantation of the canine heart. Surg Forum 11: 18
5. Barnard CN (1967) The operation. South African Medical Journal, 41: 1271
6. Stinson EB, Payne R, Griepp RB, Dong E Jr, Shumway NE (1971) Lancet 2: 459
7. Brumbaugh J, Baldwin JC, Stinson EB, Oyer PE, Jamieson SW, Beaver CP, Henley W and Shumway NE (1985) Quantitative analysis of immunosuppression in cyclosporine-treated patients with lymphoma. Heart Transplantation. In press
8. Webb WR, Howard HS (1957) Cardiopulmonary transplantation. Surg Forum 8: 313
9. Lower RR, Stofer RC, Hurley EJ and Shumway NE. Complete homograft replacement of the heart and both lungs (1961) Surgery 50: 840–845
10 Reitz BA, Burton NA, Jamieson SW, Pennock JL, Stinson EB, Shumway NE. Heart and lung transplantation. Auto and allo transplantation in primates with extended survival (1980) Jour of Thoracic and Cardiovascular Surgery 80: 360–371
11. Oyer PE, Stinson EB, Jamieson SW, Hunt SA, Reitz BA, Beiber CP, Schroeder JS (1982) One-year experience with cyclosporin A and clinical heart transplantation. Heart Transplantation 1: 285–290
12. Jamieson SW, Stinson EB, Oyer PE, Baldwin JC and Shumway NE (1984) Operative technique for heart/lung transplantation. Jour of Thor and Cardvascular Surg 87: 930–935
13. Burke CM, Morris AJ, Dawkins KD, Yousem SN, McGregor CGA, Baldwin JC, Theodore J, Jamieson SW. In press. Obliterative bronchiolitis in chronic pulmonary rejection, abstract presented at International Society for Heart Transplantation – 1985.

# III. Chronic coronary heart disease

# Emergency medical treatment in acute coronary insufficiency

P.R. LICHTLEN

Acute coronary insufficiency (ACI) is defined as a syndrome of new and abrupt onset of ischemia. ACI often consists of one single ischemic episode progressing directly into acute myocardial infarction. More common are multiple episodes of prolonged ischemia, repeated attacks of angina pectoris occurring usually at rest, but also at low lewels of exercise [1–4]. When typical, the attacks have a crescendo-character both with regard to their intensity as well as frequency. However, as was shown by continuous monitoring of the electrocardiogram and hemodynamic parameters, not all ischemic attacks are accompanied by angina pectoris [5–7], whereas ischemic ST-segment changes are always present, either ST-depression or ST-elevation depending on the degree and location of ischemia (transmural or endocardial). It is important to note that this syndrome not only includes unstable angina pectoris but also preinfarction angina as well as the acute stage of myocardial infarction [2].

## Pathophysiology of ACI

Medical treatment of ischemia must be oriented on the underlying pathophysiological process. The basic event of ACI always consists in an abrupt decrease of the lumen size of a coronary obstruction in a large coronary artery going from a subcritical stage (e.g. degree of stenosis less than 70%, most stenotic diameter greater than 2 mm) to a clinically critical stage (degree of stenosis between 75 and 95%, most stenotic diameter less than 1 mm or total occlusion) [2, 8] (Fig. 1). This in a minority of cases is due purely to functional changes i.e. a sudden increase in smooth muscle tone in the remaining wall segment of an eccentric stenosis, leading to a critical reduction in lumen size or even complete occlusion, i.e. coronary spasm. Usually, these 'vasospastic' changes of coronary obstructions are reversible, either spontaneously or under the administration of vasorelaxing drugs, mainly Ca-antagonists or nitrates. The abrupt increase in the degree of stenosis, however, more often is due to anatomical changes, i.e. a rapid

172

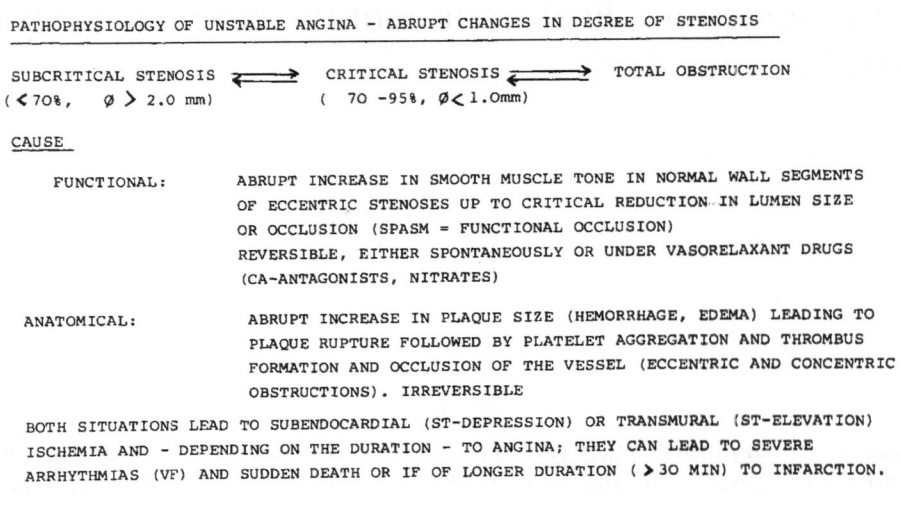

PATHOPHYSIOLOGY OF UNSTABLE ANGINA - ABRUPT CHANGES IN DEGREE OF STENOSIS

SUBCRITICAL STENOSIS ⇌ CRITICAL STENOSIS ⇌ TOTAL OBSTRUCTION
( < 70%,   Ø > 2.0 mm)        ( 70 -95%, Ø< 1.0mm)

CAUSE

FUNCTIONAL:     ABRUPT INCREASE IN SMOOTH MUSCLE TONE IN NORMAL WALL SEGMENTS
                OF ECCENTRIC STENOSES UP TO CRITICAL REDUCTION IN LUMEN SIZE
                OR OCCLUSION (SPASM = FUNCTIONAL OCCLUSION)
                REVERSIBLE, EITHER SPONTANEOUSLY OR UNDER VASORELAXANT DRUGS
                (CA-ANTAGONISTS, NITRATES)

ANATOMICAL:     ABRUPT INCREASE IN PLAQUE SIZE (HEMORRHAGE, EDEMA) LEADING TO
                PLAQUE RUPTURE FOLLOWED BY PLATELET AGGREGATION AND THROMBUS
                FORMATION AND OCCLUSION OF THE VESSEL (ECCENTRIC AND CONCENTRIC
                OBSTRUCTIONS). IRREVERSIBLE

BOTH SITUATIONS LEAD TO SUBENDOCARDIAL (ST-DEPRESSION) OR TRANSMURAL (ST-ELEVATION)
ISCHEMIA AND - DEPENDING ON THE DURATION - TO ANGINA; THEY CAN LEAD TO SEVERE
ARRHYTHMIAS (VF) AND SUDDEN DEATH OR IF OF LONGER DURATION ( > 30 MIN) TO INFARCTION.

*Figure 1.* Pathophysiological concept of unstable angina pectoris. Functional and anatomical changes leading to a sudden increase in the degree of an obstruction in an epicardial coronary artery. (for details see text)

increase in size of an atherosclerotic plaque due to plaque haemorrhage or edema, eventually leading to the rupture of the plaque followed by adhesion and aggregation of platelets at the now rough surface of the plaque; normally this leads to rapid platelet thrombus formation and occlusion of the coronary artery [9, 10]. This usually irreversible process occurs both in eccentric as well as concentric obstructions and independent of their degree, although it is observed more often in high grade obstructions [11, 12]. Both, functional and anatomical changes of stenoses lead to either subendocardial or transmural ischemia, and, depending on the duration of the ischemic event, also to angina; they can result in severe arrhythmias [1, 8], in rare cases in ventricular fibrillation and sudden coronary death [8]; if of longer duration (for instance more than 30 minutes) they can also lead to myocardial infarction. It should be emphasized that in many cases functional and anatomical changes are combined, an abrupt increase in vasomotor tone leading to plaque rupture and platelet thrombus formation and eventually to complete occlusion and acute myocardial infarction [3].

The clinical equivalents of ACI are listed on Figure 2. Unstable angina pectoris concerns mainly angina at rest, especially if it is of the 'spastic' type (variant angina), but also cases with angina at rest and during exercise or in rare cases only during exercise. In angina occurring only at rest, especially when attacks are frequent, a sudden increase in vasomotor tone, coronary spasm is usually present, with or without underlying coronary artery disease, i.e. low or high grade eccentric obstructions [13]; angina at effort usually is accompanied by a marked decrease in exercise capacity and a low anginal threshhold, either due to an

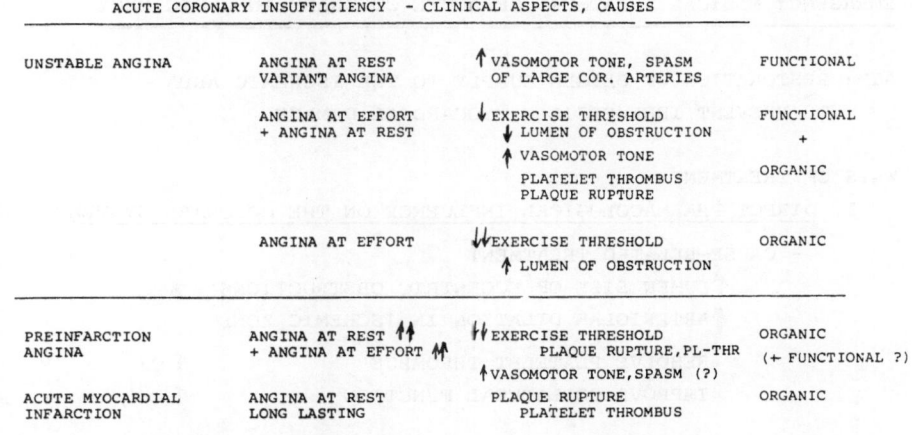

ACUTE CORONARY INSUFFICIENCY - CLINICAL ASPECTS, CAUSES

| UNSTABLE ANGINA | ANGINA AT REST<br>VARIANT ANGINA | ↑ VASOMOTOR TONE, SPASM<br>OF LARGE COR. ARTERIES | FUNCTIONAL |
| | ANGINA AT EFFORT<br>+ ANGINA AT REST | ↓ EXERCISE THRESHOLD<br>↓ LUMEN OF OBSTRUCTION<br>↑ VASOMOTOR TONE<br>PLATELET THROMBUS<br>PLAQUE RUPTURE | FUNCTIONAL<br>+<br>ORGANIC |
| | ANGINA AT EFFORT | ↓↓ EXERCISE THRESHOLD<br>↑ LUMEN OF OBSTRUCTION | ORGANIC |
| PREINFARCTION<br>ANGINA | ANGINA AT REST ↑↑<br>+ ANGINA AT EFFORT ↑↑ | ↑↑ EXERCISE THRESHOLD<br>PLAQUE RUPTURE,PL-THR<br>↑ VASOMOTOR TONE,SPASM (?) | ORGANIC<br>(+ FUNCTIONAL ?) |
| ACUTE MYOCARDIAL<br>INFARCTION | ANGINA AT REST<br>LONG LASTING | PLAQUE RUPTURE<br>PLATELET THROMBUS | ORGANIC |

*Figure 2*. Clinical aspects of acute coronary insufficiency, underlying pathophysiological changes.

increase in vasomotor tone and/or plaque rupture and formation of platelet thrombi, partially occluding the lumen, these thrombi being, however, washed away at various intervals and by this spontaneously reopening the vessel [9]. In preinfarction angina and especially in acute myocardial infarction the cause is usually mainly organic, the rupture of an atherosclerotic plaque leading to a platelet thrombus definitely occluding the vessel. During the last years several reports suggested that also in the majority of patients with classical unstable angina rapid progression of coronary artery disease is the primary underlying process, subtotal obstructions and even sudden occlusions in so-called 'complicated plaques' [8, 14, 15], the increase in vasomotor tone being an associated phenomenon; in these cases myocardial infarction is often prevented due to extensive collateralization which took place at an earlier time, i.e. before complete occlusion of the major coronary artery [2].

**Emergency medical treatment**

The aim of drug treatment is the restauration of oxygen supply to the ischemic area and the prevention of irreversible damage. The various possibilities of drug therapy are summarized in Figure 3.

*Direct pharmacological influence on the coronary system*

Today a variety of drugs is known to lead to vascular smooth muscle relaxation and to coronary artery dilatation and by this to an increase in lumen size,

EMERGENCY MEDICAL TREATMENT OF ACUTE CORONARY INSUFFICIENCY

AIM: RESTORATION OF OXYGEN SUPPLY TO THE ISCHEMIC AREA
     TO PREVENT IRREVERSIBLE MYOCARDIAL DAMAGE

WAYS OF TREATMENT:
  1. DIRECT PHARMACOLOGICAL INFLUENCE ON THE CORONARY SYSTEM

     - CAUSE-RELATED TREATMENT
          ↑LUMEN SIZE OF ECCENTRIC OBSTRUCTIONS)  ↑CF
          ↑ARTERIOLAR DILATION IN ISCHEMIC ZONE)

          RESOLVE PLATELET THROMBUS              ↑ CF
          IMPROVE COLLATERAL FUNCTION            ↑ CF

     - INDIRECT EFFECTS,  OXYGEN DEMAND
          ↓LVEDP,↓LVEDV  ( ↓PRELOAD), RELIEF ENDOCARDIUM
          ↓ BLOOD   PRESSURE   ( ↓ AFTERLOAD)

  2. MYOCARDIAL PROTECTION
          - AFTERLOAD REDUCTION, ↓WALL TENSION, ↓ STRESS
          - PREVENTION OF CA-OVERLOAD
          - PRESERVATION OF MITOCHONDRIAL STRUCTURAL DAMAGE
            OF ATP-BREAKDOWN, OF GLUCOSE-DEPLETION

*Figure 3*. Possible ways of medical treatment of acute coronary insufficiency and expected effects.

especially in eccentric obstructions possessing still enough normal vascular smooth muscle cells able to relax [13, 16]. Marked smooth muscle relaxation is achieved especially by two types of drugs, nitrates and Ca-antagonists. Sublingual administration of nitrates results in an approximately 20 to 30% increase in lumen size of normal epicardial coronary arteries; a similar degree of dilation is also observed in most of the eccentric stenoses [8, 13, 17]. It is of importance to note, however, that nitrates – when administered by the sublingual or oral route – have no effect on coronary arterioles, coronary resistance remaining unchanged and coronary blood flow showing an autoregulatory decrease following the drop in myocardial oxygen consumption [18]. Only when injected directly into a coronary artery does nitroglycerin lead to a short transient increase in coronary blood flow, that is a decrease in coronary resistance [18, 19]. Nitrates, introduced into the treatment of angina pectoris more than 100 years ago, act within the smooth muscle cell, where they are transformed into nitro sothioles and stimulate guanylate cyclase which catalyzes the transformation of GPT to cGMP; the latter, in a so far unknown way leads to profound smooth muscle relaxation [20].

Ca-antagonists were brought into the treatment of ischemic heart disease only during the last 20 years. Today, 3 Ca-antagonists are mainly used, verapamil, diltiazem, and nifedipine, the latter representing the strongest arterial vasodilator among them. Nifedipine, a dihydropyridine, leads to long-standing approximately 30% dilation of normal segments of epicardial coronary arteries as well as of eccentric coronary stenoses [8, 13, 21, 22, 23, 24]. When given sublingually, a slowly progressing dilatation of the epicardial coronary arteries up to 30 minutes and longer can be observed [23, 24, 25, 26]. Furthermore, in contrast to nitroglycerin, nifedipine – as well as diltiazem and verapamil – leads to a mild increase in myocardial blood flow due to coronary arteriolar dilatation which, however, is not strong enough to block autoregulation [27, 28]. Both, nitroglycerin and nifedipine can be administered acutely as intravenous infusions [29] (Fig. 4). Under these conditions, nitroglycerin leads to a transient increase in heart rate and drop in blood pressure, both changes, however, being rapidly corrected by physiological counterregulation (pseudo-tolerance). Nifedipine, in contrast, leads to a mild but long-lasting decrease in systolic blood pressure and increase in cardiac output [29]. Pulmonary wedge pressure on the other hand is reduced only by nitroglycerin. In unstable angina, both drugs lead to a significant reduction in the number of anginal attacks over more than 24 hours [29].

Coronary artery vasorelaxation is enhanced under the combination of nitrates and Ca-antagonists; critical eccentric obstructions often dilate by 50% and more, and the most stenotic diameter often reaches more than 2 mm and by this is well outside the clinically critical range [13, 26] (Fig. 5). This behaviour is based on the

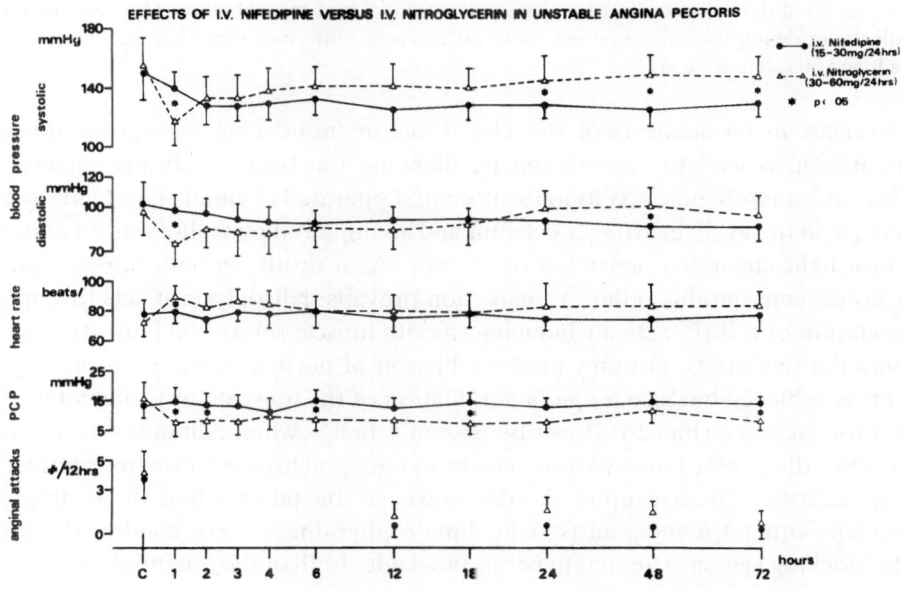

*Figure 4.* Intravenous infusion of Nifedipine (15–30 mg/24 hours) versus Nitroglycerin (30–60 mg/24 hours) over 72 hours in 10 patients with unstable angina pectoris.

EFFECT OF 20mg NIF + .8 mg NTG ON CORONARY ARTERY STENOSES
(n = 50)

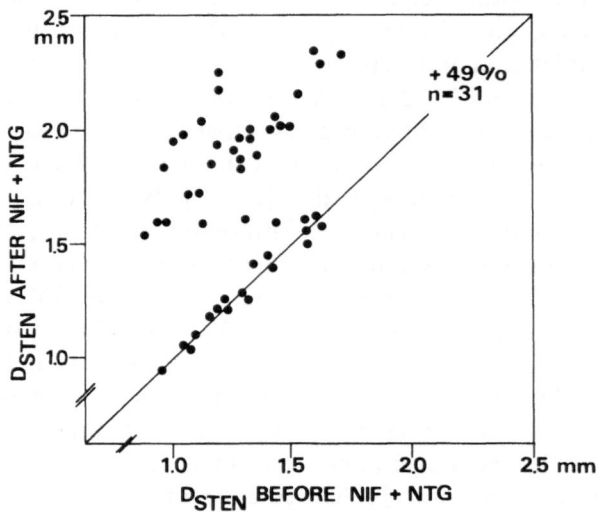

*Figure 5.* Dilation of most stenotic diameter of highgrade coronary obstructions located mainly in the proximal left anterior descending artery. Measurements were performed approx. 10 min. after sublingual administration of the two drugs from coronary angiograms taken in at least 4 different projections, using a vernier caliper with an accuracy of 0.05 mm (interobserver variability less than 7%). The tip of the catheter (diameter approx. 1.8 mm) was used for calibration. Obstructions not dilating were identified as concentric ones, those dilating as eccentric ones with a few exceptions. (for details and literature see text)

differences in mechanisms of the two drugs in influencing vasomotor tone. Ca-antagonists lead to vasodilation by blocking the transmembrane calcium-influx into smooth muscle cells in the potential operated channel. This leads to a decrease in the available trigger-calcium and an impaired phosphorylation of the myosin light chain and activation of myosin. As a result, smooth muscle contraction is considerably reduced, relaxation prevails. Nitroglycerin acts through stimulation of cGMP, actively inducing smooth muscle relaxation [20]. By combining the two drugs, not only marked dilation of normal coronary artery segments is achieved but also a significant dilation of the most stenotic diameter of eccentric stenoses (Fig. 5). It can be assumed that – when administered as an infusion – the effect of the two drugs can be maintained for the entire time of their administration. Great caution should, however, be taken when these drugs, especially other Ca-antagonists than dihydrophyridines – are combined with beta-blocking agents. The simultaneous blockade, both of the potential operated as well as the beta-receptor operated channel leaves the alpha-receptor-operated channel as the only one to influence vasomotor tone; under these circumstances, vasoconstricting stimuli will remain unbalanced by vasodilatation and coronary

BEHAVIOUR OF VASOMOTION OF CORONARY ARTERIES DEPENDING ON
PHARMACOLOGICAL REGULATION OF   POC  AND ROC

| DRUG | POC<br>VC | ROC-$\beta_2$<br>VD | ROC-$\alpha_1$<br>VC | VASOMOTION<br>VC  VD |
|------|------|------|------|------|
| NO DRUG | + | + + | + | ↑   ↑ |
| Ca-ANT-<br>AGONIST | ∅ | + + ( + ) | + ( + ) | ↑  ⇑ |
| Ca-ANT-<br>AGONIST<br>+<br>$\beta$-BLOCKER | ∅ | ∅ | + | ↑  – |

POC = POTENTIAL OPERATED CHANNEL, ROC = RECEPTOR OPERATED
CHANNEL, VC = VASOCONSTRICTION, VD = VASODILATION

*Figure 6.* Vasomotion of coronary arteries in relation to Ca-flux inhibition on the potential and receptor operated channels. (for details see text)

artery spasm may result more easily, especially in patients with a mild tendency to variant angina (typical example in Figure 6). Figure 7 summarizes these effects: if one assumes that under normal conditions smooth muscle vasomotor tone in large epicardial coronary arteries is midway between relaxation and constriction and if vasoconstriction is provided by two other channels, the potential operated channel as well as the alpha-receptor-operated channel whereas active vasodilation is possible only through one channel, the beta 2-receptor channel, it follows that blockade of one constrictor channel (the potential operated channel using a Ca-antagonist) and one dilating channel (the beta 2-receptor operated channel by a beta-blocking agent) leaves the alpha 1-constrictor channel unopposed. In addition, it seems that also in human coronary arteries the alpha-receptor mediated tone is low in comparison to the beta-receptor tone as derived from the absence of vasoconstriction under normal circumstances. However, during blockade of the two channels, any increase in alpha 1-tone can easily lead to massive vasoconstriction, that is coronary artery spasm, especially when additional constricting stimuli are present.

Hence, *prevention of unstable angina pectoris* due to increased vasomotor tone and spasm is best achieved by oral treatment with high doses of Ca-antagonists, if necessary combined with nitrates [30, 31] (Fig. 8). The *acute situation* of unstable angina is preferably managed by intravenous infusion of Ca-antagonists, eventually combined with nitroglycerin until complete suppression of anginal attacks

178

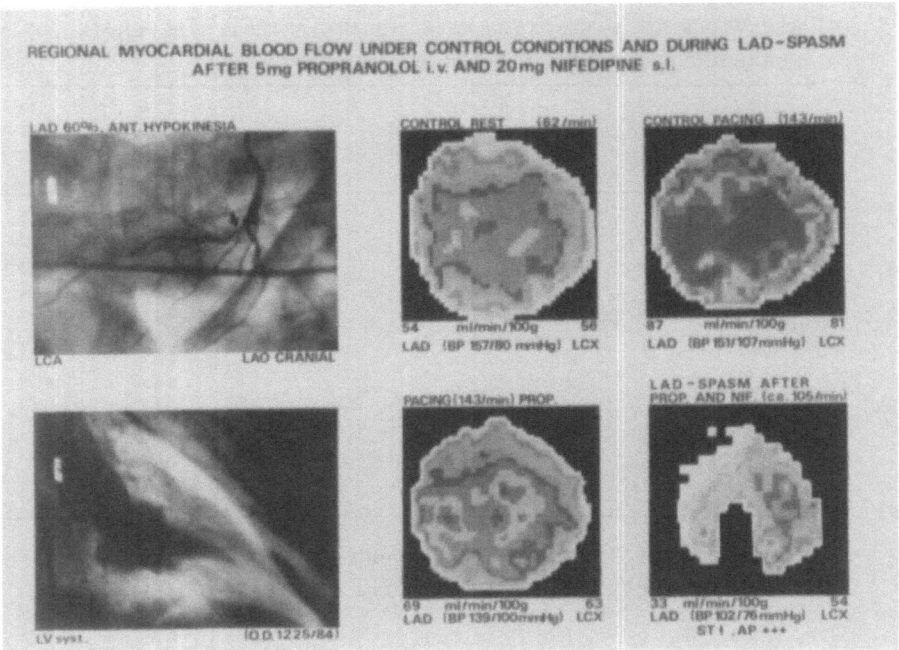

*Figure 7.* Coronary artery spasm after combined administration of Nifedipine (20 mg sublingually) and Propranolol (5 mg i.v.) On the left: coronary and left ventricular angiogram, the former demonstrating a highgrade obstruction in the proximal left anterior descending branch. In the middle and on the right: flow images after intracoronary injection of 20 mCi 133 Xe into the left coronary artery. At rest (middle upper panel) flow was identical in the normal circumflex and the poststenotic LAD-area; during control pacing up to ST-depressions of 0.1 mV in leads V5 and V6 and angina pectoris flow increased in both areas, in the poststenotic area probably due to an increase mainly in the epicardial region; after Propranolol and identical heart rate and duration of pacing flow was lower in both region than during control pacing; 2 minutes after pacing under Propranolol and Nifedipine, ST-elevations in V5 and V6 occurred and the patient suffered from severe angina. Flow decreased to 33 ml/min/100 gr in the poststenotic region, seen also in the loss of colors in the flow image. ECG and flow were only normalized after administration of several capsules of nitroglycerin.

is achieved; this treatment has to be followed by oral administration of these drugs for a longer period of time. In the rare situation of *acute myocardial infarction provoked by coronary artery spasm*, similar treatment as in acute attacks of unstable angina should be instituted. For the reasons mentioned above, beta-blockers should be withhold in this situation.

In presence of platelet thrombus formation following rupture of a plaque, medical treatment has to focus on the prevention or lysis of this clot. During the last years prevention of arterial platelet thrombus formation was attempted mainly by administering acetylsalicylic acid (ASA). Whether large (more than 300 mg/day) or small doses (30 mg/day) should be used, is still an open question.

EMERGENCY MEDICAL TREATMENT IN ACUTE CORONARY INSUFFICIENCY
RELATION BETWEEN CAUSE OF ACI, AIM OF TREATMENT AND CLINICAL EVENT

| | PREVENTION | | ACUTE TREATMENT | |
|---|---|---|---|---|
| | UNSTABLE ANGINA | ACUTE MI | UNSTABLE ANGINA | ACUTE MI |
| INCREASED VASOMOTOR TONE SPASM | ORAL: CA-ANT (+)NITRATES | ---------+ | CA-ANTAGONISTS I.V. ev. oral + i.v. or s.l. NTG  Ø BETABLOCKERS ! | i.v. CA-ANT. + i.v. NTG  Ø BETABLOCKERS ! |
| PLAQUE RUPTURE PLATELET THROMBUS | ASA LOW DOSE! ASASANTIN | ---------+ | ASA ev. TPA ? SK ?? CA-ANTAG. I.V./po | SHORT INTERVAL: SK  IV ± IC TPA ! CARDIOPROTECTION: CA-ANTAGONIST GIK, BBL ? |
| SWELLING RUPTURE OF PLAQUE | ?? CA-ANTAG.? ASA ? | ---------+ | CA-ANT. (HIGH DOSE) ev. NTG | ?? |

OFTEN COMBINATION OF DRUGS IS NECESSARY, OFTEN DRUGS CAN ONLY ASSIST INVASIVE REPERFUSION-TREATMENT

*Figure 8.* Emergency medical treatment of acute coronary insufficiency, preventions and acute treatment (see text).

The rationale to use small doses is based on the observation that high doses of ASA would block not only thromboxane A2 but also prostaglandine formation as ASA through acetylation irreversibly inhibits cyclo-oxygenase and affects both legs of the arachidonic pathway blocking the production of cyclic endoperoxides [10, 31]. It would therefore seem that with regard to thromboxane A2, which causes vasoconstriction and platelet aggregation, the administration of ASA leads to a beneficial effect, whereas with regard to prostacycline (PGI2) causing vasodilation and inhibition of platelet aggregation [32], an unwanted effect would result. Whether low doses of ASA block only the thromboxane pathway without influencing the prostacycline pathway, is, however, still unclear at the present time.

In the rare event of ACI due to plaque rupture and platelet thrombus formation not yet developing to acute myocardial infarction – as in the presence of good collateral function – an attempt to lyse the clot should be made either using streptokinase or tissue plasminogene activators (TPA), the latter due to its higher specificity being more suitable for that treatment. In these cases, however, thrombolytic therapy should only be instituted when platelet thrombus formation as the cause of unstable angina pectoris has been clearly demonstrated by coronary angiography [14]. Ca-antagonists and eventually nitrates should always be added for additional vasodilation.

Treatment of *acute myocardial infarction* today often includes thrombolysis. Up to now plasminogen activators, especially streptokinase were used, administered either directly into the occluded coronary artery [33, 34], a procedure necessitating coronary catheterization or they were given systemically by intravenous infusion [35, 36]. Most recently, tissue plasminogene activators, especially from the recombinant type, were introduced [37–40]. This treatment has the advantage that fibrinolysis takes place mainly at the location of the clot and by this avoids a massive decrease of systemic fibrinogen as observed under streptokinase. In addition, it is also free from immunological reactions. Multicenter studies using TPA in acute myocardial infarction are underway [39, 40].

Thrombolysis in acute myocardial infarction should – whenever possible – be accompanied by measures for *myocardial protection*. It was shown very clearly, that during ischemia there is extensive Ca-overload of the cytosole and especially of the mitochondria leading to irreversible membrane and mitochondrial damage [41, 42]; animal experiments showed that this can be avoided by administration of Ca-antagonists and LV-function can be preserved to a great deal [42, 43]. Both measures, thrombolysis as well as cardioprotection through administration of Ca-antagonists are, however, only effective, when the time of ischemia is kept short, i.e. reperfusion takes place before complete irreversible damage has occurred [42]. The fact that animal experiments showed a clear cardioprotective effect when these drugs were given before coronary occlusion is promising, however, is only of limited value with regard to the human situation. Nevertheless, it can be said that today there is a positive trend throughout the medical community towards acceptance of early reperfusion through clot lysis by intravenous administration either of streptokinase or TPA in acute myocardial infarction; it is also felt that angioplasty of the remaining high degree obstruction should be performed soon after clot lysis. This type of treatment is especially recommendable in younger people and whenever the interval between the onset of anginal pain and the possible administration of thrombolytic agents is short (less than 3 hours). Nevertheless, at the present time, reperfusion is not yet 'a must'. Most of the studies published so far are still equivocal with regard to limitation of infarct size as well as reduction of early and late mortality, especially when complications of thrombolysis are included. On the other hand, the present data from several centres also suggest that mortality of acute myocardial infarction is considerably increased if no early or late lysis of the clot is achieved and the infarct-related vessel remains completely occluded [34, 44].

## Conclusions

Emergency medical treatment of acute coronary insufficiency became a reality today and should always preceed the invasive treatment. Often it is mandatory that medical treatment is prolonged during the time of invasive treatment and even beyond.

# References

1. Lichtlen PR (1980) Klinik, Diagnostik und Therapie der Unstabilen Angina pectoris. Internist 21: 636–645
2. Lichtlen PR (1983) Klinik und medikamentôse Therapie der koronaren Herzkrankheit. Dtsch Ärztebl 80: 17–31, 32–36
3. Maseri A (1982) Active and quiescent phases in coronary disease: Role of varied and changing susceptability to dynamic obstructions. Circulation 63: II-B
4. Chierchia S (1985) Unstable Angina pectoris: Pathophysiologic concepts derived from clinical observations. In: Hugenholtz P, Goldman BS (eds) Unstable angina, current concepts and management. Stuttgart-New York: Schattauer, p 49–54
5. Deanfield JE, Maseri A, Selwyn AP, Ribeiro P, Chierchia S, Krikler S, Morgan M (1983) Myocardial ischemia during daily life in patients with stable angina. Relation to symptoms and heart rate changes. Lancet Vol 2 (Oct 1): 753–758
6. Deanfield JE (1984) Assessment of transient myocardial ischemia in daily life. In: Hammersmith Cardiology Workshop Series, Vol. I, A. Maseri, J.F. Goodwin (eds), Raven Press, New York, p 113–117
7. Selwyn A (1985) Value of continuous ECG in detecting ST-depression and arrhythmias. Eur Heart J (in press)
8. Lichtlen PR, Rafflenbeul W, Freudenberg H (1985) Pathoanatomy and function of coronary obstructions leading to unstable angina pectoris, anatomical and angiographic studies. In: Unstable angina, current concepts and management, P.G. Hugenholtz, B.S. Goldman (eds), Schattauer, Stuttgart-New York, p 81–93
9. Folts JD, Crowell EB, Row GG (1976) Platelet aggregation in partially obstructed vessels and its elimination with aspirin. Circulation 54: 365–377
10. Born GVR (1985) Pathogenetic possibilities of unstable angina. In: Unstable angina, current concepts and management. P.G. Hugenholtz, B.S. Goldman (eds), Schattauer, Stuttgart-New York, p 13–18
11. Davies MJ, Thomas A (1984) Thrombolysis and acute coronary artery lesions in sudden cardiac ischemic death. New Engl J Med 310: 1137–40
12. Davies MJ, Thomas A (1981) The pathological basis and microanatomy of occlusive thrombus formation in human coronary arteries. Phil Trans R Soc London B294: 225–29
13. Rafflenbeul W, Lichtlen PR (1982) Zum Konzept der dynamischen Koronarstenose (The concept of dynamic coronary stenoses). ZfK 71: 439–444
14. Théroux P, Moise A, Waters DD (1985) Coronary angiography in unstable angina. In: Unstable angina, current concepts and management, P.G. Hugenholtz, B.S. Goldman (eds), Schattauer, Stuttgart-New York, p 39–47
15. Moise A, Théroux P, Taeymans Y, Waters DD, L'Espérance J, Fines P, Descoings B, Robert P (1984) Clinical and angiographic factors associated with progression of coronary artery disease. JACC 3: 659–667
16. Freudenberg H, Lichtlen P (1981) The normal wall segment in coronary stenoses – a postmortal study. ZfK 70: 863–869
17. Rafflenbeul W, Urtaler F, Russell RO, Lichtlen P, James TN (1979) Dilatation of coronary artery stenoses after isosorbide dinitrate in man. Br Heart J 43: 546–549
18. Lichtlen PR, Halter J, Gattiker K (1974) The effect of isosorbide dinitrate on coronary flow, coronary resistance, and left ventricular dynamics under exercise in patients with coronary artery disease. Basic Res in Cardiol 69: 402–420
19. Bernstein L, Friesinger GC, Lichtlen PR, Ross RS (1966) The effect of nitroglycerin on the systemic and coronary circulation in man and dogs. Myocardial blood flow measured with 133-Xenon. Circulation 33: 107–
20. Kukovetz WR, Holzmann S (1983) Mechanism of nitrate-induced vasodilation and tolerance.

182

ZfK 72, Suppl III: 14–19
21. Schulz W, Anderten W, Reiber JHC, Bernauer R, Kaltenbach M, Kober G (1983) Active and passive coronary vasodilation after intracoronary and sublingual nitroglycerin. ZfK 72, Suppl III: 82–86
22. Lichtlen PR, Rafflenbeul W (1985) Effects of Calcium-antagonists on fixed and dynamic obstructions in patients with severe coronary artery disease. In: Proceedings of the meeting on dihydropyridines, R. Gross (ed), Springer-Verlag, Heidelberg (in press)
23. Nellessen U, Daniel W, Rafflenbeul W, Reil G, Raude E, Hecker H, Lichtlen P (1985) Dilation of human epicardial coronary arteries after nifedipine in relation to blood levels. In: 6th International Adalat-Symposium, P.R. Lichtlen (ed), Excerpta Medica, Amsterdam (in press)
24. Schulz W, Kraus G, Kaltenbach M, Kober G (1981) Einfluß von intrakoronarem und intravenösem Nifedipine auf die allgemeine und lokale Weite von epikardialen Koronararterien bei stabiler Angina pectoris – ein anti-anginöser Wirkaspekt. ZfK 70: 809–815
25. Rafflenbeul W, Lichtlen PR (1983) Quantitative coronary angiography: evidence of a sustained increase in vascular smooth muscle tone in coronary artery stenoses. ZfK 72: Suppl III, 87–91
26. Rafflenbeul W, Lichtlen PR (1983) Release of residual vascular tone in coronary artery stenoses with nifedipine and glyceryl-trinitrate. In: 5th International Adalat Symposium, M. Kaltenbach, H.N. Neufeldt (eds), Excerpta Medica, Amsterdam-Oxford-Princeton, p 300–308
27. Lichtlen PR, Daniel WG, Engel HJ (1985) Effects of the calcium-entry blocking agents nifedipine, verapamil and diltiazem on regional myocardial blood flow in patients with severe coronary artery disease. (in prep)
28. Lichtlen PR (1975) Coronary and left ventricular dynamics under nifedipine in comparison to nitrates, beta-blocking agents and dipyridamole. In: 2nd International Adalat Symposium, W. Lochner, W. Braasch, K. Kroneberg (eds), Springer, Berlin-Heidelberg-New York, p 212–224
29. Rafflenbeul W, Bossaller C, Lichtlen P (1985) Intravenous infusion of nifedipine in patients with unstable angina pectoris. In: 6th International Adalat Symposium, P.R. Lichtlen (ed), Excerpta Medica, Amsterdam (in press)
30. Antman E, Muller J, Goldberg S, McAlpin R, Rubenfier M et al. (1980) Nifedipine therapy for coronary artery spasm, experience in 127 patients. New Engl J Med 302: 1269–73
31. Goldman GJ, Pitchard AD (1983) The natural history of coronary artery disease: Does medical therapy improve the prognosis? Progr in Cardiovasc Dis 25: 513–522
32. Dustin GJ, Moncada S, Vane JR (1979) Prostaglandines, their intermediate and precursor: Cardiovascular actions and regulatory roles in normal and abnormal circulatory systems. Progr in Cardiovasc Dis 21: 405–430
33. Schwarz F, Schuler G, Katus H, Hofmann M, Manthey J, Tillmann H, Mehmel H, Kübler W (1982) Intracoronary thrombolysis in acute myocardial infarction: duration of ischemia as a major determinant of late results after recanalization. Am J Cardiol 50: 933–937
34. Kennedy JW, Ritchy JL, Davis KB, Stadius ML, Maynord CH, Fritz JK (1985) The Western Washington randomized trial of intracoronary streptokinase in acute myocardial infarction. A 12 months follow-up report. New Engl J Med 312: 1073–78
35. Ganz W, Geft I, Shah PK, Lew AS, Rodriguez L, Weiss T, Maddahi J, Behrman DS, Charuzi Y, Swan HJC (1984) Intravenous streptokinase in evolving acute myocardial infarction. Am J Cardiol 53: 1209–1216
36. Schröder R, Biamino G, von Leitner ER, Linderer TH, Heitz J, Vôhringer HF, Wegscheider K, Andresen D, Arndts HR, Brüggemann Th, Grassot A, Lichey J, Oeff M, Brocain E, Schäfer JH, Sörensen R (1982) Systemische Thrombolyse mit Streptokinase – Kurzzeitinfusion bei akutem Myokardinfarkt. ZfK 71: 709–718
37. Tiefenbrunn AJ, Robinson AK, Kurnick PB, Ludbrook PA, Sobel BE (1985) Clinical pharmacology in patients with evolving myocardial infarction of tissue-type plasminogene activator produced by recombinant DNA technology. Circ 71: 110–116
38. Collen D, Topol EJ, Tiefenbrunn AJ, Gold HK, Weisfeldt MN, Sobel BE et al. (1984) Coronary

thrombolysis with recombinant human tissue-type plasminogen activator: a prospective, randomized, placebo-controlled trial. Circ 70: 1012–1017

39. The TIMI Study Group (1985) The thrombolysis in myocardial infarction (TIMI) trial. New Engl J Med, April 4th: 932–936

40. Verstraete M, Borg M, Cullen D, Erbel R, Lennane RJ, Mathey D, Michels HR, Scharff M, Kebis R, Bernard R, Brower RW, de Bono DP, Huhmann W, Lubsen J, Meyer J, Rutsch H, Schmidt W, von Essen R (1985) A randomized trial of intravenous recombinant tissue-type plasminogen activator versus intravenous streptokinase in acute myocardial infarction. Lancet, April 13th: 842–847

41. Nayler WG (1983) The role of calcium in myocardial ischemia and cell death. In: Calcium channel blocking agents in the treatment of cardiovascular disorders, P.H. Stone, E.M. Antman (eds), Futura Publishing Comp, Mount Kisko, New York, p 81–105

42. Reimer KA, Jennings RB (1985) Effects of calcium channel blockers on myocardial preservation during experimental acute myocardial infarction. Am J Cardiol 55: 107B–115B

43. Henry PD, Schuchleib R, Burda LJ (1978) Effects of nifedipine on myocardial perfusion in ischemic injury in dogs. Circ Res 43: 372–379

44. Trappe HJ, Hartwig CA, Wenzlaff P, Lichtlen PR (1985) Arrhythmia profile and sudden cardiac death in patients with isolated stenoses or occlusions of the left anterior descending branch. ZfK 74: 165–175

# Percutaneous transluminal coronary angioplasty

P. LEIMGRUBER and A.R. GRÜNTZIG

## Introduction

In the United States, atherosclerotic coronary vascular disease remains the most common cause of death. Despite tremendous emphasis on diagnosis and disease prevention, most advances have come in the form of palliative therapy of overt disease.

The medical treatment of coronary artery disease has improved due to the introduction of beta blockers and calcium blockers. In addition, bypass graft surgery has undergone numerous refinements since Favaloro first implanted an aortic coronary saphenous vein graft in 1967 [1]. This procedure has been tremendously effective in providing symptomatic relief for most patients with obstructive coronary disease.

The origin of percutaneous transluminal coronary angioplasty (PTCA) can be traced to the work of Dr. Dotter who in 1964 introduced a catheter technique for therapeutic intervention in peripheral vascular disease [2]. This technique was improved to include a distensible (balloon) tip in 1974 [3]. Further changes led to its experimental use in the coronary circulation in 1976 [4]. Finally, on September 16, 1977 in Zurich, Switzerland, PTCA was first performed on a patient with obstructive coronary artery disease by Dr. Gruentzig [5]. Since then, PTCA has undergone tremendous change and improvement in material and technique, with a corresponding drop in morbidity and mortality. Today it is considered the therapy of choice in selected patients with coronary artery disease and is an alternative for patients who would otherwise require bypass graft surgery.

## Indications

Indications for PTCA have changed considerably during the past several years because of procedure refinements and technical advances.

Single vessel disease: well-defined, hemodynamically significant single vessel disease remains the classic indication for PTCA. Patients in this group would otherwise require bypass graft surgery because of severe symptoms refractory to medical treatment. Patients should be selected for PTCA whose anatomy is favorable for dilatation. Stenosis length should not exceed 15–20 mm. Patients with left main stenosis are excluded due to the potential hazard of life-threatening dissection of this vital vessel as well as possible unfavorable long term results. Patients who have had prior bypass graft surgery can also be candidates for PTCA. However, this group of patients has a higher morbidity and mortality rate when emergency bypass surgery is required following PTCA [6]. Though initial success is comparable to single vessel angioplasty, the recurrence rate in dilated vein grafts is higher than when angioplasty is performed in native coronary arteries. One exception to this rule is stenosis in vein grafts involving a distal anastomcsis site. These have excellent long-term prognosis.

Double vessel disease: High success rates and low complication rates have led to the inclusion of patients with double vessel disease as acceptable candidates for PTCA. Criteria for selection of patients in this group is stricter than that outlined for single vessel disease since these patients have an increased potential of having complications. Further work still needs to be done regarding the timing and strategy of dilatation in patients with multivessel diseases.

Other indications: Recent advances in PTCA have shown it to be a concomitant modality of treatment to streptokinase in patients with acute myocardial infarction. Also, in a small group of patients requiring bypass graft surgery, intraoperative angioplasty can be used to dilate small vessels otherwise not amenable to bypass grafting.

**Procedure**

PTCA demands more concise angiographic information than that possible in many catheterization laboratories. High resolution and rapid visualization of multiple projections is necessary for catheter manipulation. Radiological capabilities considered optimal for performing PTCA include 1) an X-ray tube image intensifier capable of multiangular projections, including cranial and caudal angulation. It should be easy to position and preferably biplanal; 2) a high resolution image intensifier and monitor chain to provide definition of the steerable 0.4 mm diameter guidewire; 3) multimode image intensification including 10–13, 15–18, 30–23 cm field sizes; 4) capacity for increasing those permitting brief periods of increased penetration and definition; 5) high resolution freeze frame video recorder so that at least 2 guide projections can be displayed simultaneously for comparison with real-time images. Four TV monitors are necessary.

Two catheters are needed to perform PTCA. A guiding catheter is available in modified Judkins, Amplatz and Brachial size #8 and #9 French. The dilatation catheter has two lumen. The central lumen is utilized for contrast injections, pressure measurements and passage of a small 0.4 mm steerable guidewire. The balloon dilatation catheter is advanced over the guidewire once it is placed in the appropriate coronary artery. The second lumen is used for balloon inflation with a mixture of contrast material in a 50/50 ratio with sterile, normal saline. This presents visualization of the balloon and prevents air embolism should the balloon rupture. The outer diameter of the balloon is predetermined and constant during a wide range of inflation pressures (5–10 atmosphores). At present, inflatable sized balloons are available in outer diameters of 2–4.2 mm.

The dilatation catheter is inserted into the guiding catheter through a Y-connector. This makes it possible to continuously monitor relative pressure at the tip of the guiding catheter and to inject contrast material into the coronary ostium for visualization of the corresponding coronary arteries.

After a patient's functional capacity has been defined by exercise testing and surgical backup arranged, informed consent is obtained. The patient is taken to the cath laboratory. Tranquilizers are given as pre-medication. Local anesthesia to the groin is accomplished with 2% Lidocaine. The femoral vein is cannulated and a pacing catheter is advanced into the right ventricular apex. This is for controling brady-arrhythmias and serves as a spatial marker between contrast injections. The femoral artery is then punctured and a sheath inserted. Using a 1.6 mm diameter guidewire, the selected guiding catheter is advanced retrogradely into the ascending aorta. Several medications are administered at this point to prevent thrombosis (10000 units Heparin intravenously) and to minimize spasm (nitrates and calcium blockers). Angiograms of the vessel are obtained to 1) define anatomy and to be certain the guiding catheter is seated properly in the coronary ostium without wedging, which prevents severe hemodynamic consequences; 2) define the lesion's geometry, including its eccentricity; 3) define the vascular path to the stenosis so that the origins of side branches are displayed; 4) identify branches at risk of closure during balloon inflation; and 5) define the distal vessel and its ramifications.

The dilatation catheter is then advanced through the guiding catheter with the movable, steerable J guidewire extending from the catheter tip about 10–15 cm. Since the guidewire can be rotated 360°, it is possible to selectively advance the wire and subsequently maneuver the balloon catheter into the appropriate coronary artery. Aortic pressure and the pressure at the distal tip of the balloon catheter are continuously and simultaneously recorded. A sharp drop in distal pressure occurs when the lesion has been crossed with the balloon catheter. When the catheter is in the desired location, the balloon is inflated for 20–30 seconds. Often several inflations are necessary to obtain satisfactory angiographic enlargement of the stenosis. The pressure gradient across the stenosis should be reduced to less than 15–20 mmHg for a satisfactory dilatation. Once an adequate result has been obtained (often with several inflations), the procedure is terminated and pull-back pressures are recorded. A post-interventional angiogram is performed in 3 different views. Residual percent diameter stenosis is measured using a digital electronic caliper system from the mean value of the 3 projections. The patient is returned to his room and the femoral sheaths are removed, approximately 3 hours later. Appropriate local hemostasis is applied. Patients are routinely monitored with telemetry after the procedure and CPK checked regularly. Post-procedure medications include nitrates, calcium blockers, and acetylsalicylic acid.

## Results

Success rates have risen and frequency of complications have lessened as experience with angioplasty increases (Table 1).

Between 1980 and 1984, 3956 patients underwent balloon dilatation at Emory University Hospital. Several patients had dilatations in more than 1 artery for a total of 4592 attempted lesions. The overall primary success rate was 90%. Emergency coronary bypass surgery was necessary in 2.7% of the patients. MI defined by Q-waves or significant R loss was present in 2.5% of the patients and mortality was 0.2%.

The primary success rate has increased steadily with a significant increase demonstrated after the advent of the steerable balloon catheter in 1982.

Recently, the National Heart, Lung and Blood Institute PTCA Registry reported the results of 3079 patients. The reported primary success rate was 67%. Emergency coronary artery bypass graft surgery was neccessary in 6.6% of the patients, MI occurred in 5.3%, and deaths related to PTCA occurred in 0.9%. In the same report, PTCA was associated with a significantly lower success rate, higher complication rate, mortality rate in women than in men. The difference was attributed to the female patients being older and more symptomatic [7].

The long-term efficacy of PTCA is very encouraging. After one year post-PTCA, 78% of the patients remained improved [8]. According to the data from the National Heart, Lung and Blood Institute PTCA Registry, successful PTCA

*Table 1.* Emory University experience.

|  | Patients N | Lesions N | Primary success | Patient (%) | | |
|---|---|---|---|---|---|---|
|  |  |  |  | CABG | MI | Death |
| 1980–81 | 518 | 540 | 82% | 5.6 | 3.7 | 0 |
| 1982 | 813 | 896 | 91% | 2.8 | 1.7 | 0.1 |
| 1983 | 1260 | 1424 | 91% | 2.1 | 2.0 | 0.2 |
| 1984 | 1365 | 1532 | 90% | 2.5 | 2.9 | 0.2 |
| Total | 3956 | 4392 | 90% | 2.7 | 2.5 | 0.2 |

188

alone results in sustained improvement in 84% of patients. The angiographic recurrence rate in our institute is currently 32%. However, this figure may be misleading since many patients who are asymptomatic refuse to undergo repeat angiogram because of their clinical well-being. Recurrence is most common within the first 6 months after PTCA. A second PTCA carries a smaller complication rate and a better primary success rate. Recurrence after the second dilatation is similar to that of the first procedure.

It is estimated that approximately 15–20% of patients requiring revascularization can be treated with PTCA. When carefully chosen, this therapeutic alternative not only has many benefits comparable with those of surgery but has additional advantages as well. These include functional outcome, reduction in physical and emotional suffering, substantial economic savings, and reduced time lost from work. In conclusion, the role of PTCA in the management of coronary artery disease has continued to evolve during the past six years as experience has grown and technical advances have been made. As has been clearly demonstrated in its relatively short history, PTCA offers an effective means of immediate palliation in symptomatic coronary artery disease. The natural history of coronary artery disease is one of progression and the ideal therapy is one which can be used repeatedly through the years. Technical advances in our diagnostic skills hopefully will enable physicians to intervene earlier in the course of the disease, prior to the compromise of ventricular function which often accompanies triple vessel disease. The main question, however, is still unanswered and that is whether PTCA is an alternative approach to coronary artery bypass graft surgery in patients with multivessel disease. Preliminary reports indicate safety and good results may be obtained when PTCA is performed in these patients. However, the true usefulness and exact role needs to be carefully determined in a randomized study comparing coronary artery bypass surgery and PTCA in patients with multivessel disease. Hopefully in the future, patients with coronary artery disease can be diagnosed early before their disease progresses to severe triple vessel disease, when it may be too late for PTCA.

### References

1. Favaloro RG (1968) Saphenous vein autograft replacement of severe segmental coronary occlusion: Operative technique. Am Thorac Surg 5: 334–339
2. Dotter CT, Judkins MP (1964) Transluminal treatment of arteriosclerotic obstruction: Description of a new technic and a preliminary report of its application. Circulation 30: 654–670
3. Grüntzig AR, Hopf H (1974) Perkutane Rekanalisation chronischer arterieller Verschlüsse mit einem neuen Dilatationskatheter: Modifikation der Dotter-Technik. Deutsch med Wschr 99: 2502–2505
4. Grüntzig A, Riedhammr H, Turina M, Rutishauser W (1976) Eine neue Methode zur perkutanen Dilatation von Koronarstenosen Tierexperimentelle Prüfung. Verh Deutsch Ges Herz Kreislaufforsch 42: 282–285

5. Grüntzig AR, Senning A, Siegenthaler WE (1979) Non-operative dilatation of coronary artery stenosis. NEJM 301: 61–68
6. Dorros G, Cowley MJ, Simpson J, Bentivoglio LG, Block PC, Bourassa M, Detre K, Gosselin AJ, Grüntzig AR, Kelsey SF, Kent KM, Mock MB, Mullin SM, Myler RK, Passamani ER, Stertzer SH, Williams DO (1983) Percutaneous transluminal coronary angioplasty: Report of complications from the National Heart, Lung, and Blood Institute PTCA Registry. Circulation 67: 730
7. Cowley MJ, Mullin SM, Kelsey S, Kent KM, Grüntzig A, Detre K, Passamani ER (1985) Sex differences in early and long-term results of coronary angioplasty in the NHLBI PTCA Registry. Circulation 71: 90
8. Kent KM, Bentivoglio LG, Block PC, Bourassa MG, Cowley M, Dorros G, Detre K, Gosselin AJ, Grüntzig A, Kelsley SF, Mock M, Mullin S, Passamani E, Myler RK, Simpson J, Stertzer SH, Williams DO (1983) Long-term efficacy of percutaneous transluminal coronary angioplasty (PTCA): Report from NHLBI-PTCA Registry. (abstr) Circ 68 (Suppl III): 6

# The role of percutaneous transluminal coronary angioplasty (PTCA) in unstable angina

J. MEYER, R. ERBEL, H.J. SCHMITZ, T. POP, K. v. OLSHAUSEN,
B. HENKEL, H.J. RUPPRECHT, H. KOPP and S. EFFERT

## Summary

Transluminal coronary angioplasty is successfully used in stable and unstable angina. Preferably the first angiography and PTCA are performed within the same cath-lab procedure. By this, the patient has not to be exposed to the cath-lab situation twice. The costs for personnel and material are reduced. In 145 patients the stenosis diameter was improved from $75.9 \pm 11.7\%$ obstruction to $23.3 \pm 17.1\%$ (improvement $52.6 \pm 17.9\%$) without significant differences between concentric and eccentric, but with differences in right and left coronary artery stenoses. The absolute diameter was improved from $0.69 \pm 0.29$ mm to $2.07 \pm 0.48$ mm (improvement $1.4 \pm 0.55$ mm), in the 1984 series from $0.58 \pm 0.31$ mm to $1.94 \pm 0.51$ mm (improvement $1.36 \pm 0.48$ mm).

In 81 successfully treated patients a control angiography has been performed after six months. The recurrence rate was significantly higher than in stable angina (36% vs. 28%). The stenoses had deteriorated from $23.7 \pm 16.2\%$ immediately after the dilatation to $40.8 \pm 28.3\%$ at the control study. There were no significant differences between the group with lasting success and that with a restenosis with respect to the degree of the initial stenosis and the immediate result after dilatation.

The number of pathologically contracting segments was diminished from $6.2 \pm 5.9$ to $3.2 \pm 4.8$ segments in patients with good results and remained constant ($7.0 \pm 5.6$ to $7.0 \pm 4.6$ segments) in those with restenosis.

PTCA can be used with good results and a low complication rate ($<3\%$) as well in unstable as in stable angina. Since the trauma for the patient and the costs for personnel and material are much lower than with bypass surgery, PTCA is an alternative in a remarkable percentage of patients.

Percutaneous transluminal coronary angioplasty (PTCA) can nowadays be regarded as an established therapy for patients with chronic stable angina pectoris [1, 2]. Since 1980 this method is also successfully applied to patients with unstable angina [3–8]. In this subgroup of angina pectoris a reasonable number of patients (approximately 30%) show localized major stenoses [9]. While some patients can be stabilized medically, others deserve emergency coronary bypass graft operation [10]. Since 1978 we regularly schedule coronary arteriographies in patients with unstable angina in such a way that PTCA can immediately be performed where necessary.

**Patients and methods**

Onehundredfortyfive patients with a clinical syndrome of unstable angina were selected for PTCA. Most of them were transferred from other institutions after having had their first coronary arteriography there. All patients had developed increasingly frequent attacks of severe pain either of recent onset or superimposed on previously milder angina within the last two to three months. In at least one instance reversible ST-segment elevations or depressions and/or negative T-waves without development of new Q-waves were recorded in each patient. Before PTCA there were no major enzyme changes indicative of a myocardial infarction.

The pretreatment consisted of 20 mg nifedipine and 500 mg acetylsalicylic acid the day before PTCA. Most of them were primarily treated with nitroglycerin infusions (2–10 mg/h), nifedipine (3–4 × 20 mg/24 h) and betablockers (50–200 mg metoprolol/24 h) in order to stabilize the crescendo angina.

Before PTCA the principal investigator explained the protocol, possible advantages and the risk of the method to the patient. All patients received a detailed written information form, which had been approved by the university's legal advisers. Written consent was obtained not only for PTCA but also for an emergency bypass operation, should this become necessary.

After the arterial punction 10000 IU of heparin were given i.v. Before withdrawing the balloon from the coronary artery 0.2 mg nitroglycerin plus another 3000 IU of heparin were injected intracoronarily via the lumen of the balloon catheter. The procedures were regularly scheduled at noon time, when a surgical team was available for an emergency bypass operation.

After PTCA all patients were monitored for 24 hours in the coronary care unit, ECGs and blood samples for enzyme analysis were taken every six hours. The introducing sheeth was left in place for 24–36 hours in order to have a quick access in case of late complications. Heparin was administered for 24 hours after the operation at a rate of 800–1200 IU/h. Additionally 3 × 20 mg of nifedipine were given.

The patients were usually discharged three days later. Until 1981 they received oral coumadine for six months. Since 1982 they regularily took 500 mg acetylsalicylic acid/die for six months plus 3 × 10 mg nifedipine/die. The routine control arteriography was scheduled six months later.

Up to now 81 of the successfully treated patients had a follow-up study. They received 10 mg nifedipine and 500 mg acetylsalicylic acid the evening before and 20 mg nifedipine and 1.6 mg nitroglycerin immediately before the control procedure.

Statistical analysis was performed using students' T-test for unpaired samples. A p-value <0.05 was considered to be significant. All numbers given represent mean values plus minus standard deviation.

## Results

### Acute results

Between 1978 and 1982 the success rate was 75%. After low profile balloon catheters with steerable guide became available, the success rate in 1983 and 1984 had risen to 80%. In 163 patients with stable angina treated 1983 and 1984 this rate has been 85%. Because of the improved catheter material the number of high-grade stenoses passed by the balloon has slightly risen between the series 1978–1983. (Fig. 1) and 1984 (Fig. 2). The degree of stenoses in unsuccessfully treated patients in both series was higher than in those with a successful approach. In the 1984 series (Fig. 2) the degree of passed stenoses was slightly higher than in the

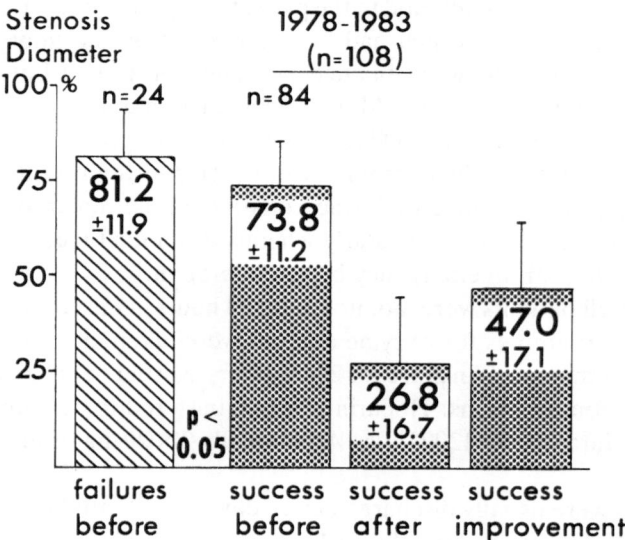

*Figure 1.* Dilatation for unstable angina, results of the series 1978–1983. Stenoses measured in percent of luminal diameter.

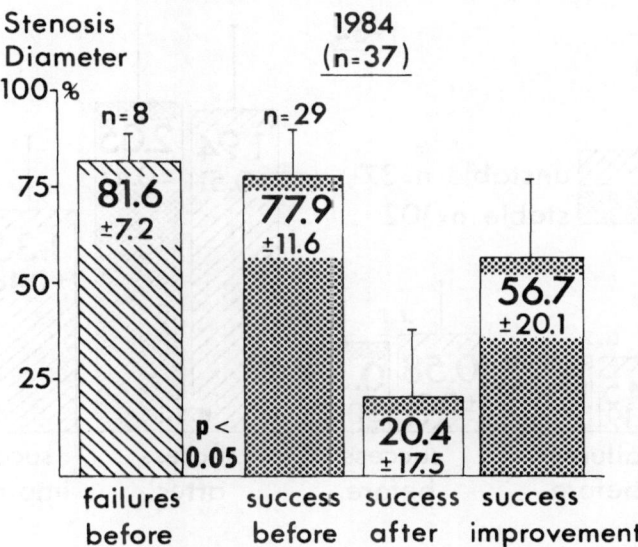

*Figure 2.* Dilatation for unstable angina, series 1984. Stenoses measured in percent of luminal diameter.

previous one. After the treatment the resting stenoses in the early series was reduced to 26.8 ± 16.7%. In the recent series the remaining stenosis was even less (20.4 ± 17.5%). The improvement of luminal diameter has risen from 47.0 ± 17.1 to 56.7 ± 20.1%.

The comparison between patients with unstable and with stable angina pectoris in the 1984 series (Fig. 3) shows no significant difference in the successfully and the unsuccessfully treated groups. There were no significant differences in the diameter of the vessels immediately after treatment in both groups. Also the rate of improvement was comparable in both groups (Fig. 3).

The patients with stenosis of the right coronary artery (RCA) had a significantly higher degree of stenoses before PTCA than those with stenoses of the anterior descending artery LAD (Fig. 4). After treatment there were no significant different residual stenoses. The degree of improvement was also comparable.

In a small group of 44 patients (27 concentric and 17 eccentric) we analized whether there was any difference in the treatment with relation to the configuration of the narrowing (Fig. 5). Patients with concentric stenoses had a slightly, however, not significantly higher rate of stenosis before and immediately after PTCA. The improvement was also slightly less than in those with eccentric stenoses. At the control study six months later these patients had gained a somewhat higher rate of restenoses than those with a previously eccentric form.

## Dilatation for Unstable vs. Stable Angina

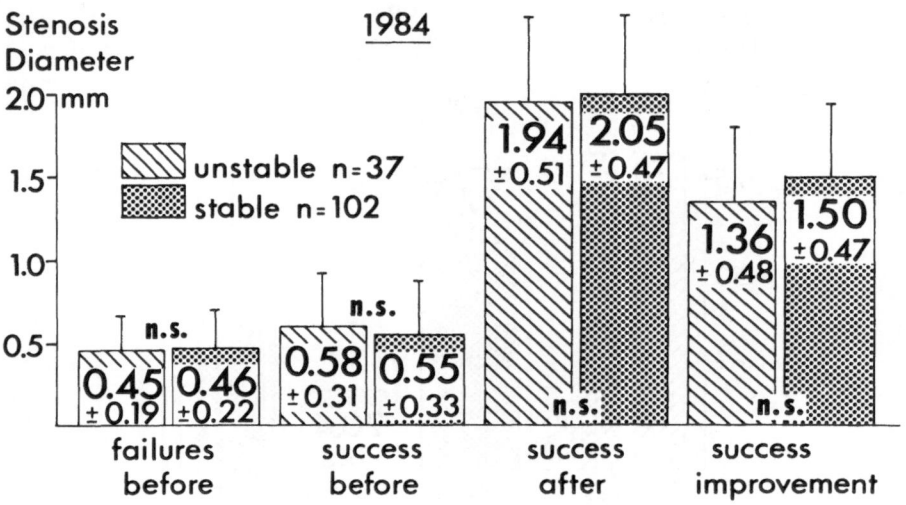

*Figure 3.* Comparison between vessel obstruction in unstable versus stable angina pectoris, series 1984. Vessel lumen measured in absolute values (mm).

## Successful Dilatation
## for Unstable Angina LAD / RCA Stenoses

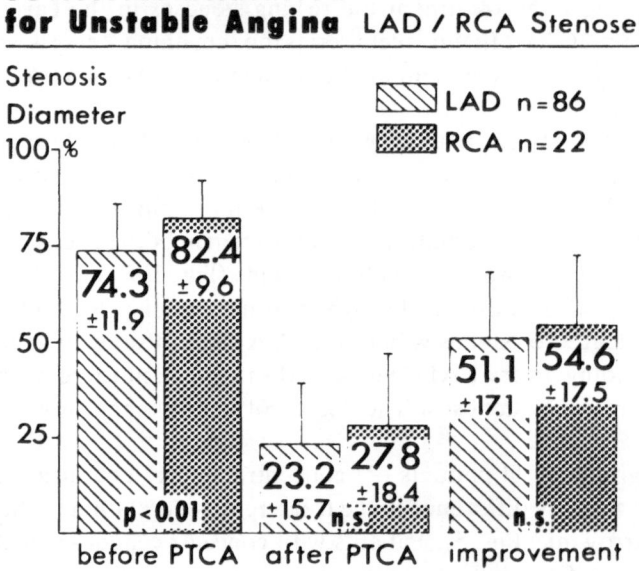

*Figure 4.* Comparison between PTCA in LAD and RCA-stenoses. Patients with unstable angina. Stenoses measured in percent of luminal diameter.

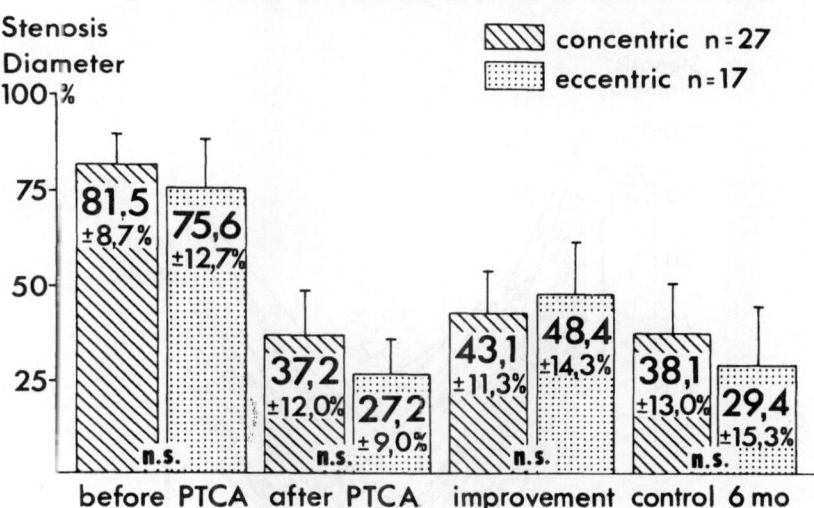

*Figure 5.* Comparison of PTCA in concentric versus eccentric stenoses. Stenoses measured in percent of luminal diameter.

*Late results*

In 81 out of 113 patients with initially successful PTCA we were able to perform a control study (Fig. 6). The diameter stenosis before PTCA in this subgroup was not significantly different from the 1984 group (77.9 ± 11.6% vs. 75.5 ± 11.1%). After PTCA the stenosis was calculated to be 23.7 ± 16.2%. The degree of improvement in all cases was at least 20% of luminal diameter. In some patients nearly no residual stenosis was detected immediately after PTCA. Six months later a wide scatter of measurements was observed. The average vessel obstruction was 40.8 ± 28.3%. While in some patients the luminal diameter was even less, a relapse has occured in others (Fig. 6).

We were not able to detect any correlation between the degree of stenosis before PTCA in the group with permanent success compared to the group with relapse (Fig. 7). Also the degree of stenosis immediately after PTCA was not different.

In 41 patients we were able to compare left ventricular angiograms before PTCA with those at the repeat study six months later. These angiograms were comparable with respect to the heart rate. There were no extrasystoles during angiography. In 27 patients with persisting improvement of the coronary artery

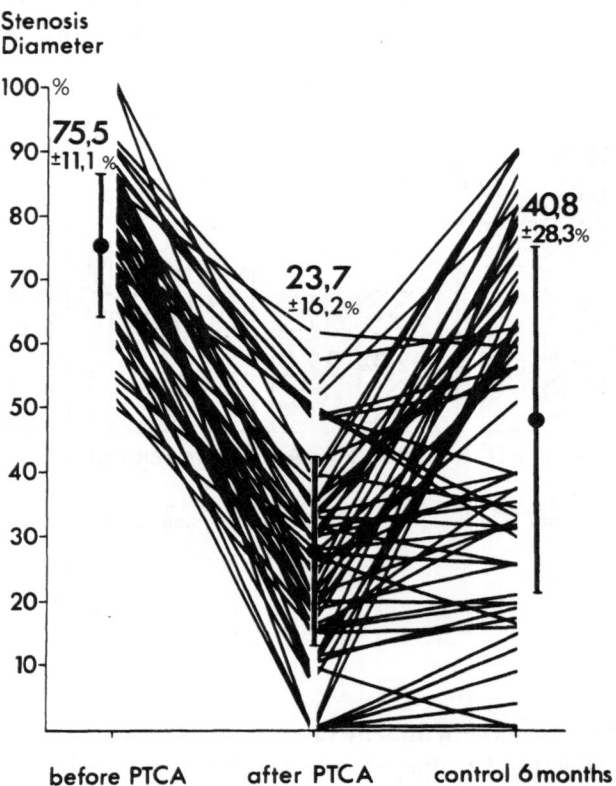

*Figure 6.* Follow up study of 81 patients with successfully treated coronary artery stenosis in unstable angina. Luminal diameter before and after PTCA as well as after six months.

stenosis the number of pathological wall segments had decreased from $6.2 \pm 5.9$ to $3.2 \pm 4.8$ segments (ns). Despite good coronary angiographic results in two patients a hypokinesia had occurred meanwhile (Fig. 8). In patients with re-stenosis there was no correlation between the early and the late results.

*Complications*

In the whole group of 145 patients with unstable angina treated between 1978 and 1984 (Table 1) two patients died, one from lung embolism and one from sudden

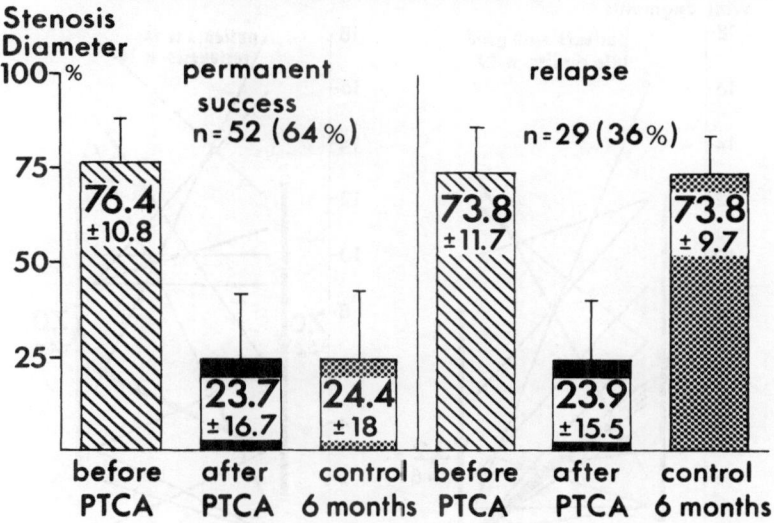

## Dilatation for Unstable Angina
### Control study 6 months, n = 81

*Figure 7.* Comparison between patients with permanent success and with relapse before, immediately after PTCA as well as at the control study six months later.

cardiac death. In both autopsy showed open coronary vessels. Three patients received emergency operation because of vessel occlusion, while in four patients new Q-waves occurred. The death rate was 1.4%, the rate of operations plus infarctions 4.8%. The results were slightly worse than those in patients with stable angina (Table 1).

*Table 1.* Complications in all patients with stable and unstable angina treated between 1978–1984 (n = 484).

| Unstable angina n = 145 | | Stable angina n = 339 | |
|---|---|---|---|
| 1 Lung embolism + 2nd day | | 1 Vessel occlusion → Op → sepsis + | |
| 1 Sudden death 3rd day | | 1 Emergency operation | |
| 3 Emergency operations | | 5 Infarctions | |
| 4 Infarctions | | | |
| Death rate: | 1.4% | Death rate: | 0.3% |
| Op. + infarctions: | 4.8% | Op. + infarctions: | 1,8% |

198

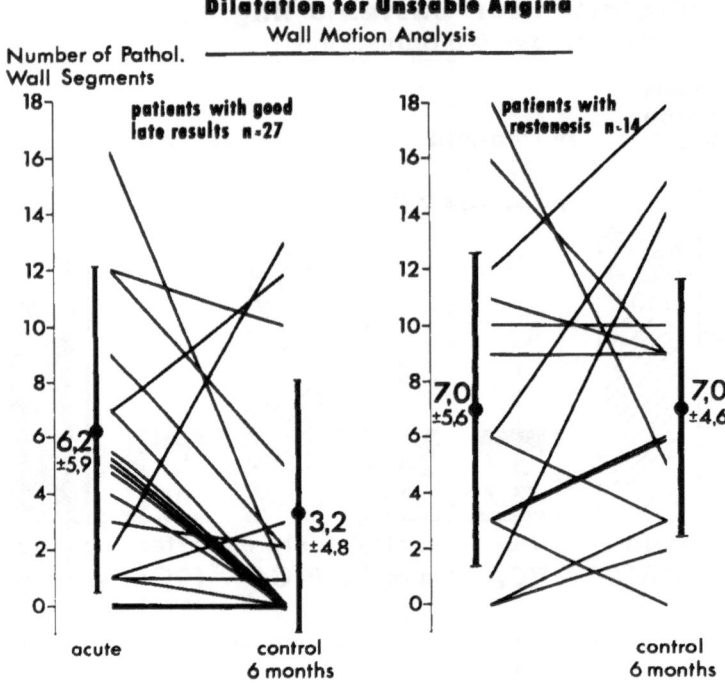

*Figure 8.* Comparison of wall motion analysis in patients with good late results after PTCA and those with restenosis. Number of pathologically contracting segments out of a total of 36 segments per ventricle.


## Discussion

The clinical syndrome of unstable angina has attracted great interest during the last ten years with respect to diagnosis, prognosis, and medical as well as surgical treatment [11, 12]. Despite initial stabilization of symptoms the rate of acute vessel occlusion leading to myocardial infarction and the mortality rate during the first year is quite high [10, 13]. At least 30% of patients with unstable angina show a single vessel disease. Another about 30% suffer from a double vessel disease with mostly isolated, proximal subtotal stenoses of the major coronary arteries [9, 13]. Such patients often between 30 and 50 years of age may be potential candidates for PTCA. In recent years the indication for PTCA has been extended from single to double, in some instances also to triple vessel diseases [14, 15].

As in our series the leading coronary artery stenoses in the majority of cases are found in the left descending coronary artery. Only patients with dominant right coronary artery obstructions may develop the clinical syndrome of unstable angina. In our series the relation between LAD and RCA was 1:4. If a stenosis in the right coronary artery occurs, it is mostly higher than in LAD obstructions. The free wall of the left ventricle and the interventricular septum show a higher oxygen demand than the posterior wall and the right ventricle. Even moderate vessel obstructions especially under physical exercise may therefore lead to earlier symptoms. Patients with isolated stenoses of the left circumflex artery seldomly show symptoms requiring angiography.

In directly admitted patients we prefer to perform PTCA within the same cath-lab procedure, in which the initial coronary arteriography is done [3–6]. All patients therefore receive the same pretreatment as in scheduled PTCA procedures. By this combination we save time, cost and equipment. The patient has not to return to the cath-lab for another intervention. Especially in patients with severe unstable angina not reacting to nitroglycerin-infusions, nifedipine and betablockers, the acute enlargement of the stenosed coronary artery by PTCA improves blood flow to the jeopardized myocardium and by this prevents ischemia and sometimes even myocardial infarction.

To exclude coronary spasms we pretreat all patients with nitroglycerin and nifedipine. For reasons not fully understood up to now the clinical symptoms and apparently also the degree of vessel obstruction often change very rapidly in patients with unstable angina. This may be the reason why in some patients during angiography the degree of vessel obstruction is only measured between 50 and 70%. Probably additional spastic components occur during the anginal phases.

Since 1978 we have extended the indication for PTCA to patients with unstable angina [3–6]. During the following years coronary angioplasty has become an established treatment for this threatening form of the coronary artery disease [7, 8, 15]. The success is depending on several factors. In patients without successful treatment the remaining luminal diameter was significantly smaller than in those with successful treatment. The average lumen was even smaller than the tip of the balloon catheter. Via the newly available steerable guides the low profile catheters can now be introduced into the stenotic area. Despite the technical improvements of the last two years, however, in about 16% of all cases we were not able to reach the stenosis with the balloon segment and to enlarge the stenosis. Because of the severe narrowing and the friction of the balloon within the coronary artery system the balloon, however, could not be advanced.

In a subgroup of our patients we analized whether there was any difference in the treatment of eccentric or concentric stenoses. Neither the pretreatment nor the post-dilatation lumen were significantly different. The amount of enlargement and the successrate were now comparable.

Patients with unstable angina pectoris seem to sufffer from an acute, rapidly progressive deterioration of their coronary artery disease [4, 5, 10, 13, 16]. It may be possible that this type of intimal plaque is different from that in patients with stable angina. The amount of vessel obstructions in patients with stable and in unstable angina treated in our clinic was not significantly different. After dilatation, however, in patients with stable angina the residual stenosis was slightly but not significantly lower than in those with unstable angina.

Opposite to patients with stable angina who have a recurrence rate within the next six months of about 25%, we found a recurrence rate in patients with unstable angina of 36% [2, 3–6, 17–19]. Those groups did not differ in the treatment before and immediately after dilatation as well as during the six months follow-up period. We were not able to detect any differences in the average degree of stenosis before and immediately after dilatation. Further studies and more detailed analysis in a larger series of patients will show, why patients with unstable angina show this high rate of restenoses.

In our whole series, despite all the early results including the learning phase in 1978 are included, the rate of infarction plus vessel obstruction was quite low. In patients with unstable angina, however, the complication rate of operations plus infarctions with 4.8% was higher than in patients with stable angina (1.8%).

Also the mortality rate in unstable angina (1.4%) was higher than in the comparison group (0.3%). In both patients dying after PTCA the autopsy showed no vessel obstruction or dissection, which might have been the cause for the lethal outcome. In one patient a lung embolism appeared after she was already mobilized. In the other patient probably an acute rhythm disturbance during sleep has led to the clinical picture of sudden cardiac death.

Only three out of seven patients with vessel obstruction during PTCA received emergency bypass operation. Despite all three of them were operated on within the first 90 minutes pathological Q-waves indicative for transmural myocardial infarction were found in all of them. This corresponds to the experience of the Frankfurt group, where in the majority of cases after emergency bypass operation for PTCA complications signs of infarctions were found [20]. Generally, the number of infarctions and the mortality rate in PTCA are quite comparable to those in good series of bypass surgery in unstable angina.

The study has shown that PTCA can effectively and economically dilate highly stenotic coronary vessels and improve coronary perfusion in unstable angina. The technique will now also be extended to suitable cases with double and triple vessel disease [14, 15].

PTCA can postpone the time of bypass graft surgery in a number of cases. It will at least gain time in critical situations until bypass surgery is available. The trauma for the patient is much less than with bypass surgery. The costs for equipment, material, and personnel staff is about 20% of that for bypass surgery [21]. After a total hospital stay of five days the patient can return to work one week later.

It is to be expected that the indications and possibilities of angioplasty will be influenced within the future by further technical developments of the catheter material [2].

# References

1. Grüntzig AR, Senning A, Siegenthaler WE (1979) Nonoperative dilatation of coronary artery stenosis: Percutaneous transluminal coronary angioplasty. N Engl J Med 301: 61–68
2. Grüntzig AR (1984) Percutaneous transluminal coronary angioplasty: 6 years' experience. Am Heart J 107: 818
3. Meyer J, Böcker B, Erbel R, Bardos P, Messmer BJ, Effert S (1980) Treatment of unstable angina with transluminal coronary angioplasty (PTCA). Circulation 62/III: 160
4. Meyer J, Schmitz H, Erbel R, Kiesslich T, Böcker-Josephs B, Krebs W, Braun PC, Bardos P, Minale C, Messmer BJ, Effert S (1981) Treatment of unstable angina pectoris with percutaneous transluminal coronary angioplasty. Cath. Cardiov Diagnosis 7: 361–371
5. Meyer J, Schmitz HJ, Kiesslich R, Erbel R, Krebs W, Schulz W, Bardos P, Minale C, Messmer BJ, Effert S (1983) Percutaneous transluminal coronary angioplasty in patients with stable and unstable angina pectoris: Analysis of early and late results. Am Heart J 106: 973–980
6. Meyer J, Erbel R, Schmitz HJ, Pop T, Meinertz T, Schreiner G, Henkel B, Henrichs KJ, Rupprecht HJ, Effert S (1984) Transluminal Angioplastik – Unstabile Angina, frischer Infarkt. 50. Jahrestg Dtsch Ges Herz-und Kreislaufforschg, Mannheim, 1984; Z Kardiol 73/II: 167–176
7. Williams DO, Riley RS, Singh AK, Gewirtz H, Most RS (1981) Evaluation of the role of coronary angioplasty in patients with unstable angina pectoris. Am Heart J 102: 1–9
8. David PR, Waters DD, Scholl JM, Crepéau J, Szlachcic J, Lespérance J, Hudin G, Bourassa M (1982) Percutaneous transluminal coronary angioplasty in patients with variant angina. Circulation 66: 695–702
9. Papapietro SE, Niess GS, Paine TD, Mantle JA, Rackley CE, Russel RO, Rogers WJ (1980) Transient electrocardiographic changes in patients with unstable angina. Relation to coronary anatomy. Am J Cardiol 46: 28
10. Borer JS (1980) Unstable angina: A lethal gun with an invisible trigger. N Engl J Med 302: 1200
11. Phillips SJ, Zeff RH, Kongtahworn C, Jannone L, Brown TM, Zeff RL, Breshani S, Gordon DF (1981) Surgical therapy for evolving myocardial infarction: Herz 6: 55
12. Hultgren HN, Pfeiffer JF, Angell WW, Lipton MJ, Bilisaly J (1977) Unstable Angina: Comparison of medical and surgical treatment. Am J Cardiol 39: 734
13. Nictor MF, Likoff MJ, Mintz GS, Likoff W (1981) Unstable angina pectoris of new onset: A prospective clinical and arteriographic study of 75 patients. Am J Cardiol 47: 228
14. Hartzler GO (1983) Percutaneous transluminal coronary angioplasty in multivessel disease. Cath Cardiov Diagn 9: 537
15. Dorros G, Stertzer SH, Cowley MJ, Myler RK (1984) Complex coronary angioplasty: Multiple coronary dilatations. Am J Cardiol 53: 126–130
16. Moise A, Theroux P, Taeymans Y, Descoings B, Lespérance J, Waters DD, Pelletier GB, Bourassa MG (1983) Unstable angina and progression of coronary atherosclerosis. N Engl J Med 309: 685
17. Kaltenbach M, Kober G, Schmidt-Moritz A, Scherer D (1983) Rezidivhäufigkeit nach erfolgreicher transluminaler Koronarangioplastik. Dtsch med Wschr 108: 1387–1390
18. Meier B, Grüntzig AR, Siegenthaler WE, Schlumpf M (1983) Long-term performance after percutaneous transluminal coronary angioplasty and coronary artery bypass grafting. Circulation 68: 796–802
19. Holmes, DR Jr, Vlietstra RE, Smith HS, Vetrovec GV, Kent KM, Cowley MJ, Faxon DP, Grüntzig AR, Kelsey SF, Detre KM, van Raden MJ, Mock MB (1984) Restenosis after percutaneous transluminal coronary angioplasty (PTCA): A report from the PTCA registry of the National Heart, Lung, and Blood Institute. Am J Cardiol 53: 77–81
20. Satter P, Scherer D (1985) Der akute aorto-koronare Bypass bei Komplikationen nach Katheterdilatation der Koronararterien. Dtsch Med Wschr 110: 540–543
21. Jang GC, Block PC, Cowley MJ, Grüntzig AR, Dorros G, Holmes Jr DR, Kent KM, Leatherman LL, Myler RK, Sjolander SME, Stertzer SH, Vetrovec GW, Willis Jr WH, Williams DO (1984) Relative cost of coronary angioplasty and bypass surgery Am J Cardiol 53: 52–55

# PTCA-success: reliability of non-invasive methods

R. VON ESSEN, R. UEBIS, B. BERTRAM, S. EFFERT,
B. VONDENBUSCH, J. SILNY and G. RAU

**Summary**

The main indication for PTCA is based on clinical symptoms. Therefore relief or improvement of angina and reduction of antianginal therapy are most important, although, subjective criteria of successful PTCA (short term and long term). As restenosis occurs in 20 to 33% (mostly within the first weeks) there is a need for an objective non-invasive indicator.

A new positive stress test is highly specific but a negative test does not exclude recurrence, as its sensitivity is only 50 to 70% and depends on the degree and location of stenosis. An increase of sensitivity can be reached by a withdrawal of antianginal therapy, if tolerated. The knowledge of a pathological stress test before PTCA makes it much easier to judge new symptoms. Therefore it is generally accepted to do a stress test in all patients before and after PTCA and to compare both with the angiographical results. Scintigraphical methods have been reported to be more sensitive. Regional perfusion disturbances assessed by thallium-201 exercise scintigraphy and no increase of left ventricular ejection fraction during exercise, measured by a gated blood pool technique with technetium-99m, indicate restenosis. Both are not available in most hospitals and expensive.

As the insufflation of the balloon produces complete coronary artery occlusion and regional well defined ischemia, we developed a mapping system with 63 x-ray transparent electrodes to detect the precordial region of ischemia according to the occluded vessel. These data provide important information of precordial regions with ischemic ECG changes and hopefully improve the sensitivity of ECG exercise tests. In conclusion, the use of clinical symptoms in conjunction with ECG and myocardial scintigram acquired during exercise provide a lot of information but can not substitute angiogram, if there is any suspicion of restenosis.

## Introduction

After successful PTCA the most striking problem is the development of restenosis. Most groups report a recurrence rate between 25 to 35%. Only the group in Frankfurt has a rate below 20% [1]. Since restenosis occurs mostly within the first few weeks after PTCA and since not all patients are willing to have a reangiography to document the long-term success, non-invasive methods are necessary to separate those with a good long-term result from those with restenosis. This paper will focus on the sensitivity of (a) the symptoms of the patients, (b) exercise performance (work load and ejection fraction measured by gated blood pool scintigraphy), (c) exercise electrocardiography and (d) exercise scintigraphy using thallium-201 in regard to detect restenosis.

Finally new developments are presented, which hopefully will improve the sensitivity of exercise ECG.

A 40-year-old man was unsuccessfully treated with almost all available antiarrhythmic drugs including amiodarone because of ventricular tachycardia and ventricular ectopic beats. When he came to our hospital at coronary angiography he had a complete proximal occlusion of the left anterior descending artery (LAD) but no anterior myocardial infarction. The LAD was perfused via collaterals from the right coronary artery (RCA). After successful PTCA the arrhythmias disappeared completely and the patient is well now 6 months later without any medication (Fig. 1).

## Angina pectoris

The main indication for PTCA is not the treatment of arrhythmias but the treatment of angina, reduction of antianginal drugs, prevention of myocardial infarction and delay of bypass operation.

Although symptoms are subjective criteria they are most important from the patient point of view.

In a consecutive series of 189 pts with an angiographically proven good long-term result 82.9% had an improvement of one or more Canadian Cardiovascular Society classes (CCS) at the time of the control angiogram 5 to 6 months later. In those 45 pts with a restenosis (loss of gain of more than 20%), however, also in this group more than 50% had an improvement of symptoms compared to the complaints before PTCA (Fig. 2).

60.1% of those patients with no restenosis were free of angina but also 21.6% of those with restenosis (Fig. 3). Three patients with a good long-term result in the dilated vessel had a new stenosis in another coronary artery.

One patient with a complete occlusion 6 months after successful PTCA was free of symptoms without myocardial infarction. These data indicate that relief of symptoms after PTCA does not necessarily mean a good angiographical long-

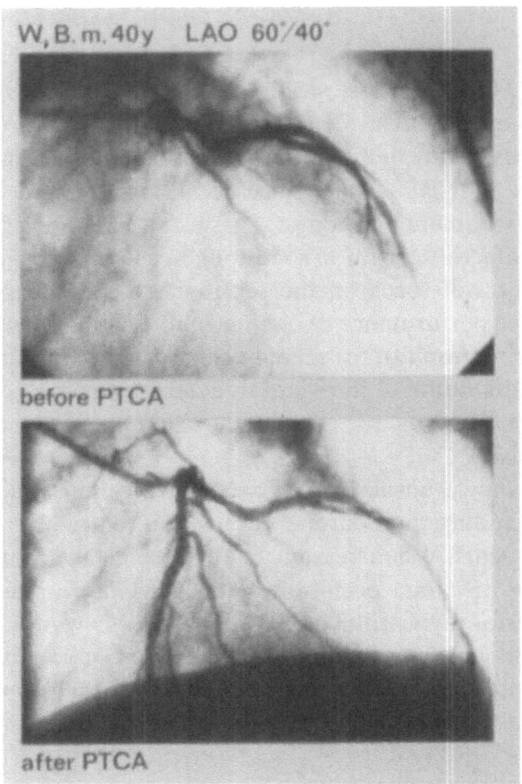

*Figure 1.* Coronary angiography (LAO 60°/40° view) of a 40 year-old man before and after PTCA of a LAD occlusion, that caused malignant arrhythmias.

term result and persisting angina can be found in patients with good angiographical results.

**Left ventricular function**

Improvement of left ventricular function during exercise after successful PTCA using gated blood pool cardiac scintigraphy with technetium-99m is a further non-invasive method to separate patients with long-term successful PTCA from those with restenosis [2, 3, 4]. After successful PTCA patients have a significant improvement of work load and duration of exercise [5] (Fig. 4).

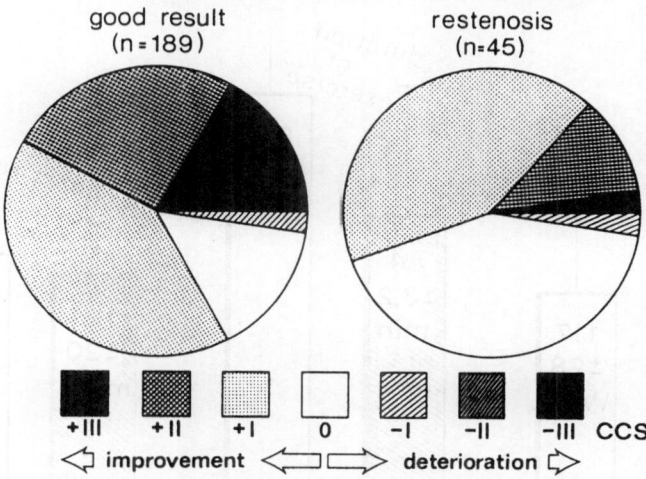

*Figure 2.* Change of angina after PTCA. Correlation between improvement or deterioration and angiographical findings at a control angiography 3 to 6 months after the PTCA procedure.

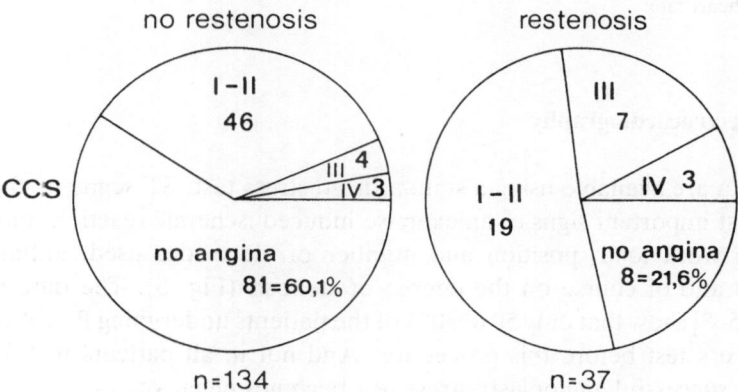

*Figure 3.* Degree of angina (Canadian Cardiovascular Society (CCS) classification) in patients with no restenosis (left) and patients with restenosis (right) at the time of control angiography.

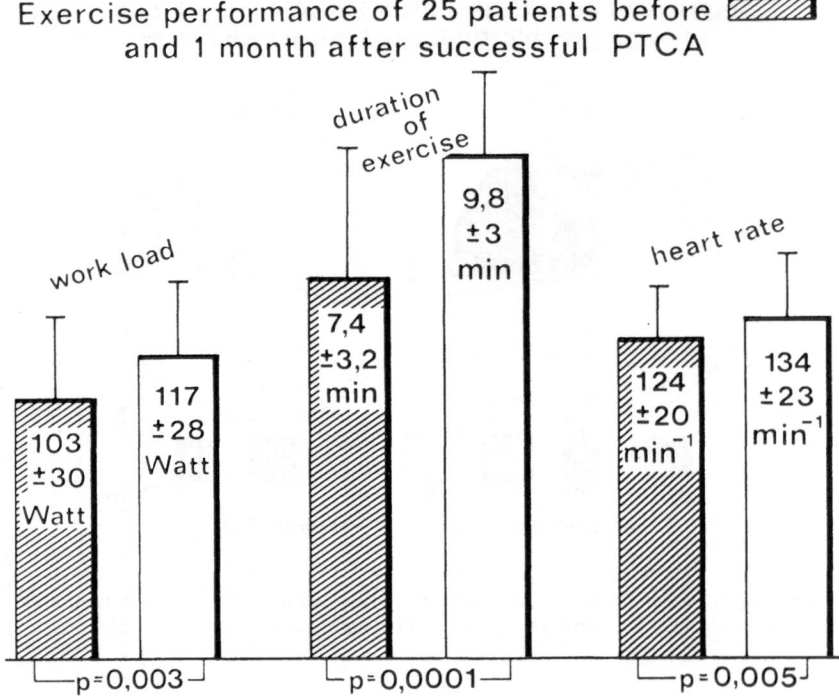

*Figure 4.* In patients with successful PTCA there is a significant increase of work load, duration of exercixe and heart rate.

### Exercise electrocardiography

Further data are available using a standardized stress test. ST-segment changes are the most important signs of an exercise induced ischemic reaction, but they depend on work load, position and number of electrodes used, antianginal medication and of course on the degree of stenosis (Fig. 5). The data in the literature [5–8] show that only 50 to 80% of the patients undergoing PTCA have a positive stress test before this procedure. And not in all patients with angiographically successful angioplasty stress test becomes negative.

However, if stress test is positive before and negative immediately after PTCA it is a very useful and valid non-invasive method for the long-term follow-up. In combination with symptoms it provides us with sufficient information and in these patients without recurrence of angina and negative stress test reangiography is not necessary.

Therefore it is generally accepted to do a stress test in all patients before and after PTCA, if possible without medication and with the same work load and to

Stress test and ST—segment changes before PTCA

|  | | n | Area Sten (%) | ST↓ | Sensitivity |
|---|---|---|---|---|---|
| | Bourassa et al | 54 | 78 ± 13 | 0,2 0,1 | 59 % |
| II | Cowley et al | 22 | 82 ± 3,5 | – | 86 % |
| | Grüntzig et al | 132 | – | 0,2 0,1 | 72 % |
| pacing | Williams et al | 6 | 74 ± 16 | – | 100 % |
| mapping | v. Essen et al | 32 | 92,4 ± 8 | 0,1 | 75 % |

*Figure 5.* Sensitivity of ECG-stress tests in relation to number of patients, degree of stenosis, criteria of pathological ST segment changes and number of electrodes. Although we used a mapping system with 48 precordial electrodes and improved the ECG signals ('averaging') and although our patients had the highest degree of stenosis, sensitivity was only 75%.

compare both with the angiographical results. If there is a good correlation further and more expensive or invasive tests are not necessary.

## Scintigraphy

Even though thallium-201 myocardial scintigraphy does not reveal morphologic changes in the dilated coronary artery, it can be used to assess the functional capacity of the vessel and to demonstrate changes in myocardial perfusion after PTCA. Hirzel et al. [9] examined the scintigraphic images obtained before PTCA, within 3 weeks after PTCA and at 5 to 6 month intervals after PTCA in a subgroup of patients.

In 43 out of 49 patients (sensitivity 88%) thallium-201 scintigraphy disclosed typical isolated zones of reduced activity after exercise that filled in as redistribution occurred. The location of this exercise-induced defect corresponded closely to the arteriographic findings.

Within 3 weeks after successful PTCA thallium scans were obtained in 31 cases. In 28 the scintigram revealed a significant increase in thallium activity in the previously ischemic region. In 3 successful cases without a clear-cut, exercise induced defect in the scintigrams obtained before PTCA, the activity in the suspected region was either identical or only slightly less but still normal after PTCA. 16 patients were followed by repeated exercise scintigraphy at 5 to 6 month intervals up to 30 months after PTCA. The relative thallium-201 activity had returned to normal and in four patients further improvement in perfusion with time was seen. In three cases a limited reduction in thallium-201 activity in the same location as before PTCA coincided with angiographically proven restenosis. These data have been confirmed by other groups [6].

It is concluded that thallium-201 exercise scintigraphy, a completely non-invasive technique, clearly provides the best documentation of ongoing changes in myocardial perfusion after PTCA but unfortunately this technique is not available in many hospitals and costs are high.

## New developments to improve the sensitivity of exercise electrocardiography

The insufflation of the balloon of the dilation catheter in the stenotic coronary artery produces a complete occlusion of the artery and a regional well defined ischemia.

In the first step we looked at the time course of the ischemic electrical reaction during PTCA using 8 precordial electrodes located adjacent to the Wilson leads V4 and V5 in patients with a proximal LAD stenosis. In some cases we saw a ST-segment depression when the non inflated balloon passes the stenosis. During 10 to 15 seconds after start of insufflation of the balloon the ST-segment depression changes into a ST-segment elevation. In each electrode the ST-elevation 60 milliseconds after S reaches an almost stable level that does not increase further, if insufflation continues. Deflation of the balloon coincides with a disappearance of the ST-segment elevation (Fig. 6).

In a second step we developed a mobile mapping system with 63 non-equidistantly positioned precordial electrodes and three limb leads (Fig. 7).

The signals of all electrodes are sampled simultaneously within a time window of 2.5 seconds and with a cycle of a minimum of 5 seconds, to register the

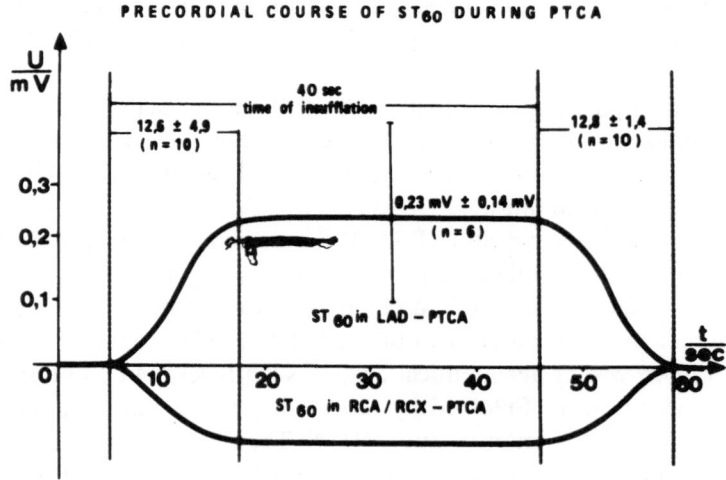

*Figure 6.* Course of the ST segment in 8 precordial leads (adjacent to $V_3$, $V_5$) (60 ms after J point) during insufflation of the balloon in patients with proximal LAD, RCA and CX stenosis.

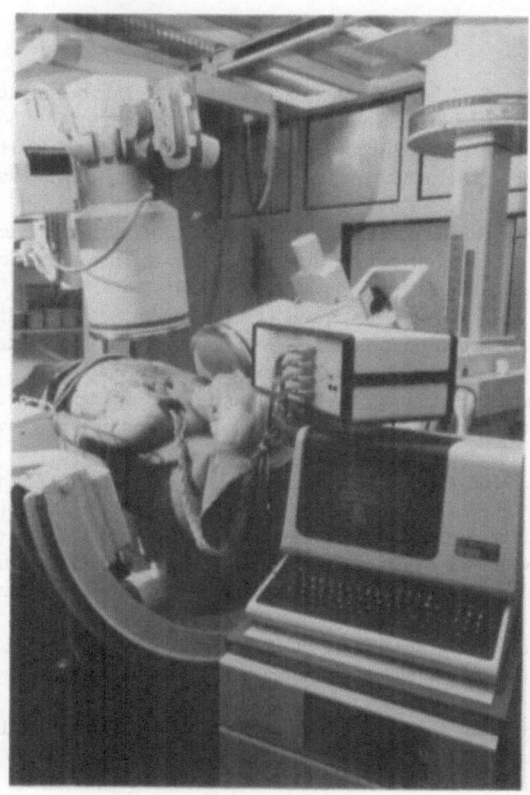

*Figure 7.* X-ray transparent electrode mapping system with 63 leads for ECG recording during the PTCA procedure.

dynamics of ST-segment elevation or depression without loss of information. The application of this method during PTCA of LAD, RCX or RCA stenoses enables us to find a relation between different phases of ischemia, the location of the stenotic or occluded vessel and the corresponding electric potential distribution on the body surface. We hope the data help to improve sensitivity of ECG stress tests by a better insight into the relation between the stenotic coronary artery and precordial location of ischemia.

In conclusion, clinical symptoms in conjunction with ECG and myocardial scintigram acquired during exercise provide a lot of information about the success of PTCA, but cannot substitute angiography, if there is any suspicion of re-stenosis.

# References

1. Kaltenbach M, Kober G, Scherer D, Vallbracht C (1984) Rezidivhaeufigkeit nach erfolgreicher Ballondilatation von Kranzarterienstenose. Z Kardiol 72 (Suppl. 2): 161–166
2. Sigwart U, Grbic M, Essinger A, Bischof-Delaloye A, Sadeghi H, Rivier JL (1982) Improvement of left ventricular function after percutaneous transluminal coronary angioplasty. Am J Cardiol 49: 651–657
3. Kent KM, Bonow RO, Rosing DR, Ewels CJ, Lipson LC, McIntosh CL, Bacharach S, Green MS, Epstein SE (1982) Improved myocardial function during exercise after successful percutaneous transluminal coronary angioplasty. N Engl J Med 306: 441–446
4. Bonow RO, Kent KM, Rosing DR, Lipson LC, Bacharach S, Green MS, Epstein SE (1982) Improvement left ventricular diastolic filling in patients with coronary artery disease after percutaneous transluminal coronary angioplasty. Circ 66: 1159–1167
5. Meier B, Gruentzig AR, Siegenthaler WE, Schlumpf M (1983) Long-term exercise performance after percutaneous transluminal coronary angioplasty and coronary artery bypass grafting. Circ 68: 796–802
6. Scholl JM, Chaitman BR, David PR, Dupras G, Brevers G, Val PG, Crepeau J, Lesperance J, Bourassa MG (1982) Exercise electrocardiography and myocardial scintigraphy in the serial evaluation of the results of percutaneous transluminal coronary angioplasty. Circ 66: 380–390
7. Cowley MJ, Vetrovec GW, Wolfgang TC (1981) Efficacy of percutaneous transluminal coronary angioplasty: technique, patient selection, salutary results, limitations and complications. Am Heart J 101: 272–280
8. Klepzig Jr H, Scherer D, Kober G, Maul FD, Kanemoto R, Standke G, Hoer G, Kaltenbach M (1981) Funktionsverbesserung nach transluminaler koronarer Angioplastik (TCA). Herz 6: 252–258
9. Hirzel HO, Nuesch K, Gruentzig AR, Luetolf UM (1981) Short- and long-term changes in myocardial perfusion after percutaneous transluminal coronary angioplasty assessed by thallium-201 exercise scintigraphy. Circ 63, 1001–1007

# Myocardial protection from PTCA-related ischemia

V. HOMBACH, H.W. HÖPP, F.M. Mc DONALD, M. FUCHS,
A. HANNEKUM, A. HEINEN, A. OSTERSPEY, T. EGGELING,
H. HIRCHE and H.H. HILGER

## Summary

Since it's introduction into clinical cardiology PTCA proved to be an effective method for reduction of coronary stenoses, thus leading to relief of angina pectoris and an increase of exercise tolerance in CHD patients. The success rates of PTCA depend on the type of lesion, catheter material, experience of the angiographer, and on the inflation pressure and inflation time used. With longer inflation times possible hazards of PTCA-induced ischemia may arise like LV pump failure or the occurrence of dangerous ventricular arrhythmias. Myocardial protection during PTCA may be achieved by means of intracoronary (ic.) administration of Nitro glycerine and/or Nifedipine (or other calciumantagonists as well) prior to inflation, or by simultaneous perfusion of the dependent myocardial area with arterial blood during the whole inflation period. Several studies using ic.-Nitroglycerine and/or Nifedipine have shown that sometimes symptoms and particularly signs of myocardial ischemia on PTCA may be delayed by these drugs and the occurence of ventricular arrhythmias decreased, thus allowing potentially longer inflation periods. On the other hand, using quantitative LV angiography we could demonstrate that the impairment of global and regional LV contraction due to PTCA-induced ischemia was considerably and significantly less pronounced when using simultaneous perfusion with arterial blood during inflation. Administration of Nitroglycerine and/or Nifedipine by ic.-route seems to be a simple, rapid and safe method of myocardial protection from PTCA-related ischemia, but it may not preserve LV global and regional performance to such a degree as could be achieved using perfusion with arterial blood. The perfusion method may, therefore, provide the opportunity to also attempt PTCA in patients with multiple vessel disease and severely impaired left ventricular perfomance, as well as in individuals with left main stenoses.

## Introduction

Since it's introduction into clinical cardiology by A. Grüntzig in 1977 [1], percutaneous transluminal coronary angioplasty (PTCA) has proved to be an effective method for reduction of degree of coronary stenoses, thus leading to relief of angina pectoris and improvement of exercise tolerance in patients with stable and unstable angina pectoris [2]. The overall success rates of PTCA range from 60–90%, depending on the experience of the cardiologist performing PTCA, on localization and pathoanatomy of the stenosis, on the catheter material used, and on inflation pressure and inflation time [2, 3]. On the other hand, with longer inflation times, e.g. 45–70–90 seconds, possible hazards of PTCA-induced ischemia like pump failure or severe life threatening ventricular arrhythmias may ensue. Therefore preservation of ischemic myocardium during PTCA seems mandatory, and we are reporting the preliminary experience with different methods of myocardial protection from ischemia during the inflation periods of PTCA.

## Modes of protection

From a theoretical view two different approaches for myocardial protection are available, a pharmacological and a more physiological type of preservation. Drugs like Nitroglycerine or calciumantagonists (Nifedipine, Verapamil, or Diltiazem) may be administered orally or intravenously, and presumably intracoronarily just prior to inflation, whereas the more physiological procedure is a simultaneous perfusion of the jeopardized area of myocardium distal to the stenosis using arterial blood as the perfusion medium [4, 5]. One might expect that with drugs like Nitroglycerine or calciumantagonists myocardial protection could be achieved by unloading the left ventricle as a whole (particularly with the administration of Nitrates) and/or by a local 'cardioprotective' effect of intracoronary (ic.) injection of calciumantagonists. On the other hand simultaneous perfusion with arterial blood through the free lumen of the dilatation catheter distal to inflation site should directly compensate for the stop of coronary blood flow by supplying the dependent myocardial area with a certain amount of oxygen. Thus, PTCA related ischemia may be partially or even completely prevented, if a sufficient amount of blood could be delivered throught the narrow lumen of the dilatation catheter.

## Clinical and experimental results

In a pilot study we have evaluated the effect of 0.2 mg ic.-Nifedipine in a cohort of 12 male patients undergoing PTCA of LAD-stenoses (n = 11), or RCA-stenosis

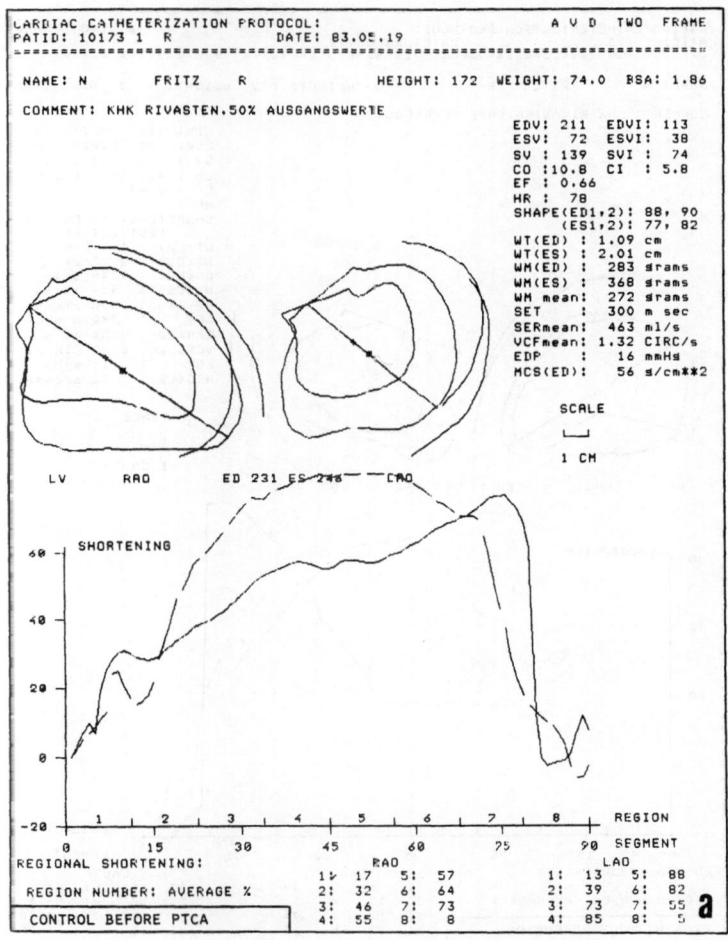

```
CARDIAC CATHETERIZATION PROTOCOL:                      A V D  TWO  FRAME
PATID: 10173 1  R              DATE: 83.05.19
===============================================================================

NAME: N      FRITZ   R              HEIGHT: 172  WEIGHT: 74.0  BSA: 1.86

COMMENT: KHK RIVASTEN.50% AUSGANGSWERTE
                                            EDV: 211   EDVI: 113
                                            ESV:  72   ESVI:  38
                                            SV : 139   SVI :  74
                                            CO :10.8   CI  : 5.8
                                            EF : 0.66
                                            HR :  78
                                            SHAPE(ED1,2): 88, 90
                                                 (ES1,2): 77, 82
                                            WT(ED) : 1.09 cm
                                            WT(ES) : 2.01 cm
                                            WM(ED) :  283 grams
                                            WM(ES) :  368 grams
                                            WM mean:  272 grams
                                            SET    :  300 m sec
                                            SERmean:  463 ml/s
                                            VCFmean: 1.32 CIRC/s
                                            EDP    :   16 mmHg
                                            MCS(ED):   56 g/cm**2

                                            SCALE
                                            L___I
                                            1 CM

    LV    RAO      ED 231 ES 248    CAO
```

SHORTENING

```
 60
 40
 20
  0
-20
       1    2    3    4    5    6    7    8    REGION
      0    15    30    45    60    75    90   SEGMENT
REGIONAL SHORTENING:          RAO              LAO
                         1:  17  5:  57   1:  13  5:  88
REGION NUMBER: AVERAGE % 2:  32  6:  64   2:  39  6:  82
                         3:  46  7:  73   3:  73  7:  55
CONTROL BEFORE PTCA      4:  55  8:   8   4:  85  8:   5    a
```

*Figure 1a.* Quantitative left ventricular angiography (LAO and RAO 45° projection) in a patient with PTCA attempt of LAD stenosis. Control angio at resting conditions. A computer program (AVD, Siemens, Erlangen, FRG) was used for evaluation (single and multi-frame technique) of global (top center and right) and regional (bottom) left centricucontraction performance. Note the normal contraction behavior of anterior and posterior wall segments of the left ventricle.

(n = 1). 4 patients had experienced a previous myocardial infarction, in 3 patients with the vessel involved that was not considered for PTCA, whereas in one patient the infarct-related vessel was considered for relief of stenosis by PTCA. On left ventricular angiography 2 patients showed anterior wall hypocinesia, 2 patients late systolic bulging, and 3 patients inferior wall hypocinesia. Left ventricular (LV) ejection fraction was equal or more than 50% in all patients studied.

Prior to PTCA a control LV and coronary angiography was performed, since

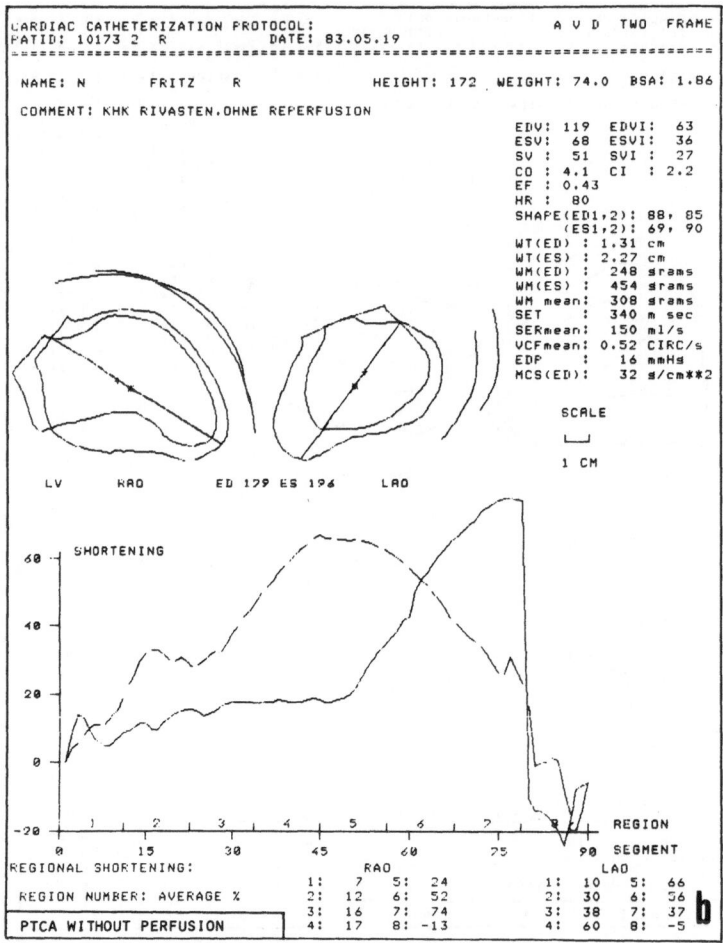

*Figure 1b.* Quantitative LV angiography during PTCA without perfusion of arterial blood during balloon inflation. Note the marked contraction defect within the anterior wall and apical region of the left ventricle (same patient as in Fig. 1a).

the initial diagnostic angios were performed several months prior to the time of the PTCA attempt. Betablocking drugs were discontinued 6 days prior to the time of the study, and long acting nitrates and/or calciumantagonists were withdrawn one day before performing PTCA. All patients gave their written informed consent, and they were studied in the post-absorptive non-sedated state. First dilatation was performed without any pre-medication, using a conventional Grüntzig G-20-30 dilatation catheter, with inflation pressures of 6–9 athmospheres and inflation times of 45–70 seconds. Following deflation of the balloon the dilatation catheter was withdrawn to allow free flow to the coronary vessel for

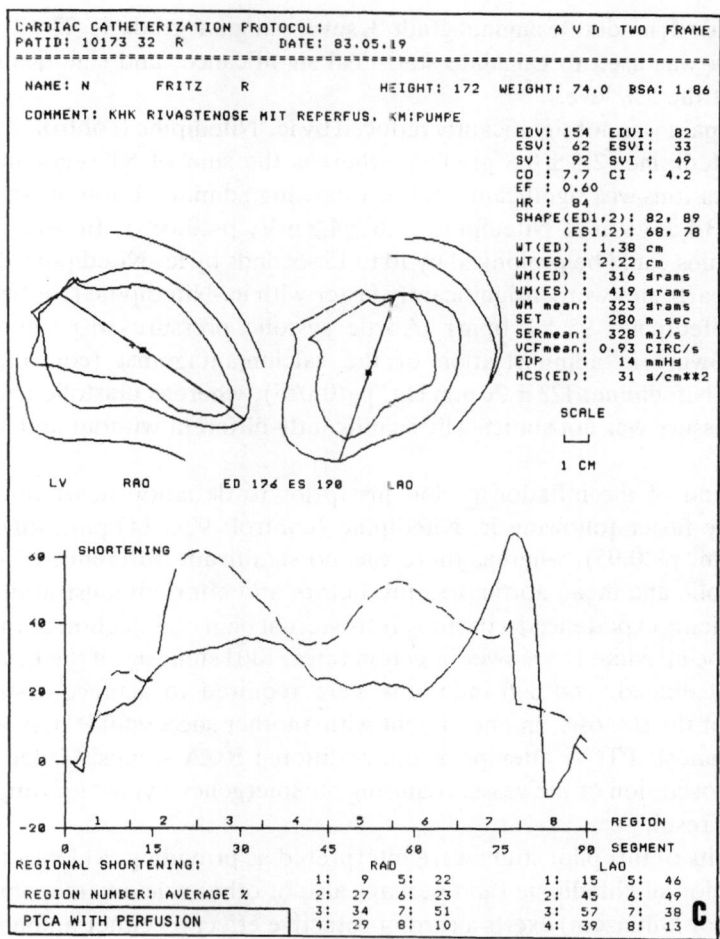

```
CARDIAC CATHETERIZATION PROTOCOL:                    A V D  TWO  FRAME
PATID: 10173 32  R              DATE: 83.05.19
================================================================

NAME: N      FRITZ   R              HEIGHT: 172  WEIGHT: 74.0  BSA: 1.86

COMMENT: KHK RIVASTENOSE MIT REPERFUS. KM:PUMPE
                                          EDV: 154   EDVI:   82
                                          ESV:  62   ESVI:   33
                                          SV :  92   SVI :   49
                                          CO : 7.7   CI  :  4.2
                                          EF : 0.60
                                          HR :  84
                                          SHAPE(ED1,2): 82, 89
                                               (ES1,2): 68, 78
                                          WT(ED) : 1.38 cm
                                          WT(ES) : 2.22 cm
                                          WM(ED) :  316 grams
                                          WM(ES) :  419 grams
                                          WM mean:  323 grams
                                          SET    :  280 m sec
                                          SERmean:  328 ml/s
                                          VCFmean: 0.93 CIRC/s
                                          EDP    :   14 mmHg
                                          MCS(ED):   31 s/cm**2

                                          SCALE
                                          L___I
                                          1 CM

    LV     RAO     ED 176 ES 190   LAO
```

SHORTENING

REGIONAL SHORTENING:

| REGION NUMBER: AVERAGE % | RAO | | LAO | |
|---|---|---|---|---|
| | 1: 9 | 5: 22 | 1: 15 | 5: 46 |
| | 2: 27 | 6: 23 | 2: 45 | 6: 49 |
| PTCA WITH PERFUSION | 3: 34 | 7: 51 | 3: 57 | 7: 38 |
| | 4: 29 | 8: 10 | 4: 39 | 8: 13 |

C

*Figure 1c.* Quantitative LV angiography during PTCA plus simultaneous perfusion with oxygenated blood to the region of jeopardized myocardium distal to the inflation site of an LAD stenosis within the first 3rd of this vessel. Global and regional LV performance is much less impaired, when compared to the status without perfusion (see Fig. 1b, same patient as in Figs. 1a and b).

3–5 minutes. Thereafter the stenosis was passed again, and 0.2 mg of Nifedipine were injected via the free lumen of the balloon catheter over a period of 30–60 seconds. After an interval of 2–4 minutes post-injection (mean: 2.5 ± 0.5 minutes) a second inflation was performed using the same inflation pressure and inflation time as before administration of the drug. The following parameters were measured: heart rate, aortic pressure (systolic, diastolic, mean), distal occlusion pressure within the coronary artery approached, sum of ST-segment alterations (depressions or elevations) within the 6 extremity leads (Einthoven and Goldberger), and grade of angina pectoris (4 grades: no angina: grade 1, mild angina: grade 2, moderate angina: grade 3, severe angina: grade 4). The T-test for paired data was used to calculate statistical significance, and significance was accepted at the 5% level.

Anginal pain was not significantly reduced by ic.-Nifedipine (control: 2.6 ± 0.8 grades, Nifedipine: 2.5 ± 0.8 grades), whereas the sum of ST-segment elevations-depressions was significantly lower following administration of Nifedipine (control: 13.1 ± 7.9 mV, Nifedipine: 7.6 ± 4.8 mV, p<0.005). In 4/12 patients inflation times could be prolonged by 10 to 15 seconds by ic.-Nifedipine. Prior to inflation heart rates were insignificantly faster with ic.-Nifedipine (control: 90 ± 16 bpm, Nifedipine: 95 ± 14 bpm). Aortic systolic pressure was significantly lower following ic.-administration of the calciumantagonist (control: 133 ± 17 mm Hg, Nifedipine: 123 ± 20 mm Hg, p<0.025), whereas diastolic and mean arterial pressure was not statistically significantly different without and with ic.-Nifedipine.

At the end of the inflation period just prior to deflation heart rates were significantly faster following ic.-Nifedipine (control: 92 ± 14 bpm, Nifedipine: 101 ± 13 bpm, p<0.05), whereas there was no significant difference of the systolic, diastolic and mean aortic pressure before and after administration of the drug. 4 patients experienced a burning retrosternal pain on injection of the drug, that could be alleviated by slower injection rates. 10/11 stenoses of the LAD were successfully dilated, and 3–6 inflations were required to achieve a sufficient reduction of the stenosis. In one patient with another successful PTCA-attempt of LAD stenosis PTCA attempt of the additional RCA stenosis failed due to spasm and occlusion of the vessel requiring an emergency bypass grafting with a favourable result.

The results of this pilot study were interpreted as providing evidence that ic.-administration of Nifedipine (and perhaps also of other calciumantagonists like Verapamil or Diltiazem) exerts a cardioprotective effect by either unloading the left ventricle, or by a local 'cardioplegic' effect when delivered to the jeopardized area of myocardium prior to inflation-induced ischemia. Moreover this type of protection seemed to be a simple, safe and effective approach that could be used as a routine procedure during everyday PTCA attempts.

In a second series of investigations the effect of simultaneous perfusion with arterial blood during balloon inflation via the free lumen of the balloon catheter was evaluated. 10 male patients, aged 46–57 years were studied, 6 with single vessel disease, 2 with double vessel disease, and 2 with triple vessel disease. Left ventricular function was normal in 7 individuals, late systolic bulging present in 3 patients, and hypocinesia seen in 3 individuals. In 9 patients PTCA was attempted for LAD stenosis, and in one patient for RCA stenosis. Betablocking drugs were discontinued 6 days prior to the time of the study, and long acting nitrates and calciumantagonists were withdrawn one day before the time of the study. An informed written consent was obtained in each of the patients, who were studied in the non-sedated postabsorptive state. In all patients a control left ventricular and coronary angiogram was performed. Thereafter two inflation periods were performed in a randomized order without and with perfusion with arterial blood, that was withdrawn from a second arterial (pigtail) catheter placed in the left ventricle via a left femoral artery approach. Following control measurements of heart rate, left ventricular and aortic pressure the balloon was inflated, and the same values obtained after 30 seconds of inflation, and LV angiography was then performed up to 45 seconds of balloon inflation before deflation. A 5 minutes interval was observed between the first and second inflation period, that was performed with exactly the same inflation pressure and time. When using the conventional Grüntzig G 20–30 balloon catheter, that catheter was withdrawn between the first and second inflation to allow free flow, and when using the late guiding catheter the guide wire was left in place whereas the balloon catheter itself was withdrawn for free flow purposes. The perfusion medium was arterial blood that was slightly diluted to a mean hematocrit value of $30 \pm 2\%$ in 7 patients, whereas in 3 patients whole blood was used as the perfusate. The injection rates obtained were 14–20 ml/min (mean: $16 \pm 2$ ml/min) using hand injection, where lower perfusion rates were feasible with the conventional G20–30 and higher perfusion rates with the steerable balloon catheters of the newer generation of balloons. LV angiograms performed during inflation without and with perfusion were analyzed using a computer program (AVD, Siemens, Erlamen, FRG). The following parameters were measured and/or calculated: angina pectoris (4 grades: grade 1: no angina, grade 2: mild angina, grade 3: moderate angina, grade 4: severe angina), the sum of ST segment elevations/depressions in the Einthoven and Goldberger leads, heart rate, LV and aortic pressures, ejection fraction (EF), LV volume indices, systolic ejection time (SET), mean systolic ejection fraction (EF), LV volume indices, systolic ejection time (SET), mean systolic ejection rate (SERmean), mean velocity of circumferential fiber shortening (VCFmean), as well as regional and long axis shortening. Statistical significance was calculated using Student's T-test for paired data, the level of significance was accepted when $p < 0.05$.

The following results were obtained: Angina pectoris grades were not significantly different in both inflation periods (without perfusion: $1.7 \pm 1.2$ grades, with perfusion: $1.9 \pm 1.1$ grades). The sum of ST segment elevations/depressions was significantly lower with blood perfusion (without perfusion: $12.2 \pm 6.7$ mV, with perfusion: $7.6 \pm 5.5$ mV, $p < 0.005$). The heart rate was insignificantly faster with perfusion, whereas LV systolic pressure was significantly lower without perfusion as compared to the values with perfusion (without perfusion: $114 \pm 14$ mm Hg, with perfusion: $124 \pm 16$ mm Hg, $p < 0.05$). LV early diastolic (without perfusion $11.2 \pm 5.9$ mm Hg, with perfusion: $7.8 \pm 5.7$ mm Hg, $p < 0.02$) and enddiastolic pressures (without perfusion: $21.4 \pm 4.6$ mm Hg, with perfusion: $16.9 \pm 5.0$ mm Hg, $p < 0.005$) were significantly lower, when arterial blood was perfused during the balloon inflation period. Systolic aortic pressure was significantly lower without perfusion (same values as LV-systolic pressure), whereas diastolic and mean aortic pressure was not significantly different between both inflation periods. LV-EF was significantly higher with perfusion as compared to the values without perfusion (without perfusion: $32.8 \pm 18.3\%$, with perfusion: $50.4 \pm 10.6\%$, $p<0.001$). The enddiastolic volume index was significantly lower (without perfusion: $100.0 \pm 26.5\,\text{ml/m}^2$, with perfusion: $96.0 \pm 18.5\,\text{ml/m}^2$, $p<0.05$), endsystolic volume index lower (without perfusion: $62.8 \pm 31.4\,\text{ml/m}^2$, with perfusion: $46.4 \pm 17.5\,\text{ml/m}^2$, $p<0.05$), and both stroke volume index (without perfusion: $38.4 \pm 14.5\,\text{ml/m}^2$, with perfusion: $53.8 \pm 17.3\,\text{ml/m}^2$, $p<0.005$) and cardiac index (without perfusion: $3.22 \pm 0.90\,\text{ml/min/m}^2$, with perfusion: $4.78 \pm 1.38\,\text{l/min/m}^2$, $p<0.01$) were significantly higher, when arterial blood perfusion was performed during balloon inflation. SET was insignificantly shorter when perfusion was used, whereas SERmean was significantly higher with perfusion (without perfusion: $239.0 \pm 81.9\,\text{ml/s}$, with perfusion: $346.0 \pm 89.0\,\text{ml/s}$, $p<0.01$). VCFmean was insignificantly better with perfusion as compared to values obtained during inflation without perfusion (without perfusion: $0.59 \pm 0.40\,\text{CIRC/s}$, with perfusion: $0.82 \pm 0.25\,\text{CIRC/s}$, $p<0.1$). When using the 90° radiant analysis method for measuring regional shortening in per cent of maximal shortening rates, the number of segments with relative shortening rates below 30% were significantly higher without perfusion, as compared to the status with perfusion (without perfusion: $51.6 \pm 23.7$ segments, with perfusion: $38.7 \pm 21.1$ segments, $p<0.025$), indicating a significantly better regional contraction pattern when arterial blood was supplied to the jeopardized myocardial area (example in Fig. 1).

In a series of experiments in 17 domestic pigs Mc Donald and coworkers [8] studied the effect of simultaneous perfusion with whole or diluted blood on LV hemodynamics, induction of ventricular arrhythmias, and on hematologic parameters of the perfusate during balloon inflation periods of 1–5 minutes with the balloon catheters placed in the middle third of the LAD. The mere presence of a 2.0 mm balloon catheter (Grüntzig steerable 2.0) within LAD without inflation led to a significant reduction of mean arterial blood pressure, peak systolic LV pressure and LV-dp/dt max, whereas LV filling pressures and percentage segment shortening did not change significantly. In 5/17 animals ventricular fibrillation occured with the presence of the balloon catheter in LAD without inflation. The perfusion medium used was heparinized blood (whole blood with a hematocrit of $33 \pm 4\%$, or diluted blood with a hematocrit value of $26 \pm 2\%$). During balloon inflations of 2, 3 and 5 minutes without perfusion significant reductions in mean arterial pressure, peak systolic LV pressure and LV-dp/dt max were seen at all times measured, whereas no significant changes of hemodynamic parameters were observed with perfusion, regardless of whether whole blood or diluted blood was used as the perfusate. The same holds true for regional contraction behavior. The mean flow rates obtained with whole blood were 14.5 as compared to 21.0 ml with diluted blood. In some experiments occlusion of the catheter due to thrombus formation was observed, when whole blood was used as the perfusate, but on no occasion with diluted blood. In 7/17 animals ventricular fibrillation occured within 1–5 minutes of inflation without perfusion, in contrast to lack of VF occurrence when simultaneous blood perfusion was used. In myocardial biopsies examined at the arteriolar-capillary level fresh thrombus formation was seen in 2/9 biopsy samples obtained after balloon inflation without perfusion, in 1/9 samples after whole blood perfusion, and in 0/9 samples after perfusion with diluted blood.

## Discussion

The results of our pilot study indicate that ic.-administration of Nifedipine may delay the occurence of signs of myocardial ischemia during PTCA, thus providing potentially longer inflation periods. Similar results were recently published by Erbel and coworkers [9] and Schreiner and associates [10], who found favourable effects of ic.-administration of both Nitroglycerine and Nifedipine. Not only could the inflation times be prolonged with regard to the occurence and degree of ST segment alterations, but also were ventricular arrhythmias be prevented by both drugs. And moreover, the effects were additive when both drugs were administered in a randomized order. Since ic.-Nitroglycerine lowered both mean arterial and left ventricular filling pressure, the authors concluded that Nitroglycerine exerted it's beneficial effect by primarily unloading left ventricular myocardium (pre- and afterload reduction), thus improving endocardial and collateral blood flow. On the other hand, Nifedipine did not significantly influence hemodynamic parameters, and consequently a certain regional 'cardioplegic' effect was discussed, as can also be derived from our data with ic.-Nifedipine. Serruys and coworkers [11, 12, 13] were able to demonstrate beneficial effects of ic.-Nifedipine on regional and global LV performance together with a reduction of myocardial oxygen consumption in studies with free coronary flow, as well as a decreased myocardial lactate release during PTCA. These authors also discuss a regional 'cardioplegic' effect of ic.-Nifedipine, the mechanism of which was interpreted as 'selective electromechanical decoupling'. In conclusion, from the above mentioned reports and also from corresponding results of animal experiments [13, 14] it may be derived that both Nitroglycerine and Nifedipine (and probably other calciumantagonistic drugs like Verapamil or Diltiazem as well) may protect jeopardized ventricular myocardium from ischemic damage to some degree. And the routine prophylactic use of ic.-Nitroglycerine plus ic.-or sublingual Nifedipine (or other calciumantagonists) seems justified, in order to increase the safety of the PTCA procedure and to allow potentially prolonged inflation periods. However, the question remains to be answered, to what degree ic.-Nitroglycerine and/or calciumantagonists will preserve global and regional LV performance during inflation periods of 45–70 seconds (and longer), since appropriate studies using quantitative LV angiography have not been reported as yet.

A more logical and physiological approach to protect ventricular myocardium from PTCA related ischemia seems to be the method of simultaneous perfusion with arterial blood through the free lumen of the balloon catheter during the whole inflation period. As can be derived from our results in humans, global and regional LV performance can be considerably and significantly preserved by this method, although only a limited amount of blood (12–20 ml/min) can be delivered to the dependent myocardial area via the small lumen of the balloon catheter. In domestic pigs perfusion flows of 15–21 ml/min as a mean were able to completely prevent deterioration of LV hemodynamics and the occurence of potentially deleterious ventricular arrhythmias, particularly of ventricular fibrillation. From these animal experiments it can be supposed, too, that the use of diluted blood with a hematocrit of about 25% may reveal the highest degree of safety, since in no instance was local thrombosis formation observed at the tip of the balloon catheter and/or embolization of thrombotic material to the arteriolar-capillary vascular bed. When specially designed 'high flow' balloon catheters will be available in the future, higher perfusion rates of about 25–30 ml/min with diluted blood may be achieved, that should be sufficient to completely prevent deterioration of LV performance during PTCA. Thus, it seems not to be utopic that, using this method of simultaneous blood perfusion, with one or two inflation periods of 2–4 minutes and inflation pressures of 6–12 athmospheres, PTCA procedures may be highly effective and safe. Therefore this method could be conveniently applied as a routine procedure in patients with normal and particularly impaired left ventricles, in those with multiple vessel disease, and perhaps also in individuals in whom PTCA of left main stenoses may be considered, all of whom being conditions with higher risks of complications like LV pump failure, when LV myocardium is not protected from severe ischemia.

## References

1. Grüntzig AR (1978) Transluminal dilatation of coronary artery stenosis. Lancet 1: 263
2. Kent KM, Mullin SM, Passamani ER (Guest Editors) (1984) Proceedings of the National Heart, Lung, and Blood Institute Workshop on the Outcome of Percutaneous Transluminal Coronary Angioplasty Amer J Cardiol 53–12
3. Faxon DP, Kelsey SF, Ryan TJ, Mc Cabe CH, Detre K (1984) Determinants of successful percutaneous transluminal coronary angioplasty: Report from the National Heart, Lung, and Blood Institute Registry Amer Heart J 108: 1019
4. Hombach V, Höpp HW, Fuchs M, Behrenbeck DW, Tauchert M, Hilger HH (1983) Preservation of ventricular myocardium during PTCA by intracoronary Nifedipine Circulation 68 (Suppl III) (abstr) 567
5. Hombach V, Höpp HW, Behrenbeck DW, Tauchert M, Fuchs M, Hilger HH (1984) Methods of myocardial protection during PTCA-Role of intracoronary blood perfusion and of Nifedipine. International Symposium 'Cardiology 84' – Pacemakers-Angioplasty-Fibrinolysis', Sevilla, Spain, 1984, 35 (abstr)
6. Busch U, Pfeiffer U, Baumann G, Sebening H, Blömer H (1984) Distal vessel perfusion via

dilatation catheter after coronary artery occlusion Europ Heart J 5, Suppl 1, 120

7. Fuchs M, Behrenbeck DW, Hombach V Die invasive Diagnostik der koronaren Herzkrankheit. In: Hombach V (ed) (1984) Kardiologie – Grundlagen-Fortschritte-Klinische Erfahrungen, Band 1: Die Koronare Herzkrankheit, Stuttgart-New York FK Schattauer-Verlag ; S 83

8. Mc Donald FM, Fuchs M, Kreuzer J, Höpp HW, Heinen A, Arnold G, Heymanns L, Hirche HJ, Hombach V (1985) Haemodynamic and anti-arrhythmic protective effects of intracoronary perfusion during percutaneous transluminal coronary angioplasty Europ Heart J, In press

9. Erbel R, Schreiner G, Henkel B, Pop T, Meyer J (1983) Improved ischemic tolerance during percutaneous transluminal coronary angioplasty by intracoronary injection of Nitroglycerin Z Kardiol 72, Suppl 3, 71

10. Schreiner G, Erbel R, Henkel B, Pop T, Meyer J (1983) Improved ischemic tolerance during percutaneous coronary angioplasty (PTCA) by antianginal drugs Circulation 68, Supp III, 389 (abstr)

11. Serruys PW, Brower RW, Ten Katen HJ, Bom AH, Hugenholtz PG (1981) Regional wall motion from radiopaque markers after intravenous and intracoronary injections of nifedipine Circulation 63, 584

12. Serruys PW, Hooghoudt TEH, Van den Brand M, Hugenholtz PG (1981) Influence of intracoronary nifedipine on left ventricular performance and myocardial oxygen consumption in human subjects Europ Heart J 2 (Suppl A) 51

13. Serruys PW, Van den Brand M, Brower RW, Hugenholtz PG (1983) Reginal cardioplegia and cardioprotection during transluminal angioplasty, which role for nifedipine? Europ Heart J, 4 (Suppl C) 115

14. Nayler WG, Slade AM (1982) The cardioprotective effect of verapamil Clin Exptl Pharmacol Physiol (Suppl 8) 75

15. Fleckenstein A: Specific inhibitors and promoters of calcium action in the excitation-contraction coupling of heart muscle and their role in the prevention or production of myocardial lesions. In: Harris P and Opie L (eds) (1971) Calcium and the Heart London New-York Academic Press, 135

# Time limits for emergency bypass grafting in preventing myocardial infarction

HANNEKUM A., G. ARNOLD, V. HOMBACH, A. KUX and B. HERSE

## Introduction

New therapeutic concepts for management of acute or evolving myocardial infarction, such as systemic or intracoronary thrombolysis and/or subsequent intra-coronary ballon dilatation, have led to an increase in emergency coronary surgical interventions as adjunct therapeutic methods. Likewise, elective percutaneous transluminal coronary angioplasty (PTCA) with the associated risk of vascular occlusion may require urgent surgical intervention. The primary aim of any invasive treatment of acute myocardial ischemia (i.e., thrombolysis, dilatation, surgery) is the *prevention* of myocardial necrosis. Early revascularization of an existing infarct, however, either may reduce the size of the infarct area by improving blood supply to the marginal zone or partially may restore the structure and function of injured myocardium. Numerous experimental *morphologic* studies in animal models have confirmed the ischemic tolerance of myocardial cells to be only 20 to 60 minutes [1–6]. In contrast, several experimental and clinical studies published during the last 10 years have demonstrated the possibility of myocardial salvage, seen by restoration of normal function, even after reperfusion later than 3 hours after onset of ischemia [7, 8]. Complete restoration of ventricular function has even been reported in cases with electrocardiographic and enzymatic manifestations of transmural infarction [9, 10]. Consequently, in the individual case, it is extremely difficult to predict whether emergency restoration of perfusion in ischemic myocardium definitively prevents cell necrosis, only reduces the size of the infarcted area, leads to restitution of the structure and function of damaged myocardial cells, or whether negative effects, such as hemorrhagic infarction or reperfusion-induced arrhythmias, are likely to occur.

## Factors influencing ischemic tolerance of myocardial cells

The wide variation in the time intervals between the onset of ischemia and the first morphologic indications of cell necrosis, on the one hand, and the presence of a positive reperfusion effect with subsequent salvage of damaged myocardium, on the other, is governed by the inhomogeneous progression of cell necrosis. The rapidity with which necrosis develops depends on the following secondary factors:

1. complete cutoff or severe reduction of blood flow,
2. permanent or temporary vascular occlusion,
3. size of ischemic zone,
4. individual type of coronary artery circulation,
5. number and caliber of collateral vessels,
6. hemodynamic changes during ischemic event,
7. general metabolic status of patient,
8. metabolic changes in affected myocardial cells,
9. metabolism-related effect on myocardial oxygen requirements.

These various influencial factors make *prospective* estimation of the extent of existing injury on the basis of time elapsed between ischemic event and surgical intervention, extremely difficult. Data on ischemic time limits for prevention of myocardial infarction vary considerably, even those obtained under experimental conditions in which some factors can be controlled.

Since ischemic myocardium losses its contractile capacity within 30 seconds, kinetic and perfusion studies of the affected area (angiography, echocardiography, perfusion scintigraphy) during the ischemic event or in the early post-ischemic phase are not suitable for differentiating between reversible injury of the myocardium and necrotic damage. Consequently, kinetic studies cannot be expected to predict the success of early revascularization. They are best employed retrospectively for semiquantitative determination of the approximate reduction achieved in the size of the infarct area on followup examination.

Likewise, myocardial cell necrosis can only be confirmed or excluded retrospectively by electrocardiography, and the extent of necrosis, at the most, estimated semiquantitatively by analysis of enzyme concentrations [11, 12]. The attempt to determine ischemic tolerance of myocardial cells and time limits for reversibility, therefore, ist restricted to experimental morphologic studies in animal models. The applicability of these findings to the human heart is limited by species-specific variations in coronary artery system and collateral blood supply.

## Morphological alterations and aspects for restoration in ischemic myocardium

Jennings and Schaper were the first investigators to conduct experimental studies on ultrastructural myocardial cell changes during ischemia and reperfusion. Reimar and coworkers quantified in experimental animals the dependent relation between extent of myocardial necrosis and duration of vascular occlusion. These researchers demonstrated a progression of myocardial cell necrosis from the subendocardial layer to the subepicardium. 38% of the transmural mass of the heart muscle was already irreversibly damaged 40 minutes after permanent vascular occlusion, 57% after 3 hours, and 71% after 6 hours. Accordingly, extensive subendocardial necrosis can be expected within one hour after occlusion of coronary artery [2]. In an earlier publication by the same team, irreversibly damaged myocardial cells were identified after only 20 minutes of ischemia. The morphologic manifestations of irrevesibility apparently become visible earlier after restoration of blood flow [3, 13]. Contrary to earlier opinions, cell damage occurs first and injury of the capillary endothelium becomes obvious up to 40 minutes later. Irreversible cell necrosis, therefore, is very probably due to intracellular metabolic changes and not to ulterastructual vascular injury [3, 4]. Reperfusion results in total disturbance of water- and electrolyte regulation. The inflow of amorphous substances into the cells, seen in electron microscopy, as a sign of irreversibility, therefore, is detectable earlier after reperfusion [1, 3, 13].

The extremely short ischemic tolerance in dogs (up to 40 mins) was, more or less, confirmed in man by Schaper and coworkers in their studies on human myocardium in the context of aortic valve surgery. Focal manifestations of irreversible cell damage were found after 50 minutes of ischemia. When the capillary endothelium is already injured, regeneration of reversibly damaged cell is more gradual and can even be delayed for several days, depending on the duration of the primary ischemia [13, 14]. The extent of the existing damage of the capillary endothelium limits the structure-salvaging effect of early postinfarction reperfusion to a few hours.

Whereas histologic studies by light microscopy are less sensitive for early diagnosis of cell necrosis and the manifestations of necrosis are often not visible for hours after the ischemic event, electron microscopy offers the possibility of early detection of irreversible cell damage and, subsequently, a more optimal definition of the actual time limits. The ultrastructural alterations develop parallel to the metabolic changes, e.g., reduction of oxydative phosphorylation, decrease of high-energy phosphates, and increase of anerobic glycolysis.

Excluding the influence of the secondary factors mentioned above, the absolute ischemic tolerance of single myocardial cells, therefore, presumably ranges from 20 to 40 minutes. This short interval should be taken into consideration not only in establishing the indication for emergency revascularization, but also in deciding to institute intracoronary thrombolytic therapy in acute myocardial infarction. Likewise, we have to consider the grave effect of late reperfusion, e.g., refractory ventricular dysrhythmias and impaired regional myocardial function in hemorrhagic infarction with a raising of mortality [15, 16].

**Electrocardiographic and enzymatic manifestations of reversible or irreversible myocardial injury**

Whereas T-wave changes on the electrocardiogram basically tend to characterize reversibility of acute ischemic damage of the myocardium, ST-segment changes can indicate reversible as well as irreversible damage. Loss of R-wave voltage or development of abnormal Q-waves are generally accepted as signs of transmural necrosis. Development of pathologic Q-waves and/or loss of R-voltage, however, does not necessarily parallel the occurrence of necrosis; such electrocardiographic manifestations often appear after a delay of several hours. Under reperfusion these manifestations of irreversible damage, however, my appear earlier [8, 9, 17]. Similarly, with persisting vascular occlusion, an elevation of the infarct-specific enzyme concentrations occurs after several hours, whereas, with reperfusion of ischemically injured myocardial regions, both the rise and the peak of serum enzyme concentations occur earlier [8, 9, 17].

Consequently, neither electrocardiogaphic nor enzymatic changes are well suited for predicting the change of successful revascularization or the extent of the existing ischemic injury, preliminary to deciding for or against an intervention in acute myocardial ischemia. The extent of necrosis and/or its prevention, therefore, can only be evaluated retrospectively.

The use of ST-segment and T-wave changes to diagnose nontransmural infarction in patients who have undergone emergency surgery may well augment the sensitivity of the electrocardiographic diagnosis of an infarction, but it also reduces the specificity, since such changes may be indicative of postoperative pericarditis or metabolic dysfunction [18]. A highly probable or confirmed cell necrosis should only be presumed when a concurrent rise of infarct-specific enzymes, expecially the heart-specific isoenzyme of creatinine kinase, is present. Radionuclide scintigraphy with technetium 99 pyrophosphat or thallium 201 may well make possible an even more reliable qualification and possibly quantification of an infarct event in connection with electrocardiographic and enzymatic changes [18]. Its wide application for patients with acute myocardial ischemia, however, seems to be less practical. Controlled preoperative and postoperative studies, however, should provide further informations about the actual ischemic tolerance of the heart.

The difficulty of estimating time limits for the prevention or the reduction in size of myocardial infarction, whether prospectively or retrospectively, prompted us to take myocardial biopsies from the presumed center of the ischemic zone during emergency coronary revascularization surgery. The histologic changes were subsequently correlated with ischemic times, state of coronary vessels, electrocardiographic and enzymatic changes as well as hemodynamic status during the ischemic event.

**Material and methods**

Between January 1982 and February 1985, 26 patients (5 women, mean age 42,8 years and 21 men, mean age 50,4 years) with temporary or permanent vascular occlusion underwent urgent coronary surgery at the University Hospital for Cardiovascular Surgery in Cologne (Fig. 1). In 18 patients, the intervention was performed following PTCA, in 3 after acute myocardial infarction and successful intracoronary thrombolysis; and in another 3 acute myocardial infarction with unsuccessful intracoronary thrombolysis. One patient with stenosis of the left main coronary artery suffered an irreversible spasm during diagnostic angiography; another patient developed a thrombotic occlusion of an aorto-coronary bypass graft and the revascularized vessel shortly after surgery. 17 patients had single vessel disease, most of them LAD stenosis, 6 two vessel disease and 3 three vessel disease.

The decision for surgery was based on extreme ST-segment elevation with concomitant chest pain (permanent vascular occlusion) or temporary ST elevation, with depression during intracoronary perfusion via a coronary catheter in 4 patients. 5 patients developed asystole or ventricular fibrillation in the catheterization suite.

The operation was performed under extracorporeal circulation and systemic hypothermia (28° C). Myocardial revascularization was achieved by aorto-coronary vein grafts in all patients. Prior to grafting, cardioplegia was induced in 20 patients by infusion of Bretschneider's cardioplegic solution and in 3 patients by Kirsch-Cardioplegia. Cardioplegia was not induced in the last 3 patients with multiple revascularization; in these cases, the occluded vessel was first anastomized by temporary aortic crossclamping and then immediately reperfused.

Sequential punch biopsies from the presumed center of the ischemic zone in the myocardium were performed intraoperatively in each of the last 16 patients. The first biopsy was taken at institution of extracorporeal circulation, shortly before aortic crossclamping, the last biopsy, as late as possible after reperfusion of the ischemic zone via aorto-coronary bypass grafts, but before discontinuation of extracorporeal circulation. To obtain tissue specimens from the subendocardial layer, the biopsy needle was put into the free ventricular cavity and then withdrawed until resistance was felt on reaching the endocardium. The biopsy material was processed for light and electron microscopy by immediate fixation in glutaraldehyde or phosphate-buffered formalin solution with following tissue preparation as described by Arnold and coworkers [19].

Clinically the diagnosis of perioperative infarction was based on the postoperative electrocardiogram and the changes in serum enzyme concentrations. Transmural infarction was determined by loss of R-wave voltage and/or development of abnormal Q-waves and elevation of the infarct-specific enzymes. The diagnosis of nontransmural infarction was based on St-segment alterations or T changes with concurrent elevation of creatinine kinase (CK-MB) the heart muscle-spe-

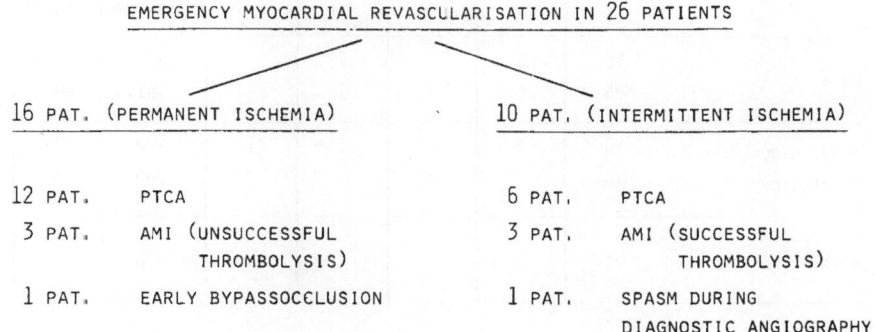

*Figure 1*. Emergency bypass grafting in 26 patients after ischemia following percutaneous transluminal coronary angioplasty (PTCA), in acute myocardial infarction (AMI) or after early postop. bypass occlusion University of Cologne (Jan. 82–Feb. 85).

cific isoenzyme of more than twice the levels considered normal at our institution. Nonspecific ST-segments and/or T-wave changes without concurrent enzyme response were considered not indicative of cell necrosis.

Postoperative followup was predominantly noninvasive since recatheterization was not possible in most patients.

## Results

In 16 of 26 patients, the indication for operation was *complete* cutoff of blood flow; 5 patients were resuscitated during transport to the operating room (3 following PTCA, 2 following unsuccessful thrombolysis). 4 of these 16 patients died 3 on the operating table. 2 patients suffered therapy refractory arrhythmias, the other 2 low cardiac output syndrome. 4 of the 12 surviving patients developed transmural infarction with subsequent left ventricular aneurysm (2 pats) or mild global left heart failure (2 pats) (Figs. 1, 2). The mean time between vessel occlusion and reperfusion of ischemic myocardium by vein graft was 126 minutes in the patients with single vessel disease following PTCA, 162 minutes in those with multiple vessel disease, and more than 210 minutes in those with acute myocardial infarction and unsuccessful thrombolysis (Fig. 2).

The poor outcome of the 8 patients who died or suffered severe complications correlated retrospectively with the extraordinarily length of ischemia until intraoperative reperfusion in the patients with single vessel disease. In those with multiple vessel disease, it correlated with the absence of angiographically demonstrable collateral blood flow to the distal part of the coronary artery (Fig. 3).

In the other 10 patients who underwent urgent surgery with temporary perfusion of the injured vessel, the indication for operation was coronary dissection

| | | N | + | TI | LVA | ISCHEMIA (MIN) |
|---|---|---|---|---|---|---|
| PTCA | 1 VD | 6 | | 1 | | 126.5 ± 27.1 |
| | MVD | 6 | 2 | 1 | | 161.5 ± 49.4 |
| ACUTE MYOCARDIAL INFARCTION | 1 VD | 2 | 1 | 1 → | 1 | 270 / 325 |
| | MVD | 1 | 1 | | | 260 |
| ACVG-OCCLUSION | 1 VD | 1 | | 1 → | 1 | 210 |

*Figure 2.* Time of ischemia and complications in 16 patients with permanent vessel occlusion before emergency revascularisation (1 VD = one vessel disease, MVD = multiple vessel disease, TI = transmural infarction, LVA = left ventricular aneurysm, ACVG = aorto-coronary-vein-graft).

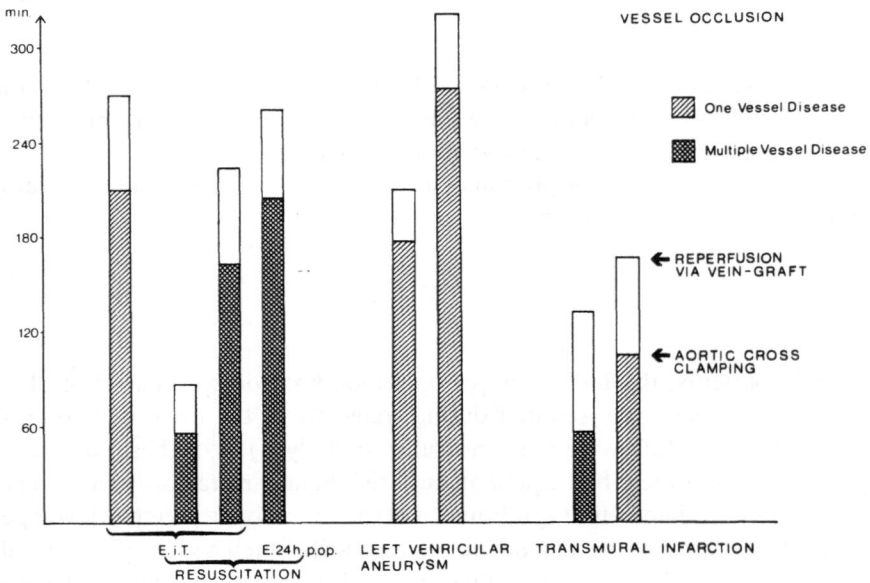

*Figure 3.* Time of ischemia, complications and extent of coronary disease in 8 patients (50%) with poor outcome after early surgical intervention.

with critical reduction of blood flow, irreversible spasm or unsuccessful dilatation of stenosis following successful intracoronary thrombolysis with concurrent temporary ST-segment elevation and severe chest pain. Reperfusion was carried out in 4 patients by infusion of oxygenated blood into the distal segment via an intracoronary catheter. This resulted in a significant diminuition of ST-segment elevation. 2 patients suffered transmural infarction without significant loss of ventricular function. Due to lack of exact information on these patients, the total ischemic time after acute myocardial infarction can only be estimated (Fig. 4). 10

| | | N | ÷ | TI | |
|---|---|---|---|---|---|
| PTCA | 1 VD | 5 | - | | PERFUSION VIA |
| | MVD | 1 | - | | PTCA-CATH. IN 4 PAT. |
| ACUTE MYOCARDIAL INFARCTION (SUCCESSFUL THROMBOLYSIS) | 1 VD | 3 | - | 2 | TIME INTERVAL BETWEEN AMI AND THROMBOLYSIS < 3 HOURS |
| IRREVERSIBLE SPASM DURING ANGIOGRAPHY | MVD | 1 | - | | |

*Figure 4*. Incidence of myocardial infarction after urgent revascularisation following temporary occlusion or intermittent reperfusion of injured vessel in 10 patients.

patients (39%) suffered transmural and 6 patients (22%) nontransmural infarcation. Another 10 patients (39%) postoperatively showed only nonspecific or no electrocardiographic changes; serum enzyme concentrations were not elevated (Table 1). No correlation could be established between the absolute height of the CK-NB concentration and the manifestations of transmural or nontransmural damage. The shortest interval between onset of ischemia and reperfusion of occluded vessels with postoperative diagnosis of transmural infarction was 88 minutes (Table 2). This patient presented an acute LAD occlusion and chronic occlusion of the circumflex branch of the left coronary artery with left circulation type. Excluding this patient, the mean ischemic time for patients with transmural infarctions after complete vascular occlusion and subsequent balloon dilatation was 172 minutes. By contrast, the mean ischemic time was 170 minutes in nontransmural infarction and 110 minutes in patients with no postoperative indications of myocardial necrosis (Table 2).

Biopsies were taken from the last 16 patients (after temporary perfusion of occluded coronary artery: 5 patients; after permanent occlusion: 11 patients). The following four types of morphologic cell damage were established which are dependent, for the most part, on the duration of ischemia and/or, in the case of multiple vessel disease, minor collateral blood flow (Fig. 5).

*Table 1*. Incidence of perioperative myocardial infarction.

| | Occlusion | | | Intermittent perfusion | | | n |
|---|---|---|---|---|---|---|---|
| | PTCA | AMI | ACVG-Occl. | PCTA | AMI | SPASM | |
| T.I. | 4 | 3 | 1 | – | 2 | – | 10 |
| NT. I | 4 | – | – | 1 | 1 | – | 6 |
| no I | 4 | – | – | 5 | – | 1 | 10 |

T.I. = Transmural Infarction, NT.I. = Non Transmural Infarction, no I. = No Infarction.

230

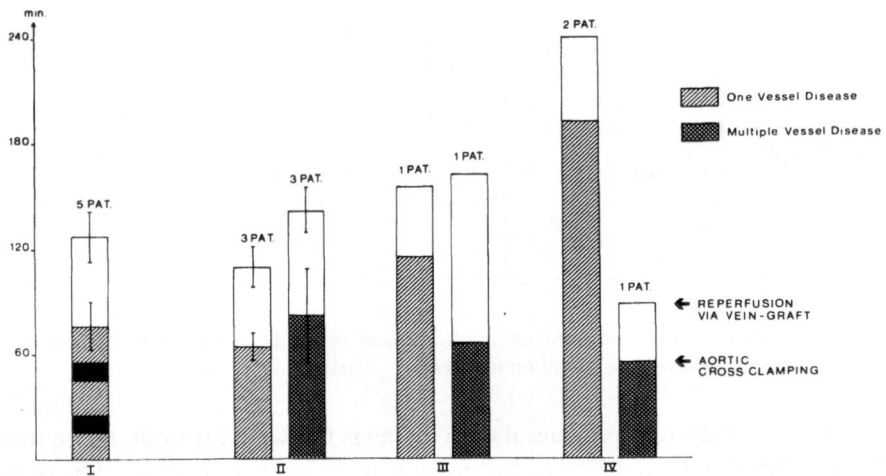

*Figure 5.* Relationship of elapsed ischemic time, multiple vessel disease and *type* of morphologic cell damage (I–IV, explanation see text).

Type I    *uncharacteristic cell edema* and nuclear swelling on first biopsy in patients with temporary reperfusion and signs of regeneration after reperfusion on final biopsy.

Type II   *myofibrillar degeneration,* characterized by crossbands, electron microscopically mitochondrial alterations of varying degree but facultative reversibility on reperfusion biopsy.

Type III  *myofibrillar degenerations,* mitochondrial degenerations but ultrastructural at least focally irreversible types of coagulation necrosis.

Type IV   early signs of *coagulation necrosis* already seen on first biopsy with tendency of deterioration on final biopsy.

*Table 2.* Relationship of elapsed ischemic time and manifestation of myocardial necrosis.

| | Occlusion | | | Intermittent perfusion | | | n |
|---|---|---|---|---|---|---|---|
| | PTCA | AMI | ACVG-Occl. | PTCA | AMI | SPASM | |
| T.I. | 152,5 ± 57,7 (88–225) | 285 (260–325) | 210 | – | ≈170 | – | 10 |
| NT. I | 170 ± 23,7 (155–205) | – | – | 136 | ≈122 | – | 6 |
| no I | 110 ± 9,1 (97–118) | – | – | 130,6 ± 19,5 (100–150) | – | 130 | 10 |

T.I. = Transmural infarction; NT. I = Non transmural infarction; no I = No infarction.

On light microscopy, the morphologic changes indicative of *reversibly damaged myocardium* are uncharacteristic intracellular and interstitial edema without blue luxol staining. These changes were found both pre- and postischemically in 5 patients with 10 minutes temporary perfusion of the injured vessel up to 3 times at the most. The mean interval between primary symptom and first biopsy after institution of extracorporeal circulation was $76 \pm 15,6$ minutes. The second biopsy was taken on the average 15 minutes after restoration of blood flow, i.e., $127,4 \pm 16.5$ minutes after the first symptom (Fig. 5). In these patients, electron microscopic assessment showed slight mitochondrial swelling, cristae fragmentation, and diminished matrix density; no amorphous densities, however, were observed in the matrix space (Fig. 6). This patient suffered LAD occlusion following PTCA with 50 minutes of cumulative ischemia, i.e., 10 minutes of ischemia, 10 minutes of temporary perfusion, and, prior to aortic crossclamping, 40 minutes of ischemia.

Direct comparison of the preischemic and postischemic specimens from this patient reflects the effect of 20 minutes of reperfusion, i.e., reduction of mitochondrial matrix density and reappearance of normal matrix granula and of tortous course of cristae (Fig. 7).

The light microscopic *reperfusion phenomenon* in ischemic myocardium is characterized by the appearance of crossbands, which are visualized by the blue staining luxol reaction [19]. This type of myofibrillar degeneration may be indicative of a cell membrane failure that is not necessarily followed by cell death. The presence of cell regeneration or cell death can be determined only by electron microscopy. Ultrastructurally, the varying extent of mitochondrial changes in biopsies taken after reperfusion may reflect the success of early reperfusion in the individual case. Obvious characteristics determining the beneficial or detrimental effect of reperfusion are the extent of mitochondrial swelling, the degree of cristae alterations, and the occurrence of amorphous densities. A biopsy taken from the left ventricular apex 130 minutes after LAD occlusion and 20 minutes after reperfusion shows moderate to severe mitochondrial damage with matrix clearing and ruptured cristae (Fig. 8). The lack of amorphous densities can be interpreted as a characteristic of reversibility. This type of ultrastructural change was observed in 6 patients (Group II) with a mean ischemic time to aortic crossclamping of 73 minutes ($\pm 19,9$) and to reperfusion via vein graft of 125,7 minutes ($\pm 20,7$). By contrast, another biopsy (Fig. 9) taken 30 minutes after reperfusion of occluded LAD with a total ischemic time of 162 minutes shows severe mitochondrial edema. Mitochondria lying between coarse crossbands exhibit vesicular cristae, multiple amorphous densities and occasional intermembraneous inclusions as indicative of irreversible cell damage at least focally. Postoperatively, this patient suffered transmural infarction with mild global left heart failure (Group III, 2 patients; mean time to reperfusion, $158,5 \pm 4.9$ min).

*Irreversible* myocardial cell damage is characterized by massive cell swelling, dilatation of sarcomere, light microscopically visible poor luxol staining. These

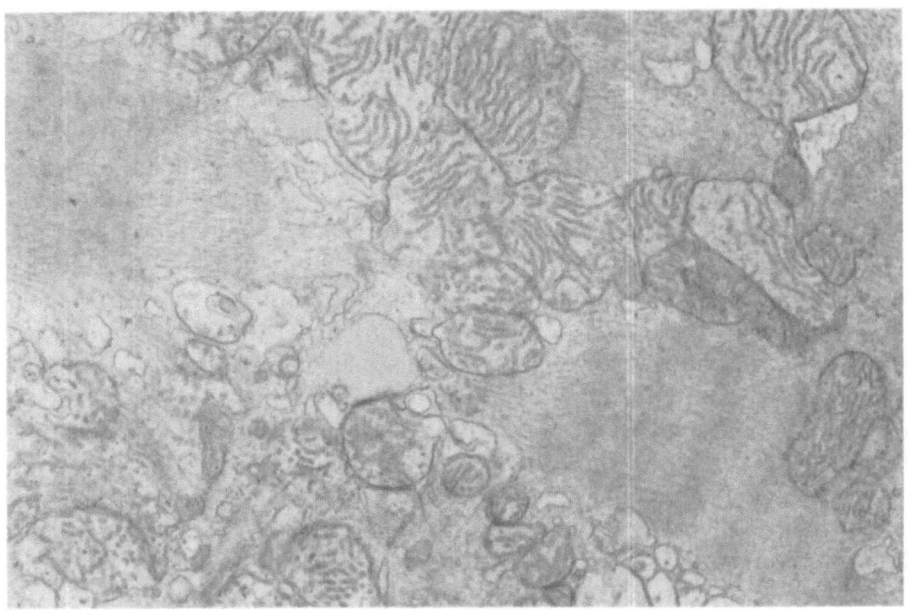

*Figure 6.* Myocardium after 50 min. of cumulative ischemia, 10 min. of ischemia, 10 min. of temporary perfusion, and prior to cardioplegia, 40 min. of ischemia. Note swollen mitochondria with cleared matrix and focally ruptured cristae. × 16.500 (reduction 70%).

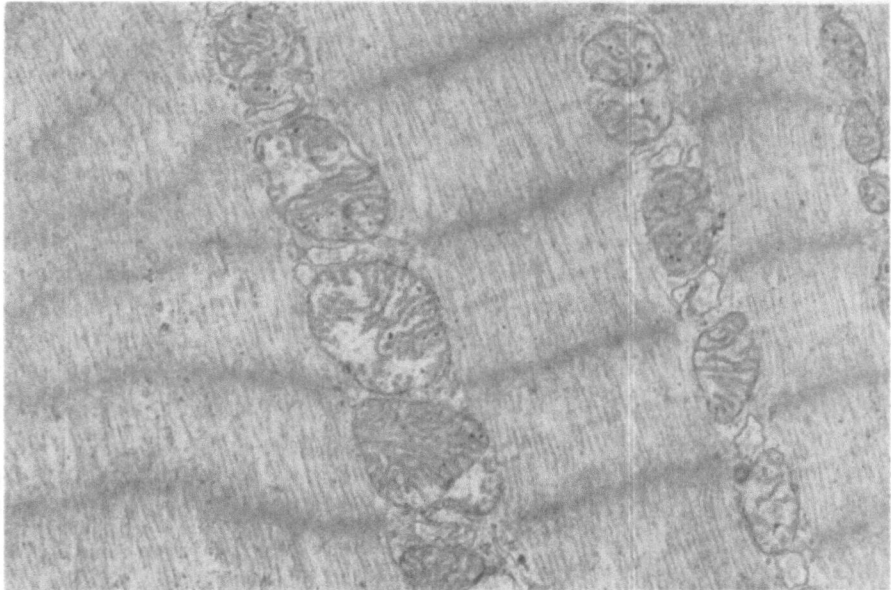

*Figure 7.* Myocardium of the same patient as in Fig. 6, following 30 min. of cardioplegic ischemia and 20 min. of reperfusion via the vein graft. Note reduction of mitochondrial matrix clearing and reappearance of normal matrix granula and of tortuous course of cristae. × 16.500 (reduction 70%).

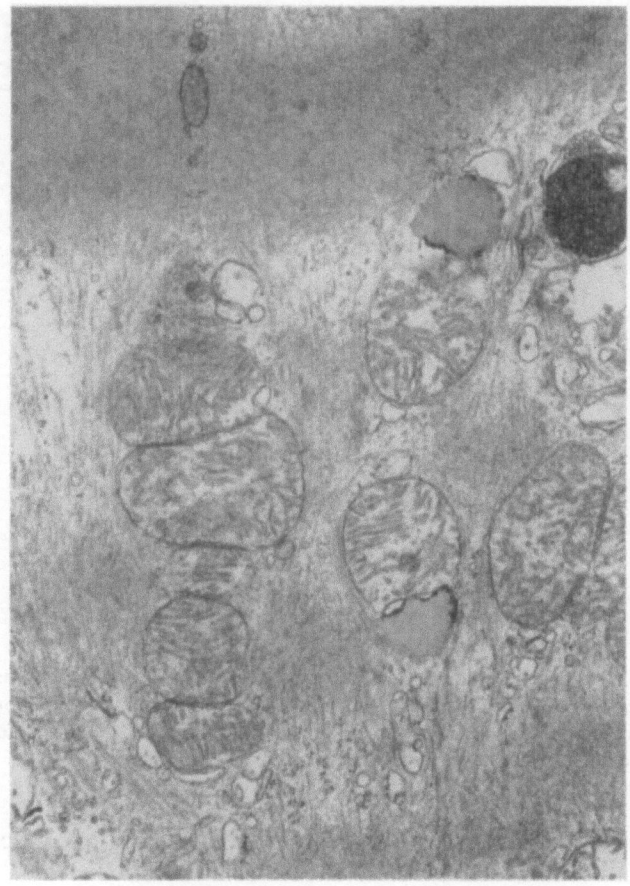

*Figure 8.* Myofibrillar degeneration 20 min. of reperfusion following 130 min. of ischemia. Moderate to severe mitochondrial damage with matrix clearing and ruptured cristae, but lack of amorphous densities. × 16.500 (reduction 70%).

manifestations are not necessarily present on the preischemic biopsy. We found ultrastructural manifestations, indicative of an early type of coagulation necrosis, e.g., massively swollen mitochondria, ruptured cristae, prominent amorphous densities within mitochondria, cell membrane defects, and capillary endothelial lesions, in 3 patients (Group IV, Fig. 10). In one of these patients, who also suffered chronic occlusion of the circumflex artery, these manifestations were apparent as early as 55 minutes after LAD occlusion. Most criteria for irreversibility were already distinctly evident on the first biopsy (Fig. 11). Reperfusion was restored by aorto-coronary vein graft 33 minutes later, i.e., 88 minutes after vessel occlusion. The patient died on the operating table of severe low cardiac output. A postischemic biopsy was taken 82 minutes after reperfusion (Fig. 12).

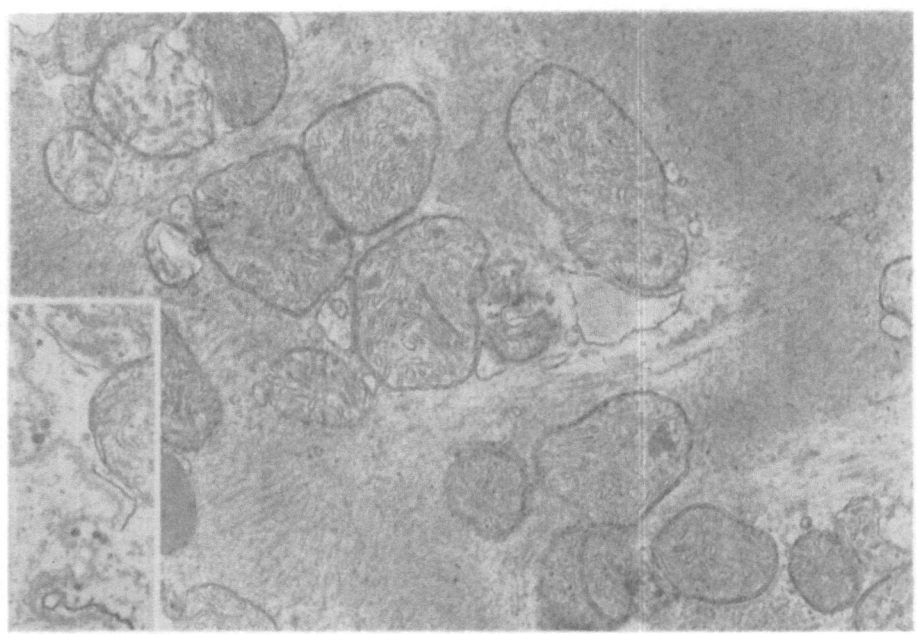

*Figure 9.* Myofibrillar degeneration; 30 min. of reperfusion following 162 min. of ischemia. Mitochondria lying between coarse cross bands exhibit vesicular cristae, multiple amorphous densities and occasional intermembranous inclusions. × 21.500. Inset: Note large sarcolemmal defects underneath the detached glycocalyx. × 26.400 (reduction 70%).

The obvious signs of irreversibility document the deteriorating effect of reperfusion in this case.

**Discussion**

Reperfusion of ischemic myocardium can affect the type and extent of myocardial cell damage and, consequently, may lead to regeneration of heart muscle cells. After a certain time interval, however, coagulation necrosis is to be expected, at least focally; its progression however can also be considerably accelerated by reperfusion. Due to the extraordinarily broad range of ischemic times, it is extremely difficult to establish a correlation to the type of morphologically visible cell damage as well as to the individual vascular status. In Figure 13, the ischemic time for each biopsied patient stands opposite to the vascular status and the postoperative extent of myocardial cell necrosis as determined by electrocardiographic and enzyme analysis. Only minor nonspecific reversible cell damage is to be expected after temporary perfusion of a vessel occluded primarily by spasm or dissection, even when the cumulative period of ischemia to surgical interven-

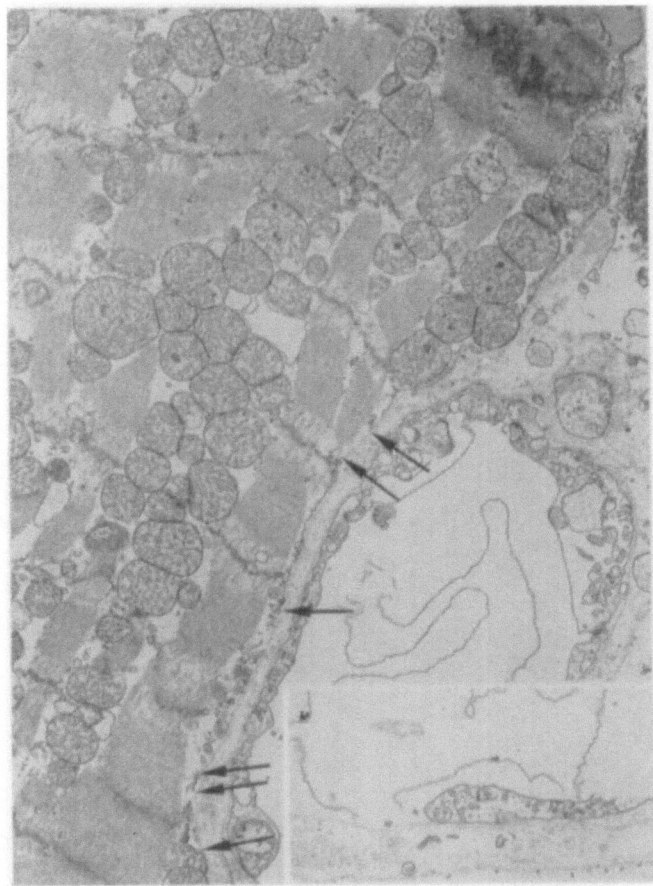

*Figure 10.* Irreversibly injured myocardium, 210 min. of ischemia and 39 min. of reperfusion. Note dilatation of sarcomeres, prominent amorphous densities within mitochondria and multifocal sarcolemmal defects (arrows). × 5.800. Inset: Damaged endothelium with membrane defects and protruding cytoplasmic blebs. × 9.600 (reduction 70%).

tion is as long as 60 minutes (pats 1–5). With single vessel disease and a total ischemic time of two hours to restoration of perfusion (pats 6–8), no clinically evident signs of infarction stand opposite to morphological myofibrillary degeneration, which tends to regenerate early in the course of reperfusion. The same morphologic changes were found in patients 9–11. In these patients, multiple vessel disease with subsequent multiple revascularization led to a longer interval between onset of ischemia and restoration of perfusion via bypass grafts. Both the longer duration of the ischemia and the possibly poorer collateral perfusion after the ischemic event could well be the cause of the electrocardiographically and enzymatically demonstrable mostly nontransmural necrosis. The extent of trans-

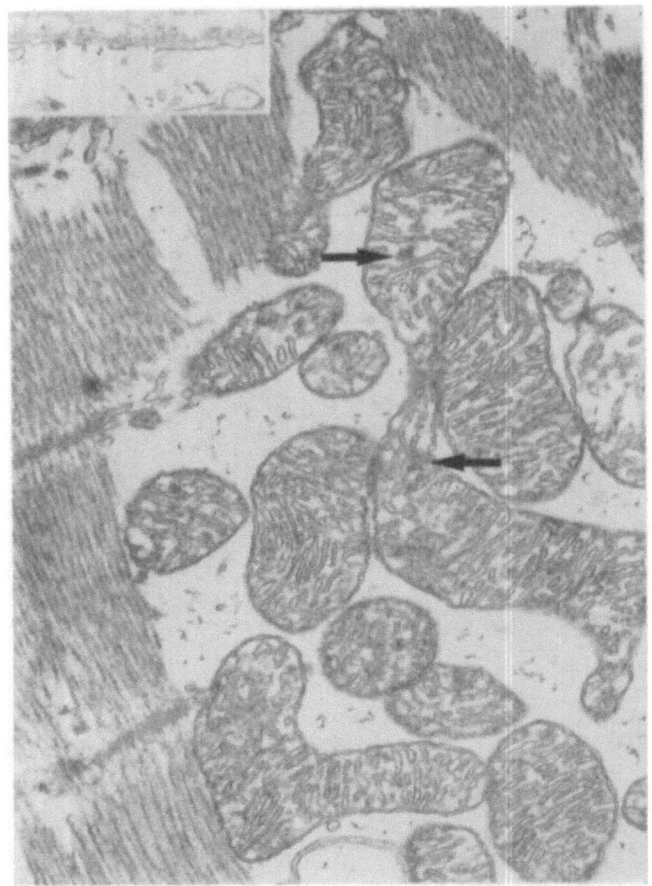

*Figure 11.* Irreversible ischemic injury (55 min. ischemia) prior to reperfusion; acute occlusion of LAD, preexistent occlusion of RX. Note vesicular, ruptured cristae and occasional amorphous matrix densities (arrows). × 5.800. Inset: Minute sarcolemmal breaks covered by the fuzzy external lamina. × 20.400 (reduction 70%).

mural necrosis in patient Nr. 11, in whom the duration of ischemia was only 2 hours, is explained by poor residual perfusion until surgery. Closed chest massage was required from occlusion of the vessel until institution of extracorporeal circulation.

Early forms of coagulation necrosis are to be expected, at least focally, with ischemic times of more than 150 minutes. In patient Nr. 12, these morphologic changes in single vessel disease (LAD) stand opposite to a long interval between onset of ischemia and surgery. Patient Nr. 13 developed a complete occlusion in the context of PTCA of the circumflex branch. Since a 50% occlusion of the right coronary artery, which also supplies the posterior wall, was present, the advanced

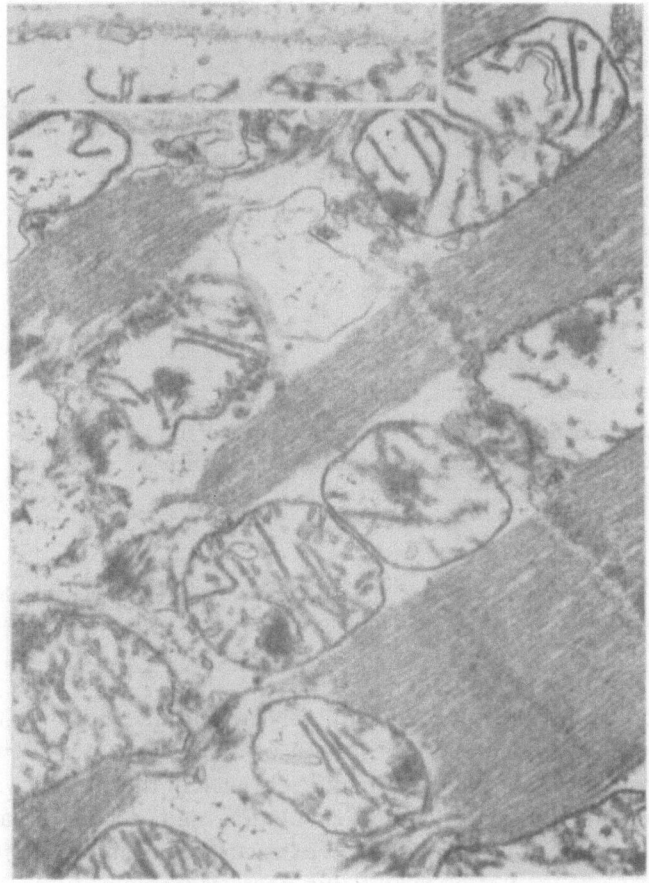

*Figure 12.* The same irreversibly injured myocardium as in Fig. 11; 88 min. of ischemia followed by 82 min. of reperfusion. Deterioration of damage: extreme mitochondrial clearing, abundant amorphous densities, multiple intracristal inclusions. × 26.400 (reduction 70%). Inset: Extensive sarcolemmal defects. × 20.400 (reduction 70%).

morphology may be explained by reduced collateral perfusion. In both patients, however, the infarction clinically was nontransmural.

Extensive coagulation necrosis was found in patients 14–16. In one case, occlusion of a LAD bypass, which was diagnosed late, with concomitant coronary artery thrombosis resulted in a period of ischemia lasting more than 3 hours. After transmural infarction, a left ventricular anteriolateral wall aneurysm developed some time after surgery. After thrombotic occlusion of a stenosed LAD and unsuccessful lysis and dilatation in patient Nr. 15, revascularization was not possible for 4 hours. The patient died on the operating table of reperfusion-induced arrhythmias. Patient Nr. 16, who has been mentioned several times, also

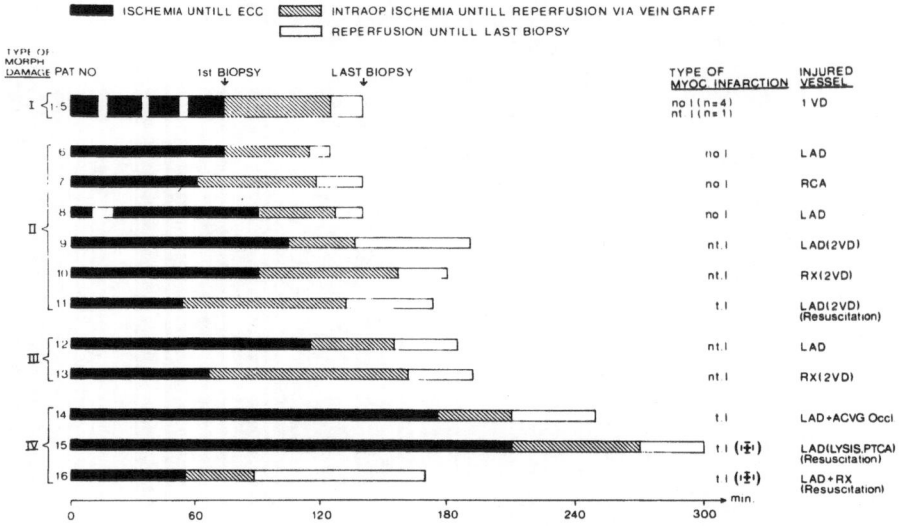

*Figure 13.* Type of morphological damage, time of ischemia and reperfusion, extent of clinically evaluated myocardial infarction and type and number of injured vessels in 16 patients who were biopsied intraoperatively.

died on the operating table of severe low cardiac output syndrome; the interval between onset of ischemia and reperfusion of the occluded LAD was only 88 minutes. Chronic occlusion of the circumflex branch of the coronary artery (Fig. 14) and subsequent poor collateral circulation and decompensated hemodynamics (reanimation until institution of extracorporeal circulation) explain the extremely early appearance of coagulation necrosis (see also Figs. 11, 12).

The upper and lower clinically relevant time limits for early revasularization to prevent myocardial infarction, as reflected by influential factors, such as complete vascular occlusion, ischemic time to cardiac relief by extracorporeal circulation, total ischemic time to reperfusion, vascular status (single or multiple vessel disease) as well as circulatory state prior to surgical intervention are best defined in patients 9–13.

After elapsed time of ischemia of more than 2 hours evidence of myocardial necrosis can be expected. Poor collateral blood flow which has to be reflected mostly in left anterior descending artery injury reduces these time limits significantly. This short period of time we have to consider when indicating urgent myocardial revascularisation after ischemia complicating PTCA or in case of decision against or for thrombolysis in acute myocardial infarction. It should be the primary aim, not only to reduce size of infarction area but to protect the ultracellular and microvascular structure to *prevent* ischemic damage.

Intraaortic balloon pumping (IABP) potentially may have a beneficial effect on ischemic tolerance by augmentation of coronary perfusion during diastole with

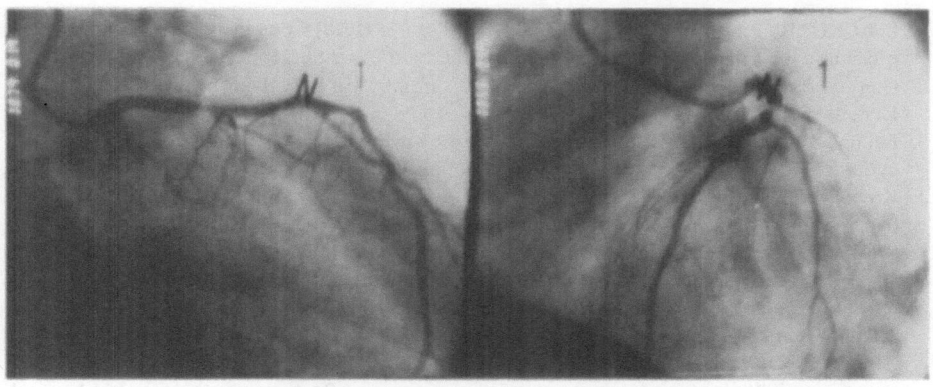

*Figure 14.* Angiography of patient number 16: Chronic occlusion of the circumflex branch and subtotal stenosis of left anterior descending artery prior to PTCA-attempt.

recruiting coronary collaterals [20]. In patients with limited collateral channels IABP may reduce the extent of myocardial necrose at best [21]. However, the absence or presence of collaterals is frequently unknown, or angiographically not visible.

Therefore operation should not be delayed by problems during insertion of intraaortic balloon in case of acute myocardial ischemia. Orthograde infusion of oxygenated blood in the distal segment of injured vessel via intracoronary catheters, at last intermittent if possible, probably is superior, decreasing the extent of myocardial necrosis as seen in four of our patients [22].

Aware of these short time limits in preventing myocardial infarction PTCA procedures with 4–6% incidence of emergency operation at present [23] should be performed under immediate availability of a surgical team in our opinion.

## References

1. Kloner RA, Ganote ChE, Whalen DA jr, Jennings RB (1974) Effect of a transient period of ischemia on myocardial cells. Am J Pathol 74, No 3: 399–422
2. Reimer KA, Lowe JE, Rasmussen MM, Jennings RB (1977) The wavefront phenomenon of ischemic cell death. Circulation 56, No 5: 786–794
3. Kloner RA, Roberts ER, Carlson N, Maroko PR, De Boer LWV, Braunwald E (1980) Ultrastructural evidence of microvascular damage and myocardial cell injury after coronary artery occlusion: Which comes first? Circulation 62, No 5: 945–952
4. Roberts CS, Schoen FJ, Kloner RA (1983) Effect of coronary reperfusion on myocardial hemorrhage and infarct healing. Am J Cardiol 52, No 6: 610–614
5. Jennings RB, Sommers HM (1960) Moycardial necrosis induced by temporary occlusion of a coronary artery in the dog. Arch Pathol 70: 68
6. Jennings RB, Baum JH, Herdson HB (1965) Fine structural changes in myocardial ischemic injury. Arch Pathol 79: 139

7. Leitz KH, Rentrop KP, Oster H, Blanke H, Kreuzer H (1980) Combined medical and surgical procedure in acute myocardial infarction. Thorac Cardiovasc Surgeon 28: 285–290
8. Ganz N, Buchbinder N et al (1981) Intracoronary thrombolysis in evolving myocardial infarction. Herz 6, 1: 37–43
9. Phillips SJ, Zeff RH (1981) Surgical therapy for evolving myocardial infarction, results in 138 patients. Herz 6, 1: 55–62
10. Krebber HF, Mathey DG, Schofer J, Rodewald G (1983) Indication for early aorto-coronary bypass surgery after successful intracoronary lysis. Thorac Cardiovasc Surgeon 31: 50–53
11. Schwarz F, Faure A, Katus H, von Olshausen K, Hofmann M, Schuler G, Manthey J, Kübler W (1983) Intracoronary thrombolysis in acute myocardial infarction: an attempt to quantitate its effect by comparision of enzymatic estimate of myocardial necrosis with left ventricular ejection fraction. Am J Cardiol 51, 10: 1573
12. Althaus K, Gurtner HO, Baur H, Hamburger S, Roos B (1977) Consequences of myocardial reperfusion following temporary coronary occlusion in pigs, effects on morphologic, biochemical and haemodynamic findings. European Journal of Clinical Investigations 7: 437–443
13. Schaper J, Schwartz F, Kittstein H, Kreisel E, Winkler B, Hehrlein FW (1980) Ultrastructural evaluation of the effects of global ischemia and reperfusion on human myocardium. Thorac Cardiovasc Surgeon 28: 337–342
14. Schaper J, Schaper W (1983) Reperfusion of ischemic myocardium, ultrastructural and histo-chemical aspects. J Am Coll Cardiol 1: 1037–1046
15. Bresnehan GF, Roberts R, Shell, Ross WE, Sobel BE (1974) Deleterious effects due to hemor-rhage after myocardial reperfusion. Am J Cardiol 33: 82
16. Wood D, Roberts CH, van Devanter StH, Kloner R, Cohn LH (1982) Limitation of myocardial infarct size after surgical reperfusion for acute coronary occlusion. J Thorac Cardiovasc Surgeon 84: 353–387
17. Murphy DA et al (1984) Surgical management of acute myocardial ischemia following per-cutaneous transluminal coronary angioplasty. J Thorac Cardiovasc Surgery 87, 3: 332–339
18. Schaff HV et al (1984) Detrimental effect of perioperative myocardial infarction on late survival after coronary artery bypass. J Thorac Cardiovasc Surgery 88, 6: 972–981
19. Arnold G, Hannekum A, Hombach V. Impending human myocardial infarction: stages of reversible and irreversible injury evidenced by sequential biopsies. Arch pathol (in press)
20. Jakobey JA, Taylor WJ, Smith GT, Gorlin R, Harken DE (1963) A new therapeutic approach to acute coronary occlusion. Opening dormant coronary collateral channels by counterpulsation. Am J Cardiol 11: 218–227
21. Margolis JR (1982) The role of the percutaneous intraaortic ballon in emergency situations following percutaneous transluminal coronary angioplasty. In: Kaltenbach M, Grüntzig A, Rentrop K, Bussmann WD (eds) Transluminalcoronary angioplasty and intracoronary throm-bolysis. Berlin-Heidelberg, New York: Springer Verlag, pp 144–150
22. Hombach V, McDonald FM, Fuchs M, Hannekum A, Höpp HW, Osterspey A, Heinen A, Hilger HH (1985) Myocardial salvage during percutaneous transluminal coronary angioplasty. International Symposium on invasive cardiovascular therapy: recent advances and future de-velopments May 5–8, Cologne/Germany (in press)
23. Dorros G, Cowley MJ, Simpson J, Bentivoglio LG, Block PC, Bourassa M, Detre K, Gosselin AJ, Grüntzig A, Kelsey SF, Kent KM, Mock MB, Mullin SM, Myler RK, Passamani ER, Stertzer SH, Williams DO (1983) Percutaneous transluminal coronary angioplasty. Report of complica-tions from the National Heart, Lung and Blood Institute PTCA Registry, Circulation 67: 723–730

# Coronary artery bypass grafting in chronic coronary heart disease

R.W. HACKER and M. TORKA

Conservative treatment as well as percutaneous transluminal coronary angioplasty (PTCA) have shifted the indication for coronary artery bypass grafting (CABG) towards more severely diseased hearts, taking away the good risk cases with proximally obstructed, but otherwise wide-calibred coronary arteries and well-preserved ventricles, and replacing them by patients with diffusely diseased vessels and scarred myocardium, not responding to medical treatment, and not amenable to PTCA.

In order to redefine the indications for CABG, two questions have to be answered

1.  How effectively has CABG so far achieved its goals of improving symptoms and prolonging life?
2.  How does the risk and success rate of CABG compare with that of medical treatment?

Results of CABG will be demonstrated, using the data of 2,700 consecutive patients, who had myocardial revascularization with saphenous vein grafts between 1974 and 1981 at the Chirurgische Universitätsklinik Erlangen/Germany, and have been followed up for 1 to 10 years postoperatively. Preoperative data are shown in table 1.

## Angina pectoris after CABG

There is no discussion, that the effect of CABG on angina pectoris is far superior to the effect of medical treatment.

Our own experience shows, that angina pectoris, which was present in 99% of all patients preoperatively, was completely abolished in 62% of patients within the first year after surgery (Fig. 1). During the following years the percentage of patients in functional class I decreased at a rate of about 2% yearly. Nevertheless,

242

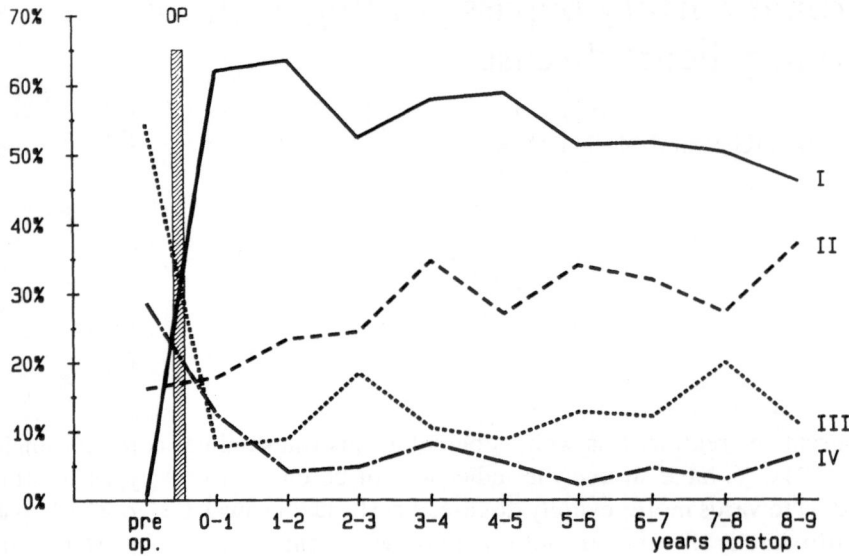

*Figure 1.* Functional class (NYHA) after CABG vs. follow-up period.

*Table 1.* Preoperative data.

|  | n | % |
| --- | --- | --- |
| Sex male | 2472/2700 | 91.6 |
|     female | 228 | 8.4 |
| Age mean | 52,9 years | (SE = 7.4 years) |
| Myocardial infarction | 1455/2664 | 54.6 |
| Functional class (NYHA) |  |  |
| I | 22/2700 | 0.8 |
| II | 438 | 16.2 |
| III | 1469 | 54.4 |
| IV | 771 | 28.6 |
| No. of >50% obstructed coronary arteries |  |  |
| 1 | 548/2700 | 20.3 |
| 2 | 793 | 29.4 |
| 3 | 1060 | 39.3 |
| left main disease | 299 | 11.1 |
| Ventricular function |  |  |
| normal | 1268/2639 | 48.1 |
|     regional hypokinesia | 906 | 34.3 |
|     regional akinesia | 465 | 17.6 |

even 10 years after surgery, almost half of the surviving patients were still without symptoms. At about the same rate, at which functional class I declined over the years, functional class II increased, while the percentage of patients in class III and IV remained almost constant.

The incidence of symptomatic improvement was significantly influenced by preoperative functional class, number of obstructed coronary arteries and graft occlusion, whereas the probability of being free of angina pectoris postoperatively was affected by sex, preoperative functional class, degree of revascularization and graft occlusion (Table 2).

## Early mortality after CABG

Early mortality after CABG used to be as high as 10% in the early years of coronary artery bypass surgery and has steadily declined since to around 1% in good surgical units nowadays.

Among our patients, early mortality until 30 days after surgery was 1.1%. This includes all patients with elective as well as emergency procedures. For different subgroups early mortality varied between 0.5% for patients in functional class I and II preoperatively and 2.5% for patients in functional class IV (Fig. 2). Only two of the preoperative parameters could be identified as having a significantly negative influence on early mortality: functional class IV and emergency procedures.

More important than preoperative parameters seems to be the institution, at which the surgery is performed: Among 15 hospitals taking part in the Coronary Artery Surgery Study, early mortality differed between 0.3% and 6.6%, this is by a factor of 22 [1]. This difference was not caused by a difference in the preoperative status of the patients, as could be shown by the ratio of observed and expected mortality. Expected mortality was calculated according to the clinical and angiographic characteristics of the patients, who received CABG. It could be demonstrated, that the actual operative mortality and the ratio of observed and expected mortality went roughly parallel, thus indicating, that high early mortality was not that much a matter of high risk patients but of inadequate surgical treatment.

## Late survival after CABG

Prolongation of life following CABG by reducing the risk of premature death due to coronary heart disease is difficult to prove, since, unlike with symptoms, it canot be judged by comparing the pre- and postoperative situation of an individual patient.

Among our patients actuarial survival was 83.4% 10 years after surgery (Fig.

3). This is equivalent to a linearized annual mortality rate of 1.8%, quite similar to that of an age and sex matched group of the general population.

It has been demonstrated, that the survival of medically treated patients with

*Table 2.* Angina pectoris after CABG vs. pre-, intra- and post-operative parameters.

| | n | Functional class I % | Improved % |
|---|---|---|---|
| Total | 2525 | 55.7 | 82.4 |
| Sex male | 2314 | 56.6 $\quad$ p<1.0 | 82.7 |
| female | 211 | 45.0 | 79.1 |
| Age ≤30 years | 6 | 66.7 | 66.7 |
| 31–40 years | 128 | 60.9 | 82.0 |
| 41–50 years | 726 | 50.6 | 77.1 |
| 51–60 years | 1316 | 55.0 | 84.0 |
| 61–70 years | 333 | 67.9 | 87.4 |
| >70 years | 16 | 50.0 | 13.8 |
| Preop. myocardial infarction | | | |
| + | 1350 | 54.5 | 82.0 |
| ∅ | 1147 | 57.4 | 80.6 |
| Preop. functional class (NYHA) | | | |
| I | 24 | 75.0 | 0 |
| II | 421 | 67.2 $\quad$ p<0.1 | 67.2 |
| III | 1376 | 55.6 | 83.8 $\quad$ p<0.1 |
| IV | 704 | 48.4 | 91.5 |
| Preop. ventricular function | | | |
| normal | 1215 | 55.7 | 80.1 |
| regional hypokinesia | 846 | 57.3 | 85.8 |
| regional akinesia | 411 | 51.1 | 81.0 |
| No. of obstructed coronary arteries | | | |
| 1 | 521 | 54.9 | 78.3 |
| 2 | 747 | 51.7 | 80.5 |
| 3 | 987 | 57.1 | 84.3 $\quad$ p<0.1 |
| left main disease | 270 | 63.3 | 88.5 |
| Revascularization | | | |
| complete | 1560 | 59.1 $\quad$ p<0.1 | 82.4 |
| incomplete | 965 | 50.3 | 82.3 |
| Grafts all patent | 579 | 51.6 | 80.0 |
| not all patent | 72 | 31.9 $\quad$ p<0.1 | 58.3 $\quad$ p<0.1 |
| all occluded | 23 | 34.8 | 60.9 |

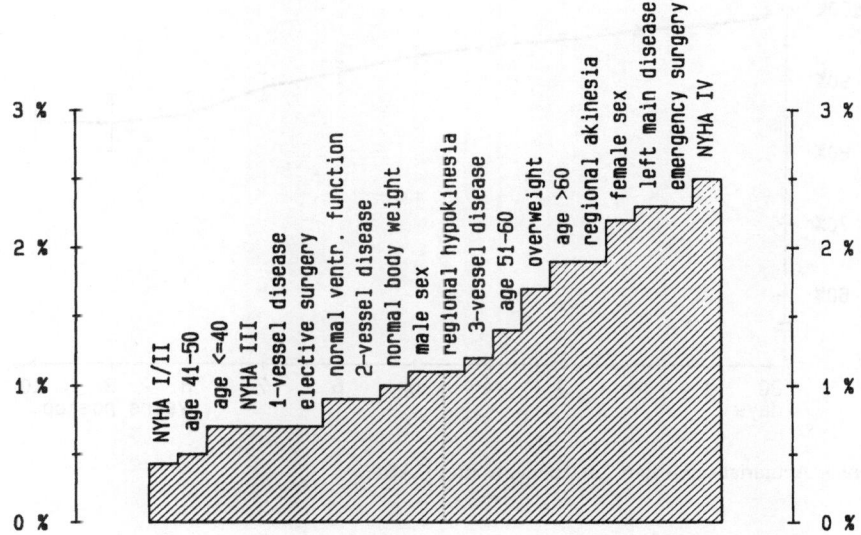

*Figure 2.* Early mortality (%) after CABG vs. pre- and intraoperative parameters.

coronary heart disease depends mainly on two angiographic parameters: the number of obstructed coronary arteries and the left ventricular function [2, 3, 4]. It is often argued, that the original data on this subject, gathered 10 to 15 years ago, are not true anymore, since the use of beta-blockers and calcium-antagonists supposedly has had a positive influence on survival under medical therapy.

In order to update these figures, we have calculated the yearly mortality of our patients, who died, while waiting for the operation, that is roughly within the time interval between coronary angiography and surgery (Fig. 4): Within an average waiting period of about 4 months, the death rate was less than 1% for patients with 1-vessel-disease, about 1.5% for patients with 2-vessel-disease, 2% for patients with 3-vessel-disease and within a somewhat shorter waiting-period of three months it was 2.5% for patients with left main disease. Provided, that this tendency remains the same until the end of one year, the estimated annual mortality would be 2% for patients with 1-vessel-disease, 5% for patients with 2-vessel-disease, 6% for patients with 3-vessel-disease and 10% for patients with left main disease. This is not much different from the figures published 10 years ago, at least not in this group of patients selected for CABG.

Theoretically the influence of the number of obstructed coronary arteries on survival should be abolished by the operation. Practically, there are still significant differences in late survival depending upon the preoperative coronary artery involvement, although less pronounced than without surgery (Fig. 5). The main reason for the remaining difference is incomplete revascularization, which has a negative influence on late survival, and which is most likely to occur in patients

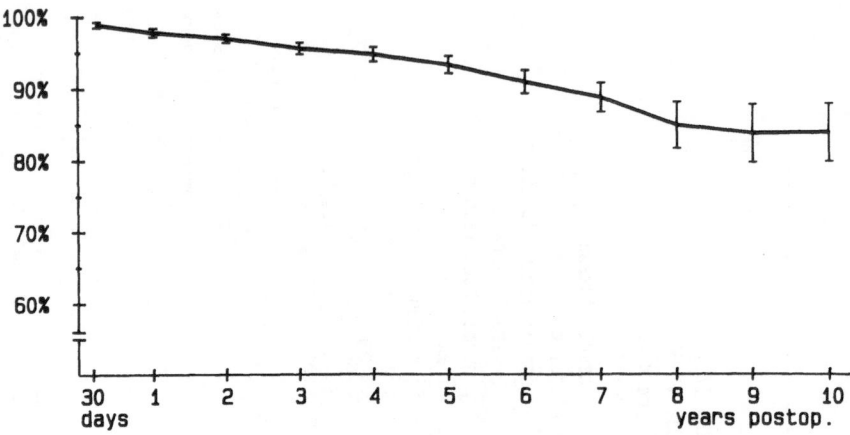

*Figure 3.* Actuarial survival of 2,700 patients after CABG.

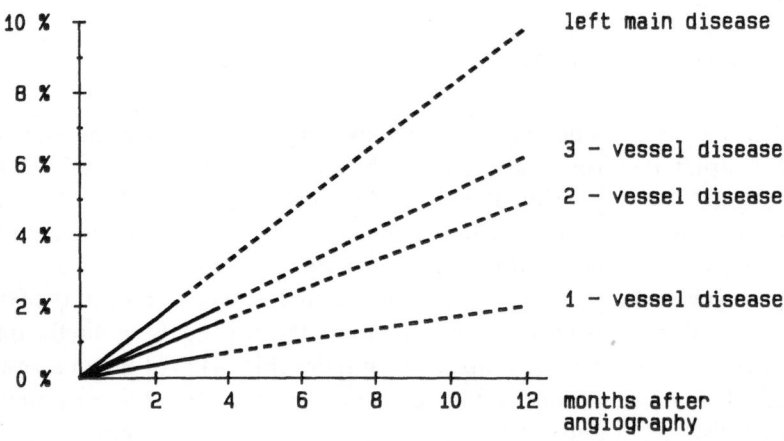

*Figure 4.* Preoperative mortality (%) vs. number of obstructed coronary arteries.

with multi-vessel disease. If this parameter is eliminated by considering patients with complete revascularization only, identical survival rates for all patients, regardless of their preoperative vessel involvement can be demonstrated (Fig. 6).

Impaired left ventricular function definitely shortens the life expectancy of patients despite of medical treatment. Among our patients waiting for the operation, the estimated annual mortality was 3% for patients with normal ventricular function and between 7 and 8% for patients with akinetic or hypokinetic segments of left ventricular myocardium (Fig. 7).

The influence of impaired left ventricular function on late survival remains after surgery, since scar tissue will not disappear following revascularization (Fig.

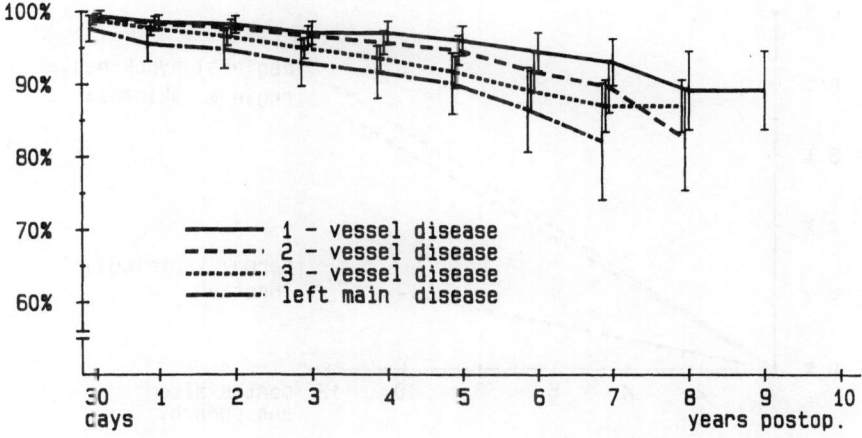

*Figure 5.* Actuarial survival after CABG vs. number of obstructed coronary arteries.

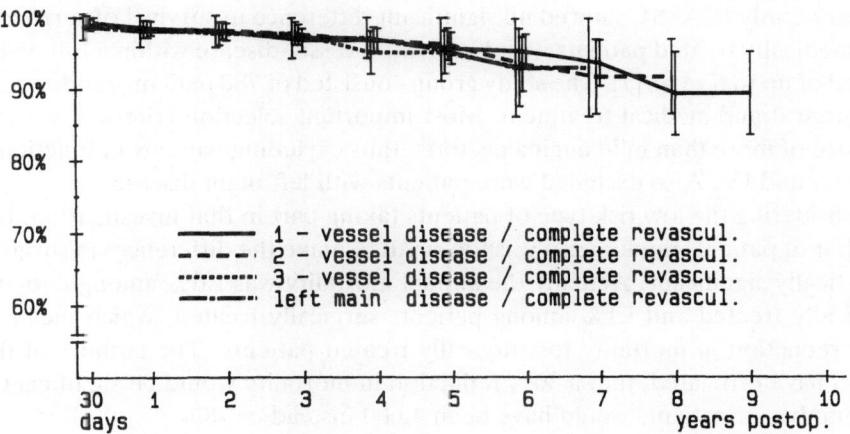

*Figure 6.* Actuarial survival after CABG in patients with complete revascularization vs. number of obstructed coronary arteries.

8). Surgical intervention before myocardial infarction therefore is most desirable.

Although the data presented so far seem to demonstrate, that in all subgroups of different vessel involvement and ventricular function the annual mortality for surgically treated patients is reduced by more than 50% as compared to medically treated patients, this is certainly no reliable proof, that surgical therapy of coronary heart disease is superior to medical therapy as far as life expectancy is concerned. Several randomized studies have failed to demonstrate a significant difference in survival under surgical and medical therapy, except for patients with left main disease [5], with 3-vessel-disease and with certain types of 2-vessel-

248

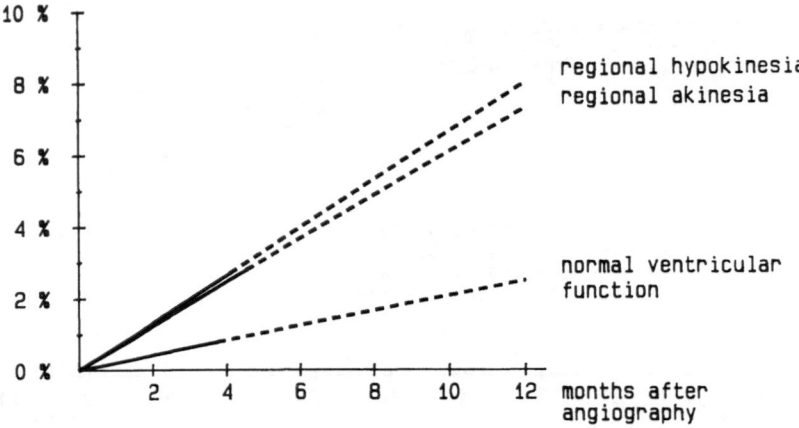

*Figure 7.* Preoperative mortality (%) vs. ventricular function.

disease [6]. The most recent of the randomized studies, the Coronary Artery Surgery Study (CASS), showed no significant difference in survival of surgically and medically treated patients with 1-, 2- and 3-vessel-disease within a follow-up period of up to 6 years [7]. The study group consisted of 780 patients randomized for surgical and medical treatment. Most important selection criterion was the absence of more than mild angina pectoris, thus excluding patients in functional class III and IV. Also excluded were patients with left main disease.

Considering the low risk type of patients taking part in that investigation, the number of patients randomized was too small to make the differences in survival statistically significant: Actually the annual mortality was 1.6% among patients medically treated and 1.1% among patients surgically treated, which means a 30% reduction in mortality for surgically treated patients. The authors of the CASS have estimated, that a 30% reduction in mortality would be significant if the number of patients would have been 4.600 instead of 780.

Another reason, why the CASS did not show any significant difference, seems to be the fact, that 23.5% of patients, originally assigned to receive medical therapy, had bypass surgery by 5 years, in most instances because of the development of worsening angina in spite of rigorous medical treatment. These patients nevertheless were considered to belong to the group, to which they were initially assigned, regardless of the subsequent therapy they received. One can expect, that these patients would have influenced the survival rate of the medically treated group negatively, had they not been operated upon, once they became functional class III and IV patients.

As to the duration of a possible beneficial effect of CABG on survival, ROSKAMM found, that during the first 5 postoperative years the survival curve of 1,000 operated patients ran parallel to that of the age- and sex-matched general population. Thereafter the annual mortality of the operated patients increased in

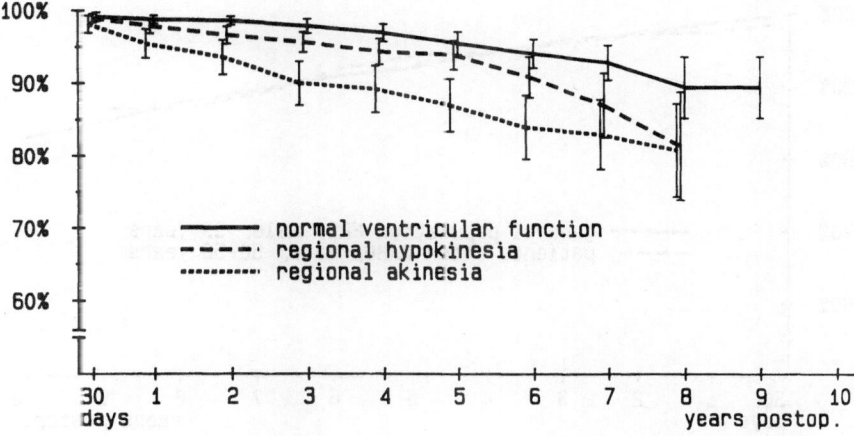

*Figure 8.* Actuarial survival after CABG vs. preoperative ventricular function.

comparison to that of the general population up to 6% at 10 years postoperatively [8].

Our own data do not support this statement: Since 53 years was the mean age of our patients at the time of operation, we constructed the survival curve for 998 of our male patients aged 53 plus/minus 3 years and compared it to the survival curve of 53 year old males of the general population (Fig. 9): There was no recognizable difference in survival within the follow-up period of 9 years postoperatively.

## Work status after CABG

What we obviously have not achieved, is getting people back to work after CABG. Among our male patients aged 60 years or younger at the time of follow-up, 48% were working postoperatively (Fig. 10). This percentage was maintained throughout the follow-up period of 9 years, although the percentage of patients with subjectively unlimited working ability declined slightly during the same period of time.

Compared to the employment rate of the general male population in the FRG, the employment rate of our patients was considerably lower (Fig. 11). The difference increased with age from 25% for patients in their early forties to 48% for patients in their late fifties. This could at least in part be due to the multimorbidity of older patients, who are cured from angina pectoris as often as their younger collegues, but nevertheless remain unfit for the demands of their job due to ailments caused by diseases other than coronary heart disease.

That medical achievements are only of limited significance for the return-to-work rate after CABG may be demonstrated by the fact that of all patients free of angina pectoris only 62% worked, while 38% had been retired.

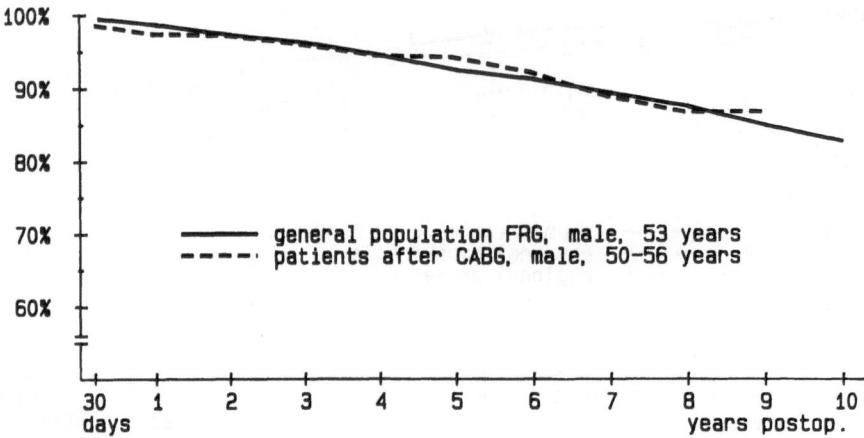

*Figure 9.* Actuarial survival of surgically treated patients (Erlangen) and patients assigned to medical or surgical therapy (CASS).

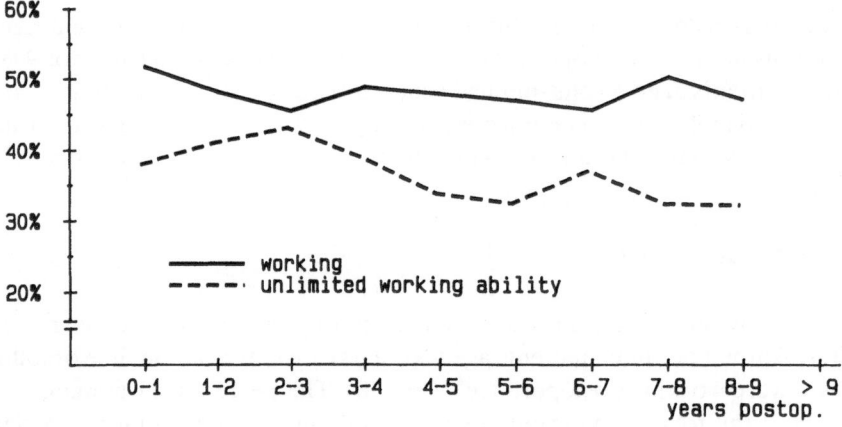

*Figure 10.* Survival rates of male patients after CABG and of males of comparable age in the general population.

## Indications for CABG

In summary then there are definite indications for CABG as far as improvement of symptoms is concerned: All patients, whose symptoms cannot be controlled properly by medical treatment are candidates for surgical treatment or PTCA, depending upon the angiographic situation. This is definitely true for all patients in functional class III and IV and for some in functional class II, whose life stiles requires more strenuous activity than can be done without provoking symptoms.

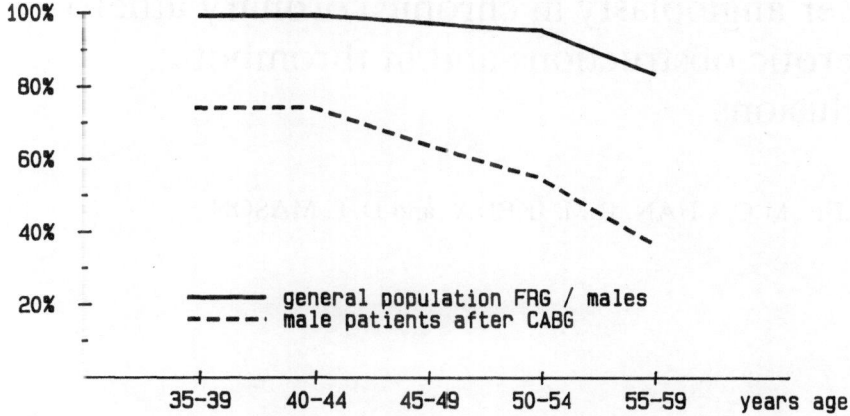

*Figure 11.* Postoperative work status after CABG vs. follow-up period.

There are less definite indications for CABG as far as prolongation of life is concerned: left main coronary artery obstruction is a definite, 3-vessel-disease a likely indication for surgery. Although for patients with 1- and 2-vessel-disease and mild or absent angina pectoris there is no proven advantage of surgical over medical therapy, PTCA or CABG should always be considered in patients with high grade proximal obstructions in dominant coronary arteries, since the consequences of myocardial infactions caused by these obstructions are often life threatening or disabling.

## References

1. Kennedy JW, Killip T, Fisher LD, Alderman EL, Gillespie MJ, Mock MB (1974–1979) The clinical spectrum of coronary artery disease and its surgical and medical management. Circulation 66 (Suppl III): (1982) III–16
2. Bruschke AVG, Proudfit WL, Sones Jr. FM (1973) Progress study of 590 consecutive nonsurgical cases of coronary disease followed 5–9 years. Circulation 47: 1147
3. Bruschke AVG, Proudfit WL, Sones Jr. FM (1973) Progress study of 590 consecutive nonsurgical cases of coronary disease followed 5–9 years. Circulation 47: 1154
4. Harris PJ, Harrell Jr FE, Lee KL, Behar VS, Rosati RA (1979) Medically treated coronary artery disease. Circulation 60: 1259
5. Read RC. Murphy ML, Hultgren HN (1978) Survival of men treated for chronic stable angina pectoris J Thorac Cardiovasc Surg 75: 1
6. European Coronary Surgery Study Group (1982) Long-term results of a prospective randomized study of coronary artery bypass surgery in stable angina pectoris. Lancet 2: 1173
7. CASS Principal Investigators and Their Associates (1983) Coronary Artery Surgery Study (CASS) a randomized trial of coronary artery bypass surgery. Circulation 68: 939
8. Roskamm H, Betz P, Schmuziger M, Stürzenhofecker P (1984) Survival and functional long-term results (5–11 years) in 1,000 patients after aorto-coronary bypass surgery Europ. Heart Journal (5, Suppl. I): 77

# Laser angioplasty in chronic coronary atherosclerotic obstructions and in thrombotic occlusions

G. LEE, M.C. CHAN, R.M. IKEDA, and D.T. MASON

## Summary

The potential use of lasers to vaporize chronic coronary atherosclerotic stenoses and thrombotic obstructions is rapidly becoming recognized. Its light energies can be focused into tiny, flexible optical fiber made of silica which can be inserted into a blood vessel and passed intravascularly to an area of obstruction. The ease of plaque penetration is largely dependent upon the absorptive characteristics of the plaque and thrombus. Argon energies (454–514 nm) are capable of vaporizing and penetrating red cell rich clots (due to the presence of hemoglobin pigment) but do not readily penetrate clots devoid of hemoglobin. In in-vivo studies, laser radiation produces a vaporized crater in the atherosclerotic plaque and this area is covered with fibrin and platelets but is rapidly endothelialized. Potential complications of recanalizing coronary obstructions include perforation, vascular wall injury, aneurysm formation, debris, and thrombogenesis. Laser recanalization on coronary or peripheral atherosclerotic arteries using a variety of methodologies has been tried in a few patients with variable reported success. Long-term patency in treated patients is still lacking. Improvements in intravascular laser delivery systems are necessary prior to further clinical application.

The laser (acronym for Light Amplification by Stimulated Emission of Radiation) is one of the brightest lights generated by man. Its first medical use occurred in the 1960's in the field of ophthalmology to photocoagulate abnormal vessels and seal retinal tears. Since then the laser has been applied to virtually all fields of medicine and new uses for clinical application are continually being explored. One of these potential areas is in the recanalization of chronic atherosclerotic and thrombotic obstructions particularly in the coronary arteries.

## Current medical lasers

The laser generates photons or energy bundles with a narrow band of wave-length (monochromatic) specific to the lasing medium. The photons are coordinated in phase with one another in time and space (coherent). Further, the laser beam is collimated with very slight divergence (collimated). These physical properties of laser make it possible to package and focus the light into a tiny beam of prodigious energy capable of destroying atherosclerotic plaque obstruction.

The most commonly used lasers in medicine are the argon, neodymium-yttrium-aluminium-garnet (Nd-YAG), and carbon dioxide ($CO_2$) lasers. The argon laser emits photons with wavelengths between 0.488 and 0.514 $\mu$m, which is within the blue-green portion of the visible electromagnetic spectrum. The Nd-YAG is a solid-state laser which emits a wavelength of 1.06 $\mu$m and the $CO_2$ laser emits a wavelength of 10.6 $\mu$m, which are both in the infra-red invisible portion of the electromagnetic spectrum. Since the infra-red beams are invisible, it is necessary to provide a second visible aiming laser beam of lower power in order to achieve precise placement during surgical manipulations.

**Existing delivery systems**

The development of flexible optical fibers has made it possible to propagate light internally into body cavities, and concomitantly to transmit images formed by optical fiber bundles within internal organs back to the viewer without open surgical exposure. Optical fiber (less than 1 mm outer diameter) made of silica quartz is small and flexible and can be passed internally into blood vessels. Due to the refractive properties of the fiber, the beam is confined internally and incident energy can be conducted to its target with very little energy loss. Both argon and Nd-YAG wavelengths can be transmitted in this manner. However, fibers used to deliver the long wavelength $CO_2$ energies are not yet readily available, since the materials that transmit the beam may not be technologically feasible at the present time, or may be toxic under physiologic conditions.

The amount of power generated by a laser and delivered by the optical fiber is measured in watts. The total energy delivered (joules) is a product of the power and duration of exposure (seconds). As laser light passes out of the fiber, the location of the focal plane where the spot diameter is smallest is the point with the greatest power of concentration. The power density determines the effect of the power delivered to the target tissue. Power density varies directly with the power and inversely with the surface area of the beam. As the distance away from the focal plane increases, the spot diameter or surface area enlarges and the power concentration falls.

**In-vitro studies on coronary atherosclerotic disease**

The immediate effects of laser radiation have been documented using human cadaver atherosclerotic coronary disease which is primarily composed of mixtures of lipoid, hyalinized and calcified materials. The atherosclerotic plaque is vaporized when exposed to argon, Nd-YAG or $CO_2$ laser radiation (1–5); surrounding the vaporized area is a charred lining. Transmitted through an optical fiber, the laser beam can be directed coaxially as close as possible along the central axis of the blood vessel, dissolving plaque adjacent to the stenotic lumen and thereby extending the diameter of the existing channel (Fig. 1). In total atherosclerotic obstruction, it may even create a newly vaporized channel.

Plaque penetration depends on the physical and thermal properties of the laser beam and on the absorptive characteristics of the plaque material. Thus, the higher the power intensity, or the longer the laser exposure, or the more focused the beam, the greater is the depth of plaque penetration. Rapid vaporization producing a cleanly incised smooth walled crater can be achieved in plaque containing materials of lower densities such as lipid-laden deposits [1–3]. However, laser penetration is relatively retarded by high density deposits such as heavily calcified plaque, producing an irregular and roughened lining around the central vaporized area [1–3]. Greater extent of charred remnants may be found in the laser-induced channel of calcified plaque than in hyalinized plaque obstruction. In lipid-laden plaque occluded coronary artery, no charred debris is found in its laser-treated passageway.

## Chronic in-vivo studies

The chronic response of laser radiation following removal of atherosclerotic disease was demonstrated in swine fed a hyperlipidemic diet [6]. $CO_2$ laser exposure produced vaporized craters (approximately 2 mm in diameter and 1 mm in depth). Two days following laser treatment, the crater was partially covered with platelet-fibrin thrombi. By two weeks, the surface of the depressed crater had mostly re-endothelialized, with some fibrin platelets remaining. Collagen had formed in the immediate subendothelial, lateral and medial portions of the crater. Eight weeks after the treatment, the lased site was still depressed and the surface of the crater had completely re-endothelialized. Moreover, thrombogenic complications did not occur under these experimental conditions. Thus, the chronic response to laser radiation following removal of atherosclerotic disease demonstrated rapid healing without thrombogenic complications and a lasting depressed vaporized crater with little or no damage to the surrounding tissue.

Further long-term studies in atherosclerotic arteries of Rhesus monkeys fed an atherogenic diet have also determined whether the effects of laser radiation can accelarate the atherosclerotic process [7]. Following several argon laser exposures upon the femoral arteries and aorta, light and electronmicroscopic examination following 2 to 60 days showed that the vaporized crater had significantly less atherosclerosis than the unlased plaque border. Thus, there was no evidence of increased atherosclerotic development following laser therapy.

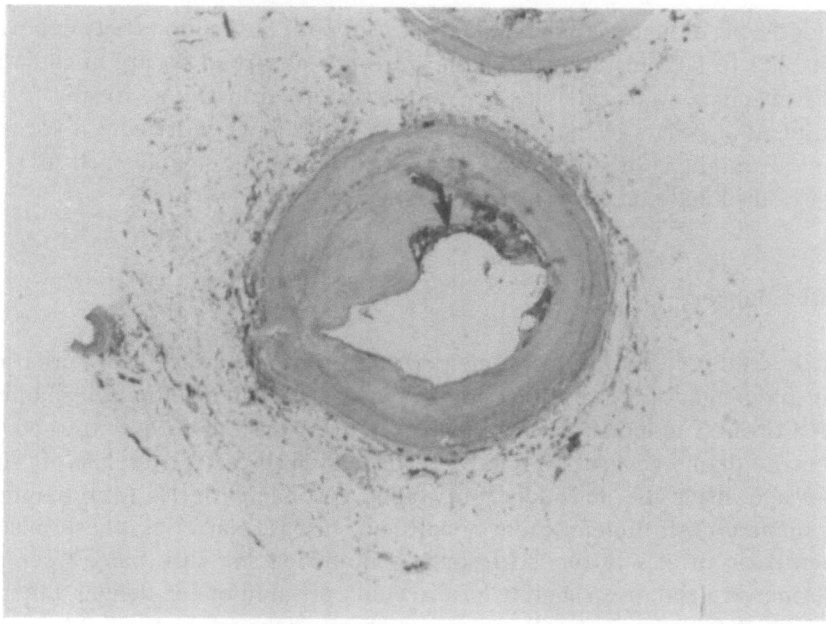

*Figure 1.* Cross-section of obstructed human atherosclerotic coronary artery. Laser energies delivered via tiny flexible optical fiber were directed coaxially along the central axis of the stenotic artery, dissolving plaque adjacent to the stenotic lumen, thereby widening the vascular channel. Note the charred lining (arrow) along the vaporized area.

## Studies on thrombotic occlusions

Since thrombosis often accompanies atherosclerotic disease, the effect of laser radiation on human thrombus has been demonstrated. In early studies, blood was obtained from normal human volunteers and allowed to clot. The clotted samples were cut to fixed lengths of 3 to 11 mm. An argon laser was selected and penetrated increased depths of thrombus in a linear dose fashion. The longer the red blood clot, the higher is the energy necessary to penetrate through that clot [8].

The thrombus is a complex aggregation of blood platelets, white cells and red cells in a fibrin network. The vaporization of each of these different substances in the obstructed vessel may differ according to the wavelength emitted by the laser [9]. The spectrophotometric scan of freshly formed thrombus demonstrated typical absorption curve for hemoglobin pigments (with major absorbent peaks between wavelengths 400 to 600 nm). Argon energies have wavelengths between 488 to 514 nm which can be transmitted down tiny flexible optical fiber and are easily absorbed by the red blood clot. Spectrophotometric scan of clots devoid of red blood cells or hemoglobin pigment showed poor absorption (between wave-lengths 350 to 600 nm) and such clots were not absorbed by argon radiation. Moreover, since argon energies are poorly absorbed in water, freshly formed thrombus that occurs in the coronary artery of patients with acute myocardial infarction, might better be dissolved with thrombolytic agents such as strep-tokinase, urokinase or tissue plasminogen activators.

**Potential dangers**

In its present state of development, perforation of the vessel wall is the most significant danger of the laser procedure. Perforation can be either mechanically induced or laser induced. Current optical delivery systems (i.e. 200 to 600 $\mu$m quartz core diameter) are still relatively stiff and their distal tip relatively sharp for passage inside the delicately thin walled coronary arteries (approximately 2 mm diameter). In human cadaver coronary diseased arteries, these mishaps frequently occur at a tortuous site or at a branched site [10]. Since laser light travels in a straight line, a slightly misdirected optical fiber can deliver a thermal burn through the atherosclerotic plaque and beyond the arterial wall. Use of high laser energies for long durations to vaporize plaque tends to increase this risk further. Thus far a laser beam wavelength that is absorbed by plaque but that spares the normal vascular wall has not been found.

Studies in animals have documented the consequences of laser catheter inter-vention into the coronary arteries [11]. Although flexible 200 to 400 $\mu$m central core quartz fiber was advanced into coronary arteries without untoward effects, laser energies approximating those used to vaporize plaque resulted in laser burns perforating the coronary artery, producing cardiac tamponade and causing hemo-dynamic and electrical instability.

Chronic risks of laser phototherapy have been demonstrated in rabbits fed an atherogenic diet and allowed to develop atherosclerotic lesions [12]. In animals examined immediately after laser treatment, low level energies produced a vaporized crater within the atherosclerotic plaque at the endothelial surface; in others, the medial layer was also injured. Interestingly, aortic aneurysms with muscular wall damage were found in half of the animals that were followed up to 14 days following the laser procedure. Consistent findings which included thin-ning or irregular dilatation of the muscularis layer were also evident in normal dog arteries exposed to laser radiation for up to 14 days [12].

Laser vaporization also produces minute particles that can effluoresce from the focal point of the concentrated beam. Phototherapy of severely calcified lesions may result in dislodged debris into the vascular channel and embolize distally. Further, disruption of subendothelial structures by laser radiation can expose collagen and induce platelet aggregation, fibrin deposition and thrombosis [10].

## Laser angioplasty in patients

Early attempts at laser angioplasty in patients with peripheral and coronary artery disease have confirmed the efficacy, difficulties and risks of the procedure in its current state of development. For the most part, the overall results were not surprisingly different from qualitative data gathered from preclinical studies. In patients with claudication and angiographically obstructed femoral and popliteal arteries, laser catheter intervention can effectively recanalize these arteries with some success [13, 14]. However, long-term patency studies are still lacking.

In a trial using 5 patients with coronary disease undergoing coronary bypass surgery, argon laser radiation delivered by flexible quartz fiber reportedly recanalized stenotic lesions of two left anterior descending and three right coronary arteries [15]. One of the patients had his right coronary artery stenotic segment excised and biopsied following the laser procedure and the histological specimen showed extensive charring, medial wall disruption and coagulation necrosis. In the remaining four patients, only one was reported to have patency of his lased native vessel within 25 days of intervention; the other three had occlusion or restenosis of their lased site. It was possible that these arteries thrombosed or closed off due to competitive flow. Mechanical and/or laser-induced coronary perforation occurred in one of the patients during the procedure.

## Future development

### Laser catheter with visualization and vaporization capabilities

Recanalization of an atherosclerotic obstruction within a blood vessel necessitates the precise placement of the laser fiber. By viewing the obstructed area, the laser beam can be directed to the diseased target for controlled thermal therapy [16, 17]. In this manner, complications such as vascular perforation and aneurysm formation may be avoided. Further, plaque and thrombus obstructions may be differentiated. The latter distinction may be noteworthy, since differing energy densities may be necessary for laser penetration.

Conceived in 1977, early prototype catheters have shown the feasibility of simultaneously visualizing and vaporizing atherosclerotic plaques implanted in living animals. Subsequent prototype catheter (outer diameter 3 mm, length 100 cm) has been tested for use in peripheral vessels in living dogs [18]. The device consisted of fiberoptic bundle for viewing, and channels for housing the laser fiber and suctioning/flushing capabilities (removal of gas, blood, particulate debris and injection of contrast dye or perfluorocarbon blood substitutes). A balloon around the distal catheter tip can be inflated to momentarily halt the flow of blood and stabilize the catheter within the vessel. Similar but smaller laser catheter systems need to be refined and tested in the coronary arteries.

258

## Laser-heated metal cap

The efficacy of a laser-heated metal cautery cap mounted at the distal end of the optical fiber has been tested in living animal vessels and in human cadaver atherosclerotic vessels [19]. Derived from work done utilizing an electrical soldering iron, the laser-heated metal cautery cap too is capable of instantaneously dissolving atherosclerotic lesions upon physical contact. The device avoids the inherent problems of direct free laser beam inadvertently straying from the target area causing vascular perforations and aneurysms. While technical improvements are being made prior to clinical application, the laser-heated metal cautery cap delivery system possesses important advantages over bare-tipped fibers, particularly in terms of safety during recanalization of atherosclerotic vascular obstructive disease.

## Excimer laser

The absorption of ultraviolet light upon atherosclerotic disease from an excimer laser results in a different ablative outcome than with absorption of visible (argon) or infra-red (Nd-YAG, $CO_2$) radiation. Ultraviolet light causes photochemical ablation of the atheroma and generally no thermal injury [20, 21]. A precisely defined incision can result without any thermal damage to the surrounding tissue. The depth of penetration varies directly with the cumulative number of ultraviolet pulses emitted while the width of the radiated channel remains unchanged. While application of ultraviolet light using excimer laser has certain advantages, the mutagenic or toxic effects of ultraviolet laser energies is still unknown and optical fiber used to deliver the ultra-short wavelength excimer light (i.e. 193 nm) is not technically feasible at the present time.

### Acknowledgements

We thank Mr. James Metcalfe, Mr. Andrew Deems, Mr. Chris Matthew and the San Francisco Laser Center for their support and Ms. Leslie Silvernail for secretarial assistance.

### References

1. Lee G, Ikeda RM, Kozina J, Mason DT (1981) Laser dissolution of coronary atherosclerotic obstruction. Am Heart J 102: 1074–1075
2. Lee G, Ikeda R, Herman I, Dwyer RM, Bass M, Hussein H, Kozina J, Mason DT (1983) The qualitative effects of laser irradiation on human arteriosclerotic disease. Am Heart J 105: 885–889

3. Lee G, Ikeda RM, Chan MC, Stobbe D, Kozina J, Jiang MC, Reis RL, Mason DT (1984) Current and potential uses of lasers in the treatment of atherosclerotic disease. Chest 85: 429–434

4. Abela GS, Normann S, Cohen D, Feldman RL, Geiser EA, Conti CR (1982) Effects of carbon dioxide, Nd-YAG and argon laser radiation on coronary atheromatous plaques. Am J Cardiol 50: 1199–1205

5. Choy DSJ, Stertzer S, Rotterdam HZ, Bruno MS (1982) Laser coronary angioplasty: Experience with 9 cadaver hearts. Am J Cardiol 50: 1209–1211

6. Gerrity RG, Loop FD, Golding LAR, Erhart LA, Argenyl ZB (1983) Arterial response to laser operation for removal of atherosclerotic plaques. J Thorac Cardiovasc Surg 85: 409–421

7. Abela G, Franzini D, Crea F, Pepine CJ, Conti CR (1984) No evidence of accelerated atherosclerosis following laser radiation. (Abstract) Circulation 70 (Suppl. II): 323

8. Lee G, Ikeda RM, Stobbe D, Ogata C, Chan MC, Seckinger DL, Vazquez A, Theis J, Reis RL, Mason DT (1983) Effect of laser radiation on human thrombus: Demonstration of a linear dissolution dose relationship between clot length and energy density. Am J Cardiol 52: 876–877

9. Lee G, Chan MC, Seckinger DL, Vazquez A, Rosenthal PK, Lee KK, Ikeda RM, Reis RL, Hanna ES, Mason DT. Argon laser radiation of human clots: Differential photoabsorption in red cell rich and red cell poor clots. Thrombosis Research (in press)

10. Lee G, Ikeda RM, Chan MC, Lee MH, Rink JL, Reis RL, Theis JH, Low R, Bommer WJ, Kung AH, Hanna ES, Mason DT. Limitations, risk and complications of laser recanalization – a cautious approach warranted. Am J Cardiol (in press)

11. Lee G, Seckinger D, Chan MC, Embi A, Stobbe D, Thomson RV, Sanchez NA, Ikeda RM, Reis RL, Mason DT (1984) Potential complications of coronary laser angioplasty. Am Heart J 106: 1577–1579

12. Lee G, Ikeda RM, Theis JH, Chan MC, Stobbe D, Ogata C, Kumagai A, Mason DT (1984) Acute and chronic complications of laser angioplasty. Vascular wall damage and formation of aneurysms in the atherosclerotic rabbit. Am J Cardiol 53: 290–293

13. Ginsburg R, Kim DS, Guthaner D, Toth J, Mitchell RS (1984) Salvage of an ischemic limb by laser angioplasty: Description of a new technique. Clin Cardiol 7: 54–58

14. Geschwind H, Boussignac G, Teisseire B, Vieilledent C, Gaston A, Becquemin JP, Mayiolini P (1984) Percutaneous transluminal laser angioplasty in man (Letters to the Editor). Lancet I: 844

15. Choy DSJ, Stertzer SH, Myler RK, Marco J, Fournial G (1984) Human coronary laser recanalization. Clin Cardiol 7: 377–381

16. Lee G, Ikeda RM, Dwyer RM, Hussein H, Dietrich P, Mason DT (1982) Feasibility of intravascular laser irradiation for in vivo visualization and therapy of cardiocirculatory diseases. Am Heart J 103: 1076–1077

17. Lee G, Ikeda RM, Stobbe D, Ogata C, Theis J, Hussein H, Mason DT (1983) Laser irradiation of human atherosclerotic obstructive disease: Simultaneous visualization and vaporization achieved by a dual fiberoptic catheter. Am Heart J 105: 163–164

18. Lee G, Ikeda RM, Stobbe D, Ogata C, Embi A, Chan MC, Reis RL, Mason DT (1984) Intraoperative use of dual fiberoptic catheter for simultaneous in vivo visualization and laser vaporization of peripheral atherosclerotic obstructive disease. Cathet Cardiovasc Diagn 10: 11–16

19. Lee G, Ikeda RM, Chan MC, Dukich J, Lee MH, Theis JH, Bommer WJ, Reis RL, Hanna E, Mason DT (1984) Dissolution of human atherosclerotic disease by fiberoptic laser-heated metal cautery cap. Am Heart J 107: 777–778

20. Grundfest W, Litvack F, Forrester J, Fishbein M, Morgenstern L, Mc. Dermid S, Pacala T, Rider D, Laudenslager J (1984) Pulsed ultraviolet lasers provide precise control of atheroma ablation. (Abstract) Circulation 70 (Suppl. II): 35

21. Isner JM, Clarke RH, Donaldson RF, Muller DF, Foxall TL, Laliberte SM, Libby R, Alroy J, Ucci AA (1984) The excimer laser: Gross, light microscopic, and ultrastructural analysis of potential advantages for use in laser therapy of cardiovascular disease. (Abstract) Circulation 70 (Suppl. II): 35

# Coronary sinus perfusion for preservation of jeopardized myocardium

W. MOHL and E. WOLNER

## Introduction

The use of the coronary sinus route to protect ischemic myocardium was proposed by PRATT as early as in 1898 [1]. Several investigators have since reported on beneficial effects of coronary sinus manipulations. During the first period of coronary sinus interventions, permanent coronary sinus ligation and arterialization were applied. Adverse effects such as engorgement of the venous system, hemorrhages and deterioration of cardiac performance contributed to a temporary demise of this method. Finally, with the enormous advancement of open heart surgery and especially coronary bypass grafting, coronary sinus manipulations completely lost their rationale. It is the result of advanced medical instrumentation and interventional cardiology that the coronary sinus route became once more an attractive access route to deprived myocardium. In the past, coronary sinus manipulation aimed at revascularization of ischemic zones by major surgery. Nowadays, percutaneous catheters are used to protect ischemic myocardium temporarily until ultimate revascularization is available.

## Differences in coronary sinus interventions

### 1. Synchronized retroperfusion (SRP)

In the early 1970s, Meerbaum et al [2] reported on a new coronary sinus retroperfusion technique allowing venous drainage during the cardiac systole and retroperfusing arterial blood during the cardiac diastole. Several authors showed the ability of this method to effectively gain access to ischemic myocardium [3].

## 2. Pressure-controlled intermittent coronary sinus occlusion (PISCO)

Another approach to the problems of retroperfusion was taken by the authors, who invented an intermittent coronary sinus occlusion technique in the late 1970s [4]. This method does not imply retroperfusion of arterial blood into the coronary veins. Its efficiency seems to be related to the redistribution of venous flow to deprived coronary circulation during the occlusion phase of the coronary sinus. This occlusion phase is limited to a certain plateau level of systolic coronary sinus pressure and venous drainage is reinstituted. This plateau level is thought to be a measure of the filled coronary venous capacitance. During the release phase, coronary venous drainage empties the surplus of perfusate, allowing reinstitution of coronary sinus occlusion within seconds. The occlusion/release cycle length varies in between individuals, but is usually about 10 sec occlusion/ 5 sec release.

## 3. Retroinfusion (RCSP)

Both methods allow to additionally retroinfuse pharmaceutical agents into the center of ischemia. Several articles showed the efficacy of retroinfusion [5, 6]. It seems, however, that the most effective form of RCSP still has to be found. Retroinfusion of cardioplegia is another valuable method used with good success in many cardiac centers [7, 8].

## Pathophysiologic considerations

The coronary venous system is a fine meshwork of coronary veins and venules connecting all parts of the coronary vasculature. The coronary sinus drains approximately 70% of venous blood. The remaining 30% are drained by small cardiac veins and the Thebesian system into virtually all cardiac chambers. One therefore can argue that retroperfused blood enters the center of ischemic areas or that most of the blood is drained during the cardiac systole through the coronary sinus and another part is lost in the small cardiac veins. The efficacy of SRP on ischemic myocardial function and the reduction of infarct size show that although part of the retroperfusate might be lost, retroperfusion per se or changes of the pressure-flow relationship in the coronary microcirculation induced by the cushion of retroperfused arterial blood act beneficially on jeopardized myocardium. The fact that PISCO seems to be as effective on myocardial ischemia as SRP is another indication that both methods, though technically distinctly different, may induce similar pathophysiologic changes within the ischemic myocardium. The mode of action and the efficacy of SRP with retroperfusion of oxygenated blood seems obvious. Recent success with PISCO, however, shows that alternating cycles of coronary sinus occlusion and release induce changes in the following manner: coronary sinus occlusion is used to redistribute flow toward underperfused areas, to force venous blood into zones where puffer systems react with acidotic tissue, and ional fluxes reverse compartimental changes. During the intermittent release of occlusion, the rapid decrease of flow impedance drains pooled venous blood and washes out scavenged metabolites. (While SRP appears to act by retroperfusion of oxygenated blood and therefore results in an increase in supply, the mode of action of PISCO is apparently based on the redistribution of venous flow and washout).

**Beneficial effects of coronary sinus interventions**

Profound reduction of infarct size as well as improvement of regional ischemic dysfunction was found in several experimental series [9, 10, 11]. Conflicting results on reduction of infarct size induced by PISCO recently showed the necessity of adaptation of the coronary sinus occlusion/release cycles, since this intervention is coronary sinus pressure controlled [12]. The challenge of today are the first human trials of coronary sinus interventions. Both SRP and PICSO have been investigated in humans [13, 14], and as far as preliminary data is available, it seems that coronary sinus interventions will mark a new era in interventional cardiology. Gore tried SRP in patients with severe unstable angina with good success [14], Mohl investigated PICSO in the early reperfusion phase after global ischemia in patients undergoing coronary artery bypass grafting. Both techniques show promising results, but further investigations, both clinically and experimentally, are clearly needed to show the clinical significance of these interventions.

Retroinfusion of pharmaceutical agents and cardioplegia both showed favorable results. Karageuzian retroinfused procainamide to improve severe arrhythmias in dogs [5]. Povzhitkov [6] and Meerbaum [15] reported on retroperfusion of prostaglandines and streptokinase, Both agents were more effective in treating ischemia and reopening occluded arteries as controls. Cardioplegic delivery is without any doubt the superior method to cool the myocardium and to prevent ischemia in certain patients with severe regional underperfusion or in patients undergoing aortic valve replacement [16].

**Hazards of the method**

As any intervention, coronary sinus manipulations entail a number of hazards. Coronary sinus catheterization, both during open heart surgery or percutaneously, seems safe. However, we have to consider that rigid catheters and inexpert handling may rupture the sinus. The technique used for SRP involves shunting blood through narrow catheters with the hazard of blood traumatization. Moreover, recent reports neglect clinically relevant changes of blood components.

SRP is synchronized by an ECG controlled pump system. PICSO techniques seem to be easier and simpler as compared to SRP. PICSO itself uses the coronary sinus pressure dynamics to effectively limit and optimize the timing of the obstruction and release period of the venous outflow. Computer modeling of the CS pressure dynamics and empiric observations on different hemodynamic variables allow assumption of the theoretically most effective pump cycle.

## Clinical implications

To evaluate experimental and clinical results, the International Working Group on Coronary Sinus Interventions [17] has been formed to standardize the methods, compare efforts, enhance communication and thus intensify cooperation within the scientific community.

## References

1. Pratt FH (1898) The nutrition of the heart through the vessels of Thebesius and coronary sinus. Am J Physiol 1: 86
2. Meerbaum S, Lang T, Osher JV, Hashimoto K, Lewis GV, Feldstein C, Corday E (1976) Diastolic retroperfusion of acutely ischemic myocardium. Am J Cardiol 37: 588
3. Maurer G, Punzengruber C, Haendchen RV, Torres MAR, Meerbaum S, Corday E (1984) Penetration of coronary venous injections into ischemic myocardium. In: Mohl W (ed) The Coronary Sinus. Darmstadt: Steinkoppf Verlag, New York Springer Verlag: pp 167
4. Mohl W (1984) Development and rationale of pressure-controlled intermittent coronary sinus occlusion – A new approach to protect ischemic myocardium Wien klin Wschr 96 (1), pp 20
5. Karagueuzian HS, Ohta M, Drury JK, Fishbein MC, Corday E, Meerbaum S, Mandel WJ, Peter T (1984) Coronary venous retroinfusion of procainamide in the management of inducible ventricular tachyarrhythmias in conscious dogs, during chronic myocardial infarction. In: Mohl W (ed) The Coronary Sinus. Darmstadt: Steinkopff Verlag, New York Springer Verlag, pp 385
6. Povzhitkov M, Haendchen RV, Meerbaum S, Fishbein M, Rit J, Corday E (1982) Protective effect of coronary venous prostaglandin E1 retroperfusion during acute myocardial ischemia. Am J Cardiol 49: 1017
7. Fabiani JN, Relland J, Carpentier A (1984) Myocardial protection via the coronary sinus in cardiac surgery: Comparative evaluation of two techniques. In: Mohl W (ed) The Coronary Sinus. Darmstadt: Steinkopff Verlag, New York Springer Verlag, pp 305
8. Chui RCJ (1984) Cold cardioplegia via retrograde coronary sinus infusion for myocardial protection. In: Mohl W (ed) The Coronary Sinus. Darmstadt: Steinkopff Verlag, New York Springer Verlag, pp 275
9. Mohl W, Glogar D, Mayr H, Losert U, Sochor H, Pachinger O, Kaindl F, Wolner E (1984) Reduction of infarct size induced by pressure controlled intermittent coronary sinus occlusion. Am J Cardiol 53: 923
10. Haendchen RV, Fishbein MC, Meerbaum S, Corday E (1984) Superiority of hypothermic vs normothermic synchronzied coronary venous retroperfusion for protection of acutely ischemic myocardium. In: Mohl W (ed) The Coronary Sinus. Darmstadt: Steinkopff Verlag, New York Springer Verlag, pp 392

11. Mohl W, Punzengruber C, Moser M, Kenner T, Heimisch W, Haendchen RV, Meerbaum S, Maurer G, Corday E (1985) Effects of pressure controlled intermittent coronary sinus occlusion on regional ischemic myocardial function. Am J Coll Cardiol 5: 939

12. Zalewski A, Goldberg S, Slysh S, Carew TE, Maroko PR (1986) Is the effect on infarct size of intermittent occlusion of the coronary sinus similar to that of arterialisation of the local cardiac vein? Circ Vol 70, Supp II/86

13. Mohl W, Glogar D, Kenner T, Klepetko W, Moritz A, Moser M, Müller M, Schuster J, Wolner E (1984) Enhancement of washout induced by pressure controlled intermittent coronary sinus occlusion (PISCO) in the canine and human heart. In: Mohl W (ed) The Coronary Sinus. Darmstadt: Steinkopff Verlag, New York Springer Verlag, pp 537

14. Gore JM: Personal communication

15. Meerbaum S, Lang T, Povzhitkov M, Haendchen RV, Uchiyama T, Broffman J, Corday E (1983) Retrograde lysis of coronary artery thrombus by coronary venous streptokinase administration. J Am Coll Cardiol 1 (5): 1262

16. Roberts AJ (1984) An overview of myocardial protection in open heart surgery. In: Mohl W (ed) The Coronary Sinus. Darmstadt: Steinkopff Verlag, New York Springer Verlag, pp 247

17. Faxon D, Mohl W (1984) Summarizing statement of the panel of working groups. In: Mohl W (ed) The Coronary Sinus. Darmstadt: Steinkopff Verlag, New York Springer Verlag, pp 549

# LDL – Apheresis for the treatment of patients with familial hypercholesterolaemia

M. TAUCHERT, A. GACZKOWSKI, H. BORBERG, K. OETTE
and W. STOFFEL

## Introduction

Familial hypercholesterolaemia is characterized by an elevation of low density lipoprotein (LDL), related to the genetic expression of a membrane receptor defect. The patients suffer mainly from coronary heart disease, established at an early age leading to longterm disability and early death. The majority of the heterozygous patients can be controlled with conventional therapy consisting of diet, exercise and cholesterol lowering drugs. However approximately 10% of the patients, including the homozygous group, cannot be suffiently treated this way and needs an additional elimination therapy.

Plasma exchange was introduced as an effective approach to control the progression of the disease, also leading to regression in some patients [5]. However the drawbacks are obvious. Being neither specific nor selective, essential plasmaproteins as for instance high density lipoprotein or immunoglobulins are equally removed, usually limiting the frequency of the treatment to one therapy per two weeks. The expenses are considerable and may at some places limit the number of patients to be treated. The transfer of infectious disease though unlikely cannot always be guaranteed.

During the last years LDL-apheresis was introduced for the specific removal of the pathogenic substrate into clinical medicine and we wish to report on our experience with this therapeutic approach.

## Materials and methods

Sterile Sepharose Cl-4b carrying an anti Apo-B antibody was prepared as described earlier [3] and transferred into columns, which after exclusion of pyrogenicity were entered into the plasma line of a Fenwal Celltrifuge II or IBM 2997 continuous flow blood cell separator. For anticoagulation 2500 units of heparin were injected as a bolus immediately at the beginning of the treatment and continued to be perfused with 40 units per minute during the first half of the procedure, replaced from ACD–B at a 1:22–1:16 ratio during the second half. A whole blood flow rate of 60–70 cc/min was generally established. As the centrifuges were run at maximal g-force (2200 rpm), plasma flow rates of 35–45 ml/min were generally established. The process of adsorption and desorption was performed as described [1, 4] and controlled from an automated Medicap AD-device, developed for both, selective and specific adsorption procedures [2].

## Treatments

The treatments were generally performed at weekly intervals, except for the early therapies, when an appropriate protocol and strategy had not yet been developed. Sometimes interruptions for holidays or other personal reasons had to be permitted, however they did usually not exceed 5 weeks. After the capacity of each column was established in vivo, each therapy was performed to obtain a posttreatment level of 150 mg/dl, which could generally be established except for the early treatments. The group of patients now being treated is shown in Table 1. It is rather heterogenous for several reasons. For instance a young homozygous boy (P. Dr.) is treated to prevent the development of coronary heart disease and to obtain regression of peripheral lipid deposits. His older sister (P. Dr.), with already established coronary heart disease and considerable xanthomas, is treated to achieve regression of both, like the majority of the seriously ill, heterozygous patients. The treatment of two patients (A. Th. and K.W.) is of interest to evaluate, whether coronary bypasses can be maintained without the development of atheromas in the walls of the implanted vessels.

LONGTERM LDL-APHERESIS IN FAMILIAL HYPERCHOLESTEROLAEMIA :

GENERAL PATIENT DATA

| | PATIENT | AGE | SEX | GENOTYPE | TOTAL CHOLESTEROL WITHOUT THERAPY (mg/dl) | FIRST APHERESIS |
|---|---|---|---|---|---|---|
| 1. | K.H. | 40 Y | F | heterozygous | 477 | I / 1981 |
| 2. | Pe.Dr. | 14 Y | M | homozygous | 644 | XI / 1981 |
| 3. | Pa.Dr. | 16 Y | F | homozygous | 660 | XI / 1981 |
| 4. | Z.S. | 29 Y | M | heterozygous | 532 | III / 1982 |
| 5. | K.W. | 56 Y | M | heterozygous | 459 | VI / 1982 |
| 6. | B.Sch. | 19 Y | F | homozygous | 924 | XII / 1982 |
| 7. | A.T. | 29 Y | F | homozygous | 764 | XII / 1982 |
| 8. | B.T. | 21 Y | F | heterozygous | 518 | III / 1984 |
| 9. | W.R | 41 Y | F | heterozygous | 363 | VII / 1984 |
| 10. | N. | Y | F | heterozygous | 491 | IV / 1984 |

## Results

The results obtained so far demonstrate, that a normalisation of the cholesterol level can be obtained for both, the single treatment (Fig. 1) as well as for the patient over time (Table 2). The rate of side effects has been published earlier and

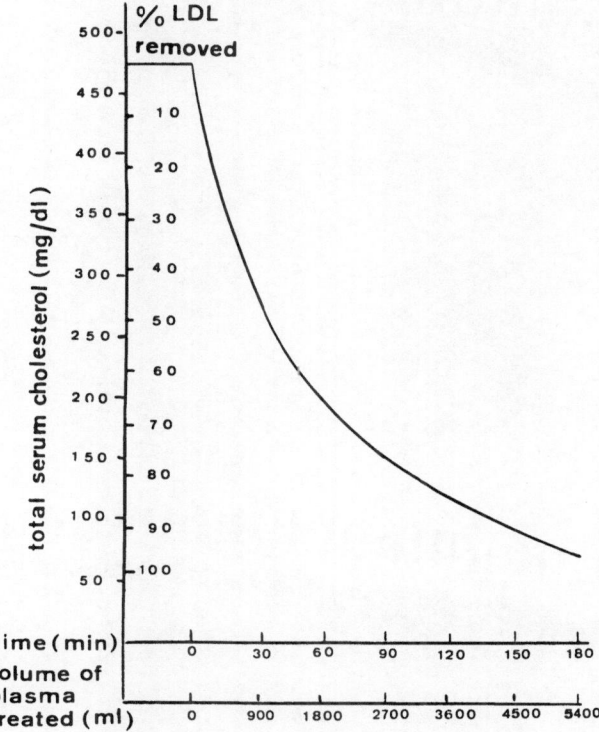

*Figure 1.* Absolute concentration change and percentage removal of LDL-cholesterol.

*Table 2.* Efficacy of LDL-Apheresis: Average total cholesterol under continuous therapy.*

| Patient | Without $T_x$ | 1981 | 1982 | 1983 | 1984** |
|---------|---------------|------|------|------|--------|
| D.P. | 644 | 245 | 231 | 256 | 246 mg/dl |
| S.Z. | 532 | – | 206 | 174 | 223 mg/dl |
| W.K. | 459 | – | 220 | 203 | 221 mg/dl*** |
| T.A. | 764 | – | 504 | 284 | 251 mg/dl |
| H.C. | 477 | 252 | 248 | 254 | 238 mg/dl |

* Mean of post – pretreatment values (Normal 130–260 mg/dl).
* * From January 1st–June 30th.
* * * Biweekly intervals in 1984.
(Haemapheresis unit, Dept. Intern. Medicine, Univ. Köln).

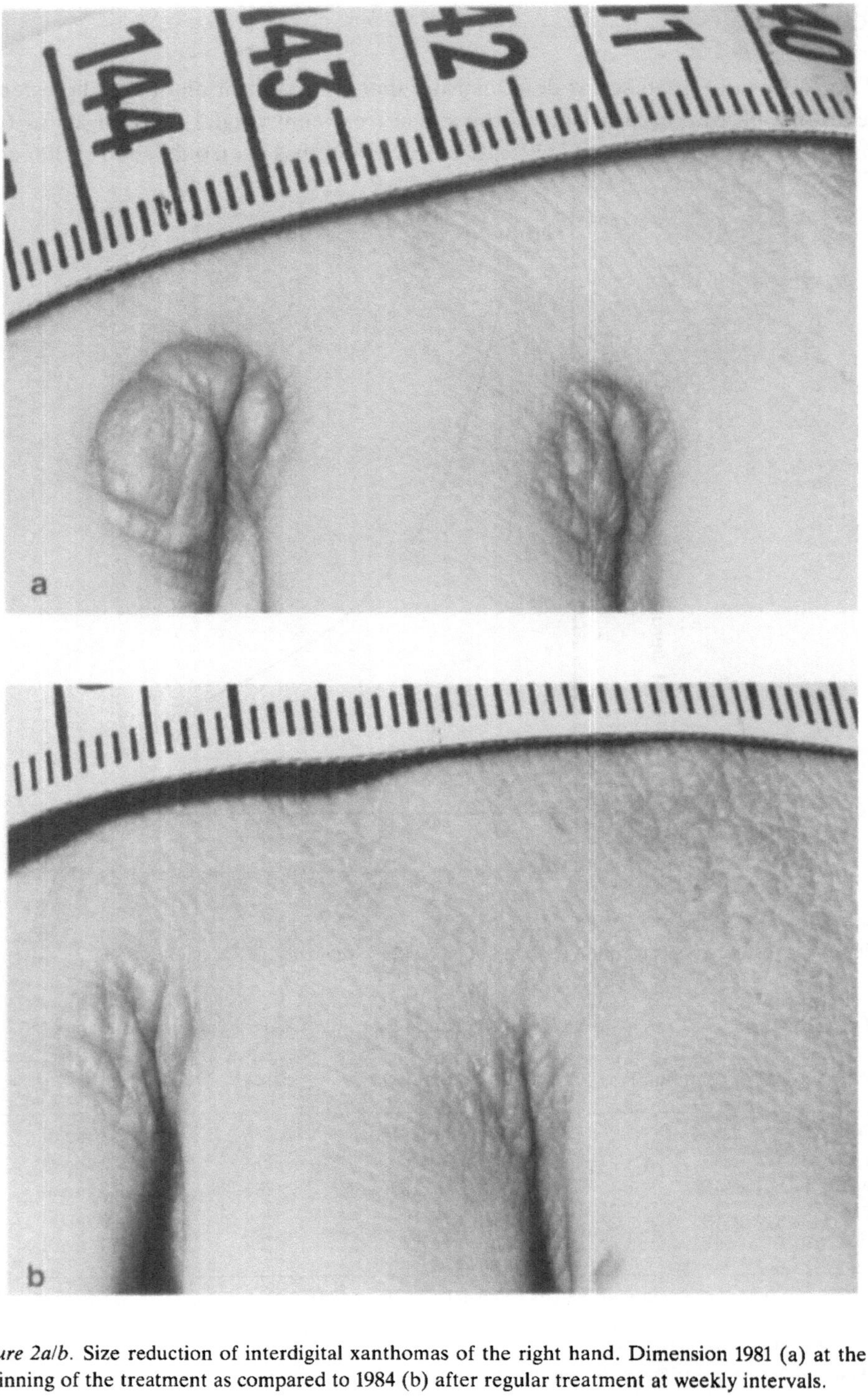

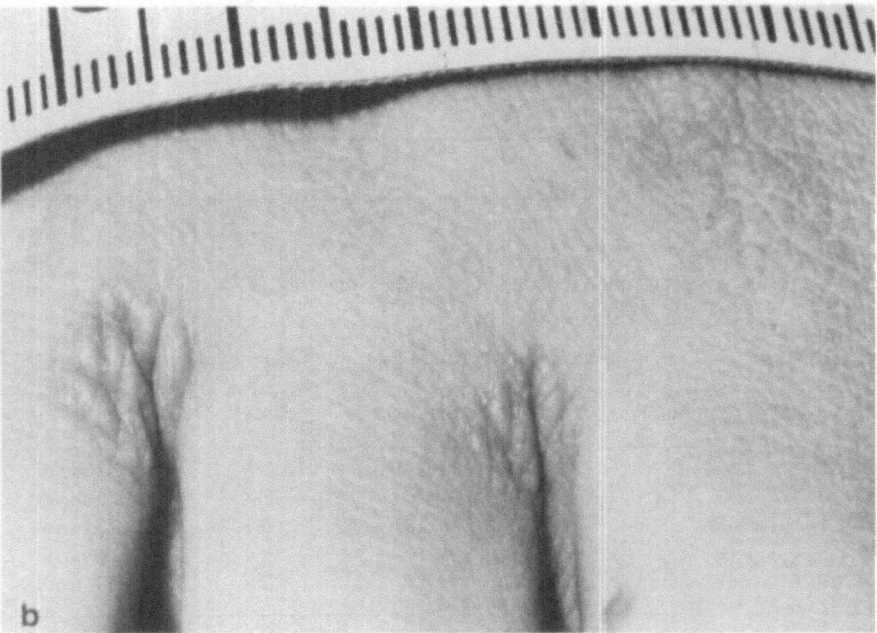

*Figure 2a/b.* Size reduction of interdigital xanthomas of the right hand. Dimension 1981 (a) at the beginning of the treatment as compared to 1984 (b) after regular treatment at weekly intervals.

could be shown to correlate with the introduction of changes of the treatment technique. It can generally be maintained at a level of less than 10% minor reactions. It is of special interest, that neither complement activation nor sensitization of any patient could be demonstrated in more than 1000 treatments performed since 1981. The dimension of peripheral xanthomas did not progress in any of the patients, but decreased in size or disappeared completely (Fig. 3). Control angiograms of coronary arteries performed in 3 patients did not show regression of stenoses so far, but demonstrated, that the disease has not progressed either. These clinical data will be published in more detail within the near future. Also a controlled multicenter trial is going to be established.

## Discussion

LDL is known to be one of the major risk factors for the pathogenesis of arteriosclerosis. This correlates with the early development of coronary heart disease in patients with familial hypercholesterolaemia. Thus, a normalization of the LDL-level has two major implications: It provides for a treatment of individuals without therapeutic alternative and it may contribute to the lipid theory of arteriosclerosis, if a long term treatment regimen either prevents the progression of the disease or leads to regression of both peripheral xanthomas as well as atheromas of the coronary arteries. The data obtained so far strongly suggest, that in our patients the progression of the disease can indeed be prevented. However due to several reasons, mainly due to the heterogeneity of the patients under treatment, regression of the coronary heart disease has not yet been demonstrated. This clearly points to the need of a controlled trial, to further elucidate, whether normalization of LDL-levels may lead to regression of coronary heart disease in these patients. One may keep in mind however, that the regression of atheromas may follow rules, which differ from those, preventing the progression of atheromatosis. Thus it is not proven, whether the atherogenicity of LDL-levels in normal individuals is comparable to the development of coronary sclerosis in these patients. Although it is generally assumed, that coronary stenoses can regress, it is not clear in which state of the disease this can still be achieved. Factors other than the LDL-level for instance the LDL/HDL ratio, local factors etc. may be equally important for the development of regression. We do not know, how much the process of regression is time dependend leading to the assumption, that years of continuous treatment are necessary. Again, many of these open questions can be answered, if this therapeutical approach is extended.

As the system described consists of reusable columns, the economy of the approach appears to be guaranteed. The columns could generally be used for 50 treatments, which means that they lasted for approximately one year. The reasons for the slow 'wearing out' process have not yet been investigated. The advantage of a specific elimination of the pathogenic substrate is obvious, as the treatment can now be tailored to the needs of the patient. A posttreatment value of 150 mg/dl is generally achieved. This is due to both, the capacity of the columns and the cycling technique developed. It refers also to homozygous patients in spite of the considerable higher LDL-levels.

## Summary

The experience with LDL-apheresis drawing from more than 1000 therapies performed since 1981 permits the following conclusions:
1.  LDL-apheresis is able to normalize the LDL titer in patients with familial hypercholesterolaemia not only during the course of one treatment but also in terms of mean values between treatments.
2.  LDL-apheresis leads to regression of peripheral lipoprotein deposits in the skin and tendons in these patients, however the process is time dependent and the extent over time differs from one patient to the other.
3.  Whether regression of coronary heart disease can be obtained, is still open. However this can be assumed, if it is permitted to transfer the observations made so far to the vascular system.

## References

1. Borberg H, Stoffel W, Oette K (1983) Plasma Ther Transfus Technol 4, 4: 459–466
2. Borberg H (1983) Europ J Clin Invest 13, II: A 39
3. Stoffel W (1981) Th Demant: Proc Natl Acad Sci (USA) 78: 611–615
4. Stoffel W, Borberg H, Greve V (1981) The Lancet ii: 1005–1007
5. Thompson GR (1981) The Lancet i: 1246

# Percutaneous transluminal angioplasty of renal artery stenoses

P.E. PETERS, V. FIEDLER, J. SCIUK, A.-R. FISCHEDICK
and H. VETTER

Percutaneous transluminal angioplasty (PTRA) is being used with increasing frequency for the treatment of renovascular hypertension and renal insufficiency caused by renal artery stenoses. The following article reviews the current status of PTRA regarding indications, technique, complications, and results of the procedure.

### Indications

Two major groups of patients are being referred for PTRA:

(1) patients with renovascular hypertension (RVH)
(2) patients with/without hypertension suffering from renal insufficiency.

In the latter group PTRA is intended to improve or salvage renal function.

In renovascular hypertension patients considered for PTRA should fulfill essentially the same generally accepted criteria for surgical revascularization. However, since PTRA carries a lower risk than renal vascular surgery, indications for balloon dilatation also include severely hypertensive patients poorly controlled on medical treatment. The proper selection of patients and the management of the blood pressure before, during, and after PTRA requires the close cooperation of a hypertension specialist. The role of renin sampling is still controversial. Levin and Tegtmeyer et al observed a higher rate of long-term cures in patients with lateralizing renal vein renin ratios, while Vetter et al were unable to confirm these data (Levin 1984, Tegtmeyer et al 1984, Vetter et al 1979).

The type of renal artery stenosis must be taken into consideration. A good long-term result can be anticipated in all types of fibromuscular dysplasia (FMD), and in short, segmental atherosclerotic lesions. Ostial lesions caused by plaques of the abdominal aorta engulfing the orifice of the renal artery are less well suited for PTRA (Tegtmeyer et al 1984). Predilatation analysis of the different types of renal artery stenoses by means of intravenous digital subtraction angiography (IV-DSA) has proven to be a reliable method of patient selection.

Renal artery stenoses with RVH occur in 1%–10% following renal transplantation (Ingrisch 1984). A great number of reasons for this complication has been discussed:

– pre-existing plaques in the iliac vessels
– trauma to the renal artery by traction or clamping
– during explantation, perfusion, or transplantation
– malrotation of the transplanted kidney
– immunologic reactions with periarteritic and subintimal fibrosis.

Ingrisch reported improvement or cure of renovascular hypertension in 7/13 patients with renal artery stenosis following transplantation by PTRA (Ingrisch 1984).

**Technique**

From a technical viewpoint, most authors use one of three variations:

(1) the guide-wire-catheter technique
(2) the use of preshaped catheters to pass the stenosis
(3) the use of coaxial systems.

In PTRA the guide-wire-catheter technique is by far the most common one. The ipsilateral femoral approach is standard procedure, excentric renal artery stenoses may require puncture of the axillary artery (Fig. 1). The renal artery is usually entered with an appropriate 5 French diagnostic catheter. A floppy-tipped guide-wire is used to traverse the stenotic segment. The catheter is then advanced over the wire into the post-stenotic arterial segment. Pressure measurements during PTRA are mandatory. Exchange is made for an angioplasty catheter the inflated balloon diameter of which is chosen by measuring the renal artery proximal and distal to the stenosis and estimating the original size of the stenotic segment. This kind of measurement does not take into account geometric magnification. Thus, the inflated balloon will overdilate by about 1 mm.

After dilatation pressure measurements are repeated. The morphologic result is being documented by arteriography. Currently digital subtraction angiography is being used during and after PTRA. The method allows the use of less concentrated contrast medium resulting presumably in less local irritation of the arterial wall following dilatation. The total amount of contrast medium can be markedly reduced which in turn may diminish the risk of renal failure due to the nephrotoxicity of contrast medium. For the same reason we are using routinely non-ionic contrast media in PTRA which have been shown to be less nephrotoxic (Scherberich et al 1985). DSA offers instant subtracted images. This feature helps to shorten the total time of the procedure. This again may reduce the inherent risks of PTRA.

## Complications

Because of the repeated catheter exchanges and the use of anticoagulants, the risk of bleeding and pseudoaneurysm formation is greater after angioplasty than in routine arteriography. Specific complications of PTRA include renal artery dissection with/without occlusion, segmental artery occlusion, transient acute renal failure or transient exacerbation of chronic renal failure (Martin et al 1985). Ingrisch collected data from the literature showing an overall complication rate of 22.6% (127 complications in 561 patients). This figure, however, includes also minor side effects such as groin hematoma. Surgery and/or hemodialysis was necessary in 30/561 PTRA cases (5.3%). there were 6 fatal complications, 4 of them myocardial infarctions occurring 2–10 days after successful dilatation of renal artery stenoses (Ingrisch 1984). Martin et al reported eleven major complications in 100 PTRA attempts, four of them required aortorenal bypass surgery. There were no secondary nephrectomies nor deaths in their collective (Martin et al 1985). Mortality during surgery in the cooperative study of renovascular disease was 5.9% (Foster et al 1975).

## Results

The results of renal angioplasty should be evaluated in the following categories:

(1) technical success rate
    complete – partial – failure
(2) blood pressure response
    cured – improved – failed
(3) response of renal function
    normalized – improved – failed

In addition, short term results must be differentiated from long-term observations. Recurrent stenoses can be anticipated in a percentage of patients not precisely known so far, mostly in those with at least 30% residual stenosis (Tegtmeyer et al 1984). Redilatation is frequently easier to perform than the initial PTRA, and the result is longer-lasting. IV-DSA was used to study 50 patients two or more years after successful renal angioplasty. Among patients with atherosclerotic stenosis, the restenosis rate was found to be 22.5% while patients with fibromuscular dysplasia showed no recurrence after PTRA (Schwarten 1984).

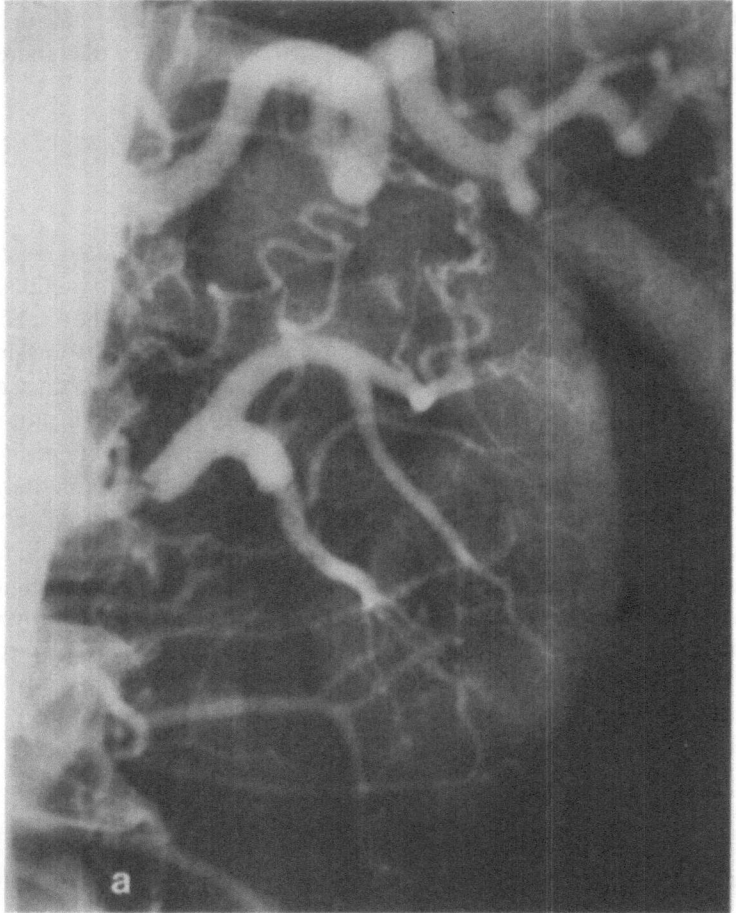

*Figure 1.* Non-ostial segmental stenosis of the left renal artery; a) pre-dilatation arteriography;
b) inflated angioplasty catheter in situ.

Technical success rate: Initial technical success rate depends on the patient
selection. In fibromuscular dysplasia the initial technical success rate may be as
high as 94% (Tegtmeyer et al 1984). Studies involving only atherosclerotic lesions
show up to 33% failures (Cohn et al 1984). The majority of reports in the
literature vary between 85% and 90% initial success rate (Ingrisch 1984, Levin
1984).

Blood pressure response: The criteria used to evaluate the results of PTRA are
as follows:

– *cured* = diastolic blood pressure of 90 mmHg or less without antihypertensive
medication and decrease of at least 10 mmHg in diastolic pressure;

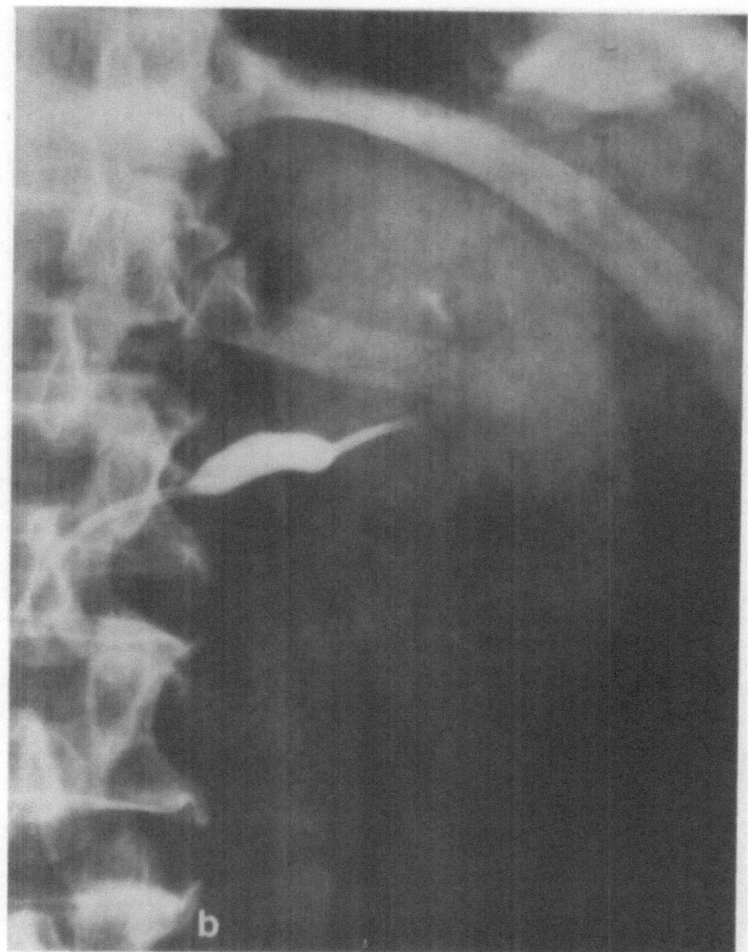

- *improved* = diastolic blood pressure between 90 and 110 mmHg with at least a 15% decrease or a marked reduction in antihypertensive medication;
- *failure* = diastolic pressure greater than 90 mmHg, or less than 15% drop in diastolic pressure.

(Foster et al 1975, Maxwell et al 1972).

Using these criteria short term cure rate in patients with fibromuscular dysplasia is 25%, 60% are improved, in 15% PTRA failed (Martin et al 1985). Tegtmeyer reported 32% cure rate, 68% improvement and 10% failures (Tegtmeyer et al 1984). Both studies showed a 85–90% benefit ratio. As mentioned earlier, the restenosis rate of FMD is very low, thus, the short term results are almost identical to long-term observations (Schwarten 1984, Tegtmeyer et al 1984).

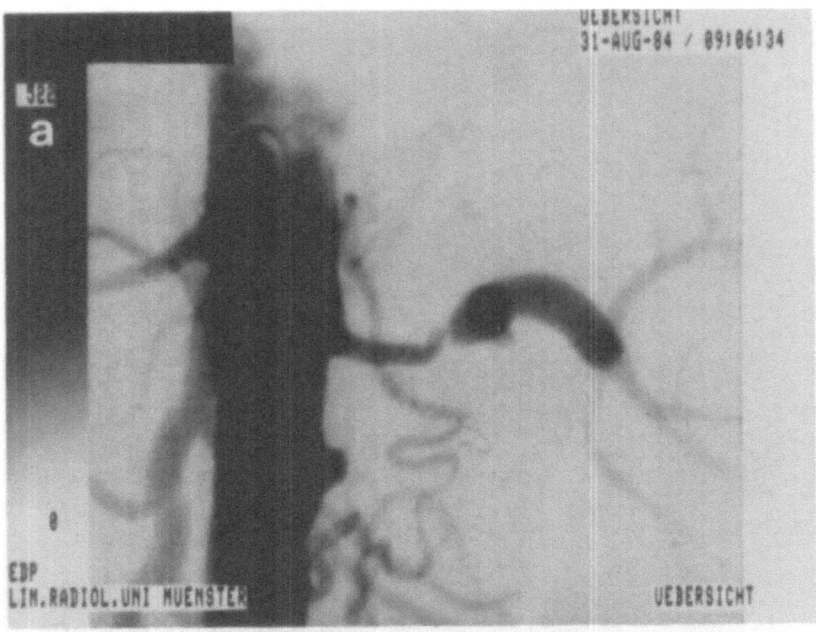

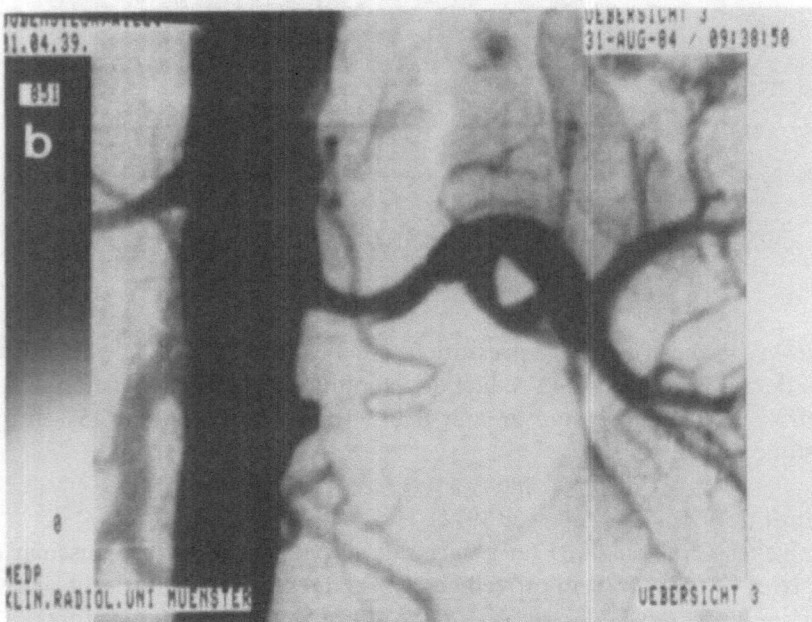

*Figure 2.* Non-ostial stenosis of the left renal artery. Agenesis of the right kidney; a) IA-DSA pre-dilatation; b) IA-DSA immediately after dilatation showing a small intimal tear; c) IV-DSA 8 weeks after dilatation; d) change in heart size following successful PTRA and cure of hypertension.

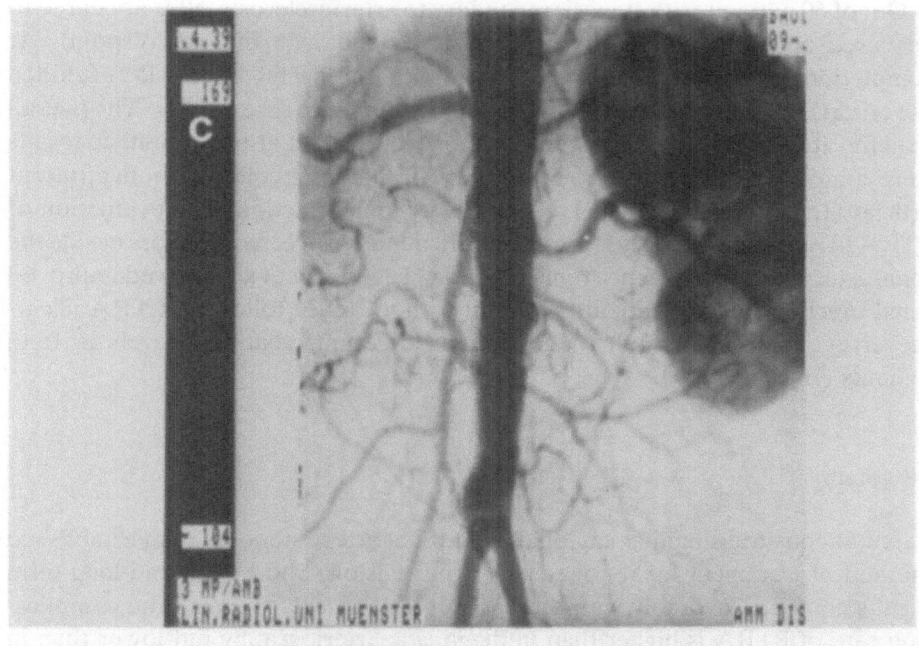

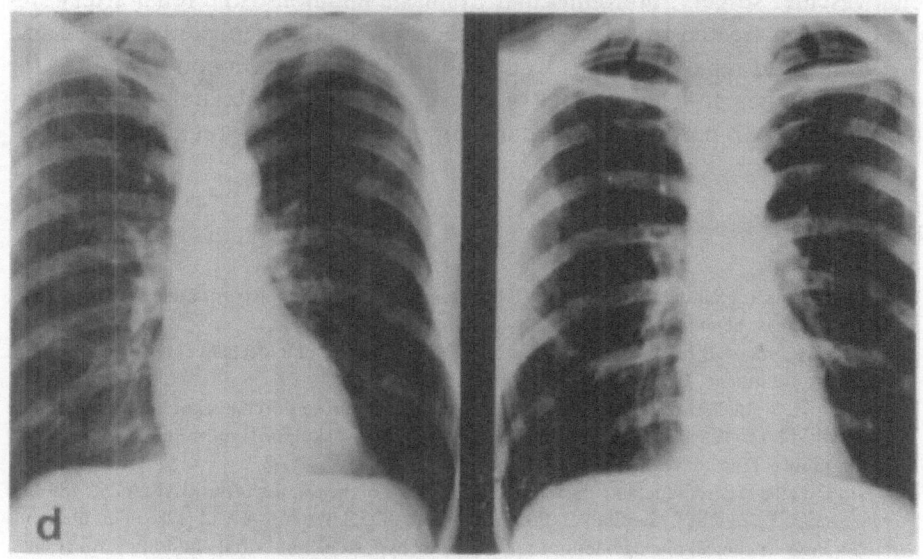

Out of 60 patients with stenosis secondary to arteriosclerosis, 50% appeared to be cured at discharge, 27% were improved, and 13% did not respond. At completion of follow-up study, i.e. 3–39 months after PTRA, only 15% fulfilled the criteria of cure, 50% were improved, the failure rate rose to 35%. The overall benefit ratio in this particular study was 65% (Martin et al 1985). Similar results were compiled by Ingrisch: 69% benefit ratio in 240 cases collected from different articles (Ingrisch 1984) (Fig. 2). Response of renal function: The evaluation of PTRA in renal insufficiency is the most difficult task since many factors beside the renal artery stenosis influence renal function. Tegtmeyer et al observed improved renal function in 13/34 patients with and without RVH following PTRA (Tegtmeyer et al 1984). Ingrisch found decreased serum creatinine levels in 15/18 patients (Ingrisch 1984).

## Summary

Percutaneous transluminal angioplasty of renal artery stenoses is an established method of treatment for renovascular hypertension. Short term and long term results compare favorably with those of surgical vascular repair. The complication rate of PTRA is higher than in diagnostic arteriography but lower than in renal vascular surgery. Fibromuscular dysplasia and non-ostial renal artery stenosis are best treated by PTRA. The procedure can be repeated if necessary. IV-DSA of the renal arteries is well suited for patient selection as well as for follow-up studies. In selected cases with severe unilateral or bilateral renal artery stenoses PTRA is performed in order to improve or salvage renal function.

## References

1. Cohn DJ, Sos TA Saddekni S, Srur MF (1984) Transluminal angioplasty for atherosclerotic renal artery stenosis. Seminars Interventional Radiology 1: 279–287
2. Foster JH, Maxwell MH, Franklin SS et al (1975) Renovascular occlusive disease: results of operative treatment. JAMA 231: 1043–1048
3. Ingrisch H. Radiologische Therapie der Nierenarterien stenose durch perkutane transluminale Angioplastik (PTA). In: Arlart IP, Ingrish H (1984) Renovaskuläre Hypertonie. Stuttgart-New York: Georg Thieme Verlag, pp 72–94
4. Levin DC (1984) Percutaneous transluminal angioplasty of the renal arteries. JAMA 251: 759–763
5. Martin LG, Price RB, Casarella WJ, Sones PJ, Wells JO, Zellmer RA et al (1985) Percutaneous angioplasty in clinical management of renovascular hypertension: initial and long-term results. Radiology 155: 629–633
6. Maxwell MH, Bleifer KH, Franklin SS, Varady PD (1972) Cooperative study of renovascular hypertension: demographic analysis of the study. JAMA 220: 1195–1204
7. Scherberich JE, Tuengerthal S, Kollath J, Riemann HE. Kontrastmitteltoxizität und Niere: Differenzierte Beurteilung durch tubulusspezifische Gewebsparameter. In: Riemann HE, Kollath J (Hrsg) (1985) Digitale Radiographie. Konstanz, Schnetztor-Verlag, pp 315–322

8. Schwarten DE (1984) Percutaneous transluminal angioplasty of the renal arteries: intravenous digital subtraction angiography for follow-up. Radiology 150: 369–373
9. Tegtmeyer CJ, Kofler TJ, Ayers A (1984) Renal angioplasty: current status. AJR 142: 17–21
10. Tegtmeyer CJ, Kellum CD, Ayers C (1984) Percutaneous transluminal angioplasty of the renal artery. Radiology 153: 77–84
11. Tegtmeyer CJ, Tegtmeyer VL, Kellum CD, Dombrowski PJ, Lledo AM (1984) Percutaneous transluminal angioplasty. The treatment of choice for vascular lesions caused by fibromuscular dysplasia. Seminars Interventional Radiology 1: 289–300
12. Vetter W, Vetter H, Tenschert W, Kuhlmann U et al (1979) Renovaskuläre Hypertonie: Prognostischer Wert der seitengetrennten Reninbestimmung im Nierenvenenblut. Klin Wochensch 57: 863

# Balloon angioplasty in peripheral vascular occlusive disease

F.-J. ROTH, P. BERLINER, W. KRINGS, I. SCHMIDTKE, B. KOPPERS and B. GRÜN

Angioplasty has become a well accepted routine method to treat peripheral arterial occlusive disease. The Dotter procedure is attempted all over the arterial system. In detail angioplasty is performed in the peripheral, the visceral, the coronary and the renal arteries and in the branches of the aortic arch including the carotid artery [1, 5, 7, 8, 10, 13, 16, 20, 21, 27, 34]. In the following the mechanism of angioplasty, the early and late results, special techniques and rare applications as well will be described treating peripheral arterial vascular disease.

## 1. Mechanism of angioplasty

In 1964 Ch. Dotter [9] thought, in atherosclerotic lesions the stenosis or the obliteration is caused by a material, which is first adhesive at the vessel wall and second unelastic compressible. Therefore by compressing the core substance the dilatation of an obliterated artery is possible without the risk of peripheral embolism [9, 10, 34].

Based on experimental work, animal and postmortem studies, on light and electron microscopic observations as well [3, 4, 6, 7, 12, 19, 36] the most important mechanism of angioplasty is believed to be a localized overstretching of the vessel wall by means of the dilatating forces of the balloon. There is observed a superficial desquamation of intimal elements, a focal splitting of the intima, and a separation of the intima from the media. A rupturing of the media and a thin overlying platelet-fibrin mural thrombus is observed. No evidence of dissection is found. The healing of the injured vessel wall is producing an additional enlargement of the balloon dilatated arterial segment [3, 4]. By experimental work there is no compression of the core substance on cadaver arteries. Therefore the theory of the mechanism of angioplasty is, the atheromatous material is incompressible and the arterial lumen is widened by a localized overstretching of the arterial wall [6, 7, 36].

In conclusion the most important mechanism of angioplasty is the overstretching of the vessel wall. The compression of the core substance, also may occur, but this mechanism is less important for a successful dilatation.

In the postangioplasty arteriogram an irregular edge of contrast column (separate margin of contrast column) correlates with splitting of the intima and the intramural cleft with the medial split [3, 4, 12]. In our own experience [10, 27] in the postangioplasty arteriogram rupturing of the intima (Table 1) occurs in 53% and medial splits in 7%. The intima split is angiographically reversible. On the other hand the intramural cleft (medial split) is irreversible. The controll arteriogram demonstrates (Fig. 1) a small defined ectasia (aneurysmatic dilatation). To avoid too much injury of the dilatated arterial segment, the balloon diameter should therefore not be larger than artery diameter measured at the arteriograph.

## 2. Early and late results and complications

The reasons, why angioplasty is well accepted, are the primary and long term results of this therapeutic principle [5, 8, 14, 21, 22, 27, 29, 33, 34]. In 1983 Gailer and co-workers [13] demonstrated in a cooperative study, that the primary results in treating iliac stenoses are 93%; treating stenoses and obliterations up to 10 cm of the femoropopliteal arteris the early success is 87%. The cure rate of the 1082 iliac patients was 85%–64% with a patency rate of 84% after three years. In the 2337 femoropopliteal patients the cure rate after 3 years was 60% with a patency rate of 75%. After 5 years the patency rate was 64%. Treating 1915 iliac artery stenoses the complications at puncture site were 1.7%. Complications requiring surgery occured in 0.8%. In the femoropopliteal segment you have to deal with 3.2% complications at puncture site and with 2.0% complications requiring surgery [13, 30]. In 1984 Rieger [22] compared long term results of angioplasty with vascular surgery in the literature using the life table. 2179 femoropopliteal angioplasties had a patency rate of 69.1% after 3 and 68.0% after 5 years. After 3 years 317 femoropopliteal angioplasties had a patency rate of 64% in stage III/IV. The patency rate of 1706 femoropopliteal venous bypass grafts was 67.5% after 3, 59%, after 5, and 44.5% after 10 years. 1945 femoropopliteal venous bypass grafts performed for limb salvage had a patency rate of 65.7% after 3, of 57.5% after 5 and 44.5% after 10 years. In this material the complications and lethality rate of

*Table 1.* Radiographic pattern of 406 consecutive postangioplasty arteriograms of iliac and femoropopliteal artery.

| | |
|---|---|
| Wall irregularities | 303 (75%) |
| Separate margin of contrast column | 214 (53%) |
| Intramural cleft | 27 (7%) |
| Smooth wall | 39 (9.6%) |
| Localized overstretching | 9 (2%) |

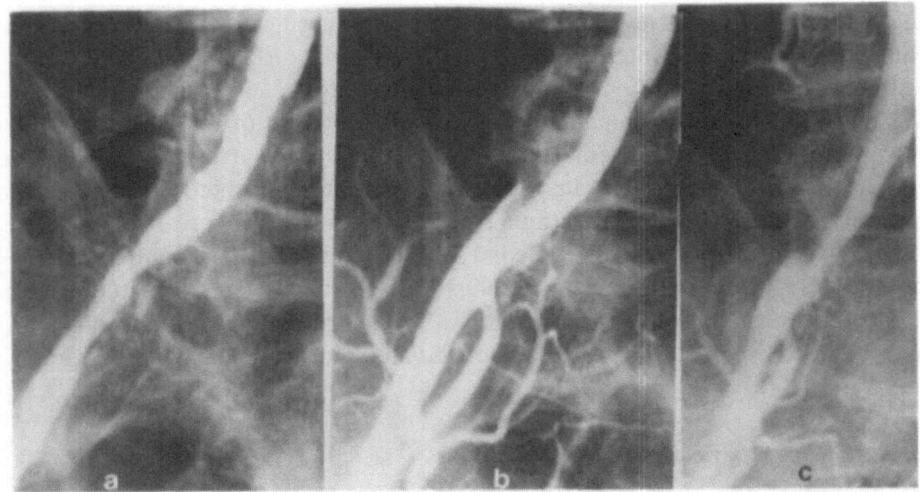

*Figure 1.* Arteriography of left iliac artery; a) stenosis of external iliac artery; b) postangioplasty arteriogram with intramural cleft (media split); c) arteriogram 27 months after PTA localized ectasia in the former stenotic segment.

vascular surgery was higher than in angioplasty. In our own experience [27] we went through 2668 of our angioplasties dividing them in two groups, patients older (A) and younger (B) than 65 ears (Tables 2 and 3). In the iliac segment we accomplished angioplasties only in stenotic lesions; in the femoropopliteal segment we recanalized stenoses and occlusions longer than 10 cm, knowing that obliterations longer than 10 cm have a high risk of acute reocclusion [1]. Mostly in stage III/IV longer occlusions were treated. In case of an occlusion of the superficial femoral artery and an additional occlusion of the lower leg arteries we again performed angioplasty for limb salvage. In group A, 2054 patients 65 years old and younger (Table 2) we technically succeeded in the iliac segment in 88% and in the femoropopliteal artery including a very small number of lower leg arteries in 74%. In 2% we had severe complications we could manage by conservative treatment (Table 4). The complication and the lethality rate were

*Table 2.* Primary results of 2054 angioplasties of iliac and femoropopliteal arteries in patients 65 years old or younger.

|  | n | + | − |
|---|---|---|---|
| Femoropopliteal artery | 1364 | 1018 (74%) | 354 (26%) |
| Iliac artery | 690 | 606 (88%) | 84 (12%) |
| Total | 2054 | 1616 (79%) | 438 (21%) |

n = number of treatments, + = technically successful, − = technically failed.

0.1%. On the other hand the 614 patients older than 65 years (Table 3), group B, had a lower primary success rate and a higher risk of complications. In detail we technically succeeded in iliaca stenoses in 83% and in femoropopliteal obliterations in 71%. The complication rate, we could conservatively manage, was 8% (Table 5). The complications requiring surgery and the lethality rate were 1%.

The reason for the lower primary success rate and the higher risk of complications in the older patient group is the multiple morbidity of these patients.

*Table 3.* Primary results of 614 angioplasties of iliac and femoropopliteal arteries in patients older than 65 years.

|  | n | + | − |
|---|---|---|---|
| Femoropopliteal artery | 471 | 335 (71%) | 136 (29%) |
| Iliac artery | 143 | 128 (83%) | 25 (17%) |
| Total | 614 | 453 (74%) | 161 (26%) |

n = number of treatments, + = technically successful, − = technically failed.

*Table 4.* Conservatively managed complications of 2054 angioplasties of iliac and femoropopliteal arteries in patients 65 years old or younger.

| | |
|---|---|
| Hemorrhage at puncture site | 7 |
| Peripheral embolism | 21 |
| Occlusions of a treated stenosis | 4 |
| Dissection of the treated segment | 5 |
| Intolerance of contrast medium | 1 |
| | 38 (1.85%) |

*Table 5.* Conservatively managed complications of 614 angioplasties of iliac and femoropopliteal arteries in patients older than 65 years.

| | |
|---|---|
| Hemorrhage at puncture site | 15 |
| Peripheral embolism | 19 |
| Occlusion of a treated stenosis | 6 |
| Dissecction of the treated segment | 5 |
| Intolerance of contrast medium | 2 |
| Stroke | 2 |
| | 49 (8%) |

## 3. Special techniques

In the last years angioplasty rapidly proceeded from the technical point of view. There is a wide spectrum of different approaches available. Usually the common femoral approach is taken [1, 7, 10, 14, 34]. Sometimes less common approaches as the axillar or seldom the brachial or even the popliteal have to be used to manage angioplasty [27]. The cross-over-technique has its own indications [2, 20, 21, 24]. The local low dose fibrinolytic therapy (catheter lysis) is a newer application [15, 16, 25, 26].

### 3.1 The axillar approach

The higher risk of complications at puncture site in the axillar approach is well known from the diagnostic arteriography. The complication rate at puncture site of femoral approach is 1.73% and of axillar approach is 3.29% [17, 31] in diagnostic arteriography. The complications at puncture site of angioplasty are even higher than of diagnostic arteriography. Therefore to cut down the complications of angioplasty the axillar approach should be strictly indicated, and only used, if there is no other technical possibility left [27]. Treating peripheral occlusive vascular disease indications for the axillar approach are angioplasty after vascular surgery (Fig. 2) and bilateral stenoses of distal iliaca or groin arteries. Of course the axillar approach sometimes has to be used to attempt angioplasty of the visceral, the renal and supraaortic arteries.

### 3.2 Popliteal approach

This application is very difficult from the technical point of view. Dotter procedure should only be attempted, if there is no other technique left and the patient unfit for surgery. The patient has to lie in the prone position. The popliteal artery has to be punctured in the popliteal fossa. We performed angioplasty twice by this advice and succeeded once (Fig. 3).

*Figure 2.* Aortography; a) patent aortobifemoral bypass graft; b) stenosis of deep femoral artery, occlusion of superficial femoral artery; patient complains pain at rest; c) postangioplasty arteriogram completely dilatated deep femoral artery stenosis in axillar approach.

*Figure 3.* Arteriography of left superficial femoral artery; a) postangioplasty arteriogram: failed PTA in common femoral approach because of direct collateral vessels; b) seond PTA in popliteal approach catheter introduced in popliteal artery, which is punctured in the popliteal fossa; c) postangioplasty arteriogram of second PTA: patent superficial femoral artery.

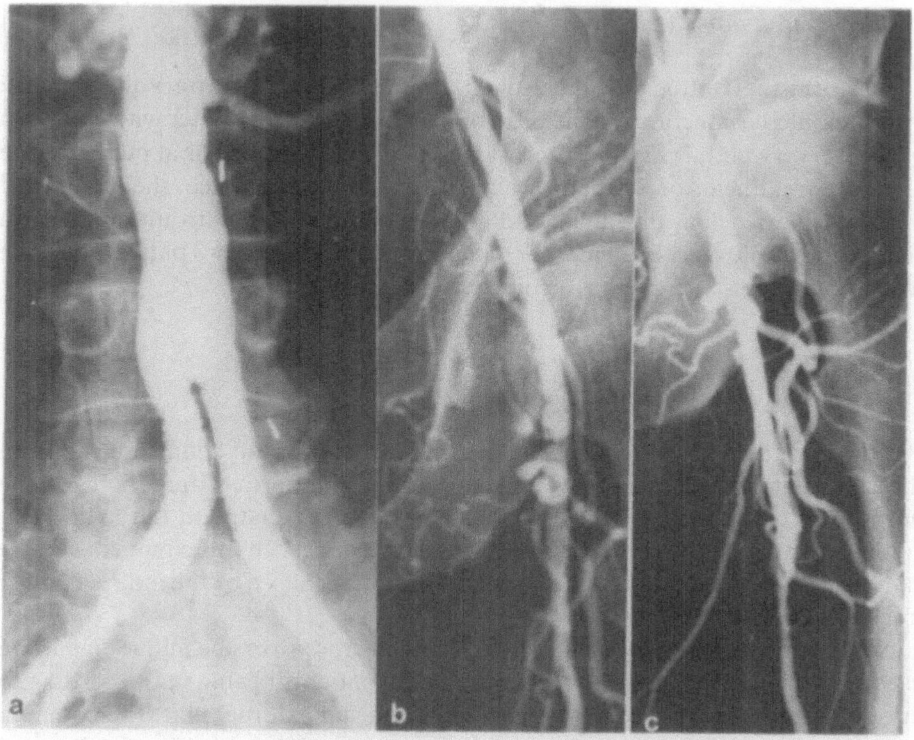

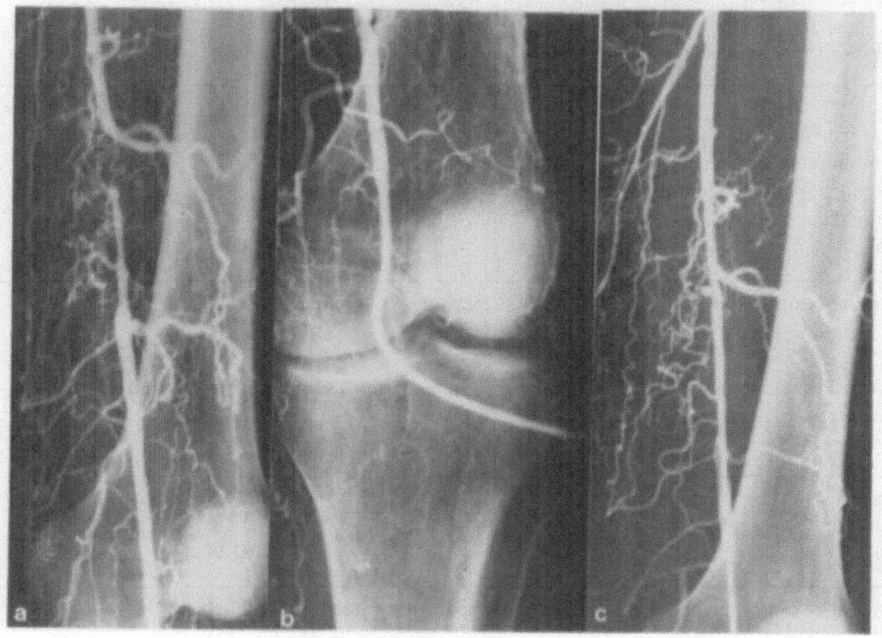

## 3.3 Brachial approach

To perform the Dotter procedure of the brachial or axillar artery the brachial artery should be punctured in the bend of the elbow. A 5 F catheter with a 4–6 mm balloon is very useful (Fig. 4). There is a risk of acute thrombosis at puncture site [27]. In 8 treatments of 5 patients we had this complication once, the patient did not deteriorate clinically at all. All our patients suffered from severe arm claudication. We succeeded in 7 our of 8 treatments. Clinically 3 patients became free of symptoms and one has significantly improved.

## 3.4 Cross over technique

Performing angioplasty in this technique the catheter has to be introduced from the contralateral side and to be advanced over the aortic bifurcation for the purpose of dilatation [2, 24]. Using the contralateral dilatation the main difficulties will arise, if the catheter tip gets some resistance. In this circumstance the catheter has the tendency to slide back into the aorta caused by the indirect power transmission [24, 27].

Attempting angioplasty of the groin arteries cross over technique has to be used. We gained our experience in treating 210 patients (Table 6). According to our definition of groin arteries we include the distal external iliac, the common femoral, the proximal superficial and deep femoral artery (Fig. 5). In total technical success is 82.9% (Tables 6 and 7). The primary success of dilatating

*Table 6.* Primary results of 210 angioplasties of groin arteries.

|  | n | + | − |
|---|---|---|---|
| Distal iliac femoral artery | 20 (10%) | 17 | 3 |
| Common femoral artery | 85 (40.5%) | 64 | 21 |
| Proximal superficial femoral artery | 28 (13%) | 25 | 3 |
| Proximal deep femoral artery | 77 (36.5%) | 68 | 9 |
| Total | 210 | 174 (82%) | 36 (18%) |

n = number of treatments, + = technically successful, − = technically failed.

*Table 7.* Primary results of 210 angioplasties of groin arteries 180 stenotic lesions and 30 occlusions.

|  | n | + | − |
|---|---|---|---|
| Stenoses | 180 | 156 (87%) | 24 |
| Occlusions | 30 | 18 (60%) | 12 |
| Total | 210 | 174 (82.9%) | 36 |

n = number of treatments, + = technically successful, − = technically failed.

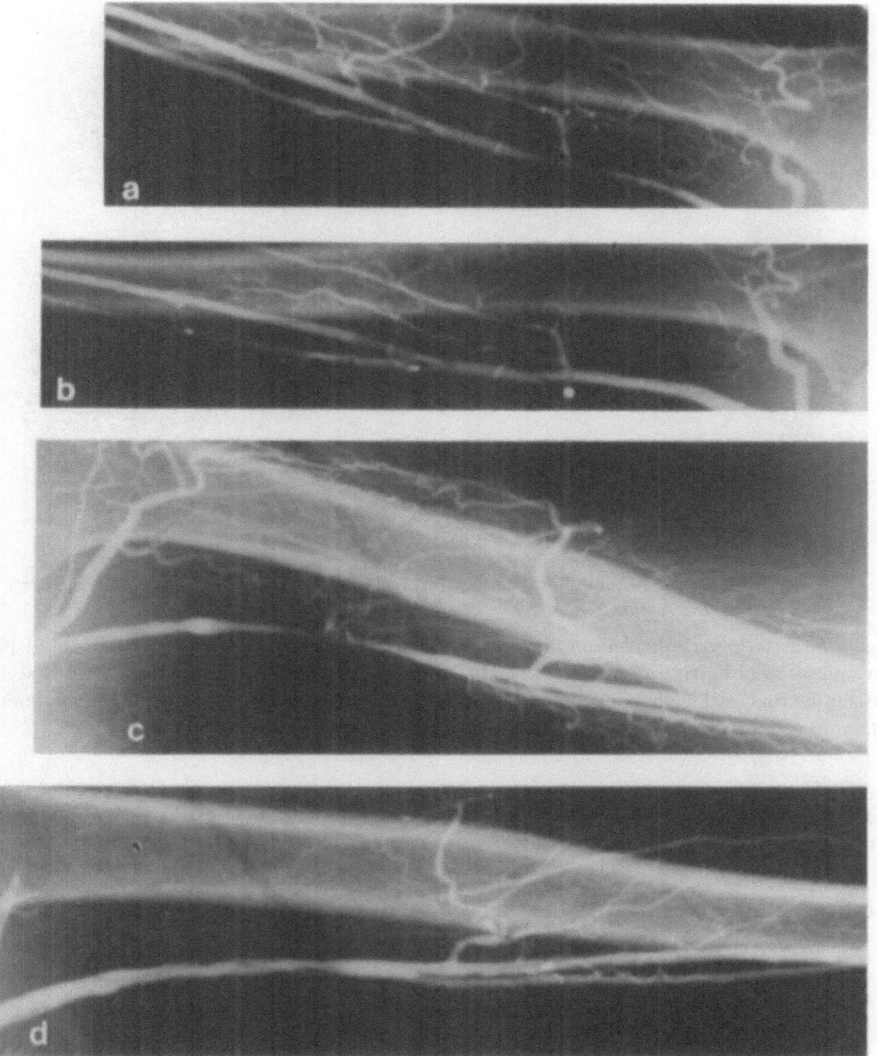

*Figure 4.* Brachial arteriogram; a) and c) both brachial arteries are duplicated in their proximal segment with stenotic lesions in the proximal portion of brachial artery; b) and d) postangioplasty arteriogram slight residual stenosis of right and left brachial artery. PTA achieved in brachial approach.

stenoses is high (87%). The recanalization of groin artery occlusion has failed in 60% (Table 7). In detail (Table 8) we failed in 50% of the common femoral artery occlusions. Therefore occlusions of the common femoral artery should be treated surgically [27]. The main reason for the low success treating occlusions is the technical difficulty in directing the guide wire and the catheter into the patent

288

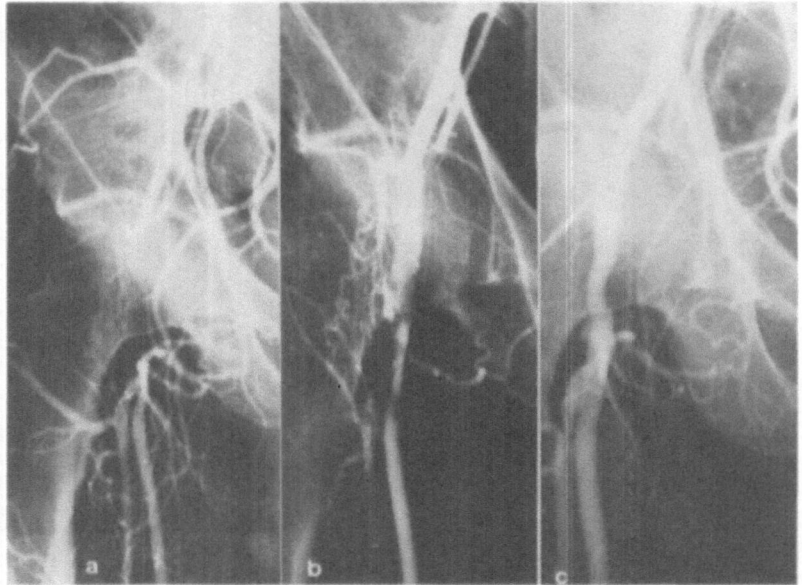

*Figure 5.* Arteriogram right groin arteries; a) occlusion of right common femoral artery; post-angioplasty arteriogram; b) significant residual stenosis of common femoral artery. PTA accomplished in cross over technique; c) controll arteriogram 3 years later patent right common femoral artery no residual stenosis.

deep femoral artery past the occlusion. In most instances the guide wire will engage the likewise occluded superficial femoral artery [24]. Complications, we could conservatively manage, occured in 6.2%. In 1% surgery (Table 9) was required [27]. In conclusion the advantage of contralateral dilatation is:

1. Angioplasty is extended to the groin arteries.
2. No haematoma in the dilatated arterial segment (important for surgery in case of failure).
3. Angioplasty is possible in obesity and postoperative scar.

*Table 8.* Primary results of 85 angioplasties of common femoral artery.

|  | n | + | − |
|---|---|---|---|
| Stenoses | 63 | 53 (84%) | 10 |
| Occlusions | 22 | 11 (50%) | 11 |
| Total | 85 | 64 (75%) | 21 |

n = number of treatments, + = technically successful, − = technically failed.

4. Right and left iliac artery stenoses or ipsilateral iliac and femoral artery stenoses may be treated in one procedure.

The main disadvantage is the risk of compliction of the healthy leg. Cross over technique is more difficult than ipsilateral dilatation from the technical point of view. Therefore the technical success is a little bit smaller compared with the ipsilateral approach (Table 10).
    Reasons for technical failure are:

1. An acute angle of the aortic bifurcation.
2. Tortuosity and elongation of the iliac arteries and
3. the indirect power transmission. Therefore stenoses and not occlusions should be treated in routine cross over technique.

Contralateral dilatation is contraindicated in case of an infrarenal aortic aneurysm, because there is a high risk of peripheral embolism, mechanically caused during the catheter manoeuvring. In the meantime we had this severe complication twice. Both patients clinically deteriorated.

## 4. PTA of infrarenal aorta

The indication for angioplasty of stenotic lesion of the infrarenal aorta is rare [10, 18, 20, 23, 34, 35]. In aortic dilatation there are risks of severe retro- or even peritonel bleeding caused by catheter perforation and of acute thrombotic occlusion of the bifurcation. In case of clinical recurrence the vascular surgeons report a periaortic induration pronounced by scarformation, which significantly makes

Table 9. Complications of 210 angioplasties of groin arteries.

| | |
|---|---|
| Occlusion of treated stenosis | 6 (2.9%) |
| Peripheral embolism | 3 (1.4%) |
| Dissection of treated segment | 2 (0.95%) |
| Large haematoma at puncture site | 2 (0.95%) |
| Surgery required | 2 (0.95%) |

Table 10. Technique and primary results of 659 angioplasties of iliac artery.

| | | | |
|---|---|---|---|
| Ipsilateral dilatation | 479 | 416 (87%) | 63 (13%) |
| Contralateral dilatation | 180 | 151 (84%) | 29 (16%) |
| Total | 659 | 567 (86%) | 92 (14%) |

n = number of treatments, + = technically successful, − = technically failed.

the bypass grafting surgery more difficult. For this reasons angioplasty of the aorta has to be indicated in close connection with the vascular surgeon. Technically angioplasty of the aorta may be performed using one, two (kissing balloons) or even three catheters in the same procedure [10, 18, 21, 23, 34, 35]. We prefer the one catheter technique. The advantage of this method is a minimal injuring (only one artery is punctured instead of 2 or 3). An optimal dilatation of the entire aortic lumen is guaranteed. Using 2 catheters the aorta is dilatated in an oval manner. Some part of the aortic wall is overstretched and the other is not dilatated satisfactorily. Angioplasty of the aorta is indicated in single atheromatous stenotic lesions. It may avoid or at least postpone vascular surgery in cases when surgery is of high risk for the patient or a patient is unfit for surgery.

## 5. Angioplasty of non-atherosclerotic lesions

Non-atherosclerotic lesions [20, 27] causing arterial obliteration are fibromusculaire dysplasia, inflammatory disease (arteriitis), trauma and miscellaneousness. We performed angioplasty of the proximal brachial artery, because of arteriitis in 5 patients. In three of them bilaterally (Fig. 4). We completely succeeded in 7 arteries and partly in two. In one patient we failed, because of an acute thrombotic occlusion at puncture site. This patient clinically did not deteriorate. The successfully treated patients became free of symptoms. The patient partly succeeded with the Dotter procedure, clinically improved.

## 6. Angioplasty of a former surgically or angioplastically treated artery

In case of clinical recurrence following angioplasty or vascular surgery the application for the Dotter procedure may be suggested [27, 28].

### 6.1 PTA after vascular surgery

We accomplished 105 angioplasties in 82 patients, 14 females and 68 males [27]. The average age was 57 years ranging from 37 to 77. In 11 patients angioplasty was performed twice or even three times (Table 11). The primary success rate was 83%, which is comparable to routine angioplasty. Because of the surgically caused change of vascular anatomy and the postoperative scar angioplasty was more difficult than usually from the technical point of view. Therefore the Dotter procedure had to be attempted in cross over technique in about 40% of the treatments. Accomplishing angioplasty of venous bypass grafts it is our policy not to puncture the graft itself, in order to avoid further damage of the venous graft (Fig 6). Injury of the vein is believed to be one of the reasons for graft's stenosis.

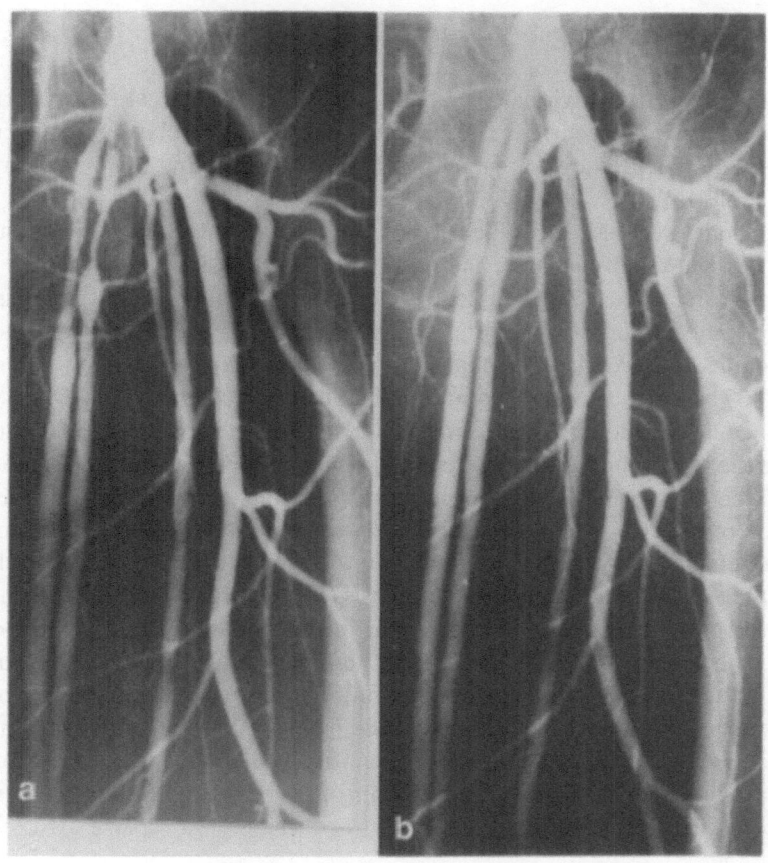

*Figure 6.* Arteriogram left femoral artery; a) occlusion of distal superficial femoral artery, femoro-popliteal venous bypass graft performed with a duplicated saphenous vein, both channels with stenotic lesions; b) postangioplasty arteriogram patent bypass graft after dilatation of both channels.

The complications are simular to those of angioplasty (Table 12). Severe complications, we could control conservatively, occured in 3.8%. One patient (1%) required surgery because of an acute thrombotic occlusion at puncture site [27]. A short time follow up of 9,9 months in average shows however a recurrence rate of 62%. This is probably caused by an acceleration of the atherosclerotic disease itself and not by an insufficiently accomplished angioplasty. Angioplasty after vascular surgery is indicated in stage II and mainly in stage III/IV for limb salvage. These patients will benefit from angioplasty, as this treatment is of low risk with an acceptable primary success. And of course a second vascular operation is more difficult and less successful than the first one. Therefore angioplasty may prevent or at least postpone a second operation.

## 6.2 Angioplasty in recurrence after the Dotter procedure

It is well known, that angioplasty may be repeated few times at the same arterial segment in case of recurrence. We went through 173 relapse treatments, 51 females, 122 males. The average age was 61,5 years ranging from 34 years to 83 years (Table 14).

The primary success for the iliac artery was 75.9%. The clinical recurrence was caused in 5 out of 25 iliac artery stenosis by a new lesion.

Our material also showed (Table 13), that 15 of 54 initial widened stenosis of the femoropopliteal segment angiographically deteriorated and became occlusions in case of clinical recurrence. The clinical recurrence angiographically was caused in 5 out of 137 cases by a new atheromatous lesion and in 12 out of the 137 patients by recurrence in the initial treated segment and a new lesion as well. In 20 out of 137 patients the recurrence was caused by recurrence of the initial treated segment. In case of recurrence in the femoropopliteal segment clinically it was found an occlusion of the artery in all patients. The arteriogram of those patients however demonstrated in 33% an unusual long stenosis in the initial successful dilatated area (Table 13). This unusual type of stenosis (Fig. 7) in case of clinical recurrence is believed to be caused by a reaction of the intima and media due to the localized injury by means of the forces of the dilating balloon. To avoid this intimal and medial fibrosis as far as possible, we recommend not to overdilate. The balloon diameter should not be larger than the vessel's diameter measured on the arteriograph, knowing that there is a slight magnification. In recurrence the primary technical success of 144 repeated treatments of the femoropopliteal artery (Table 14) was 72.2%.

Table 11. Initial results of 105 angioplasties in case of recurrence after vascular surgery.

| Operation | n | + | − |
|---|---|---|---|
| Thrombendarteriectomy | 61 | 52 (85%) | 9 |
| Embolectomy | 5 | 4 (80%) | 1 |
| Angioplasty of deep femoral artery | 9 | 5 (55%) | 4 |
| Bypass graft | 30 | 26 (87%) | 4 |
| Total | 105 | 87 (83%) | 18 |

n = number of treatments, + = technically successful, − = technically failed.

Table 12. Conservatively managed complications of 105 angioplasties after vascular surgery.

| | |
|---|---|
| Peripheral embolism | 3 (2.9%) |
| Large haematoma at the puncture site | 1 (0.9%) |
| Total | 4 (3.8%) |

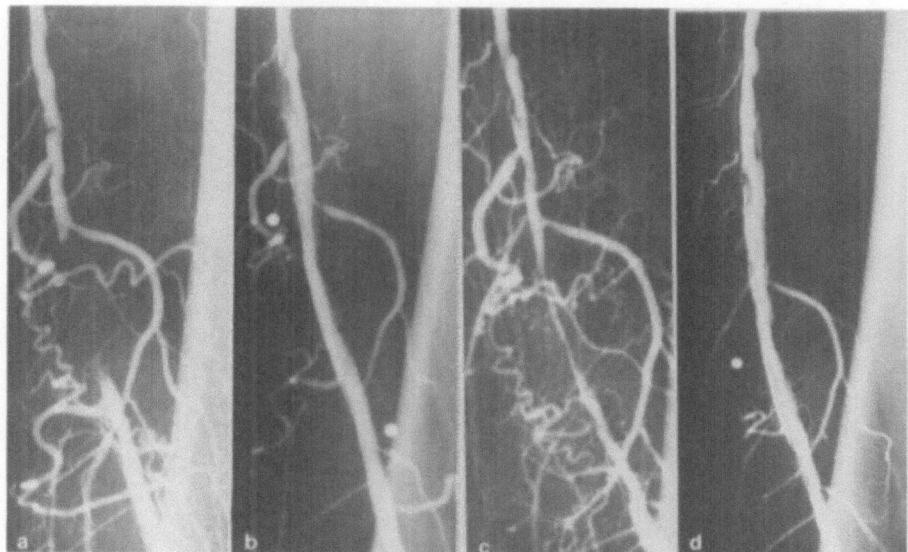

*Figure 7.* Arteriogram left superficial femoral artery; a) occlusion of superficial femoral artery; b) postangioplasty arteriogram patent femoral artery; c) clinical recurrence 7 months later. Unusual long stenosis in area of the former occlusion; d) postangioplasty arteriogram after second PTA patent superficial femoral artery.

## 7. Catheter lysis

Catheter lysis – local low dose fibrinolytic therapy – is a combination between routine angioplasty and local fibrinolysis [11, 15, 16, 25, 26]. This therapeutic principle was recommended by Hess and co-workers [15, 16] in 1980. From the technical point (26) of view one may start with low dose fibrinolysis (Lysis-PTA) using a catheter and if necessary add an angioplasty (Fig. 8). Or one performs

*Tabe 13.* Radiographic pattern of 137 patients in case of clinical recurrence after angioplasty of femoropopliteal artery.

| Angiomorphology of initially treated segments | n | Radiographic pattern in case of clinical recurrence | |
|---|---|---|---|
| | | Occlusion | Stenosis |
| Occlusion | 83 | 56 (67%) | 27 (33%) |
| Stenosis | 54 | 15 (28%) | 39 (72%) |

n = number of initial treatments of femoropopliteal artery.

294

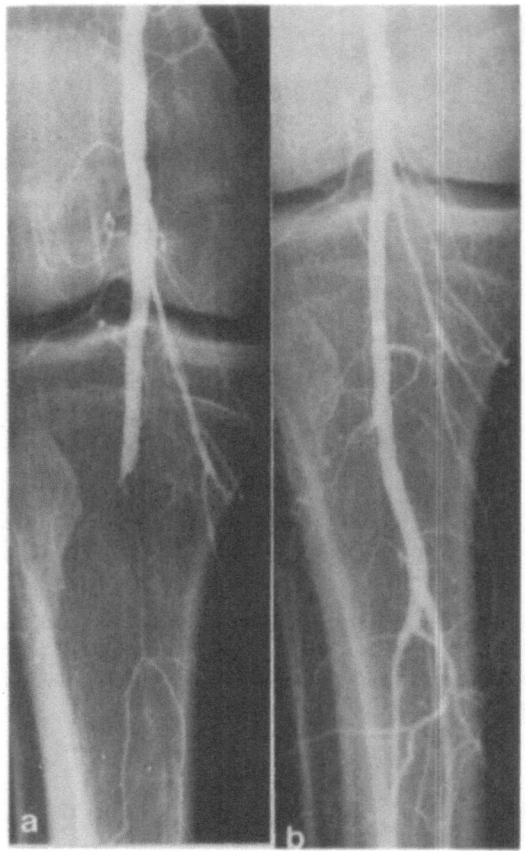

*Figure 8.* Arteriogram of right popliteal artery; a) acute occlusion of popliteal artery; b) patent artery after catheter lysis.

routine angioplasty (PTA-Lysis) first and than add low dose fibrinolytic therapy [9]. In detail, attempting the first method (Lysis-PTA) by fluroscopy, the beginning of the occlusion is located and the catheter is advanced into the core of the occluding substance in order to inject repeated single doses of the fibrinolytic drug. Five to ten minutes after each injection the catheter is pushed 1–2 cm further through the occlusion and repeated low dose of the fibrinolytic drug are administered [15, 16]. Using Streptokinase the single dose is 1000 to 2500 units and the total dose is limited to 250.000 units. In rare cases you may go up to 500.000 units. Giving Urokinase a higher dose is necessary up to four times as much. The single dose of Urokinase ranges from 2500 to 20.000 units. Mostly 5000 units are applied. The total dose is limited to 1.000.000 units.

If more than the limited total dose is given, one has to be aware of achieving a systemic fibrinolytic therapy with intra-arterial administration. In this circumstances the same complication like in systemic fibrinolytic therapy may occur, therefore the same contraindications as in systemic fibrinolysis exist.

Some times these techniques mentioned above will be changed particularly in long occlusions with a poor run off (obliteration of all 3 lower leg arteries). In these cases a 7 F catheter is advanced into the beginning of the occlusion and a second 3 F catheter is advanced into the occlusion as distal as possible. The fibrinolytic drug is applied by an injector. Mechanically 25.000 units Streptokinase or 50.000 units Urokinase are injected through each catheter per hour.

We gained our experience in 214 catheter lyses performed in 202 patients, 151 males and 51 females with the average age of 62 years, ranging from 60–70 years. In 156 out of 214 (73%) treatments the patients were clinically in stage III/IV according to Fontaine.

The primary success was 69% (Table 15). The complications and the lethality are higher than those of routine angioplasty. In particular bleeding at the puncture site and peripheral embolisation have an higher incidence (Table 16).

In 1983 and 1985 Hess and co-workers [15, 16] described in 205 treatments a

Table 14. Primary results of 173 angioplasties achieved because of clinical recurrence arteriographically demonstrated.

| | PTA | n | + | | − |
|---|---|---|---|---|---|
| Iliac artery | I | 25 | 18 (72%) | 22 75.9% | 7 (28%) |
| Iliac artery | II | 4 | 4 (100%) | | 0 |
| Femoropopl artery | I | 114 | 75 (65.8%) | 144 72.2% | 39 (34.2%) |
| Femoropopl artery | II | 30 | 29 (96.7%) | | 1 (3.3%) |
| Total | | 173 | 126 (72.8%) | | 47 (27.2%) |

PTA I = second PTA, PTA II = third PTA, n = number of treatments, + = technically successful, − = technically failed.

Table 15. Primary results of 214 catheter lysis.

| | n | + | − |
|---|---|---|---|
| Iliac artery | 14 | 8 (57%) | 6 |
| Common femoral artery | 15 | 9 (60%) | 6 |
| Femoropopliteal artery | 184 | 131 (71%) | 54 |
| Subclavian artery | 1 | 0 | 1 |
| Total | 214 | 148 (69%) | 67 |

n = number of treatments, + = technically successful, − = technically failed.

technical success rate of 71% and a clinical one of 53% observed 2 weeks after catheter lysis.

Peripheral embolisation occurred in 16% micro- and in 9% as macroembolism. This is higher than in our experience. The bleeding complications and lethality are lower than in our material [15, 16]. Hess is using only aggregation inhibitors following catheter lysis to cut down the bleeding complications [15, 16].

We treat our patients with standard intravenous Heparin therapy following catheter lysis [25, 26] to avoid acute reocclusion. We lost 3 patients. Two died because of bleeding at puncture site starting one or three days after catheter lysis. Therefore it is recommended that all patients undergoing local low dose fibrinolytic have to be kept under intensive care for three days, if Heparin therapy is added. The third patient, we lost, developed at the beginning of the catheter lysis a cardiac arrest and died.

## 7.1 Indications for catheter lysis

Catheter lysis is indicated mainly for limb salvage and less common in stage II because of the higher incidence of complications than routine angioplasty. When amputation is otherwise the last resort, this technique is strongly recommended. Low dose fibrinolytic therapy is indicated in:

1. Acute and subacute occlusions up to three months duration.
2. Occlusions longer than 10 cm and
3. acute reocclusions and peripheral embolism during routine angioplasty.

From the technical point of view one should start with local lysis and add an angioplasty if it is necessary (Lysis-PTA) in (Fig. 8):

1. Acute and subacute occlusion up to three months duration.
2. Occlusions longer than 10 cm. In these circumstances the idea is to change a long occlusion into a short one or into a stenotic lesion, which allows to accomplish angioplasty with good initial and late success.

Table 16. Complications of 214 catheter lysis.

| | |
|---|---|
| Embolisation | 28 (13%) (deterioration in one case 0.5%) |
| Bleeding at puncture site | 16 (7.5%) |
| Dissection | 1 (0.5%) |
| Exitus | 3 (1.4%) |

One should begin with routine angioplasty and, if necessary, add an catheter lysis in:

1. Hard occlusions longer than 10 cm, if the catheter can not be advanced into the occluding atheromatous material. The idea is to change an old occlusion into an acute one, which can be managed by low dose fibrinolytic therapy.
2. In case of acute reocclusion and
3. in peripheral embolisation (Fig. 9 and 10) during routine angioplasty [25, 26].

The disadvantages of catheter lysis are:

1. The treatment is time consuming, it takes 3 to 6 hours.
2. The patients are restless and uncomfortable complaining pain at rest.
3. The patients are in poor general conditions, therefore enough personal must be available to take care of them.

The advantage of this treatment is high with a low risk for the patient.

1. Systemic reaction is minimal, if the maximal total dose of the fibrinolytic drug is limited as mentioned above.

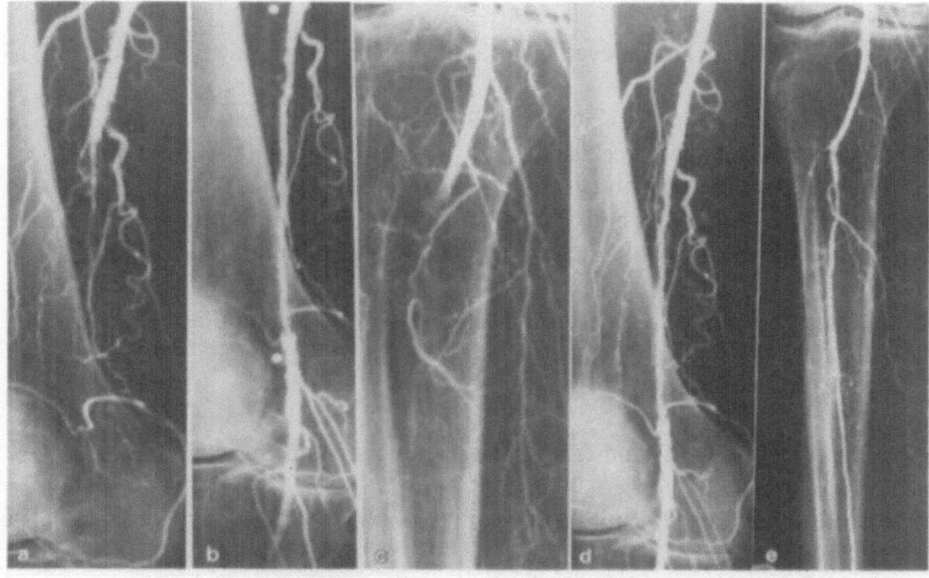

*Figure 9.* Arteriogram right femoropopliteal artery; a) occlusion of distal femoral artery; b) post-angioplasty arteriogram patent distal femoral artery; c) occlusion distal popliteal artery caused by peripheral embolisation during angioplasty; d) and e) patent superficial femoral and popliteal artery after catheter lysis.

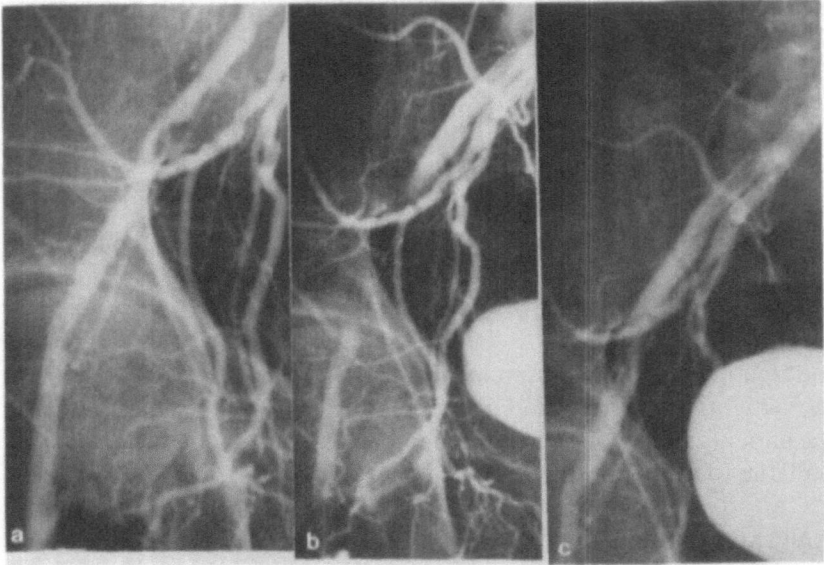

*Figure 10.* Arteriogram of right iliac artery; a) stenosis of external iliac artery; b) acute occlusion of external iliac artery during angioplasty; c) patent external iliac artery after catheter lysis in cross over technique.

2. Catheter lysis can be achieved in patients, in whom systemic lysis is contraindicated.
3. Indications for routine angioplasty can be extended to cover
   a) acute and subacute occlusions
   b) occlusions longer than 10 cm.
4. Acute reocclusions and peripheral embolism during routine angioplasty can be handled satisfactorily by means of low dose fibrinolytic therapy.

Catheter lysis should at least be used in stage III/IV when amputation is suggested [25, 26].

## 8. Indications and contraindications for angioplasty and catheter lysis

The wide spectrum of applications of angioplasty offers very differentiated indications.

Angioplasty of iliac and groin arteries is indicated in stenotic lesions in stage II up to IV. Occlusions of iliac and groin arteries are failed in about 40%, therefore occlusions in these segments should be treated surgically.

In the femoropopliteal segment angioplasty is indicated in stenoses and occlusions up to 10 cm in stage II. The Dotter procedure may be extended to occlusions longer than 10 cm and to occlusions with a poor run off (additional occlusion of all lower leg arteries) for limb salvage, in particular if there is no possibility for reconstructive vascular surgery left and amputation suggested.

Angioplasty and catheter lysis are absolutly contraindicated in severe haemorrhagic diathesis and in known severe reaction to contrast media. Relative contraindications are mostly caused by technical problems. Significant calcification of the artery, direct collateral vessels, an occlusion of an artery at its origin or obesity and postoperative scar may be reasons for technical failures. The patients will mostly benefit from this therapeutic principle, if the indication for angioplasty and catheter lysis is made together by the Radiologist and angiologically interested clinician.

## Summary

Angioplasty is a well accepted treatment of peripheral vascular disease in our days. This therapeutic principle is of low risk for the patients with good initial and late results, which are a little bit less than those of vascular surgery. The patients have to pay for this benefit with a higher complication and lethality rate. Angioplasty proceeded rapidly. There are different techniques suggested including catheter lysis. A lot of experience is gained in the meantime recommending a wide spectrum of applications all over the arterial system including non-atherosclerotic lesions as well. Performing angioplasty in peripheral vascular disease, the main indication will be limb salvage. The patients will benefit most, if the Radiologist, who usually performs angioplasty, works close together with the angiologically interested clinician, an Internist and Surgeon as well. The Radiologist has to be familiar with the different techniques and indications for angioplasty.

## References

1. Andel van GJ (1976) Percutaneous transluminal angioplasty. The Dotter procedure. Amsterdam-Oxford: Excerpta Medica
2. Bachmann DM, Casarella WJ, Sos TA (1979) Percutaneous iliofemoral angioplasty via the contralateral femoral artery. Radiology 130: 617–621
3. Block PC, Baughman KL, Pasternak RC, Fallon JT (1980) Transluminal angioplasty: Correlation of morphologic and angiographic findings in an experimental model. Circulation 61: 778–785
4. Block PC, Fallon JT, Elmer D (1980) Experimental angioplasty: Lessons from the laboratory. AJR 135: 907–912
5. Bollinger A, Schneider E (1982) Perkutane und transluminale Angioplastie peripherer und renaler Arterien. VASA 11: Heft 4
6. Castaneda-Zuniga WR, Formanek A, Tadavarthy M, Vlodaver Z, Edwards JE, Zollikofer Ch, Amplatz K (1980) The mechanism of balloon angioplasty. Radiology 135: 565–571
7. Castaneda-Zuniga WR (1983) Transluminal angioplasty. Stuttgart-New York: Georg Thieme-Verlag

300

8. Cumberland DC (1982) Percutaneous angioplasty in complete iliac occlusions. VASA 11: 297–300
9. Dotter CT, Judkines MP (1964) Transluminal treatment of arteriosclerotic obstruction. Description of a new technique and a preliminary report of its application. Circulation 30: 654
10. Dotter CT, Grüntzig AR, Schoop W, Zeitler E (1983) Percutaneous transluminal angioplasty. Technique, early and late results. Berlin-Heidelberg-New York-Tokyo: Springer-Verlag
11. Dotter CT, Rösch J, Seaman HI (1974) Selective clot lysis with low-dose streptocinase. Radiology 111: 31–37
12. Fallon JT (1980) Pathology of arterial lesions amenable to percutaneous transluminal angioplasty. AJR 135: 913–916
13. Gailer H, Grüntzig AS, Zeitler E, Late results after percutaneous transluminal angioplasty of iliac and femoropopliteal obstructive lesions – a cooperative study. In: Dotter CT, Grüntzig AR, Schoop W, Zeitler E (eds) (1983) Percutaneous transluminal angioplasty. Berlin-Heidelberg-New York-Tokyo: Springer-Verlag, p 215
14. Grüntzig A, Hopff H (1974) Perkutane Rekanalisatioin chron. arterieller Verschlüsse mit einem neuen Dilatationskatheter. Modifikation der Dotter-Technik. Deutsch Med Wochenschr 99: 2502
15. Hess H, Clot lysis in peripheral arteries. In: Dotter CT, Grüntzig A, Schoop W, Zeitler E (eds) (1983) Percutaneous transluminal angioplasty. Berlin-Heidelberg-New York-Tokyo: Springer-Verlag, p 145
16. Hess H (1985) Thrombolytic therapy and its combination with transluminal catheter dilatation. Wiener Klin Wochenschr 97: 61–64
17. Hessel SJ, Adams DF (1981) Complications of angiography. Radiology 138: 273
18. Ingrisch H, Seyferth W, Küffer G, Percutaneous transluminal angioplasty in cases of stenosis in the region of the infrarenal abdominal aorta and the aortoiliac bifurcation. In: Dotter CT, Grüntzig A, Schoop W, Zeitler E (eds) (1983) Percutaneous transluminal angioplasty. Berlin-Heidelberg-New York: Springer-Verlag, pp 127–130
19. Leu HJ, The morphological concept of percutaneous transluminal angioplasty. In: Dotter CT, Grüntzig AR, Schoop W, Zeitler E (eds) (1983) Percutaneous transluminal angioplasty. Berlin-Heidelberg-New York-Tokyo: Springer-Verlag, p 46
20. Novelline RA (1980) Percutaneous transluminal angioplasty: Newer applications. AJR 135: 983–988
21. Olbert F, Muzika N, Schlegel A (1985) Transluminale Dilatation und Rekanalisation im Gefäßbereich. Verlag; D.E. Wachholz, K.,G. Nürnberg
22. Rieger H (1984) Perkutane Katheter-Rekanalisation bei Verschlüssen und Stenosen der Becken-Beinschlagadern. Medwelt 35: 959–963
23. Roth FJ (1982) Seltene Indikationen zur Angioplastie. Röntgenpraxis 35: 308–311
24. Roth FJ, Cappius G (1982) Cross-over-Technik zur Behandlung der Leistenarterien. VASA 11: 291–296
25. Roth FJ, Krings W, Cappius G, Schmidtke I, Köhler M (1984) Die lokale, niedrig dosierte, fibrinolytische Therapie. Technik und Resultate. VASA (Suppl 12): 52–58
26. Roth FJ, Cappius G, Krings W, Schmidtke I (1984) Local fibrinolytic therapy: Indications, technique and results. Angioplasty (Vecht RJ) London: Pitman Publishing limited London: 62–71
27. Roth FJ, Krings W, Cappius G (1984) Die perkutane transluminale Angioplastie bei der Behandlung der arteriellen Verschlußkrankheit. Innere Medizin 11: 239–253
28. Schmidtke I, Roth FJ, Relapse treatment by percutaneous transluminal dilatation. In: Dotter CT, Grüntzig A, Schoop W, Zeitler E (eds) (1983) Percutaneous transluminal angioplasty. Berlin-Heidelberg: Springer-Verlag
29. Schneider E, Grüntzig A, Bollinger A (1982) Langzeitergebnisse nach perkutaner transluminaler Angioplastie (PTA) bei 882 konsekutiven Patienten mit ilikalen und femoro-popl. Obstruktionen. VASA 11: 322–326
30. Seyferth W, Ernsting M, Grosse-Vorholt R, Zeitler E, Complications during and after per-

cutaneous transluminal angioplasty. In: Dotter CT, Grüntzig AR, Schoop W, Zeitler E (eds) (1983) Percutaneous transluminal angioplasty. Berlin-Heidelberg-New York-Tokyo: Springer-Verlag. p 161

31. Stücker FJ (1985) Periphere, neurologische Komplikationen nach perkutaner transaxillärer Aortographie. Chirurg 56: 332–336

32. Zajko AB McLean GK, Freimann DB, Oleaga JA, Ring EJ (1981) Percutaneous puncture of venous bypass grafts for transluminal angioplasty. AJR 137: 799–802

33. Zeitler E, Schmidtke I, Schoop W, Giessler R, Dembski J, Mansjoer H (1976) Ergebnisse nach perkutaner transluminaler Angioplastie bei über 700 Behandlungen. Röntgenpraxis 29: 78

34. Zeitler E, Grüntzig A, Schoop W (1978) Percutaneous vascular recanalization. Technique, Application, Clinical results. Berlin-Heidelberg-New York: Springer-Verlag

35. Zorn-Bopp E, Ingrisch H, Mietaschk A, Frey W (1981) Transluminale Gefäßdilatation der distaler Bauchaorta, der A. iliaca communis und externa. Fortschr Röntgenstr 134, 5: 471–475

36. Zollikofer Ch L, Salmonowitz E, Sibley R, Chain J, Bruehlmann WF, Castaneda-Zuniga WR, Amplatz K (1984) Transluminal angioplasty evaluated by Electron Microscopy. Radiology 153: 369–374

# IV. Acute myocardial infarction

# Medical measures for reduction of myocardial infarct size

H.H. KLEIN and H. KREUZER

**Summary**

Most of our knowledge about biology of myocardial infarction were obtained in animal studies. About 30 min after occlusion of a coronary artery infarcts started to develop in the jeopardized subendocardium and spread towards the ischemic subepicardium like a wave front. The speed at which ischemic myocytes die depends on the amount of collateral and/or residual blood flow and the left ventricular oxygen consumption. Experimental animal studies suggest that early reperfusion is the most potent measure to reduce infarct size. Under certain circumstances a reduction of left ventricular oxygen consumption may reduce myocardial infarct size even in the absence of reflow. Early reperfusion seems to be associated with the treatable reperfusion injury. The interpretation of studies in man are difficult because we lack accurate means to clinically determine the risk region and the corresponding infarction. The best treatment to reduce infarct size in man is still unknown. At the present time we favor the administration of nitroglycerin, heparin, and analgetics combined with early reperfusion.

The fate of patients who survived the acute event of a myocardial infarction is in part determined by the extent of the necrotic region. Patients with larger infarctions are at a greater risk to die due to heart failure [1] or on account of ventricular fibrillation [2]. Besides the control of rhythm disturbances in a treatment aimed to reduce myocardial infarct size is highly desirable to improve the prognosis and quality of life in these patients. During the last two decades we have learnt a great deal about the biology of myocardial infarction, especially by experimental animal research. In the first part of this paper we will therefore review some important aspects obtained in experimental studies. In the second part we will evaluate clinical trials to reduce infarct size in man.

## Biology of experimental myocardial infarction

About 20–40 min after occlusion of a coronary artery in dogs the transition from reversible injury to necrosis starts in the jeopardized subendocardial layer [3]. Neither the biochemical process nor the structural alteration which are responsible for the step from reversible to irreversible cell damage are yet defined [4]. Infarcts spread like a wave front from the subendocardium towards the subepicardium [5]. The speed at which ischemic myocytes die is mainly determined by the collateral blood flow and probably to a lesser extent by the left ventricular oxygen consumption ($MVO_2$) at the onset and during ischemia [6, 7]. In dog hearts which dispose of a significant subepicardial collateral blood flow, ultimate infarct size is almost reached after 3 to 6 h of ischemia. In this species final infarct size occupies about 75% of the area at risk of necrosis. The remainder of the risk region which consists of the subepicardial layer is protected from ischemic cell death by a sufficient amount of collateral blood flow. In hearts without significant collaterals (pig, rat, rabbit) the development of infarcts proceeds much faster. In this species ultimate infarct size becomes almost as large as the perfusion bed of an occluded coronary artery after 45–90 min of ischemia [8, 9]. On the other hand occlusion of a coronary artery in the well collateralized guinea pig heart does not result in an infarction at all [8] (Fig. 1).

## Determination of infarct size

The dimensions of infarctions are always within the boundaries of the risk region, an infarct can only become as large as the corresponding ischemic regions. It is therefore obvious that occlusion of a small coronary artery can only result in a small infarct. In experimental studies we have the possibility to normalize the infarct size. This can be achieved by relating the ultimate infarction to the risk region. Normalization of infarct size allows a statistical evaluation between a treated and control group even if the number of animals enrolled in a study is rather low compared to clinical studies. Determination of the risk region can be obtained in several ways, e.g. by autoradiography [10], post mortem angiography [6], or by means of a dye [9]. Electron microscopy, histology and histochemistry are applied to assess the infarcted tissue. Although electron microscopy is a very useful tool to diagnose irreversible ischemic injury it is rather difficult to use this method for evaluation of large ischemic regions. This can be easier achieved by histological or histochemical means.

## Reperfusion injury

The term reperfusion injury describes the fact that ischemic cell death can be

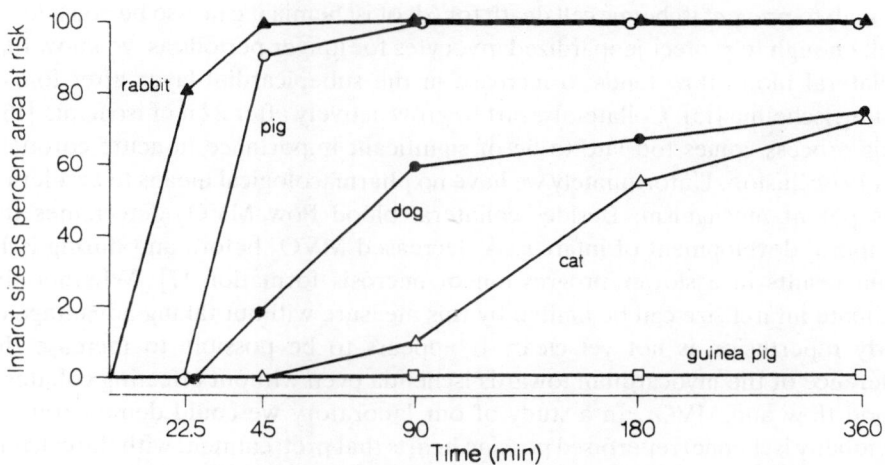

*Figure 1.* Temporal development of infarcts in different species. Species with a low collateral blood flow (rabbit, pig) exhibit the fastes evolution of infarcts. Reproduced with permission, from Schaper W (1984) Experimental infarcts and the micro circulation. In: Hearse DJ, Yellon DM (eds) Therapeutic approaches to myocardial infarct size limitation. Raven Press, New York: pp 79–90.

diagnosed by electron microscopy earlier when reperfusion has occurred. At the present time it is still unresolved wether reperfusion only unmasks already necrotic cells or wether it really causes cellular damage. There are some hints that generation of oxygen free radicals [11] and the invasion of leukocytes [12] may do some harm in the presence of early reperfusion. On the other hand reperfusion supplemented with mannitol [13] or with a calcium antagonist [14] did not decrease infarct size. The expression reperfusion injury is misleading. It is more or less generally accepted that in most instances infarct size can only be reduced if a sufficient blood flow is restored in time. Therefore, most of the myocytes at risk can only be salvaged if reperfusion occurs in time.

## Medical measures to reduce experimental infarct size

Up to now more than fifty agents have been described being able to reduce experimental infarct size. A great number of these positive results were demonstrated in questionable models and fortunately did not get access to clinical treatment. Only a few medical measures which offer the possibility to limit the extent of myocardial necrosis are generally accepted. The most effective treatment is early reperfusion of the ischemic myocardium. Reperfusion after 20–30 min of ischemia is able to salvage all jeopardized myocytes even in hearts without significant collaterals [3, 9]. In almost all experimental models ultimate infarct size is reached within 6 h of ischemia, i.e. reperfusion after this time does not appear to exhibit a substantial beneficial effect. If collateral blood flow is high enough to prevent ischemic cell death for 6 h of ischemia it can also be considered high enough to protect jeopardized myocytes for longer periods as we know that collateral blood flow tends to increase in the subepicardial layer after longer lasting ischemia [15]. Collaterals start to grow actively after 22 h of ischemia [16]. This process comes too late to be of significant importance in acute coronary artery occlusion. Unfortunately we have no pharmacological means to accelerate this potent mechanism. Besides collateral blood flow $MVO_2$ determines the temporal development of infarcts. A decreased $MVO_2$ before and during ischemia results in a slower progression of necrosis formation [7]. Whether the ultimate infarct size can be limited by this measure without taking advantage of early reperfusion is not yet clear. It appears to be possible to increase the tolerance of the myocardium towards ischemia even without affecting collateral blood flow and $MVO_2$. In a study of our laboratory we could demonstrate in regionally ischemic, reperfused porcine hearts that pretreatment with the calcium antagonist diltiazem delayed the development of infarcts although the calculated $MVO_2$ between the treated and control group did not differ and collateral blood flow is almost absent in this species [14] (Fig 2). The exact metabolic mechanism of protection remains to be clarified. When reperfusion is initiated before ultimate infarct size is reached, reperfusion injury may occur. The group of Lucchesi found that early reperfusion in leukopenic dogs or treatment with the lipoxygenase blocker BW 755C (Wellcome, U.K.) which suppress leukocyte infiltration decreased ultimate infarct size more than reperfusion without this agent [12, 17]. The same group reported that treatment with superoxid dismutase and catalase aimed to prevent oxygen free radical formation was superior to reperfusion only with blood [11]. The messages of the experimental studies can be summarized as follows:

a) time dependent development of infarcts is determined by the amount of collateral blood flow and $MVO_2$ before and during ischemia.
b) early reperfusion is the most potent measure to reduce infarct size.
c) a reduction of $MVO_2$ can delay or under certain circumstances (high collateral blood flow) even reduce myocardial infarct size.
d) pretreatment with the calcium antagonist diltiazem delays the development of infarcts even without taking advantage of a reduced $MVO_2$ or an increased collateral blood flow. This may also hold true for verapamil but not for nifedipine.
e) early reperfusion supplemented which agents which are able to limit reperfusion injury may be better than reperfusion without these compounds.

## Measurement of infarct size in patients

In contrast to experimental animal studies we do not dispose of accurate clinical methods to determine the risk region and the corresponding infarction in man. To

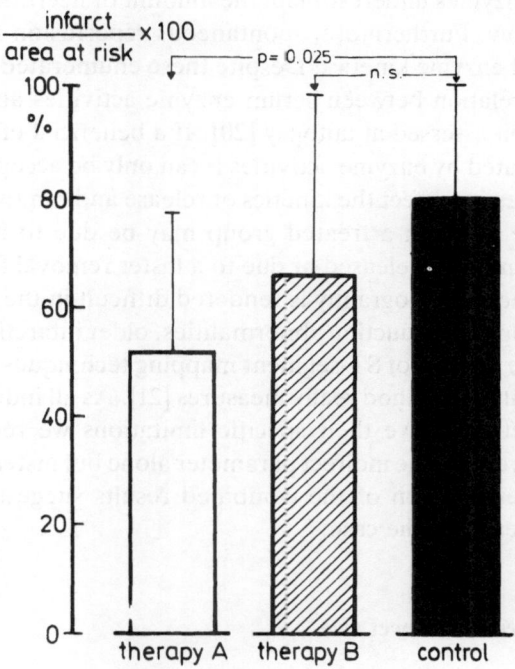

*Figure 2.* Effect of two different diltiazem treatments on infarct size in ischemic reperfused porcine hearts. Only pretreatment with diltiazem significantly reduced infarct size after 75 min of ischemia. Reproduced, with permission from Klein HH, Schubothe M, Nevendahl K, Kreuzer H (1984) The effect of two different diltiazem treatments on infarct size in ischemic, reperfused porcine hearts. Circulation 69: 1000–1005.

measure infarct size by segmental wall motion abnormalities assessed by echocardiography or ventriculography is inappropiate because these methods cannot distinguish ischemic from infarcted myocardium. In order to demonstrate a reduction of infarct size in patients, at the present time we have to rely on indirect parameters like serum enzyme kinetics, electrocardiographic indices, or mortality. Unfortunately more than 3000 patients must be enrolled in a study to prove a reduced infarct size of 15% if mortality is chosen as endpoint [18]. Determination of plasma emzyme activities like creatine kinase (CK), creatine kinase isoenzyme MB (CK-MB), or lactate dehydrogenase (LDH) can be performed without much technical effort, however the limitations to predict infarct size from enzyme activity levels must be taken into account. Serum enzyme activities can only reflect the amount of the infarcted tissue and not the extent of the risk region. There is a gap of at least several hours between the onset of infarction and the washout of myocardial enzyme activities. The level of serum enzyme activities is determined by the release from infarcted myocardium and the removal from blood. The washout of enzymes appears to be flow dependent [19]. Therefore, we expect that serum enzymes underestimate the amount of necrotic tissue if collateral blood flow is low. Furthermore, spontaneous reperfusion may complicate the interpretation of enzyme kinetics. Despite these enumerated problems there is a reasonable correlation between serum enzyme activities and the extent of myocardial infarction assessed at autopsy [20]. If a beneficial effect of an intervention is demonstrated by enzyme activities it can only be accepted as proven if this intervention does not effect the kinetics of release and removal. Otherwise a decrease in enzyme levels in a treated group may be due to an effect during autolysis when enzymes are released or due to a faster removal from blood. The interpretation of electrocardiography is rendered difficult in the presence of left ventricular hypertrophy, conduction abnormalities, older infarctions or posterior located infarcts. The validity of ST-segment mapping techniques is not proven as we do not know what this method really measures [21]. As all indirect parameters to determine infarct size have their specific limitations we recommand for a clinical study not to rely on one indirect parameter alone but instead to use several of them. If the interpretation of the combined results suggests a decrease in infarct size it may really be the case.

**Clinical studies to reduce infarct size**

In this part we do not want to discuss thrombolytical or mechanical induced reperfusion as these techniques are reviewed in detail in the following communications. Therefore, we will focus on those treatments which are not associated with reperfusion.

*a) β-blocker therapy in acute myocardial infarction*

Several randomized studies using β-blockers in the treatment of acute myocardial infarction have been carried out (22–27). Most of the trials assessed the efficacy of treatment by measurement of serum enzyme activities. Four of the six studies demonstrated a decreased level of CK, CK-MB, or LDH respectively suggesting a reduction of infarct size, although only a small number of patients were treated within 4 h after the onset of chest pain. As pointed out earlier decreased serum levels of the enzymes are not a real proof of a reduced infarct size, nevertheless treatment with β-blockers within 12 h of ischemia may result in smaller infarcts in some patients. Because of significant side-effects we hesitate to recommend the routine use of β-blockers in patients with acute myocardial infarction.

*b) nitroglycerin*

Bussmann et al [28] enrolled 60 patients with acute myocardial infarction to treatment with intravenous nitroglycerin or to a control group. CK-MB was determined to assess the efficacy of therapy. It was reported that nitroglycerin was able to reduce infarct size even in those patients in whom treatment was initiated as late as 12.8 h after the onset of symptoms. Although this result is really encouraging we have difficulty to interprete this beneficial effect. This means that the tolerance of human hearts towards ischemia is much better than that of the animals used in experimental studies or that the collateral blood flow of the patients was extremely high. In another trial Jaffee et al [29] randomized 85 patients with acute myocardial infarction to treatment with nitroglycerin or placebo. In this study only patients with inferior infarctions profited from nitroglycerin treatment. Because nitroglycerin can be safely administered in patients with acute myocardial infarction and because of its favorable hemodynamic effects (decrease in preload, slight reduction in afterload, vasodilatation of epicardial coronary arteries and increase in collateral blood flow provided the collaterals are well developed) nitroglycerin can be accepted as standard therapy in acute myocardial infarction. If this treatment alone really reduces infarct size in a substantial amount of patients remains to be clarified.

*c) Calcium antagonists*

Bussmann et al [30] performed a randomized study with verapamil in patients with acute myocardial infarction. This treatment decreased plasma CK-MB levels like nitroglycerin in the previously mentioned study. Muller et al [31] investigated the effect of oral nifedipine on the infarct size in 68 patients. In this trial nifedipine did not exhibit any beneficial effect at all. Concerning the use of calcium antagonists in patients with acute myocardial infarction we believe it is too early to come to a sound statement.

**Medial measures to reduce infarct size in man**

Although we did not discuss thrombolytical or mechanically induced reperfusion in the previous part this treatment cannot be neglected when we summarize experimental and clinical studies to support our point of view on infarct size reduction in man. We consider nitroglycerin and heparin at a sufficient dose to extend thrombin time as basic treatment. The reason to use nitroglycerin is given above. As most infarctions occur due to a thrombus formation in a coronary artery the administration of heparin should prevent further thrombus formation. To delay or even reduce infarct size it is important to decrease myocardial oxygen consumption. The best and safest way to achieve this goal is not yet clarified. We prefer the use of sedatives and analgetics to β-blockers. This treatment may be able to reduce infarct size in those patients with well developed collaterals. Although the discussion about the value of reperfusion in man is still controversial we believe that it will be of beneficial effect at least if it is initiated very early, i.e. within one to two hours after the onset of ischemia. In most instances reperfusion is the only means which is able to salvage those jeopardized myocytes which were protected from cell death by a low $MVO_2$. As we lack the clinical proof of a favorable effect of reperfusion at the present time we do not recommand this treatment for general use.

## Future trends

The interpretations of clinical studies is hampered by the lack of accurate means to determine the risk region and the corresponding infarction. In this regard improved technology of positron emission tomography and NMR may render these methods useful tools in clinical trials. The medical treatment of patients with coronary artery disease may be altered if we are able to find agents which can increase the tolerance of the heart towards ischemia that early reperfusion can salvage a greater amount of jeopardized myocardium. Furthermore treatment of reperfusion injury may be introduced into clinical trials. As the gap between onset of ischemia and reperfusion is of paramount importance instruction of the population about the symptoms of acute myocardial infarction and instruction of the general practitioners about the biology of myocardial infarction must be intensified. We do not expect to be able to limit infarct size in all patients, therefore prevention of coronary artery disease remains our most important aim.

## Acknowledgment

The cited studies of our laboratory were supported by a grant from SFB 89 Kardiologie Goettingen.

## References

1. Page DL, Caulfield JB, Kaster JA, De Sanctis RW, Sanders CA (1971) Myocardial changes associated with cardiogenic shock. N Eng J Med 285: 133
2. Bethge KP (1982) Langzeitelektrokardiographie. Berlin, Heidelberg, New York: Springer Verlag
3. Jennings RB, Reimer KA (1979) Biology of experimental acute myocardial ischemia and infarction. In: Hearse DJ, De Leiris J (eds) Enzymes in Cardiology. Chichester, New York: John Wiley and Sons, pp 21–57

4. Poole-Wilson PA (1984) What causes cell death. In: Hearse DJ, Yellon DM (eds) Therapeutic approaches to myocardial infarct size limitation Raven Press, New York: pp 43–60
5. Reimer KA, Lowe JE, Rasmussen MM, Jennings RB (1977) The wave front phenomenon of ischemic cell death. I. Myocardial infarct size in duration of coronary occlusion in dogs. Circulation 56: 786–794
6. Müller KD, Klein H, Schaper W (1980) Changes in myocardial oxygen consumption 45 minutes after experimental coronary occlusion do not alter infarct size. Cardiovasc Res 14: 710–718
7. Nienaber CH, Gottwick M, Winkler B, Schaper W (1983) The relation between the perfusion deficit, infarct size and time after experimental cornary artery occlusion. Basic Res Cardiol 78: 210–226
8. Schaper W (1984) Experimental infarcts and the micro circulation. In: Hearse DJ, Yellon DM (eds) Therapeutic approaches to myocardial infarct size limitation. Raven Press, New York: pp 79–90
9. Klein HH, Schubothe M, Nebendahl K, Kreuzer H (1984) Temporal and spatial development of infarcts in porcine hearts Basic Res Cardiol 79: 440–447
10. De Boer LWV, Strauss HW, Kloner RA, Rude RE, Davis RF, Maroko PE, Braunwald E (1980) Autoradiographic method for measuring the ischemic myocardium at risk. Effects of verapamil on infarct size after experimental coronary artery occlusion. Proc Natl Acad Sci USA 77: 6119–6123
11. Jolly SR, Kane WJ, Bailie MB, Abrams GD and Lucchesi BR (1984) Canine myocardial reperfusion injury. Its reduction by the combined administration of superoxide dismutase and catalase. Circ Res 54: 277–285
12. Romson JL, Hook BG, Kunkel SL, Abrams GD, Schork MA, Lucchesi BR (1983) Reduction of the extent of ischemic myocardial injury by neutrophil depletion in the dog. Circulation 67: 1016–1023
13. Klein HH, Nebendahl K, Schubothe M, Kreuzer H (1985) Intracoronary hyperosmotic mannitol during reperfusion does not effect the infarct size in ischemic, reperfused porcine hearts. Basic Res Cardiol – in press
14. Klein HH, Schubothe M, Nevendahl K, Kreuzer H (1984) The effect of two different diltiazem treatments on infarct size in ischemic, reperfused porcine hearts. Circulation 69: 1000–1005
15. Hirzel HO, Nelson GR, Sonnenblick EH, Kirch ES (1976) Redistribution of collateral blood flow from necrotic to surviving myocardium following coronary occlusion. Circ Res 39: 214-222
16. Schaper W, De Brabander M, Lewi P (1971) DNA-synthesis and mitosis in coronary collateral vessels of the dog. Circ Res 28: 671–679
17. Jolly SR, Lucchesi BR (1983) Effect of BW 755C in an occlusion-reperfusion model of ischemic myocardial injury. Am Heart J 106: 8–13
18. Sobel BE, Braunwald E (1980) The management of acute myocardial infarction. In: Heart Disease (ed. E. Braunwald), Saunders, Philadelphia p 1373
19. Swain JL, Cobb FR, AcHale PA, Roe CR (1980) Non-linear relationship between creatine kinase estimates and histologic extent of infarction in conscious dogs: Effects of regional myocardial blood flow. Circulation 62: 1239–1247
20. Hackel DB, Reimer KA, Ideker RE, Mikat EM, Hartwell TD, Parker CB, Braunwald EB, Buja M, Gold HK, Jaffe AS, Muller JE, Raabe DS, Rude RE, Sobek BE, Stone PH, Roberts R and the MILIS study group (1984) Comparison of enzymatic and anatomic estimates of myocardial infarct size in man. Circulation 70: 824–835
21. Holland RP, Brooks H (1977) TQ-ST segment mapping: critical review and analysis of current concepts. Am J Cardiol 40: 110–129
22. Peter T, Norris RM, Clarke ED, Heng MK, Sing BN, Williams B, Howell DR, Ambler PK (1978) Reduction of enzyme levels by propranolol after acute myocardial infarction. Circulation 57: 1091–1095
23. Johnsson BW (1980) Comparative study of cardio-selective beta-blockade and diazepam in

patients with acute myocardial infarction and tachycardia. Acta Med Scand 207: 47–53

24. Jurgensen HJ, Frederiksen H, Hansen DA, Pedersen-Bjergaard O (1981) Limitation of myocardial infarct size in patients less than 66 years treated with alprenolol. Br Heart J 45: 583–588

25. Yusud S, Sleight P, Rossi P, Ramsdale D, Peto R, Furze L, Sterry H, Pearson M, Motwani R, Parish S, Gray R, Bennet D, Bray C (1983) Reduction in infarct size, arrhythmias and chest pain by early intravenous beta-blockade in suspected acute myocardial infarction. Circulation 67: I–32–41

26. McIlmoyle L, Evans A, McBoyle D, Cran G, Barber JM, Elwood H, Salathia K, Shanks R (1982) Early in intervention in myocardial ischaemia. Br Heart J 47: 189 (abstract)

27. Hjalmarsen A, Herlitz J, Holmberg S, Rydent S, Swedberg K, Vedin A, Waagstein F, Waldenstrom A, Waldenstrom J, Wedel H, Wilhelmsen L, Wilhelmsson C (1983) The Goteborg metoprolol trial. Effects on mortality and morbidity in acute myocardial infarction. Circulation 67: I–26–32

28. Bussmann W, Passek D, Seidel W, Kaltenbach M (1981) Reduction of CK and CK-MB indexes of infarct size by intravenous nitroglycerin Circulation 63: 615–622

29. Jaffee AS, Geltmann EM, Tiefenbrunn AJ, Ambos HD, Strauss HD, Sobel BE, Roberts R (1983) Reduction of infarct size in patients with inferior infarction with intravenous glyceryl trinitrate. A randomized study. Br Heart J 49: 452–460

30. Bussmann WD, Seher W, Grungras M, Klepzig H (1982) Reduktion der CK und CK-MB Infarktgröße durch intravenöse Gabe von Verapamil. Z Kardiol 71: 164 (abstract)

31. Muller JE, Morrison J, Stone PH, Rude RE, Rosner B, Roberts R, Pearle DL, Turi ZG, Schneider JF, Serfas DH, Tate C, Scheiner E, Hennekens CH, Braunwald E (1984) Nifedipine therapy for patients with threatened and acute myocardial infarction: a randomized, double-blind placebo-controlled comparison. Circulation 69: 740–747

# Mechanical complications of acute myocardial infarction: ventricular septal defect and papillary muscle rupture

A. D. HILGENBERG and W. M. DAGGETT

Ventricular septal rupture and papillary muscle rupture are unusual complications of acute infarction, and they are associated with extremely high mortality rates without aggressive treatment. Significant advances in the surgical management of these entities have been made in recent years, allowing both acute and long term survival of many of the affected patients.

## Ventricular septal defect

### Incidence and pathogenesis

Postmortem studies from 1942 to 1979 reveal a steady incidence of septal perforation in 1.3% to 2% of acute infarcts, with no indication of a declining rate as anti-anginal medical therapy has improved [6]. The infarct associated with septal rupture is the patient's first infarction in 85% of the cases, and is typically transmural and quite extensive, involving a mean of 26% of the left ventricular wall [6, 10]. The septal rupture generally occurs within the first two weeks after acute infarction; one study found the average time of perforation to be 2.6 days after the infarct, and in our experience 77% of the septal perforations occurred within the first week after infarction [6, 12]. A large, abrupt reduction of coronary flow, in the absence of septal collateral development, results in the infarct responsible for septal rupture in most cases. Anterior-apical infarcts and infero-posterior infarcts occur with equal frequency, and the location of the perforation in the ventricular septum correlates highly with the electrocardiographic localization of the infarct [5, 12]. Our experience with patients who had undergone angiographic or autopsy analysis of the extent of coronary artery disease indicates that 23% of the patients have single vessel disease, and the remainder have occlusive disease of two or more coronary arteries [12].

*Natural history*

The poor outcome of most untreated patients with ventricular septal rupture is illustrated by two studies. Sanders, et al found a 54% mortality within the first week after diagnosis of the ventricular septal defect (VSD), and a 92% mortality at one year [13]. Oyamada and Queen reported a 24% mortality within 24 hours of development of the VSD, 65% within two weeks, and 81% mortality at eight weeks [10]. In both series, approximately 7% of medically treated patients survived greater than one year, illustrating the variation in the severity of the insult in any individual patient, and explaining in part the dramatic differences in response to surgical treatment in patients operated upon at various time intervals after septal perforation.

*Diagnosis*

The diagnosis of post-infarction VSD is a straightforward bedside procedure based upon physical examination and a right heart catheterization. Several hours or days after an acute infarction, the patient typically deteriorates abruptly with congestive heart failure and/or cardiogenic shock. The deterioration is accompanied by the development of a harsh parasternal systolic murmur in almost all of the patients and a palpable systolic thrill in approximately half of them. Signs of right heart failure are much more frequent than pulmonary congestion and left heart failure. Sixty percent of the patients develop arterial hypotension and the other peripheral manifestations of cardiogenic shock, and development of cardiogenic shock correlates more with evidence of right ventricular dysfunction than with left ventricular ejection fraction [12].

Insertion of a Swan Ganz pulmonary artery catheter will confirm the suspected diagnosis and allow proper hemodynamic monitoring to guide subsequent therapy. Blood samples for oxygen saturation are drawn from the right atrium and pulmonary artery, and a VSD is diagnosed by noting a stepup in the oxygen saturation between the two samples. The pulmonary artery pressure is usually moderately elevated, with mean pressures approximately 30 mmHg, and pulmonary wedge pressures approximately 20 mmHg. Small to moderate V waves may be noted in the wedge tracing due to mild to moderate amounts of mitral valve incompetence. The pulmonary to systemic flow ratio can be calculated, and in our patients averaged 3.7 to 1 [12].

We have advocated cardiac catheterization, coronary arteriography, and left ventriculography in patients with postinfarction VSD. In patients with cardiogenic shock, we have learned to treat them as true surgical emergencies, and have immediately inserted the intra-aortic balloon pump in order to stabilize the hemodynamics, then proceeded directly to the cardiac catheterization laboratory, and from there to the operating room [4]. We treat the patients without cardiogenic shock medically with vasodilators in order to attempt to reduce the pulmonary to systemic flow ratio, and cardiac catheterization is performed on a slightly less urgent basis.

*Preoperative preparation*

In view of the poor natural history of patients who are not treated surgically, confirmation of the diagnosis of post-infarction septal rupture is a clearcut indication for operation. The only important issue to be addressed at this point is the timing of surgical intervention. Ideally, the operation should be timed to achieve the lowest risk of mortality and morbidity for any given patient. It is clear that patients who undergo operation later than three weeks after their septal perforation have a lower operative risk than those undergoing early operation, but it seems that this is almost entirely due to less severe illness and the absence of cardiogenic shock in those patients undergoing later operation [4, 5]. Those requiring early operation are more severely ill and are usually in cardiogenic shock, with a higher operative risk, but facing the probability of almost certain death in the absence of surgical treatment.

For the patients with severe hemodynamic derangements and cardiogenic shock, the intra-aortic balloon pump offers the most important available means of temporary hemodynamic support. The balloon pump reduces left ventricular afterload, thus increasing systemic cardiac output, and decreasing the pulmonary to systemic flow ratio. In our experience, the pulmonary to systemic flow ratio was reduced an average of 23% by the intra-aortic balloon pump [1]. The use of the balloon pump in these cases leads to transient reversal of the clinical deterioration and maintains stability for cardiac catheterization and transportation to the operating room. The balloon pump does not provide a long term substitute for urgent operation, and its insertion for cardiogenic shock should be followed by *immediate* operation. Patients with septal rupture do not die of cardiac failure directly, but rather of end organ failure as a consequence of shock. Shortening the duration of shock by operating immediately is the only therapeutic solution for this group of patients, and it can yield dramatic results [4]. Thus, as long as the duration of shock has not been allowed to persist to the point of irreversible end organ failure, such as sustained anuria, no patient need be considered 'too sick' for emergency operation.

For those patients with less severe hemodynamic disturbances and in the absence of cardiogenic shock, an attempt at medical management with vasodilators can be undertaken hoping to decrease the left to right shunt and thus increase cardiac output. Both intravenous nitroprusside and nitroglycerin have been utilized for this purpose. Inotropic agents alone may increase cardiac output, but may not change the pulmonary to systemic flow ratio, therefore increasing left ventricular work and myocardial oxygen consumption. Vasopressor agents will increase the systemic afterload and further increase the pulmonary to systemic flow ratio thereby lowering cardiac output and greatly increasing myocardial oxygen consumption. If patients can be stabilized medically and end organ function is not deteriorating, operation may be delayed, but if stabilization with normal end organ function does not occur, prompt operative therapy must be undertaken. When this management plan is followed, over 60% of patients can be expected to require operation within the first three weeks after septal rupture.

*Operative management*

Continuing improvements in the intraoperative management of patients with ventricular septal rupture appear to have contributed greatly to enhanced survival. Important operative principles as practiced in our institution include: 1) cold potassium cardioplegic protection of the myocardium, 2) saphenous vein aortocoronary grafts to severely obstructed major coronary arteries outside of the zone of infarction, 3) opening the heart through the infarcted zone, 4) liberal use of prosthetic patches to close the defects without tension, and liberal use of teflon felt bolstering material to minimize the risk of sutures tearing through friable myocardium, and 5) prosthetic graft closure of inferior wall ventriculotomies to avoid suture line tension. In general, the septal perforation will be located in one of three areas and the details of the repair differ somewhat for each location.

*Apical septal rupture* is repaired by the technique of apical amputation which involves removing the infarcted apex of both the left and right ventricles. (Fig. 1) The myocardium is then re-approximated with heavy sutures reinforced by strips of teflon felt placed on both sides of the ventricular septum as well as on the epicardial surfaces of the right and left ventricles. This repair utilizes the principles of a left ventricular transinfarct approach, excision of paradoxically expanding infarcted myocardium, and placement of buttressed mattress sutures in the rim of viable muscle surrounding the infarcted area.

An *anterior septal rupture* is approached through the infarction in the anterior left ventricular wall with excision of the most severely infarcted muscle in the ventricular free wall as well as in the septum. (Fig. 2) Large defects will require closure with a prosthetic patch and direct closure of the left ventriculotomy with heavy sutures reinforced with teflon felt strips. Small anterior defects can sometimes be repaired by direct approximation of the posterior rim of the defect to the anterior left and right ventricular walls.

Repair of *posterior septal rupture* is the most challenging of the three types, and has been associated with the greatest number of technical failures in the past. A transinfarct approach is made through the posterior wall of the infarcted left ventricle with sufficient excision of the infarct to afford exposure of the defect, clear definition of its margins, and excision of necrotic septum. (Fig. 3) Most patients with a large acute inferior septal defect will require insertion of a

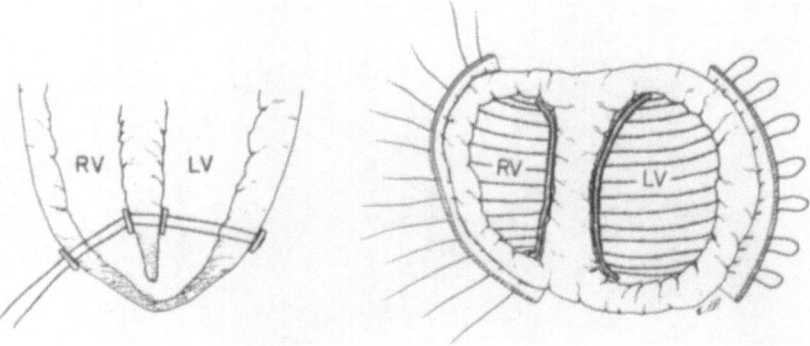

*Figure 1.* Surgical repair of an apical ventricular septal defect by apical amputation. The infarcted apices of both left and right ventricles are removed, and reconstruction accomplished by direct suture closure of the ventricles with teflon felt reinforcement.

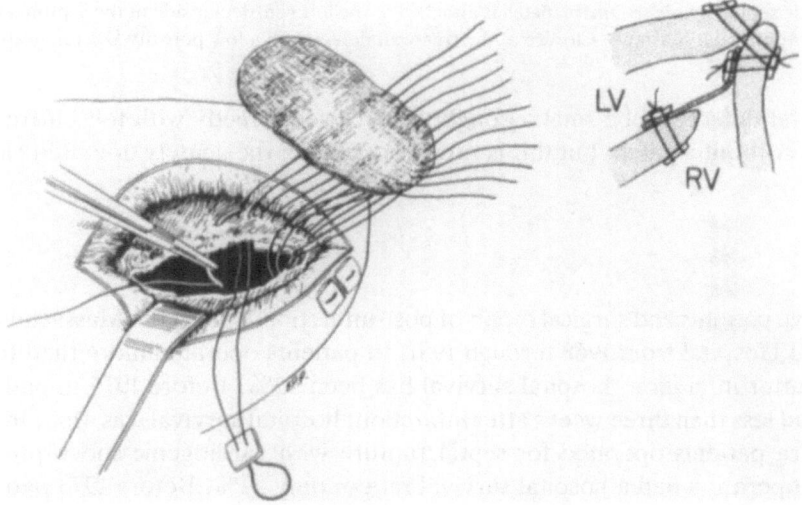

*Figure 2.* Surgical repair of a large anterior septal rupture. Exposure of the VSD by an anterior left ventricular transinfarct incision with excision of the infarcted myocardium. After excision of necrotic septal muscle, the defect is closed with a Dacron patch anchored on the left side of the septum. The left ventriculotomy is closed directly with sutures reinforced by teflon felt strips.

prosthetic patch in order to accomplish closure without tension, and the patch is anchored along the superior edge of the defect and to the right ventricular side of the free wall infarctectomy. After the septal defect is patched, closure of the free wall infarctectomy is best accomplished by suturing a low porosity Dacron graft to the inferior wall incision, in order to avoid undue tension on the closure which has been the site of suture line rupture in several of our earlier cases. Occasionally

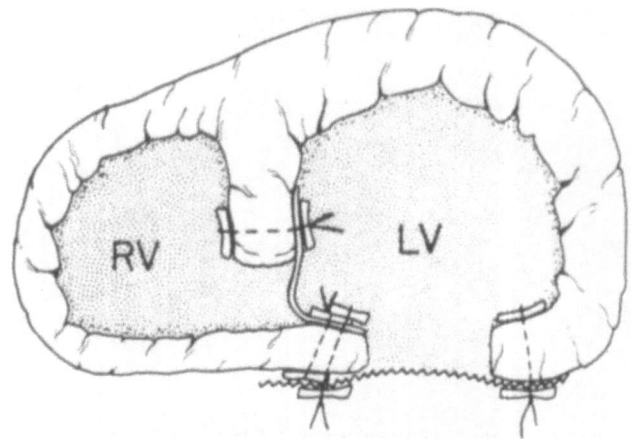

*Figure 3.* Surgical repair of large inferior-posterior septal defect. Exposure via a left ventricular inferior wall transinfarct incision with excision of the infarcted free wall myocardium. After removal of necrotic septal muscle, a Dacron patch is attached to the left ventricular side of the septum and to the right ventricular free wall. Closure of the free wall defect with a low porosity Dacron graft.

the septal defect will be small enough to be closed directly with felt buttressed sutures without a patch, but this is rarely possible in the acutely operated cases.

## Results

Fifty-five patients had surgical repair of post-infarction VSD at the Massachusetts General Hospital from 1968 through 1981. In patients operated more than three weeks after infarction, hospital survival has been 93%. Before 1975 in patients operated less than three weeks after infarction, hospital survival was 41%. In this same era patients operated for septal rupture with cardiogenic shock present before operation had a hospital survival rate of only 27%. Before 1975 patients with cardiogenic shock were supported with intra-aortic balloon pumping and vasopressors, and operation deferred pending hemodynamic stabilization. Before 1975 patients with anterior septal rupture had a hospital survival rate of 64% while patients with posterior septal rupture had a hospital survival rate of only 38%. This difference in survival according to the location of septal rupture occurred despite comparable numbers of patients in each group requiring early operation, as well as incidence of cardiogenic shock. Since 1975 patients operated less than three weeks after infarction have had an overall hospital survival rate of 70%. In patients with anterior defects 85% survived while in patients with posterior defects 67% survived. In patients operated with cardiogenic shock present before operation, survival has been 67%. Changes in management leading to improved results include: 1) immediate operation for patients with cardiogenic shock, 2) cold cardioplegic protection of the myocardium, and 3) prosthetic replacement of the posterior left ventricular free wall defect, after infarctectomy and septal repair in patients with posterior septal rupture. (4) Perioperative survival was independent of the extent of coronary artery disease and independent of left ventricular function.

Long term survival occurred in 76% of the hospital survivors after a minimum of four years of followup. All of the long term survivals of post-infarction VSD repair are in New York Heart Association Class I or II.

*Future trends*

It is possible that the incidence of post-infarction VSD will be reduced by the current aggressive practice of early reperfusion of the artery to the zone of infarction. In the absence of septal collaterals, this would appear to be the only method of eliminating this complication of acute infarction.

A new therapy which may possibly be useful in the management of patients with post-infarction VSD and right heart failure is prostaglandin E1 infusion. Our group has successfully treated five patients with refractory right heart failure after mitral valve replacement with prostaglandin E1 which acts as a potent pulmonary vascular dilator [7]. This modality may be useful in the early postoperative management of patients with substantial right ventricular infarctions and right heart failure immediately after surgical closure of the VSD.

**Papillary muscle rupture**

There are some similarities in the clinical presentation, diagnostic evaluation, and timing of treatment in patients with papillary muscle rupture when compared to those with post-infarction VSD. The infarct responsible for papillary muscle rupture is the patient's first infarction in over 90% [9]. Inferior infarctions are associated with papillary muscle rupture much more commonly than anterior infarctions, infero-posterior infarctions occurring in over 70% of the patients [9, 11]. Mitral regurgitation developed at a mean interval of 6 days after the acute infarct in a series reported by Nishimura et al [9]. Patients with ruptured papillary muscle and mitral regurgitation typically have more striking evidence of pulmonary edema and left heart failure than patients with VSD's, and cardiogenic shock with sudden deterioration and early death is more common than in the VSD patients.

Bedside diagnosis is possible by insertion of a Swan Ganz catheter and observation of large V waves in the pulmonary wedge tracing. In one reported series of patients with papillary muscle rupture, the mean pulmonary wedge pressure was 21 and the mean value of the peak V waves was 55 mmHg [9].

We advocate an identical aggressive approach to stabilization, diagnosis, and surgical treatment in patients with papillary muscle rupture as in those with VSD. For the patients in cardiogenic shock, immediate insertion of an intra-aortic balloon pump will usually improve the hemodynamic derangements. In those patients without cardiogenic shock, cautious use of vasodilating drugs can diminish the amount of pulmonary congestion and left ventricular failure. We advocate urgent cardiac catheterization, left ventriculography, and coronary arteriography in these patients in order to confirm the diagnosis and establish the degree of coronary artery disease, since approximately 50% of the patients have occlusive disease in more than one coronary artery. A majority of patients with papillary muscle rupture have a small infarction, and well preserved left ventricular function.

The timing of operative intervention in patients with papillary muscle rupture should precisely parallel the timing previously discussed for patients with VSD's. In the patients with cardiogenic shock and severe pulmonary edema, *immediate* operation is advised. In those who can be easily stabilized with medical measures, operation can be undertaken on a slightly less urgent basis.

In our institution, mitral valve replacement and coronary artery bypass grafting to major obstructed coronary arteries is the surgical treatment for patients with ruptured papillary muscle. Since the mitral regurgitation is acute and the left heart is typically of normal size, a low profile prosthesis is selected in the majority of cases. Interrupted mattress sutures with Teflon felt pledgets are utilized to minimize the possibility of paravalvular leakage. We also usually bypass the occluded coronary artery responsible for the infarction, as well as other obstructed major coronary arteries. Conservation of the mitral valve with repair of the ruptured papillary muscle would be the ideal operative procedure, but it has not been utilized in any of the patients operated early after their infarction, but it has been described in a patient operated two months after infarction [8].

Survival of patients undergoing mitral valve replacement less than two months after infarction has been 60%. Long term survival correlates significantly with left ventricular ejection fraction (EF) with 73% 4 year survival in those with EF>.35, and only 38% survival at 4 years with EF<.35 [11].

## References

1. Buckley MJ, Mundth ED, Daggett WM et al (1973) Surgical management of ventricular septal defects and mitral regurgitation complicating acute myocardial infarction. Ann Thorac Surg 16: 598
2. Daggett WM (1978) Surgical management of ventricular septal defects complicating myocardial infarction. World J Surg 2: 753
3. Daggett WM (1982) Surgical technique for early repair of posterior ventricular septal defect rupture. J Thorac Cardiovasc Surg 84: 306
4. Daggett WM, Buckley MJ, Akins CW et al (1982) Improved results of surgical management of

postinfarction ventricular septal rupture. Ann Surg 196: 269

5. Daggett WM, Guyton RA, Mundth ED et al (1977) Surgery for post-myocardial infarct ventricular septal defect. Ann Surg 186: 260

6. Daggett WM, Johnson RG Postinfarction ventricular septal rupture. In: Glenn WC (ed) (1982) *Thoracic and Cardiovascular Surgery*, 4th ed. Appleton-Century Cofts Prentice Hall: pp 1457–1470

7. D'Ambra MN, LaRaia PJ, Philbin DM et al (1985) Prostaglandin E1 (PGE1): A new therapy for refractory right heart failure and pulmonary hypertension after mitral valve replacement. J Thorac Cardiovasc Surg 89: 567

8. Gula G, and Yacoub MH (1981) Surgical correction of complete rupture of the anterior papillary muscle. Ann Thorac Surg 32: 88

9. Nishimura DA, Schaff HV, Shub C et al (1983) Papillary muscle rupture complicating acute myocardial infarction: Analysis of 17 patients. Am J Cardiol 51: 373

10. Oyamada A, Queen FB (1961) Spontaneous rupture of the interventricular septum following acute myocardial infarction with some clinico-pathologic observations on survival in five cases. Presented at the Pan Pacific Pathology Congress, Tripler US Army Hospital, October 12

11. Radford MJ, Johnson RA, Buckley MJ et al (1979) Survival following mitral valve replacement for mitral regurgitation due to coronary artery disease. Circulation 60: (Suppl I): 39

12. Radford MJ, Johnson RA, Daggett WM et al (1981) Ventricular septal rupture: A review of clinical and physiologic features and an analysis of survival. Circulation 64: 545

13. Sanders RJ, Kern WH, Blount SG (1956) Perforation of the interventricular septum complicating myocardial infarction. Am Heart J 51: 736

# History of systemic intravenous streptokinase therapy in acute myocardial infarction

J.C.W. VAN DE LOO

Historical reviews on the development of a clinical treatment method may be worthwhile if such an analysis can be made profitable for present research activities and for the design of future clinical studies. The history of thrombolytic treatment of acute myocardial infarction is now 36 years old: Since the first report appeared in 1959 in the United States it was followed by a big number of anecdotical studies. But it stimulated also the initiation of the first controlled clinical trials in the United Kingdom and in Central Europe. The results of the last of those 15 controlled clinical trials appeared in 1981 in the New England Journal of Medicine [31], just one year after the first experiences with the intracoronary application of the drug were published. The development has since speeded up with recent studies on the intravenous application of high doses of streptokinase in a few minutes and with the first experiences to replace streptokinase by human tissue plasminogen activator.

## Anecdotical studies

It is interesting to see how drug regulations and industrial manufacturing have influenced the progress of the matter: Most of the very early observations (Table 1) were made with a mixture of activated human plasminogen and a crude streptokinase which was available in the United States but not in Europe. In 1961 Behringwerke, Marburg, produced the first highly purified streptokinase and KABI, Stockholm, followed later on. The drug was licenced in Europe and numerous reports appeared in Europe but not in the States anymore (Table 2).

## Early controlled trials

The 15 controlled clinical trials on the intravenous application of a conventional streptokinase dose – what means 2.5 million units per 24 hours – have collected a total patient sample of more than 5,000 infarct patients followed up according to protocols of controlled clinical trials. The results (Table 3) were inconclusive as far as hospital mortality is concerned: 6 out of those trials, which are comparable, demonstrated a positive trend for thrombolytic treatment, 3 showed a negative and 2 no trend. The cumulative analysis of the haemorrhagic complications (Table 4), which is obviously the main limitation of the method, revealed 30 major bleedings with interruption of the treatment which corresponds to about 1%. Two deaths attributable to the thrombolytic intervention have been reported.

*Table 1.* Fibrinolytic drugs used in early trials on acute myocardial infarction (1959–1965).

| Authors | Year | No. of patients | | Fibrinolytic drugs used |
|---|---|---|---|---|
| | | Test | Control | |
| Fletcher et al (1) | 1959 | 22 | – | (SK) |
| de Leon et al (2) | 1959 | 30 | – | PL + SK |
| Boucek et al (3) | 1960 | 8 | – | PL + SK |
| Richter et al (4) | 1960 | 45 | – | PL + SK |
| Dewar et al (5) | 1961 | 17 | 16 | PL + SK |
| Datey et al (6) | 1962 | 15 | – | PL + SK |
| Richter et al (7) | 1962 | 52 | 52 | PL + SK |
| Dewar et al (8) | 1963 | 38 | 37 | PL + SK SK |
| Chazow (9) | 1965 | 100 | – | PL + SK UK |
| Boyles (10) | 1965 | 23/62/119 | | PL + SK |
| Lippschutz et al (11) | 1965 | 43 | 41 | PL + UK |

(SK): Crude streptokinase preparation. PL + SK: Mixture of human plasmin and streptokinase. UK: Urokinase

*Table 2.* Early anecdotical studies (1963–1968) using purified streptokinase in acute myocardial infarction.

| Authors | Year | N | Fibrinolytic drug used | Conclusion |
|---|---|---|---|---|
| Poliwoda et al (12) | 1963 | 20 | SK | + |
| Schmutzler (13) | 1963 | 31 | SK | + |
| van de Loo et al (14) | 1963 | 22 | SK | + |
| Körtge et al (15) | 1963 | 23 | SK | + |
| Heinrich (16) | 1965 | 23 | SK | + |
| Sauerwald (17) | 1965 | 15 | SK | + |
| Remy et al (18) | 1966 | 55 | SK | + |
| Fischer et al (19) | 1966 | 14 | SK | + |
| Sailer et al (20) | 1968 | 58 | SK | + |

326

An interesting observation was made in the Second German Swiss Trial [24] where the complaint of anginal pains and the consecutive need of analgesics were registered (Table 5). Patients treated with streptokinase had a significantly quicker relief of pains at 8, 24 and 72 hours after onset of treatment.

*Table 3.* Total hospital mortality in controlled clinical trials on intravenous streptokinase in acute myocardial infarction.

| Trial | Death rate (%) | | Trend in favour of |
|---|---|---|---|
| | Streptokinase | Controls | |
| European Working Party I (21) | 24 | 18 | Control |
| European Working Party II (22) | 18.5 | 26.3 | SK* |
| Italian Study (23) | 11.6 | 11.5 | – |
| German Swiss Trial II (24) | 14.5 | 26 | SK* |
| Australian Study (25) | 7.4 | 9.5 | SK |
| Frankfurt Trial (26) | 12.7 | 27.9 | SK* |
| European Urokinase Study (27) | 16.9 | 13.9 | Control |
| British Trial II (28) | 12.6 | 13.7 | – |
| Hannover Study (29) | 25.3 | 21.8 | Control |
| Austrian Study (30) | 10.5 | 17.3 | SK* |
| European Cooperative Study (31) | 11.7 | 17.8 | SK |

SK*): Statistically significant difference in favour of streptokinase treatment.

*Table 4.* Bleeding complications of streptokinase treated patients in controlled clinical trials on intravenous streptokinase in acute myocardial infarction.

| Trial | SK-treated patients | Bleeding without or with interruption | | Death |
|---|---|---|---|---|
| German Swiss Trial I (32) | 297 | 8 | 1 | – |
| European Working Party I (21) | 83 | 21 | – | – |
| European Working Party II (22) | 373 | 26 | 6 | – |
| Finnish Study (33) | 219 | 12 | 3 | – |
| Italian Study (23) | 164 | 17 | 6 | – |
| German Swiss Trial II (24) | 138 | 14 | – | – |
| Danish Study (34) | 67 | 3 | – | – |
| Australian Study (25) | 230 | ? | – | – |
| Frankfurt Trial (26) | 102 | 4 | – | – |
| British Trial II (28) | 302 | 36 | 6 | – |
| Austrian Study (30) | 352 | 21 | ? | – |
| Hannover Study (29) | 249 | ? | ? | ? |
| European Cooperative Study (31) | 156 | 31 | 5 | 1 |
| Total | 2.731 | 193 | 30 | 1 |

## Severity degree of the infarct and thrombolytic therapy

One experience made in a British [28] and especially in the Australian Study [25] turned out to be of particular significance: The outcome of streptokinase treated patients was different in dependence of their initial disease state. This means that the differences of mortality in favour of streptokinase were the higher the more severely ill the patients were. Table 6 provides a retrospective allocation of the died patients to selected baseline variables. All patients showed only a small insignificant difference in hospital mortality. However, patients with a previous infarction and patients above 60 years of age and those with a high Peel-index showed marked differences of mortality in favour of the streptokinase treatment. These differences were statistically significant for mortality at 3 months. The follow-up of the survived patients for 1 year [35] confirmed these figures but the differences were not statistically significant anymore.

The inconclusive situation as described above and this particular pattern of mortality in dependence of the severity of the disease were the reasons to design a new last multicentre European trial whose results were finally published in 1981 [31]. I want to comment on this in more detail because its design, conduction and evaluation are strongly affiliated to the University Department of Internal Medicine here in Cologne where the editors of this volume are working. The eleven

*Table 5.* Frequency (%) of chest pain before and after experimental treatment in patients of the II. German Swiss Trial (24) on intravenous streptokinase treatment in acute myocardial infarction.

| Time | SK treated patients (138 = 100%) | Control patients (131 = 100%) | p< |
|---|---|---|---|
| before treatment | 90 | 88 | |
| after end of infusion | | | |
| − 8 hrs | 23 | 51 | 0.01 |
| − 24 hrs | 16 | 46 | 0.01 |
| − 72 hrs | 9 | 23 | 0.01 |

*Table 6.* 3-months mortality rate by risk factors at admission in patients of the Australian Study of intravenous streptokinase in acute myocardial infarction [25].

| Risk factor at admission | Streptokinase N (%) | Controls N (%) |
|---|---|---|
| Reinfarction | 8:66 (12) | 15:62 (24) |
| Age above 60 | 7:43 (17) | 15:47 (32) |
| Peel Index ≥21 | 4:16 (25) | 8:16 (50) |
| All patients | 25:230 (11) | 29:227 (13) |

participating centres recruited 2.338 patients with an acute MI of less than 12 hours duration (Table 7). After many exclusions according to the rules of the protocol 512 patients were finally admitted to the trial. It was then the particular feature of this trial that the patients were stratified according to the severity of the disease before randomisation. The low risk patients were not submitted to the experimental intervention because it was concluded from the earlier trials that low risk patients do apparently not profit from thrombolytic treatment. The medium and severe grade patients were pooled and randomized into control or streptokinase treatment. The objectives of the trial were: May streptokinase reduce 6-months-mortality in patients of a definite pattern of increased risk and: may streptokinase improve haemodynamic and cardiac functions? The second question could not be answered because the study failed to recruit enough patients in the different centres undergoing regular measurements of left ventricular function. It turned out that the prestratification procedure was in fact able to select the low risk patients (Table 8). Their 6-months-mortality was 7%. The 6-months-mortality of the randomized patients with an increased pattern of risk at base-line was three times higher. It differed significantly between the 2 treatment groups: 50 patients died in the control group and 25 in the streptokinase treated group. Side-effects and especially bleeding complications were much more frequent in streptokinase treated patients: Most of them occured at the puncture sites. One out of the two patients with cerebral haemorrhages recovered ad integrum, the second died.

The authors of this European Cooperative Trial have drawn the following conclusions: (1) Streptokinase given intravenously for 24 hours to infarct patients

Table 7. Selection, pre-stratification and randomisation of patients in the European Cooperative Study on intravenous streptokinase in acute myocardial infarction [31].

| | | |
|---|---|---|
| *All* patients admitted with a suspected AMI | | 2.338 |
| – excluded | | 1.826 |
| Major reasons for exclusion: | | |
| born before 1900 | 13% | |
| interval >12 hours | 38% | |
| Hypertension | 33% | |
| Included in the trial | | 512 |
| Stratified according to severity | | 512 |
| – slight | 197 | |
| – medium | 307 | |
| – severe | 8 | |
| Randomised | | 315 |
| – into control group | | 159 |
| – into streptokinase group | | 156 |

of increased severity degree reduces 6 months mortality. (2) The rate of bleeding complications was low. Two cerebral haemorrhages, however, mark the treatment in this form as of potential harm. (3) It remains unclear, whether the effect on mortality is due to coronary thrombolysis or to the systemic hypofibrinogenemia.

## Summary of early experiences

If one summarizes the experiences of these earlier trials the following messages may be learnt from the intravenous streptokinase treatment in conventional doses for acute myocardial infarction:

1. A reduction of mortality is possible.
2. Higher risk patients appear to profit more than low risk patients.
3. Dosage and duration of SK-infusion are arbitrary. Essentially shorter application may still be effective and less harmful.
4. The effect on cardiac function is not yet established. It is a reasonable assumption that the final myocardial necrosis may be limited by thrombolytic treatment.

A recent retrospective and cumulative analysis [38] of 24 randomized trials on intravenous SK in acute myocardial infarction came to the conclusion that a significant reduction in mortality is evident.

The methods of thrombolytic treatment in acute infarction have meanwhile proceeded. The first comparative trial on long-term mortality after intracoronary streptokinase, published a few weeks ago from the Western Washington Study

Table 8. 6-months-mortality of patients in the European Cooperative Trial [31] on intravenous streptokinase in acute myocardial infarction.

| Patient group | No. of patients | Patients died No. (%) |
|---|---|---|
| All patients admitted (group I + II + III) | 512 | 88 (17) |
| Low risk patients (group III) | 197 | 13 (7) |
| Higher risk patients (group I + II) | 315 | 75 (24) |
| SK | 156 | 25 (16) |
| Control | 159 | 50 (31)* |

* $p \leqslant 0.02$

Group [36], revealed an interesting observation. The difference of total 1-year-mortality (8.2% in streptokinase treated patients vs. 14.7% in controls) was marked but not statistically significant as it was after the first 30 days. However, a retrospective analysis of the mortality rates according to selected base-line variables revealed marked differences between the 2 groups. Patients with a stable haemodynamic status before catheterisation had an almost identical mortality. But hypotensive or shock patients had a markedly higher difference of the mortality rate in favour of streptokinase. The same was true for patients with a low ejection fraction and for patients with previous infarction although this latter difference is not statistically significant. I admit that these were retrospective analyses of particular subgroups and not a prestratification as in the European Cooperative Study. But, also from this data the question should be put forward: Does it make sense to treat patients thrombolytically with a stable haemodynamic situation at admission or with a normal ejection fraction or with other criteria of a good prognosis?

**Is systemic activation of the fibrinolytic system only harmful or an advantage?**

The early experiences with systemic intravenous streptokinase in acute myocardial infarction allow for a critical analysis of the haematological changes which were and are presently observed in patients treated with the more recent thrombolytic treatment schedules. Streptokinase or urokinase activate the fibrinolytic system of the circulating blood. This effect is markedly less pronounced when the drug is applied locally in a reduced amount. Streptokinase exerts its local thrombolytic effect (a) through a SK-plasminogen-activator-complex and through the plasmin formed. Both will reach the surface and the inner structures of a throm-

*Table 9*. Mortality and base-line variables in the Western Washington Study on intracoronary streptokinase in acute myocardial infarction [36].

| Variables | Streptokinase treated patients No. (%) | Control patients No. (%) | Δ (%) |
|---|---|---|---|
| Blood pressure | | | |
| stable | 9 : 116 (8) | 9 : 91 (10) | 20 |
| hypotensive + shock | 2 : 18 (11) | 8 : 25 (32) | 66 |
| Reinfarction | | | |
| No | 7 : 114 (6) | 12 : 97 (12) | 50 |
| Yes | 3 : 17 (18) | 5 : 16 (31) | 42 |
| Ejection fraction | | | |
| >40 | 5 : 105 (5) | 6 : 88 (7) | 0 |
| ≤40 | 5 : 24 (21) | 11 : 24 (46) | 54 |

bus to a small extent only, but obviously they do. The (b) systemic plasmin effect leads to a dramatic fall of fibrinogen and other coagulation factors and thus to a bleeding tendency. However, this hypofibrinogenaemia decreases blood viscosity to a marked degree and may influence the microcirculation in a positive way. Furthermore, this coagulation defect leads to a strong anticoagulative activity through the inhibition of thrombin and Factor Xa by the fibrinogen degradation products. This effect may last for hours and may be more effective than any other induced anticoagulation.

Tissue-type plasminogen-activator, however, activates the fibrinolytic system of the circulating blood only to a small extent. It exerts its thrombolytic effect through the specific binding of tissue-type plasminogen-activator to fibrin-bound plasminogen and not to circulating plasminogen. Fibrin-bound plasminogen occurs almost exclusively in thrombi and so it seems justified to call tissue-type plasminogen-activator a thrombus- or fibrin- specific activator. If, moreover, tissue-plasminogen-activator does not produce systemic plasmin activity, it will induce less bleeding tendency.

However, fibrin-specific thrombolysis neither exerts any effect on blood viscosity and, thus, on microcirculation nor does it have any anticoagulative potency. This should be kept in mind when discussing about long-term survival on the one hand and the rate of early reocclusions on the other in patients with non-systemic thrombolytic treatment.

Summarizing these considerations, it would be highly desirable that future clinical trials combine their cardiological studies with a sophisticated analysis of the haemostatic system. It appears not yet clear whether systemic activation of the fibrinolytic system is an advantage for the patient or only of harm due to possible bleeding complications.

## References

1. Fletcher AP, Sherry S, Alkjaersig N et al (1959) The maintenance of a sustained thrombolytic state in man. II. Clinical observations on patients with myocardial infarction and other thrombotic disorders, J Clin Invest 38: 1096
2. De Leon AC, Bellet S, Tsitouris G et al (1960) The fibrinolytic system and use of fibrinolysis in myocardial infarction. Preliminary report, Amer J Cardiol 5: 674–679
3. Boucek RJ, Murphy WP jr (1960) Segmental perfusion of the coronary arteries with fibrinolysin in man following a myocardial infarction, Amer J Cardiol 0: 526–532
4. Richter IH, Musacchio F, Cliffton EE et al (1960) Experiences with clot-lysing agents in coronary thrombosis, Amer J Cardiol 6: 534
5. Dewar HA, Horler AR, Cassells-Smith AJ (1961) Fibrinolytic treatment of coronary thrombosis. A pilot study, Brit med J 2: 671–675
6. Datey KK, Hansoti RC, Pandya VN (1962) Value of fibrinolysin in managment of myocardial infarction. A preliminary report, JAMA 182: 1078–1081
7. Richter H, Cliffton E, Epstein S et al (1962) Thrombolysin therapy in myocardial infarction, Amer J Cardiol 9: 82–85

8. Dewar HP, Stephenson A, Horler A et al (1963) Fibrinolytic therapy of coronary thrombosis, Brit Med J 1: 915

9. Chazov EI (1965) Plasmin und Streptokinase zur Behandlung des Myokardinfarktes, Z ges inn Med 20: 727

10. Boyles PW (1965) Improved long-term survival following myocardial infarction with fibrinolytic therapy, Angiology 16: 346–350

11. Lippschutz EJ, Ambrus JL, Ambrus CM et al (1965) Controlled study of the treatment of coronary occlusion with urokinase activated human plasmin, Amer J Cardiol 16: 93–98

12. Poliwoda H, Schröder R, Heckner F (1963) Erste Erfahrungen mit der fibrinolytischen Therapie beim akuten Myocardinfarct, Dtsch med Wschr 88: 218–224

13. Schmutzler R (1963) Neuere Erkenntnisse der therapeutsche Fibrinolyse, Helv med Acta 30: 608–614

14. Van de Loo J (1963) Möglichkeiten und Grenzen der kombinierten Fibrinolyse-Antikoagulantien-Therapie des Myokardinfarktes, Med Klin 58: 1527–1529

15. Körtge P (1963) The value of streptokinase-induced fibrinolysis in the treatment of acute myocardial infarction, IX. Congr Soc europ Haemat, Lissabon

16. Heinrich HG (1965) Die Therapie des Myokardinfarktes mit Streptokinase, Z ges inn Med 20: 730

17. Sauerwald PH (1965) Über die fibrinolytische Behandlung des frischen Herinfarktes mit Streptase, Medizin heute 14: 228–232

18. Remy D, Gebauer D (1966) Die fibrinolytische Behandlung des Herzinfarktes, Med Klin 61: 220–223

19. Fischer EJ (1968) Über die fibrinolytische Therapie des Herzinfarktes, Dtsch med J 3: 84–91

20. Sailer S, Wehrschutz E, Tilz GP (1968) Die thrombolytische Behandlung der frischen Herzinfarktes, Wiener med Wschr 118: 283–285

21. Amery A, Roeber G, Vermeulen HJ et al (1969) Single-blind randomized multicentre trial comparing heparin and streptokinase treatment in recent myocardial infarction, Acta Med Scand Suppl 505: 5–35

22. European Working Party (1971) Streptokinase in recent myocardial infarction: a controlled multicentre trial, Br Med J iii: 325–31

23. Dioguardi N, Mannucci PM, Lotto A et al (1971) Controlled trial of streptokinlase and heparin in acute myocardial infarction, Lancet ii: 891–5

24. Schmutzler R, Fritze E, Gebauer D et al (1971) Fibrinolytic therapy in acute myocardial infarction, Thrombos Diathes haemorrh (Stuttg.) Suppl 47: 211

25. Bett JHN, Biggs JC, Castaldi PA et al (1973) Australian multicentre trial of streptokinase in acute myocardial infarction, Lancet i: 57–60

26. Breddin K, Ehrly AM, Fechler L et al (1973) Die Kurzzeitfibrinolyse beim akuten Myokardinfarkt, Dtsch Med Wochenschr 98: 861–73

27. Duckert F, Burkart F, Hecker S et al (1975) Controlled trial of urokinase in myocardial infarction, Lancet ii: 624–625

28. Aber CP, Bass NM, Berry CL et al (1976) Streptokinasse in acute myocardial infarction: a controlled multicentre study in the United Kingdom, Br Med J 2: 1100–4

29. Poliwoda H, Schneider B, Avenarius HJ (1977) Untersuchungen zum klinischen Verlauf des akuten Myokardinfarktes. Gemeinschaftsstudie an 26 Krankenhäusern in Nord-Deutschland, Med Klin 72: 451–8

30. Benda V, Haider M, Ambrosch P (1977) Ergebnisse der Österreichischen Herzinfarktstudie mit Streptokinase (Results of the Austrian myocardial infarction study of the effects of streptokinase) Wien Klin Wochenschr, 89: 779–83

31. European cooperative study group (1979) Streptokinase in acute myocardial infarction, New Engl J Med 301: 797

32. Schmutzler R, Heckner F, Körtge P et al (1966) Thrombolytic therapy of recent myocardial infarction, Dtsch Med Wochenschr 91: 581

333

33. Heikinheimo R, Ahrenberg P, Honkapohja H et al (1971) Fibrinolytic treatment in acute myocardial infarction, Acta Med Scand 189: 7–13
34. Gormsen J, Tidstrom B, Feddersen C et al (1973) Biochemical evaluation of low dose of urokinase in acute myocardial infarction. A double blind study, Acta Med Scand 194: 191–8
35. Bett JHN, Biggs JC, Chesterman CN et al (1977) Australian multicentre trial of streptokinase in acute myocardial infarction, Med J Aus 1: 553
36. Kennedy JW, Ritchie JL, Davis KB et al (1983) Western Washington randomized trial of intracoronary streptokinase in acute myocardial infarcation, New Engl J Med 309: 1477–82
37. Kennedy JW, Ritchie JL, Davis KB et al (1985) The Western Washington randomized trial of intracoronary streptokinase in acute myocardial infarction. A 12-month follow-up report, New Engl J Med 312: 1073–8
38. Yusuf S, Collins R, Peto R et al (1985) Intravenous and intracoronary fibrinolytic therapy in acute myocardial infarction: Overview of results on mortality, reinfarction and side effects from 33 randomized controlled trials, Europ Heart J 6 556–585

# Recent developments in intracoronary thrombolysis during acute myocardial infarction

M. COHEN and K. RENTROP

Treatment of acute myocardial infarction with intracoronary infusion of thrombolytic agents such as streptokinase or urokinase has received considerable attention over the last several years. Many investigations have appeared evaluating such different aspects as recanalization rates, efficacy in limiting infarct size, reduction in peri-infarct mortality, and treatment associated complications.

## Complications associated with intracoronary thrombolysis

There is a significant 'complication', rate associated with acute myocardial infarction in the absence of any experimental intervention. Therefore, it is difficult to pinpoint complications occurring during the acute infarct phase that are the result of early therapeutic interventions. Intervention related complication rates can be assessed only by randomized trials that include a control group not subjected to angiographic examination during the acute stage of infarction. In one such a trial, fatal cardiogenic shock occurred in two patients after manipulation of the catheter resulted in dislodgement of clot from the infarct-related left anterior descending artery to the circumflex artery [1]. In two additional patients, fatal pump failure after injection of dye was attributed to the negative inotropic properties of the contrast medium. In addition, recanalization of the right coronary artery with thrombolytic therapy, was frequently associated with hypotension, bradycardia, and conduction delays caused by activation of the Bezold-Jarisch reflex.

Reocclusion of coronary arteries after recanalization by intracoronary infusion of streptokinase has been associated with reinfarction and death [2]. It has been suggested that patency can be maintained by anticoagulation with heparin [3, 4]. However, anticoagulation with intravenous heparin is associated with a finite number of bleeding complications. This risk of bleeding may be increased if infusion of streptokinase has resulted in a drop in the fibrinogen concentration below 100 mg/dl [5]. Angioplasty [2, 6] and coronary bypass surgery [4] have been performed after intracoronary infusion of streptokinase to prevent complications arising from reocclusion and to augment flow to the reperfused myocardium [2]. These procedures may be particularly beneficial in patients with more than a 90% residual stenosis and a large segment of jeopardized myocardium [2]. Although they can be performed with minimal risk within a few days after infusion of streptokinase, the optimal timing of their use has not been established.

## Efficacy in reestablishing antegrade flow

Intracoronary infusion of streptokinase reestablishes antegrade flow in approximately 75% of completely occluded infarct-related vessels, (Table 1) [7, 8]. Modifications of the technique, such as superselective infusion of streptokinase via small infusion catheters advanced to the site of occlusion, increased infusion rate, or injection of a bolus at the initiation of therapy, have not resulted in significantly higher recanalization rates, (Table 1) [3, 4, 9–16].

## Efficacy in reducing peri-infarct mortality

Statistically significant improvement in mortality after infusion of streptokinase was reported in only one trial [12]. The mechanism of improved survival in this study remains unclear, since there was no significant improvement in left ventricular ejection fraction in the streptokinase treated group which showed the lower 30-day mortality. Furberg [17] pooled the survival data of eight prospective

*Table 1.* Recanalization rates of total obstruction with intracoronary infusion of streptokinase.

| Study | SK dose (U/min) | Bolus (USK)[a] | Subselective[b] | Recanalization rate[c] | |
|---|---|---|---|---|---|
| | | | | n/n | % |
| Khaja et al [9] | 5,000 | 15,000 | – | 12/20 | 60 |
| Anderson et al [10] | 5,000 | – | – | 15/20 | 75 |
| Ganz et al [5] | 4,000 | – | Yes | 17/18 | 94 |
| Serruys et al [1] | 4,000 | – | Yes | 30/36 | 83 |
| Kennedy [11] | 4,000 | – | Yes | 73/108 | 68 |
| Leiboff et al [12] | 2,000–4,000 | – | – | 15/22 | 68 |
| Mathey et al [13] | 2,000 | Plasminogen | – | 39/39 | 77 |
| Rentrop et al [4] | 2,000 | 10,000 | – | 17/20 | 85 |
| Smalling et al [14] | 2,000 | 10,000 | – | 73/100 | 73 |
| Rentrop et al [15] | 2,000 | – | – | Σ314/426 | 74 |

SK = streptokinase
[a] Application of a bolus of streptokinase into the infarct-related vessel before infusion.
[b] Subselective infusion of streptokinase via special catheter into the infarct-related vessel.
[c] Recanalization rate documented by sequential angiography during infusion of streptokinase.

randomized trials, including the one that showed significant improvement, and calculated a mortality of 11.0% in 382 patients treated with intracoronary infusion of streptokinase compared with 12.4% in 364 control patients; this difference was not statistically significant. In the absence of corroborative data from other investigative groups, it would seem prudent to suggest that the influence of intracoronary infusion of streptokinase on mortality remains unknown.

## Efficacy in limiting infarct size: effect on left ventricular ejection fraction

The influence of intracoronary infusion of streptokinase on ejection fraction has been assessed in five controlled trials, (Table 2) [9, 10, 12, 13, 16]. Anderson et al [10] were the only investigators to observe a significant improvement in left ventricular function from the acute of the chronic stage of infarction in patients treated with streptokinase. Lack of functional improvement in the majority of trials has been attributed to a delay of more than 4 hours between onset of infarction and commencement of therapy. However, Leiboff et al [13] found no improvement of function in patients treated with streptokinase, inspite of initiating therapy within 4 hours. It should be stated that a relatively high reocclusion rate in Leiboff's study may make the results relating to effect on left ventricular ejection fraction difficult to interpret. The published data suggest, but do not prove, that sustained early reperfusion may be associated with improvement of left ventricular function. Additionally, reperfusion after more than 4 hours may be beneficial in some subgroups of patients, as suggested, but not proven, by the functional improvement associated with infusion of streptokinase after 6 hours in

Table 2. Change in ejection fraction after intracoronary infusion of streptokinase.

| Study | IC SK (n) | Control (n) | Time to infusion (hr)[a] | Recanalization rate (%)[b] | Reocclusion (%) | ΔEF ICSK (%) | ΔEF control (%) | P value |
|---|---|---|---|---|---|---|---|---|
| Anderson et al [10] | 24 | 26 | 4.00 ± 0.75 | 75 | 0 | 3.9 ± 4.6 | − 3.0 ± 8.4 | <.001 |
| Leifboff et al [12] | 20 | 17 | 4.03 | 68 | 45 | − 2.8 | − 0.8 | NS |
| Kennedy et al [11] | 134 | 116 | 4.57 ± 2.15 | 68 | | 1.0 | 0 | NS |
| Khaja et al [9] | 20 | 20 | 5.40 ± 1.50 | 60 | | 3.0 | 2.0 | NS |
| Rentrop et al [15] | 23 | 24 | 5.90 ± 2.80 | 74 | 17 | 2.1 ± 1.1 | − 1.4 ± 9.5 | NS |

ΔEF = change in ejection fraction; ICSK = streptokinase group; Control = control group.
[a] Time interval from onset of infarction of streptokinase
[b] Recanalization rate documented by sequential angiography during infusion of streptokinase.
[c] Reocclusion rate as assessed by repeat angiography in the chronic stage of infarction.

the Mount Sinai/NYU Bellevue randomized trial [16]. To test these hypotheses, a much larger trial is being conducted.

## Other benefits and limitations

Analysis of data collected during acute phase angiography followed by intra-coronary infusion of thrombolytic agents has greatly enhanced our understanding of the pathogenesis and pathophysiology of acute myocardial infarction. In addition, it facilitates the analysis of benefits and limitation of reperfusion in general. In clinical practice, however, the value of this method is limited by several factors. Since the majority of hospitals are not equipped with cardiac catheterization laboratories, or not sufficiently staffed to perform intracoronary infusion of streptokinase on a 24-hour basis, substantial investments would be necessary to make this therapy available to all patients with acute myocardial infarction. In addition, there is always an inherent delay in initiation of any intracoronary therapy while the cardiac catheterization laboratory is prepared and baseline angiographic studies are performed [18, 19].

## Intracoronary thrombolysis with urokinase

Intracoronary thrombolysis has been attempted with urokinase. Infusion rates between 2000 and 24,000 U/min resulted in recanalization rates of 62 to 94% [5, 20, 21]. Tennant et al [5] observed that intracoronary infusion of urokinase was comparable to streptokinase with respect to reestablishment of antegrade flow. Urokinase infusion however, was associated with less marked reduction in serum fibrinogen and fewer bleeding complications.

## References

1. Serruys PW, Van Den Brand M, Hooghoudt TEH, Simoons ML, Fioretti P, Ruiter J, Fels PW, Hugenholtz PG (1982) Coronary recanalization in acute myocardial infarction: immediate results and potential risks. Eur Heart J 3: 404
2. Gold HK, Cowley MJ, Palacios IF, Vetrovec GW, Akins CW, Block PC, Leinbach RC (1984) Combined intracoronary streptokinase infusion and coronary angioplasty during acute myocardial infarction. Am J Cardiol 53: 122C
3. Ganz W, Buchbinder N, Marcus H, Mondkar A, Maddahi J, Charuzi Y, O'Connor L, Shell W, Fishbein M, Kass R, Miyamoto A, Swan HJC (1981) Intracoronary thrombolysis in evolving myocardial infarction. Am Heart J 101: 4
4. Rentrop P, Blanke H, Karsch KR, Kaiser H, Kostering H, Leitz K (1981) Selective intracoronary thrombolysis in acute myocardial infarction and unstable angina pectoris. Circulation 63: 307
5. Tennant SN, Dixon J, Venable TC, Page HL, Roach A, Kaiser AB, Frederiksen R, Tacogue L, Kaplan P, Babu NS, Anderson EE, Wooten E, Jennings HJS, Breinig J, Cambell WB (1984)

338

Intracoronary thrombolysis in patients with acute myocardial infarction: comparison of the efficacy of urokinase with streptokinase. Circulation 69: 756

6. Hartzler GO, Rutherford BD, McConahay DR, Johnson WL, McCallister BD, Gura GM, Conn RC, Crokett JE (1983) Percutaneous transluminal coronary angioplasty with and without thrombolytic therapy for treatment of acute myocardial infarction. Am Heart J 106: 965

7. Rentrop P, Smith H, Painter L, Holt J (1983) Changes in left ventricular ejection fraction after intracoronary thrombolytic therapy. Circulation 68 (Suppl I): 1–55

8. Kennedy JW and the Registry Committee, Society for Cardiac Angiography (1983) Intracoronary streptokinase in acute MI: report from the society for cardiac angiography registry. Circulation 68 (suppl III): 111–121

9. Khaja F, Walton JA, Brymer JF, Lo E, Osterberger L, O'Neill WW, Colfer HT, Weiss R, Lee T, Kurian T, Goldberg AD, Pitt B, Goldstein B (1983) Intracoronary therapy in acute myocardial infarction. N Engl J Med 303: 1304

10. Anderson JL, Marshall HW, Bray BE, Lutz JR, Frederick PR, Yanowitz FG, Datz FL, Klausner SC, Hagan AD (1983) A randomized trial of intracoronary streptokinase in the treatment of acute myocardial infarction. N Engl J Med 308: 1312

11. Kennedy JW, Ritchie JL, Davis KB, Fritz JK (1983) Western Washington randomized trial of intracoronary streptokinase in acute myocardial infarction. N Engl J Med 309: 1477

12. Leiboff RH, Katz RJ, Wasserman AG, Bren GB, Schwartz H, Varghese PJ, Ross AM (1984) A randomized angiographically controlled trial of intracoronary streptokinase in acute myocardial infarction. Am J Cardiol 53: 404

13. Mathey DG, Kuck KH, Tilsner V, Krebber HJ, Bleifeld W (1981) Non-surgical coronary artery recanalization in acute transmural myocardial infarction. Circulation 63: 489

14. Smalling RW, Fuentes F, Matthews MW, Freund GC, Hicks CH, Reduto LA, Walker WE, Sterling RP, Gould KL (1983) Sustained improvement in left ventricular function and mortality by intracoronary streptokinase administration during evolving myocardial infarction. Circulation 68: 131

15. Rentrop KP, Feit F, Blanke H, Stecy P, Schneider R, Rey M, Horowitz S, Goldman M, Karsch K, Meilman H, Cohen M, Siegel S, Sanger J, Slater J, Gorlin R, Fox A, Fagerstrom R, Calhoun WF (1984) Effects of intracoronary streptokinase and intracoronary nitroglycerine infusion on coronary angiographic patterns and mortality in patients with acute myocardial infarction. N Engl J Med 311: 1464

16. Furberg C (1984) Clinical value of intracoronary streptokinase. Am J Cardiol 53: 626

17. Anderson JL, Marshall HW, Askins JC, Lutz JR, Sorensen SG, Menlove RL, Yanowitz FG, Hagan AD (1984) A randomized trial of intravenous and intracoronary streptokinase in patients with acute myocardial infarction. Circulation 70: 606

18. Taylor GJ, Mikell FL, Moses HW, Dove JT, Batchelder JE, Thull A, Hansen S, Wellons HA, Schneider J (1984) Intravenous versus intracoronary streptokinase therapy for acute myocardial infarction in community hospitals. Am J Cardiol 54: 54: 256

19. Yasuno M, Saito Y, Ishida M, Suzuki K, Endo S, Takashashi M (1984) Effects of percutaneous transluminal coronary angioplasty: intracoronary thrombolysis with urokinase in acute myocardial infarction. Am J Cardiol 53: 1217

20. Cernigliaro C, Sansa M, Campi A, Bongo AS, Rossi P (1983) Efficacy of intracoronary urokinase in acute myocardial infarction. Circulation 68 (Suppl III) III–407

# Intravenous thrombolysis in acute myocardial infarction

R. SCHRÖDER

Until 1980, there was only one report about two cases, where angiography was performed before intravenous infusion of urokinase. At a second angiogram 13 and 16 days later, the coronary blood flow was found restored in the previously obstructed arteries [1]. When in 1980 I first reported about angiographically proven successful early recanalization of a thrombotically occluded coronary artery by high-dose brief duration intravenous streptokinase infusion [2], there was considerable scepticism and even criticism. Nowadays the effectiveness of intravenous streptokinase is generally accepted. However, although to my mind we are by now fairly well cognizant of the effectiveness of this regimen as far as recanalization of an occluded infarct-related coronary artery and restoration of coronary blood flow is concerned, there are still – or again – papers or reviews quoting for iv STK recanalization rates as low as 10% only.

Quoted is just an abstract of Rogers et al [3]. 5000.000 units of streptokinase were infused intravenously on average 8 hours after symptom onset. At angiography within 45 minutes (!) there was a recanalization in 1 of 10 patients. Interestingly enough, in none of the remaining 9 patients recanalization could be achieved by subsequent intracoronary streptokinase infusion. Actually, when the paper was presented at the American College of Cardiology 1983, the authors reported about additional 14 patients, who got 1 million units of streptokinase and in whom recanalization was achieved in 44%. In the same year, comprehensive data were published in Circulation and, seriously, these should have been quoted [4].

The same authors then started a randomized trial comparing intravenous and intracoronary streptokinase, with initiation of treatment less than 6 hours after symptom onset. The intravenous group did not have baseline angiography, thus treatment was initiated 66 minutes earlier than in the intracoronary group. A premature peaking of the serial serum CK-MB activity curve suggested early restoration of coronary blood flow in 9 of 14 patients in both treatment groups [5]. Ten days post myocardial infarction the patency rate in the iv group was 12 of 14, and in the ic group 9 of 14.

**Streptokinase**

Already in our initial studies we have shown that recanalization or restoration of coronary blood flow of the infarct-related coronary artery occurs in most patients after intravenous streptokinase [6].Angiography was performed in 75 patients three weeks later. Six patients with post intervention reinfarction and probably reocclusion are excluded. In the remaining 69 patients the infarct-related coronary artery was found patent in all 36 patients, in whom intravenous streptokinase infusion was started within 3 hours after onset of symptoms and in 27, that is 82%, of the patients with initiation of treatment 3–6 hours after symptom onset.

Table 1 shows data from 5 authors who compared recanalization rates achieved by intracoronary and intravenous streptokinase. In the intravenously treated group no coronary angiography was performed before initiation of streptokinase infusion, but treatment was started as soon as possible. At angiography 1 hour to some days later patent infarct-related coronary arteries were found more often in the iv treated groups, i.e. in 75–94% of the patients. The only exception was a patency rate of only 64% in the study of Valentine et al. They performed angiography as soon as possible, that means 1 hour or so after initiation of iv streptokinase. All data reported so far from patients in whom treatment was initiated within 6 hours after symptom onset are included in this table. Ganz et al started treatment within 3 hours after symptom onset. From the uniform results of all these studies it can be concluded that restoration of coronary blood flow

*Table 1.* Comparison of restoration of coronary blood flow in patients with evolving myocardial infarction treated with intravenous or intracoronary streptokinase.

|  |  | Patent IRA | Symptom onset to STK (min) | Angiography performed |
|---|---|---|---|---|
| Ganz et al [7] | IC-STK | 65/78 (84%) | $207 \pm 61$ | |
| | IV-STK | 78/81 (96%) | $130 \pm 41$ | 3–7 days later |
| Taylor et al [8] | IC-STK | 44/63 (70%) | $217 \pm 82$ | |
| | IV-STK | 99/121 (82%) | $190 \pm 117$ | 1 to 36 hours later |
| Valentine et al [9] | IC-STK | 63/98* (72%) | IV 67 min | |
| | IV-STK | 42/66 (64%) | earlier | as soon as possible |
| Rogers et al [5] | IC-STK | 9/14 (64%) | IV 66 min | |
| | IV-STK | 12/14 (86%) | earlier | 10 days post MI |
| Anderson et al [10] | IC-STK | 13/18 (72%) | $246 \pm 90$ | |
| | IV-STK | 15/20 (75%) | $162 \pm 66$ | Pre-discharge |

Abbreviation: IRA = infarct-related artery.
* 13 of 98 (13%) of IRA were patent at the initial angiogram and 50 of 85 (59%) opened with the IC-STK.

actually can be achieved by iv streptokinase in most patients, if treatment is initiated early.

The decisive question, however, which remains is how fast restoration of coronary blood flow does occur. If this would happen hours after initiation of treatment, it probably would be almost useless. Table 2 comprises without exception* all reported studies with angiographically proven recanalization success rates of a totally occluded coronary artery with intravenous streptokinase infusion initiated less than 6 hours after symptom onset. There was a proven recanalization success rate between 49 and 70% – on the average 57%. Although this is a high percentage of early recanalization, this figure is smaller than that reported for intracoronary streptokinase – here 77%, and less than that percentage of patent infarct-related coronary arteries found at angiography hours or days later (Table 1). This is because lysis of an intracoronary clot lasts somewhat longer with the intravenous approach as with intracoronary streptokinase, and in some patients recanalization may occur up to 3 hours after initiation of treatment. Naturally, during the acute phase of infarction the angiographic observation time was limited, mostly 1 hour or 90 minutes. Therefore, those recanalizations occurring somewhat delayed were not detected.

There is increasing evidence that for substantial salvage of jeopardized myocardium restoration of coronary blood flow must be achieved early, i.e. within about 3 hours after onset of myocardial infarction, no matter how restoration is

*Table 2.* Angiographically confirmed recanalization rates of completely occluded coronary arteries in patients with acute myocardial infarction treated with brief duration high-dose intravenous streptokinase within 6 hours after symptom onset. Comparison with intracoronary streptokinase by four authors.

|  | IV STK recanalization no. of pts | Time to recanalization minutes | IC STK recanalization no. of pts | Time to recanalization minutes |
|---|---|---|---|---|
| Schröder et al [11] | 8/15 (53%) | 38 | – | – |
| Neuhaus et al [12] | 24/38 (63%) | 48 | 28/37 (76%) | 28 |
| Blunda et al [13] | 7/10 (70%) | 54 ± 28 | 10/12 (80%) | 27 ± 14 |
| Huhmann et al [14] | 13/22 (59%) | 105 ± 68 | 20/26 (77%) | 55 ± 28 |
| Spann et al [15] | 21/43 (49%) | 30–60 | – | – |
| Alderman et al [16] | 8/13 (62%) | 39 | 11/15 (73%) | 28 |
|  | 81/141 (57%) |  | 69/90 (77%) |  |

* Just recently there was one additional abstract at the International Symposium on Cardiovascular Pharmacotherapy; Geneva, Switzerland, April 22–25, 1985. With 0.5–1.5 mio.units of STK iv, on average 4.4 h after symptom onset, there was an angiographically proven recanalization in 10/22 (45%) patients. (Saltups A. et al: Streptokinase in Myocardial Infarction. Does Late Infarct-Artery Patency mean Early Reperfusion?)

achieved. The need of prior catheterization for intracoronary administration takes time, 60–90 minutes at least in the usual clinical setting. Intravenous thrombolysis can be initiated immediately after the diagnosis, or the probable diagnosis, of myocardial infarction has been established, even in the ambulance or in the patient's home. Today the prevailing opinion is, that the somewhat longer lasting clot lysis with the intravenous approach probably can be more than balanced by the earlier begin of treatment, which should lead to an earlier restoration of coronary blood flow in many patients. Furthermore, time to lyse an intracoronary clot largely depends on the age, and thus probably the size of the thrombus. There are large differences, even if treatment is initiated early after symptom onset. We have shown this already in our first comprehensive report [17]. If intravenous streptokinase was initiated between 1–3 hours after symptom onset, there was a recanalization rate within 60 minutes after begin of the infusion of 78% as compared to only 33% if treatment was initiated 3–6 hours after symptom onset. In this respect I like to remind you that successful restoration of coronary blood flow in terms of salvage of jeopardized myocardium most probably has to be achieved within 3–4 hours after onset of myocardial infarction.

Consequently, those groups who attempted early recanalization by intracoronary streptokinase today begin intravenous pre-treatment with streptokinase or urokinase as soon as possible. It was probably Schwarz et al from Heidelberg who first compared the functional improvement in 35 patients, pretreated with 1.5 million units of streptokinase intravenously before intracoronary streptokinase application, with 34 patients treated with intracoronary streptokinase only [18]. Before institution of intracoronary streptokinase, 16 out of 35 pretreated patients showed patency of the infarct-related artery with good run-off of the contrast material, but only 1 of 34 patients without pre-treatment. Time until reperfusion was 3.2 hours in the intravenously pretreated group as compared to 4.5 hours in the group with intracoronary streptokinase only. Infarct size estimated from serial serum MB-CK activity curves and changes in the regional ejection fraction from before and 4 weeks after treatment revealed significant improvement only in the intravenously pretreated group.

Similar experiences have been made in the ongoing randomized controlled Rotterdam Intracoronary Trial. Dr Hugenholtz will deliberate on this in his presentation [19]. During the course of this trial the design was changed by adding pretreatment with intravenous streptokinase as soon as possible. Now there is a significant difference in early mortality in favor of the intracoronary group as compared to the control group. However, this significant difference originated only from that group pretreated with iv streptokinase. Without this early initiation of intravenous treatment there was no difference in the mortality rate between intracoronary streptokinase and control. It is a provocative question, how much the additional subsequent catheterization and intracoronary streptokinase after intravenous STK had actually added to the beneficial effect. Clearly, neither in the study of Schwarz et al nor in the Rotterdam Trial all patients needed this additional support, including early PTCA. It will be an important question for further research, how to identify those – may be about 30–40% – of the patients, who might get additional benefit from early catheterization, intracoronary streptokinase and/or PTCA.

## Urokinase

The other thrombolytic agent used for a long time for intravenous thrombolysis is urokinase. It is more expensive than streptokinase and relatively untested as far as treatment of myocardial infarction is concerned. In a prospective randomized, double-blind study with intracoronary infusion, the efficacy of 6.000 U/min urokinase was compared with 2.000 U/min streptokinase in 80 patients [20]. Treatment was initiated within 12 hours after symptom onset. The frequency of a successful opening of the infarct-related artery was similar for patients receiving urokinase (27 of 45, 60%) or streptokinase (20 of 35, 57%). Patients receiving urokinase had less systemic fibrinolysis and less perioperative bleeding with early surgery. In our earlier investigations we also did not find any apparent differences in the effectiveness of 500.000 units of streptokinase or 1 million units of urokinase intravenously [21]. We even had somewhat more bleeding complications with intravenous urokinase. This may have been just by chance and due to the fact that bleeding complications are more closely correlated with heparinization after thrombolysis rather than with streptokinase or urokinase itself [16, 21].

Mathey et al have treated 50 patients with an intravenous bolus injection of 2 million units urokinase, on the average 1.85 hours after onset of myocardial infarction. At angiography about 1 hour later, the infarct-related artery was found patent in 60% of the patients. There was a significant reduction in the infarct size in reperfused patients as compared to those, where the artery remained occluded [22].

## Thrombolysis in the absence of a lytic state?

Although streptokinase or urokinase can lyse coronary artery thrombi in the early hours of myocardial infarction, they are certainly no ideal agents for such a therapy. Thus, one of the most rapidly advancing areas of research in the field of thrombolytic therapy has been the search for new thrombolytic agents, particularly well-suited for use in evolving myocardial infarction. The first of these agents is the tissue-type plasminogen activator, which appears to be able to lyse clots rapidly without creating a severe systemic lytic state. Collen et al have identified a human melanoma all line that produced relatively large quantities of a biologically active tissue-type plasminogen activator [23]. In the experimental animal thrombolysis of a coronary clot was achieved within 10 minutes after intravenous injection of plasminogen activator, significantly faster than with either intracoronary or intravenous streptokinase or intravenous urokinase [24, 25]. A systemic lytic state was not observed. In a prospective randomized, placebo-controlled pilot trial patients with acute coronary thrombosis were treated with either intravenous recombinant human tissue-type plasminogen activator (rt-PA) or placebo two for one [26]. Time interval from onset of pain to iv rt-PA was 284 ± 99 minutes. Twentyfive of 33 patients (75%) receiving 0.5 to 0.75 mg/kg of rt-PA over 30 to 120 minutes had angiographically proven recanalization within 90 minutes of initiation of therapy. However, of those 25 patients with restoration of vascular patency, 5 (20%) exhibited reocclusion during the 30 minutes after discontinuation of infusion. Two other categories of compounds, acylated streptokinase-plasmin complex and pro-urokinase, which binds to fibrin only, show similar promise as agents that can affect discrete thrombolysis. The adantage of the streptokinase-plasmin complex is that it can be injected as a bolus intravenously. However, preliminary data suggest that considerable systemic fibrinolysis may occur and some severe bleeding complications have already been reported [27]. Clinicl trials will be needed to determine which, if any, of these new thrombolytic agents is preferable to streptokinase or urokinase for treatment of acute myocardial infarction.

**Recombinant human tissue-type plasminogen activator (rt-PA)**

The rt-PA is already somewhat more fully studied (Table 3). Recent results of a double-blind pilot study – TIMI A – are published, in which the effects of a 1 hour intravenous infusion of 1.5 million units of streptokinase are compared with a 3 hour intravenous infusion of 80 mg of rt-PA [28]. Angiography was performed prior and up to 90 minutes after the start of infusion. Within this time limit, in 60% of the patients treated with plasminogen activator a totally occluded infarct-related coronary artery was recanalized as compared to only 35% of the patients

Table 3. Data of two prospective randomized trials, in which the efficacy of iv rt-PA and iv STK (1.5 million units in 60 minutes) is compared.

| | rt-PA versus STK | |
| --- | --- | --- |
| | TIMI A | Europ. cooperat. |
| Onset MI to infusion | 4.8 h | 2.6–3.0 h |
| Angio | Prior and 90 min post-infusion | 75–90 min post-infusion |
| Patent | rt-PA 59/99 (60%) | 43/62 (70%) |
| IRA | STK 40/115 (35%) | 34/62 (55%) |
| Including | rt-PA _?_ | 48/62 (77%) |
| Subtotal | STK | 46/62 (75%) |

treated with streptokinase. There was no difference in bleeding complications between the two groups, that means, there are bleeding complications also in the rt-PA group. This is because with this high dose of 80 mg and a prolonged infusion of 3 hours, probably necessary to prevent early rethrombosis, a systemic lytic state also occurs with rt-PA. Early clinical reinfarction or extension, as assessed by the recurrence of chest pain and electrocardiographic and enzyme changes, was not different between the two groups. According to these data, plasminogen activator has almost twice the thrombolytic effectiveness of intravenous streptokinase with the same incidence of side-effects. The low recanalization rate of a totally occluded coronary artery of only 35% with intravenous streptokinase is at variance to the data of Table 2. The authors – the TIMI Study Group – who discussed some possible explanations for this, did not mention the most likely one. In the TIMI trial treatment was initiated rather late, up to 9 hours after myocardial infarction – on average 4.8 hours after symptom onset, and in only a very few patients within the first 3 hours. As discussed before, after such a time delay a higher recanalization rate cannot be expected within the 90 minutes of angiographic observation. A recanalization rate of 35% is exactly what we have found in our first studies, when treatment was initiated within 3–6 hours after symptom onset [17]. However, restoration of coronary blood flow in an infarct-related coronary artery 5–6 hours after onset of myocardial infarction is not what we are striving for. Substantial salvage of jeopardized myocardium can no longer be expected. For a fairer comparison of the effectiveness of iv streptokinase and rt-PA earlier initiation of treatment is needed (Table 3). The European Cooperative Study Group published results of such a study [29]. In this single-blind randomized trial patients with acute myocardial infarction of less than 6 hour duration were randomly treated with either 0.75 mg per kilogram of rt-PA over 90 minutes or with 1.5 million units of intravenous streptokinase over 60 minutes without pre-intervention angiography. Treatment was initiated on the average 2.6–3 hours after symptom onset as compared to 4.8 hours in the TIMI trial. Coronary angiography was performed 75–90 minutes after institution of treatment. Patent infarct-related coronary arteries were found in 70% of the plasminogen activator group as compared to 55% in the streptokinase group. There was no difference between the two treatment groups if still subtotally occluded coronary arteries at angiography 75–90 minutes post infusion were included, 77% versus 75%. It can be expected that after another 30 minutes or so these patients with still subtotal occlusion will have further lysis of the thrombus with substantial improvement of coronary blood flow. Thus, although undoubtedly rt-PA is superior to streptokinase, the differences are not as striking as suggested in the TIMI trial, if treatment is initiated early. And early treatment is of utmost importance in any case.

In the European Cooperative Study activation of the systemic fibrinolytic system was far less pronounced with rt-PA than with streptokinase. Until discharge there was a definite reinfarction in 2 patients of the rt-PA group as compared to 4 STK-patients. However, during the first 48 hours after end of infusion 14 in the rt-PA group had chest pain without reinfarction as compared to 5 patients in the STK group. At discharge there was a slight or definite limitation in their functional status in 27 versus 19 patients.

## Conclusion

Actual restoration of coronary blood flow will occur in most patients with either intravenous infusion of rt-PA or iv or ic streptokinase (or urokinase, respectively). Expeditious initiation of treatment with either thrombolytic agent is of major importance. Lysis with tissue-type plasminogen activator is faster, and in so far it appears to represent a major advance in thrombolysis. However, early and late mortality, reinfarction and reocclusion rate used to be assessed and compared in trials of sufficient scope. Some trials, which can be expected to have sufficient power to demonstrate efficacy and safety of thrombolysis in acute myocardial infarction are in progress or in the planning phase.

## Large controlled trials in progress

ISAM – intravenous streptokinse in acute myocardial infarction – is a prospective placebo-controlled double-blind multicenter trial. It was started in March 1982 in Germany, Switzerland and Toronto, Canada. 1.741 patients were included at the end of the recruitment phase in March 1985. Patients of both sexes up to the age of 75 years inclusive, with typical myocardial infarction symptoms and signs, until maximally 6 hours after onset of the acute event are treated with either 1.5 million of streptokinase or matching placebo. The primary endpoint is short-term, that means 21 days, and long-term mortality. Secondary endpoints are comparison of the functional results between the two groups by serial serum CK-MB activity curves, cardiac catheterization and angiography after 3–4 weeks with determination of patency of the infarct-related coronary artery, global ejection fraction, regional ejection fraction, left ventricular hemodynamics during rest and exercise as well as ECG follow-up and exercise ECG after 7 months. The results obtained in patients treated within 3 hours and 3–6 hours after onset of myocardial infarction will be compared. Data about early mortality will be available in late summer this year.

GISSI – a large Italian trial, has been started in January 1984. It is directed only to compare the effect of 1.5 million units of streptokinase intravenously or matching placebo given within 12 hours after onset of pain on hospital- and 1 year mortality. There are 177 hospitals participating. 12.000 patients shall be recruited and about 8.000 patients have already been included in 1984. The assumption is a 20% reduction in mortality.

Recruitment has just started for ISIS-2 – Second International Study of Infarct Survival. About 20.000 patients shall be recruited worldwide with the Coordinating Center located in Oxford. More than 500 hospitals are expected to start recruitment within the next two months or so. The trial also has a relatively simple design. It is expected that the 20.000 patients are recruited within 12 to 15 months. Patients will be included up to 24 hours after onset of pain, because there might be – although without salvage of jeopardized myocardium – a more benign long-term course in patients with a patent infarct-related coronary artery as compared to those, where the infarct artery remains occluded.

ISIS-2 has a 4-group design. Patients will be treated with 1.5 million units of STK and 160 mg of aspirin per day. 5.000 patients will get placebo STK and placebo aspirin, 5.000 patients placebo STK and active ASA, 5.000 active STK and placebo ASA, and 5.000 patients active STK and active ASA. Thus, one will have a subtotal of 10.000 patients with placebo STK and 10.000 patients with active STK as well as 10.000 patients with placebo ASA and 10.000 patients with active ASA. Whether the patients will get in addition heparin and/or anticoagulation is up to the discretion of the responsible physician.

After finalizing the pilot study TIMI A it is planned to start a large study in the U.S.A. summer of 1985, sponsored by the NIH, where the effects of a 3 hour intravenous infusion of 80 mg of rt-PA shall be compared with matching placebo. As in the three other trials, there will be no baseline angiography. Only patients presenting within 4 hours after onset of myocardial infarction will be included. About 3.500 patients shall be recruited and mortality assessed during 1–3 years of follow-up.

These large trials are expected to ascertain the true impact of intravenous thrombolysis upon short- and long-term morbidity and mortality as well as the complications rates introduced by such treatment. They may also recognize different outlooks according to anatomic and functional subsets, for example inferior and anterior myocardial infarction, large and small myocardial infarction, and on the relationship of possible beneficial effects on the time interval from symptom onset to initiation of treatment.

## References

1. Mazel MS, Parsa F, Riera R (1975) The use of urokinase in acute myocardial infarction: Report of two cases. J Am Geriatrics Soc XXIII: 419–25
2. Schröder R, Biamino G, von Leitner ER, Linderer T, Prokein E, Schäfer JH, Sörensen R, Grassot A (1980) Comparison of the effects of intracoronary and systemic streptokinase infusion in acute myocardial infarction: Preliminary results. In: Unstable Angina Pectoris, Rafflenbeul W, Lichtlen PR, Balcon R (eds), Georg Thieme Verlag Stuttgart-New York, 167–75
3. Rogers WJ, Baxley WA, Hood WP, Mantle JA (1983) Prospective randomized trial of intravenous vs intracoronary streptokinase in myocardial infarction. J Am Coll Cardiol 1 (2): 629 (abstr)

348

4. Rogers WJ, Mantle JA, Hood WP, Baxley WA, Whitlow PL, Reeves RC, Soto B (1983) Prospective randomized trial of intravenous and intracoronary streptokinase in acute myocardial infarction. Circulation 68: 1051–61

5. Rogers WJ, Hood WP, Reeves RC, Whitlow PL (1984) Randomized trial of intracoronary versus intravenous streptokinase in acute myocardial infarction. JACC 3 (2): 525 (abstr)

6. Schröder R, Biamino G, von Leitner ER, Linderer T, Heitz J, Vöhringer HF, Wegscheider K, Andresen D, Arntz HR, Brüggemann T, Grassot A, Lichey J, Oeff M, Prokein E, Schäfer JH, Sörensen R (1982) Systemische Thrombolyse mit Streptokinase-Kurzzeitinfusion bei akutem Myokardinfarkt. Z Kardiol 71: 709–18

7. Ganz W, Geft I, Shah PK, Lew AS, Rodriguez L, Weiss T, Maddahi J, Berman DS, Charuzi Y, Swan HJC (1984) Intravenous streptokinase in evolving myocardial infarction. Am J Cardiol 53: 1209–16

8. Taylor GJ, Mikell FL, Moses HW, Dove JT, Batchelder JE, Thull A, Hansen S, Wellons HA, Schneider JA (1984) Intravenous versus intracoronary streptokinase therapy for acute myocardial infarction in community hospitals. Am J Cardiol 54: 256–60

9. Valentine RP, Pitts DE, Brooks-Brunn JA, Williams JG, Van Hove E, Schmidt PE (1985) Intravenous versus intracoronary streptokinase in acute myocardial infarction. Am J Cardiol 55: 309–12

10. Anderson JL, Marshall HW, Lutz JR, Sorensen SG, Askins JC, Hagen AD (1984) A randomized trial of intracoronary versus intravenous streptokinase in myocardial infarction. JACC 3 (2): 526

11. Schröder R, Biamino G, von Leitner ER, Linderer T (1981) Intravenöse Streptokinase-Infusion bei akutem Myokardinfarkt. Dtsch Med Wschr 106: 294–301

12. Neuhaus KL, Kreuzer H, Sauer G, Thiemann U, Köstering H (1983) Intravenöse Streptokinase-Kurzinfusion beim akuten Myokardinfarkt. Hämostaseologie 2: 38–43

13. Blunda M, Wolf NM, Singh S, Mandelkorn J, Kersh R, Pickering N, Shechter J, Rodgers D, Workman M, Meister SG (1983) Intravenous vs intracoronary streptokinase to reopen occluded coronary arteries: Preliminary results. Circulation 66: II-184

14. Huhmann W, Nieht H (1983) Was leistet die systemische Lyse beim akuten Herzinfarkt? Z Kardiol 72: 67

15. Spann JF, Sherry S, Carabello BA, Denenberg BS, Mann RH, McCann WD, Gault JH, Gentzler RD, Belber AD, Mauerer AH, Cooper EM (1984) Coronary thrombolysis by intravenous streptokinase in acute myocardial infarction: Acute and follow-up studies. Am J Cardiol 53: 655–61

16. Alderman EL, Jutzy KR, Berte LE, Miller RG, Friedman JP, Creger WP, Eliastam M (1984) Randomized comparison of intravenous versus intracoronary streptokinase for myocardial infarction. Am J Cardiol 54: 14–19

17. Schröder R, Biamino G, von Leitner ER, Linderer T, Brüggemann T, Heitz J, Vöhringer HF, Wegscheider K (1983) Intravenaous short-term infusion of streptokinase in acute myocardial infarction. Circulation 67: 536–48

18. Schwarz F, Hofmann M, Schuler G, Kübler W (1983) Combined intravenous and intracoronary versus intracoronary streptokinase therapy in acute myocardial infarction. J Am Coll Cardiol 3 (2): 615

19. Hugenholtz P, et al (in this issue)

20. Tennant SN, Dixon J, Venable TC, Page HL, Roach A, Kaiser AB, Frederiksen R, Tacogue L, Kaplan P, Babu NS, Anderson EE, Wooten E, Jennings HS, Breinig J, Campbell WB (1984) Intracoronary thrombolysis in patients with acute myocardial infarction: comparison of the efficacy of urokinase with streptokinase. Circulation 69: 756–60

21. Schröder R, Biamino G, von Leitner ER (1982) Systemic short-time thrombolysis in acute myocardial infarction. In: Transluminal Coronary Angioplasty and Intracoronary Thrombolysis; Coronary Heart Disease IV, Kaltenbach M, Grüntzig A, Rentrop K, Bussmann WD (eds), Springer-Verlag Berlin, Heidelberg, New York, 322–40

22. Mathey DG, Schofer J, Sheehan FH, Tilsner V (1985) Die intravenöse Urokinase-Bolusinjektion beim akuten Herzinfarkt. Frühjahrstg. d. Dtsch. Ges.f. Herz-u. Kreislauff, 107 (abstr. no. 387)

23. Collen D, Rijken DC, Van Damme J, Biliau A (1982) Purification of human tissue-type plasminogen activator in centigram quantities for human melanoma cell culture fluid and its conditioning for use in vivo. Thromb Hemostas 48: 294–60

24. Bergman SR, Fox KAA, Ter-Pogossian MM, Sobel Be, Collen D (1983) Clotselective coronary thrombolysis with tissue-type plasminogen activator. Science 220: 1181–83

25. Van de Werf F, Bergmann SR, Keith A, Fox A, De Geest H, Hoyng CF, Sobel BE, Collen D (1984) Coronary thrombolysis with intravenously administered human tissue-type plasminogen activator produced by recombinant DNA technology. Circulation 69: 605–10

26. Collen D, Topol EJ, Tiefenbrunn AJ, Gold HK, Weisfeldt ML, Sobel BE, Leinbach RC, Brinker JA, Ludbrook PA, Yasuda I, Bulkley BH, Robison AK, Hutter AM, Bell WR, Spadaro JJ, Khaw BA, Grossbard EB (1984) Coronary thrombolysis with recombinant human tissue-type plasminogen activator: a prospective, randomized, placebo-controlled trial. Circulation 70: 1012–17

27. Been M, De Bono DP, Muir AL, Boulton FE, Hillis WS, Hornung R (1985) Coronary thrombolysis with intravenous anisoylated plasminogen-streptokinase complex BRL 26921. Br Heart J 53: 253–59

28. The TIMI Study Group (1985) The thrombolysis in myocardial infarction (TIMI) trial: Phase I fingings. New Engl J Med 312: 932–36

29. Verstraete M Bernard R, Bory M, Brower RW, Collen D, De Bono DP, Erbel R, Huhmann W, Lennane RJ, Lubsen J, Matthey D, Meyer J, Michels HR, Rutsch W, Schartl M, Schmidt W, Uebis R, von Essen R (1985) Randomized trial of intravenous recombinant tissue-type plasminogen activator versus intravenous streptokinase in acute myocardial infarction. Lancet, April 13: 842–47

# Percutaneous transluminal coronary angioplasty associated with thrombolysis in acute myocardial infarction: evaluation by angiographic, scintigraphic and enzymatic data

F. SCHWARZ, H.C. MEHMEL, G. SCHÜLER, M. HOFMANN, J. MANTHEY, and W. KÜBLER

## Summary

All patients who received percutaneous transluminal coronary angioplasty (PTCA) immediately after thrombolysis of acute transmural myocardial infarction (AMI) during the last 12 months (n = 26, group 1) were evaluated. Indications for PTCA were (1) ineffective thrombolysis (n = 10), and (2) high grade residual stenosis with symptoms and signs of ischemia after thrombolysis (n = 16). A group of patients with AMI treated previously and revealing similar coronary anatomy and symptoms after thrombolysis (which today are indications for PTCA but to that time did not receive it, n = 26, group 2) was retrospectively selected for comparison (matched pairs). Left ventricular and coronary angiography were carried out acutely and 4 weeks after AMI, thallium-201 scintigraphy was performed before and 24 hours after the procedure, and serum creatine kinase activity was measured every 8 hours for 3 days. Before treatment, group 1 and group 2 showed comparable stenosis of infarct vessel (96 vs 97%, NS), ejection fraction (49 vs 49%, NS), regional ejection fraction of infarct areas (26 vs 25%, NS), thallium-201 perfusion defect (39 vs 40%, NS), and serum creatine kinase activity (56 vs 56 U/l, NS). Primary successful recanalization was achieved in 23 of 26 patients (88%) of group 1 as compared to only 16 of 26 patients (62%) of group 2 (p<0.05). Stenosis immediately after treatment was 50% in group 1 and 92% in group 2 (p<0.001), stenosis after 4 weeks averaged 34% in group 1 and 84% in group 2 (p<0.001). Four weeks after treatment, ejection fraction (57 vs 45%, p<0.01), and regional ejection fraction of infarct area 37 vs 24%, p<0.001) were higher in group 1 than in group 2. Thallium-201 perfusion defect 24 hours after treatment was lower in group 1 than in group 2 for patients with anterior AMI (32 vs 45%, p<0.05) but not for patients with inferior AMI (15 vs 13%, NS). Peak serum creatine kinase activity was lower in group 1 than in group 2 (1267 vs 1843 U/l, p = 0.07, NS).

We conclude, PTCA associated with thrombolysis in AMI increased the rate of primary success as compared to a control group. PTCA reduced the stenosis of infarct vessel and improved contractile function as well as perfusion of infarct areas in selected patients in whom thrombolysis failed.

## Introduction

Data have been presented in individual patients which show dramatic improvement of symptoms, left ventricular function and myocardial perfusion after successful reperfusion of acute transmural myocardial infarction (AMI), however, controlled clinical trials elicited conflicting results [1–5]. From these observations it can be concluded that reperfusion may limit infarct size in man but the procedure and the selection process of patients are still not perfectly developed. Before final evaluation of the procedure it seems necessary (1) to find therapeutic measures to shorten the ischemic period, (2) to establish clearcut indications for subsequent revascularization as a prevention against reocclusion, and (3) to identify those patients who may benefit from the procedure [6, 7]. Several attempts have been made to improve the therapeutic procedure by surgical revascularization [8] and by percutaneous transluminal coronary angioplasty (PTCA) [9–12]. The results of previous studies are difficult to interprete (1) since a comparable control group is lacking [8], (2) because no clearcut indications for PTCA were established, and (3) since salvage of jeopardized myocardium was not demonstrated [10, 11, 12].

The purpose of the present study was therefore (1) to establish indications for PTCA in association with thrombolysis of AMI, and (2) to present angiographic, scintigraphic, and enzymatic data (characterizing infarct size) after PTCA in comparison with a control group which had thrombolysis without PTCA.

## Methods

### Patients

Between may 1982 and may 1983, 58 patients with acute transmural myocardial infarction (AMI) underwent thrombolysis to recanalize the obstructed coronary artery. Twenty-six patients thereof had immediate percutaneous transluminal coronary angioplasty (PTCA) (group 1) because of (1) unsuccessful thrombolysis ($n = 10$), and (2) high grade residual stenosis (>75% diameter reduction) of the infarct vessel ($n = 16$) with continuing or recurring chest pain and ST segment elevation. A control group was established as follows: between may 1981 and may 1982, 63 patients with AMI underwent thrombolysis without PTCA. Their coronary cineangiograms were retrospectively reviewed and on the basis of coronary morphology at the end of thrombolysis 29 patients were found who fullfilled indications for PTCA. From these 29 patients, 26 patients were selected as 'matched pairs' (group 2). Unsuccessful thrombolysis was present in 10 patients and high grade residual stenosis was found in 16 patients at the termination of thrombolysis. Diagnosis of AMI was based on (1) acute chest pain lasting longer than 30 minutes, and (2) persistent ST-segment elevation of more than 2 mm in at least 3 leads of the standard 12 lead electrocardiogram progressing to new Q-waves. Not accepted to the study were (1) patients with symptoms of more than 4 hours at entry into the coronary care unit, (2) patients over 75 years of age, and (3) patients with contraindications to streptokinase therapy. Clinical status before treatment was categorized according to Killip [13]. Before treatment, patients gave written informed consent after detailed explanation of the procedure, its possible hazards, and possible beneficial effects.

*Treatment*

Patients received 250 mg prednisolone intravenously and were treated with continuous intravenous infusion of streptokinase (1.5 million U in 50 ml saline over a period of 90 minutes) which was started in the coronary care unit immediately after consent. Intracoronary infusion of streptokinase followed after completion of left ventricular and coronary angiography [1, 2]. In 5 patients of group 1 and in 10 patients of group 2 only intracoronary infusion of streptokinase was performed. Patients were catheterized by the femoral percutaneous technique (Cordis 8F introducing sheath). Monoplane left ventricular cineangiograms were performed (30° right anterior oblique projection). After occlusion (total or subtotal) of the infarct vessel had been confirmed, intracoronary injection of 0.2 mg nitroglycerin was given, and contrast material injection was repeated. Neither nitroglycerin nor contrast agent led to recanalization. Streptokinase was continuously infused through the coronary catheter (2000–4000 U/min) until a maximal dose of 200 000 U. Contrast material injections were repeated every 15 minutes. If streptokinase infusion was ineffective in group 1, a 8F guiding catheter (Schneider-Medintag) was placed in the coronary ostium. The dilatation catheter was advanced into stenosis under fluoroscopic and pressure control [14]. Usually, a 3 mm balloon was used and several inflations were performed (20 to 30 seconds, 5 to 10 atmospheres). The sheath was left in place for 24 to 36 hours. In 19 patients of group 1 PTCA was performed within the same session after thrombolysis, in the remaining 7 patients PTCA followed 1 to 2 days later. If streptokinase infusion was ineffective in group 2 the procedure was given up at maximum dose of 200 000 U (intracoronary infusion).

Blood coagulation was checked twice daily. Fibrinogen was measured by the Clauss method [15]. Heparin was administered to maintain the partial thromboplastin time at 2 to 3 times the control value for at least 3 days. Administration of aspirin (330 mg twice daily) and dipyridamole (75 mg twice daily) was then started and continued for at least 6 months. Creatine kinase activity was determined from venous blood which was sampled in 8 hourly intervals for 3 days ([16], normal range up to 80 U/l). Left ventricular and coronary angiography were repeated 4 weeks after AMI before discharge of the patient from hospital.

## Analysis of angiograms

The angiograms were evaluated independently by 2 experienced observers. From 2 angiographic views coronary obstructions were measured and averaged (percent diameter reduction). Successful angioplasty was defined as at least 20% increase in the diameter of the lumen [17]. The angiographic ejection fraction (EF) was calculated and the regional EF was determined with the area method of Gelberg et al [18] as previously described [19]. The area system measured systolic area reduction in % of enddiastolic area. Areas corresponding to the perfusion area of the infarct vessel (anterior AMI: areas 1, 2, and 3; inferior AMI: areas 3, 4, and 5) and normal areas were averaged. Interobserver variability was 6% for EF and 4% for regional EF.

## Thallium-201 scintigraphy

Details of the technique used in our institution were previously described (20). After initial evaluation 2.0 mCi of thallium-201 were injected intravenously. Imaging was performed with a mobile gamma camera (Picker Dyna Mo) equipped with a seven pinhole collimator (aperture size 5.5 mm) immediately before and 24 hours after catheterization. The camera head was positioned over the cardiac apex in a 40–45° left lateral projection to align it with the long axis of the left ventricle. A 30% symmetric energy window centered on the 80 KeV peak was used. A total number of 2.5 million counts was collected. Twenty-four hours later, another dose of thallium-201 was injected and a second image was recorded. All data were transferred on line to a computer (DEC PDP 11/34). Eight cross-sectional planes through the left ventricular myocardium, perpendicular to the long axis, were reconstructed using a commercially available computer algorithm [21, 22]. To define area with decreased thallium-201 uptake, all reconstructed myocardial cross sections were analysed by a semiquantitative program described by Vogel et al [22]. The results are displayed as a circumferential plot over 360°. Abnormal myocardial sections are identified by comparing each circumferential plot to the lower limits of normal. The mean of all cross sections was calculated and expressed as a fraction of left ventricular circumference (% perfusion defect). Interobserver variability of analysis was 9%.

354

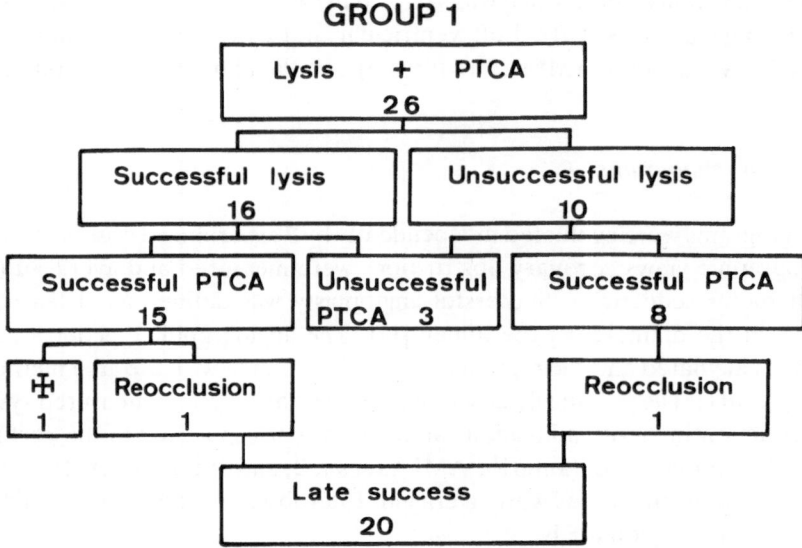

*Figure 1.* Follow-up results of patients of group 1 treated with thrombolysis (lysis) and percutaneous transluminal coronary angioplasty (PTCA).

## Statistics

Averaged data are presented as means ± SD. Student's t-test was used to compare 2 groups. Chi-square analysis was performed for data 2 × K contingency tables (Brandt-Snedecor test) [23].

## Results

### Clinical and angiographic characteristics

Before treatment, no significant differences were noted between the 2 groups with respect to sex, age, Killip class at entry into coronary care unit, location of infarction, incidence of previous infarction, and localization of infarct vessel (Table 1). Total coronary occlusion at first coronary injection was observed in 18 of 26 patients (69%) of group 1 and in 19 of 26 patients (73%) of group 2 (NS). No patient had recanalization after intracoronary nitroglycerin administration. The time interval between onset of symptoms and catheterization was 3.1 hours in group 1 and 3.3 hours in group 2 (NS, Table 1).

Primary successful recanalization was achieved in 23 of 26 patients (88%) of group 1 as compared to only 16 of 26 patients (62%) of group 2 (p<0.05).

Figure 1 illustrates the follow-up results of group 1. It is evident that successful thrombolysis occurred in 16 patients but unsuccessful thrombolysis was seen in 10 patients. From the latter 10 patients 8 had immediate successful PTCA but in 2 patients PTCA was unsuccessful. In this subgroup one late reocclusion (with clinical signs of reinfarction) was seen (Fig. 1). In the 16 patients with successful thrombolysis but high grade residual stenosis PTCA was successful in 15 patients but was unsuccessful in 1 patient in whom the infarct vessel became occluded during PTCA. Among the 15 patients with successful PTCA 1 patient died and one patient had reocclusion of the infarct vessel (without clinical signs of reinfarction).

Figure 2 displays the follow-up results of group 2. Sixteen patients had successful thrombolysis but in 10 patients thrombolysis was ineffective. In the latter subgroup 2 patients died. Among the 16 patients with successful thrombolysis 4 patients had reocclusion of the infarct vessel (3 with clinical signs of reinfarction).

*Table 1.* Clinical and angiographic characteristics of patients in the 2 groups of treatment.

| | Group 1 | Group 2 | p-value |
|---|---|---|---|
| Number of patients | 26 | 26 | |
| Male sex | 23 (88%) | 25 (96%) | NS |
| Age (years), mean ± SD | 52 ± 8 | 54 ± 12 | NS |
| Killip class (mean ± SD) | 1.4 ± 0.6 | 1.2 ± 0.4 | NS |
| Location of infarction | | | |
| Anterior | 15 (58%) | 15 (58%) | NS |
| Inferior | 11 (42%) | 11 (42%) | NS |
| Previous infarction | 5 (19%) | 2 (8%) | NS |
| Infarct vessel | | | |
| Anterior descending coronary artery proximal to first septal branch | 8 (31%) | 9 (35%) | NS |
| Anterior descending coronary artery distal to first septal branch | 7 (27%) | 6 (23%) | NS |
| Left circumflex coronary artery | 1 (4%) | 1 (4%) | NS |
| Right coronary artery | 10 (38%) | 10 (38%) | NS |
| Type of occlusion at first coronary injection | | | |
| total | 18 (69%) | 19 (73%) | NS |
| subtotal | 8 (31%) | 7 (27%) | NS |
| Hours (mean ± SD) to catheterization from onset of symptoms | 3.1 ± 1.0 | 3.3 ± 0.9 | NS |
| Successful recanalization | 23 (88%) | 16 (62%) | <0.05 |
| Occlusion due to PTCA | 1 (4%) | – | – |
| Hours (mean ± SD) to reperfusion from onset of symptoms 3.8 ± 1.1 (n = 23) 3.9 ± 0.9 (n = 16) NS | | | |
| Angiographic reocclusion after recanalization within 4 weeks | 2 (9%) | 4 (25%) | NS |
| Deaths in hospital | 1 (4%) | 2 (8%) | NS |

## GROUP 2

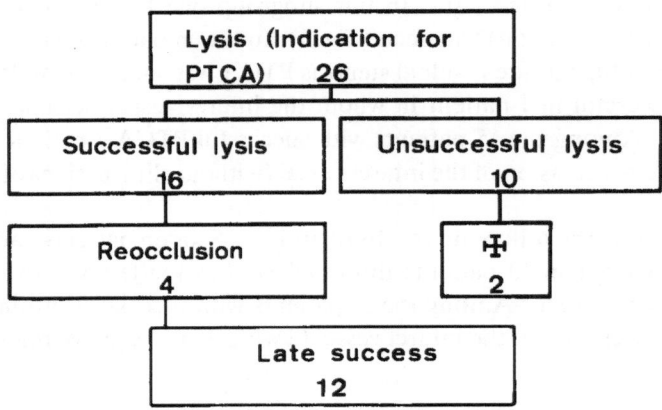

*Figure 2.* Follow-up results of patients of group 2 (treated with thrombolysis (lysis) who today would represent candidates for percutaneous transluminal coronary angioplasty (PTCA) but did not receive it at the time of their intervention.

The time interval from onset of symptoms to reperfusion was 3.8 hours in group 1 and 3.9 hours in group 2 (NS, Table 1).

The number of the late successes (primary success and no evidence of reocclusion) was 20 of 26 patients (77%) in group 1 (Fig. 1) as compared to only 12 of 26 patients (46%) in group 2 (Fig. 2, p = 0.05).

*Follow-up data*

Figure 3 shows that the degree of stenosis of infarct vessel was comparable before and immediately after thrombolysis among groups. After PTCA, however, stenosis was significantly reduced in group 1 as compared to group 2 and this difference persisted after 4 weeks (Fig. 3). An angiographic restudy could be performed in 20 patients of group 1 and in 21 patients of group 2. The following reasons account for lack of a restudy in group 1: one patient died during AMI (successful PTCA), and 5 patients refused restudy (2 patients after successful PTCA and 3 patients after unsuccessful thrombolysis and PTCA). In group 2, a restudy could not be performed in 5 patients: two patients refused restudy after successful thrombolysis (1 without and 1 patient with clinical signs of reocclusion). Two other patients died during AMI (unsuccessful thrombolysis) and 1 patient refused (unsuccessful thrombolysis). It is evident that the number of patients without angiographic restudy was similar in group 1 and group 2, furthermore, the type of AMI in dropouts (successful vs unsuccessful recanalization) was also comparable.

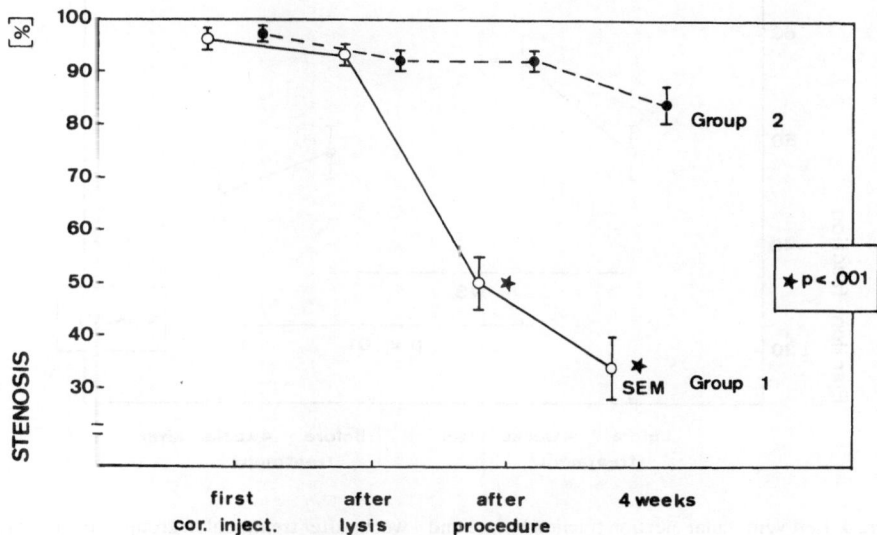

*Figure 3.* Diameter stenosis of infarct vessel at first coronary injection, after thrombolysis (lysis), after procedure (i.e. in group 1: PTCA; in group 2: thrombolysis), and 4 weeks after infarction. Significant differences existed after procedure and at 4 weeks.

Left ventricular EF increased significantly from 49 to 57% in group 1 but fell slightly in group 2 (49 to 45%). As depicted in Figure 4 EF was higher 4 weeks after treatment in group 1 than in group 2. This difference was due to changes of regional EF of infarct area as illustrated in Figure 5: regional EF of infarct area increased in group 1 but remained unchanged in group 2. Four weeks after AMI regional EF of infarct area was higher in group 1 than in group 2. Regional EF of normal area remained essentially unchanged in both groups (Table 2).

Before treatment, the thallium-201 perfusion defect was similar in both groups, 24 hours after treatment a significant reduction occurred in both groups. The perfusion defect 24 hours after treatment was smaller in group 1 than in group 2 (but the difference was not significant. Complete thallium-201 data were obtained in 18 patients of group 1 and in 21 patients of group 2. In group 1 eight patients had either no (n = 5) or only incomplete (n = 3) thallium-201 scintigrams, in group 2, 5 patients had no thallium-201 scintigrams.

Serum creatine kinase activity before treatment was within normal limits in both groups. The peak creatine kinase activity was lower in group 1 (1267 U/l) than in group 2 (1843 U/l) but the difference was not significant (p = 0.07, NS).

Table 3 lists the perfusion defects in the 2 groups subdivided according to location of AMI. Before treatment, perfusion defects were comparable between groups in patients with anterior and in patients with inferior AMI. The defects in

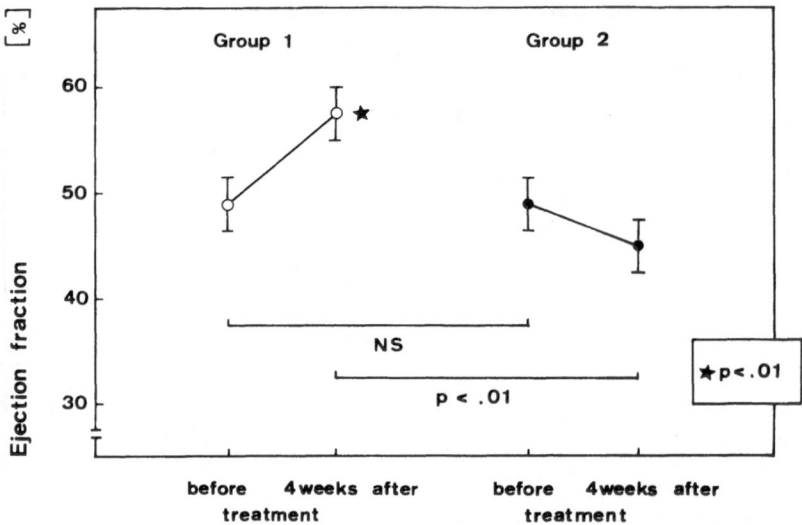

*Figure 4.* Left ventricular ejection fraction before and 4 weeks after treatment in group 1 and in group 2. Patients of group 1 revealed improvement after 4 weeks but patients of group 2 showed no significant change. Baseline values were not different between groups but at 4 weeks ejection fraction was higher in group 1 as compared to group 2.

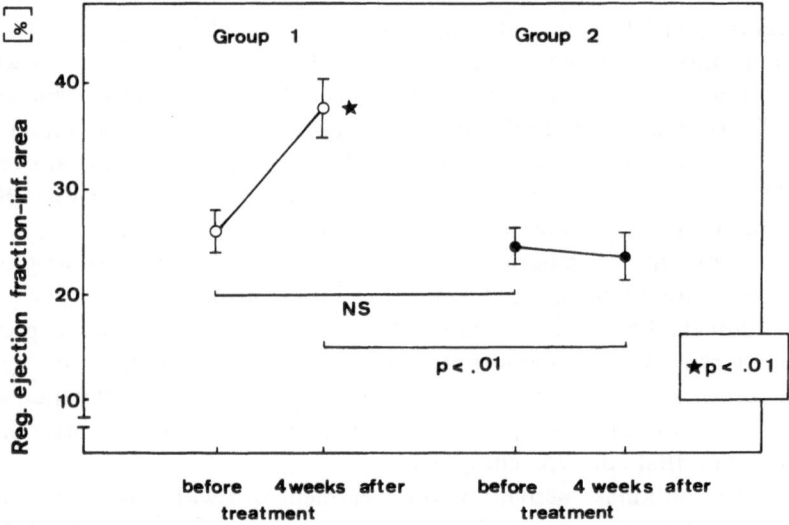

*Figure 5.* Regional ejection fraction of infarct area before and 4 weeks after treatment in group 1 and in group 2. Patients of group 1 showed improvement after 4 weeks but patients of group 2 did not. Baseline values did not differ between groups but at 4 weeks regional ejection fraction was higher in group 1 than in group 2.

anterior AMI measured nearly twice the defects in inferior AMI. Twenty-four hours after treatment, the perfusion defects in patients with anterior AMI were smaller in group 1 as compared to those in group 2 (Fig. 6). In contrast, in patients with inferior AMI no significant difference of perfusion defects 24 hours after treatment was found between groups (Table 3).

## Hospital course and complications

Cause of death was cardiogenic shock in one patient of group 1. This patient had old inferior infarction 3 years before and aortocoronary bypass operation (2 grafts) 2 years preceding the present episode. The bypass grafts to the right

Table 2. Follow-up data of patients in the 2 groups of treatment.

|  | Group 1 | Group 2 | p-value |
|---|---|---|---|
| Number of patients | 26 | 26 | |
| Stenosis of infarct vessel (%) | | | |
| at first coronary injection | $96 \pm 8$ | $97 \pm 6$ | NS |
| after thrombolysis | $93 \pm 8$ | $92 \pm 8$ | NS |
| immediately after procedure | $50 \pm 26$ | $92 \pm 8$ | <0.001 |
| 4 weeks after procedure | $34 \pm 28$ | $84 \pm 21$ | <0.001 |
| | (n = 20) | (n = 21) | |
| Hemodynamic data (mean $\pm$ SD) | | | |
| Left ventricular ejection fraction (%) | | | |
| before treatment | $49 \pm 10$ | $49 \pm 10$ | NS |
| 4 weeks after treatment | $57 \pm 11$ xx | $45 \pm 12$ | <0.01 |
| | (n = 20) | (n = 21) | |
| Regional ejection fraction of infarct area (%) | | | |
| before treatment | $26 \pm 9$ | $25 \pm 8$ | NS |
| 4 weeks after treatment | $37 \pm 12$ xx | $24 \pm 11$ | <0.001 |
| | (n = 20) | (n = 21) | |
| Regional ejection fraction of normal area (%) | | | |
| before treatment | $44 \pm 18$ | $46 \pm 18$ | NS |
| 4 weeks after treatment | $45 \pm 18$ | $42 \pm 16$ | NS |
| | (n = 20) | (n = 21) | |
| Thallium-201 perfusion defect (%) | | | |
| before treatment | $39 \pm 18$ | $40 \pm 15$ | NS |
| 24 hours after treatment | $25 \pm 16$ xx | $33 \pm 18$ xx | NS |
| | (n = 18) | (n = 21) | |
| Serum creatine kinase activity (U/l) | | | |
| before treatment | $56 \pm 33$ | $56 \pm 34$ | NS |
| peak value | $1267 \pm 884$ | $1843 \pm 1238$ | NS |
| | (n = 24) | (n = 25) | |

xx = p<0.01 as compared to before treatment (paired t-test), numbers in brackets indicate number of patients in whom paired data were obtained.

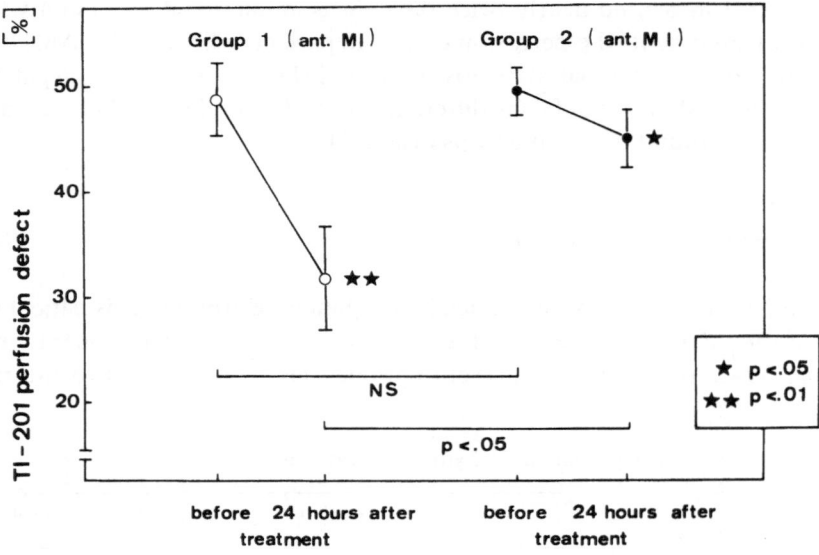

*Figure 6.* Thallium-201 perfusion defects before and 24 hours after treatment for patients with anterior myocardial infarction (ant.MI) in group 1 and in group 2. Before treatment, no significant change was seen between groups but 24 hours later the average perfusion defect was smaller in group 1 than in group 2.

coronary artery and to the left anterior descending artery were documented to be occluded by angiography 5 months after operation. The patient presented with extensive transmural anterior AMI and the left anterior descending coronary artery was acutely occluded proximal to the first septal branch. After thrombolysis a 95% stenosis was seen and PTCA was performed because of persisting pain and ST-segment elevation. Despite primary successful PTCA the patient

*Table 3.* Thallium-201 perfusion defects in the 2 groups subdivided according to location of infarction.

|  | Group 1 | Group 2 | p-value |
|---|---|---|---|
| Thallium-201 perfusion defect (%) |  |  |  |
| Anterior infarction |  |  |  |
| number of patients | 11 | 13 |  |
| before treatment | 48 ± 12 | 50 ± 8 | NS |
| 24 hours after treatment | 32 ± 16 | 45 ± 10 | <0.05 |
| Inferior infarction |  |  |  |
| number of patients | 7 | 8 |  |
| before treatment | 27 ± 20 | 24 ± 8 | NS |
| 24 hours after treatment | 15 ± 7 | 13 ± 7 | NS |

died 2 hours after the procedure. Autopsy revealed 65% stenosis at the site of PTCA without residual thrombus and a large fresh transmural anterior necrosis as well as an old inferior scar. Two patients of group 2 died in hospital: one of cardiogenic shock after large anterior AMI with extension of infarction (unsuccessful thrombolysis), the other patient died suddenly 3 weeks after anterior AMI (unsuccessful thrombolysis). The latter patient had suffered an inferior infarction 3 years ago.

A 62 years old female patient with single vessel disease and inferior AMI had reocclusion of infarct vessel due to PTCA 2 days after initially successful thrombolysis. She developed an uncomplicated reinfarction.

Bleeding complications were observed in 3 patients. Two patients had upper gastrointestinal bleeding (one in group 1 and the other in group 2) which was treated medically and 1 patient had groin hematoma (not requiring surgical therapy).

The fibrinogen level fell below 50 mg% after treatment in the majority of cases while partial thromboplastin time was prolonged to 2 to 5 times control value. No patient of group 1 but 2 patients of group 2 underwent coronary bypass surgery within 3 months after AMI.

## Discussion

PTCA was used in this study as a complementary therapeutic approach to thrombolysis. The indications for PTCA were (1) ineffective recanalization by thrombolysis, and (2) high grade residual stenosis with continuing or recurring chest pain and ST-segment elevation.

PTCA was attempted although stenosis of infarct vessel was very severe (group 1 = 96%). Furthermore, PTCA was successfully performed in 8 of 10 cases with complete vessel occlusion resistant to thrombolysis. From these data it is evident that group 1 consisted of a selected population of patients not indentical with the usual population treated by thrombolysis: a major subgroup (38%) had primary unsuccessful thrombolysis. The data show that PTCA can be safely performed in these cases with total occlusion of infarct vessel who failed to respond to thrombolysis. Thus, ineffective recanalization by thrombolysis is suggested as a major indication for PTCA in patients with AMI.

A second indication for PTCA was the presence of high grade residual stenosis after thrombolysis with continuing or recurring chest pain and ST-segment elevation. Pain was taken as an indicator of myocardial ischemia, it was anticipated that ischemic myocardial tissue could be salvaged after recanalization by PTCA. Since revascularization of necrotic tissue would be a procedure of doubtful value, PTCA was not attempted in cases without symptoms. It has been suggested to treat residual coronary stenosis after successful thrombolysis routinely by PTCA [11]. Whether this approach is justified remains to be clarified: no evidence of reduction of infarct size was presented when patients with AMI and PTCA were compared to patients without PTCA after thrombolysis. Futhermore, the rate of reinfarction was not significantly reduced after PTCA, although the symptomatic state of patients seemed to be improved [11]. In summary, our present approach needs clearcut indications for PTCA in AMI.

The rate of primary successful recanalizations was significantly higher in group 1 (23 of 26 patients, 88%) as compared to group 2 (16 of 26 patients, 62%). The rate of late successes (primary succes + lack of reinfarction up to 4 weeks) was again higher in group 1 (20 of 26 patients, 77%) than in group 2 (12 of 26 patients, 46%). The latter difference is mainly due to primary successful recanalizations by PTCA in occlusions resistant to thrombolysis.

Reocclusion of infarct vessel due to PTCA after initially successful thrombolysis was seen in 1 patient. This patient developed an uncomplicated reinfarction with uneventful recovery. Spontaneous reocclusion of infarct vessel occurred in 2 patients of group 1 and 4 patients in group 2 (the difference between groups was not significant). The 2 patients of group 1 had 75 and 64% residual stenosis of infarct vessel and the 4 patients of group 2 had 88, 92, 91, and 94% residual stenosis after thrombolysis. Hence the problem of reocclusion after thrombolysis is a problem of high grade residual stenosis.

The late hemodynamic results show that regional myocardial function of AMI recovered significantly in group 1 but not in group 2. Similarly, thallium-201 scintigraphy revealed more reduction of the perfusion defect in group 1 than in group 2, at least when anterior AMIs were considered. Finally, serum creatine kinase activity reached a lower peak in group 1 than in group 2 (although this difference did not reach a significant level). The reduction of the perfusion defect after 24 hours suggests recovery of hypoxic but still viable myocardium. Similar observations have been published by other laboratories and our own institution [20, 24, 25].

The time interval between symptom onset and reperfusion was 3.8 hours in group 1. These data are consistent with previous observations in experimental studies which revealed that the critical time interval after onset of ischemia during which reperfusion was beneficial was far below 6 hours [6]. In patients with AMI recovery of regional function of AMI was seen when reperfusion was instituted within 4 hours after onset of symptoms but no change occurred after longer time periods of ischemia [2, 19]. Thus, late thrombolysis may be ineffective or even may exacerbate myocardial injury [6, 26].

A limitation of the study is the retrospective analysis of data. Since PTCA was only used in a minority of patients who underwent thrombolysis and selection was mainly based on the angiographic and clinical response to thrombolysis it was impossible to conduct a controlled trial. The control group was treated before the routine use of PTCA in this catheterization laboratory, but thrombolysis was carried out similarly and by the same cardiologists in both groups. As shown in Table 1 and 2, baseline clinical and angiographic characteristics were similar in both groups. Patients in the control group were selected according to angiographic and clinical criteria only. Since it was carefully noted to compare patients with equal amount of myocardium at risk (perfusion area of compromised coronary artery) we used 'Matched pairs' for comparison.

## Clinical implications

It is still dicussed which approach offers the best results and the lowest rate of complications in thrombolytic therapy [6, 7]. The present study is a retrospective analysis of patients treated with PTCA associated with thrombolysis. PTCA improved markedly the primary success rate of recanalization procedure without increasing complications when clearcut indications were considered. PTCA seems to be indicated when thrombolytic therapy fails to recanalize the artery or when residual stenosis of infarct vessel produces symptoms. Under these conditions hemodynamic, scintigraphic, and enzymatic results suggest salvage of jeopardized myocardium as compared to a similar group treated with thrombolysis without PTCA

## Acknowledgement

This study was supported by a grant from the Deutsche Forschungsgemeinschaft, Bonn-Bad Godesberg, within the SFB 90, Kardiovaskuläres System, University of Heidelberg.

## References

1. Rentrop P, Blanke H, Karsch KR, Wiegand V, Köstering H, Rahlf G, Oster H, Leitz K (1979) Wiedereröffnung des Infarktgefäßes durch transluminale Rekanalisation und intrakoronare Streptokinase-Applikation. Dtsch Med Wschr 104: 1438
2. Ganz W, Buchbinder N, Marcus H, Mondkar A, Maddahi J, Charuzi Y, O'Connor L, Shell W, Fishbein MC, Kass R, Miyamoto A, Swan HJC (1981) Intracoronary thrombolysis in evolving myocardial infarction. Am Heart J 101: 4
3. Smalling RW, Fuentes F, Matthews MW, Freund GS, Hicks CH, Reduto LA, Walker WE, Sterling RP, Gould KL (1983) Sustained improvement in left ventricular function and mortality by intracoronary streptokinase administration during evolving myocardial infarction. Circulation 68: 131
4. Khaja F. Walton JA, Brymer JF, Lo E, Osterberger L, O'Neill WO, Colfer HT, Weiss R, Lee T, Kurian T, Goldberg D, Pitt B, Goldstein S (1983) Intracoronary fibrinolytic therapy in acute myocardial infarction. Report of a prospective randomized trial. New Engl J Med 308: 1305
5. Anderson JL, Marshall HW, Bray BE, Lutz JR, Frederick PR, Yanowitz FG, Klausner SC, Hagan AD (1983) A randomized trial of intracoronary streptokinase in the treatment of myocardial infarction. New Engl J Med 308: 1318

6. Sobel BE, Bergmann SR (1982) Coronary thrombolysis: some unresolved issues. Am J Med 72: 1
7. Swan HJC (1982) Thrombolysis in acute myocardial infarction: treatment of underlying coronary artery disease. Circulation 66: 914
8. Mathey DG, Rodewald G, Rentrop P, Leitz K, Merx W, Messmer BJ, Rutsch W, Bücherl ES 1981) Intracoronary streptokinase thrombolytic recanalization and subsequent surgical bypass of remaining atheroclerotic stenosis in acute myocardial infarction: Complementary combined approach effecting reduced infarct size, preventing reinfarction, and improving left ventricular function. Am Heart J 102: 1194
9. Meyer J, Merx W, Dörr R, Lambertz H, Bethge C, Effert S (1982) Successful treatment of acute myocardial infarction shock by combined percutaneous transluminal coronary recanalization (PTCR) and transluminal coronary angioplasty (PTCA). Am Heart J 103: 132
10. Goldberg S, Urban PL, Greenspon A, Lebenthal M, Walinsky P, Maroko P (1982) Combination therapy for evolving myocardial infarction: intracoronary thrombolysis and percutaneous transluminal angioplasty. Am J Med 72: 994
11. Meyer J, Merx W, Schmitz H, Erbel R, Kiesslich T, Dörr R, Lambertz H, Bethge C, Krebs W, Bardos P, Minale C, Messmer BJ, Effert S (1982) Percutaneous transluminal coronary angioplasty immediately after intracoronary streptolysis of transmural myocardial infarction. Circulation 66: 916
12. Meltzer RS, v d Brand M, Serruys PW, Fioretti P, Hugenholtz PG (1982) Sequential intracoronary streptokinase and transluminal angioplasty in unstable angina with evolving myocardial infarction. Am Heart J 104: 1109
13. Killip T, Kimball JT (1967) Treatment of myocardial infarction in a coronary care unit. Am J Cardiol 20: 457
14. Grüntzig AR, Senning A, Siegenthaler WE (1979) Nonoperative dilatation of coronary-artery stenosis. Percutaneous transluminal coronary angioplasty. New Engl J Med 301: 61
15. Clauss A (1957) Gerinnungsphysiologische Schnellmethode zur Bestimmung des Fibrinogens. Acta hematol 12: 237
16. Creatin-kinase EC 2.7.3.2. CK-NAC-monotest. Mannheim: Boehringer Mannheim Diagnostika, 1979
17. Kent KM, Bonow RO, Rosing DR, Ewels CJ, Lipson LC, McIntosh CL, Bacharach S, Green M, Epstein SE (1982) Improved myocardial function during exercise after successful percutaneous transluminal coronary angioplasty. New Engl J Med 306: 441
18. Gelberg HJ, Brundage BH, Glantz S, Parmley WW (1979) Quantitative left ventricular wall motion analysis: a comparison of area, chord, and radial methods. Circulation 59: 991
19. Schwarz F, Schuler G, Katus H, Hofmann M, Manthey J, Tillmanns H, Mehmel HC, Kübler W (1982) Intracoronary thrombolysis in acute myocardial infarction: duration of ischemia as a major determinant of late results after recanalization. Am J Cardiol 50: 933
20. Schuler G, Schwarz F, Hofmann M, Mehmel H, Manthey J, Mäurer W, Rauch B, Herrmann HJ, Kübler W (1982) Thrombolysis in acute myocardial infarction using intracoronary streptokinase: assessment by thallium-201 scintigraphy. Circulation 66: 658
21. Vogel RA, Kirch DL, LeFree MT, Rainwater JO, Jensen DP, Steele PP (1979) Thallium-201 myocardial perfusion scintigraphy: results of standard and multi-pinhole tomographic techniques. Am J Cardiol 43: 787
22. Vogel RA, Kirch D, Le Free M, Steele PP (1978) A new method of multiplanar emission tomography using a seven pinhole collimator and an anger scintillation camera. J Nucl Med 19: 648
23. Sachs L (1972) Statistische Auswertungsmethoden. Berlin, Heidelberg, New York: Springer Verlag, p 357, p 386, p 410
24. Markis JE, Malagold M, Parker JA, Silverman KJ, Barry WH, Als AV, Paulin S, Grossman W, Braunwald E (1981) Myocardial salvage after intracoronary thrombolysis with streptokinase in acute myocardial infarction: Assessment by intracoronary thallium-201. New Engl J Med 305: 777

25. Maddahi J, Ganz W, Ninomiya J, Fishbein MC, Mondkar A, Buchbinder N, Marcus H, Geft I, Shah PK, Rozanski A, Swan HJC, Berman DS (1981) Myocardial salvage by intracoronary thrombolysis in evolving acute myocaredial infarction: evaluation using intracoronary injection of thall.um-201. Am Heart J 102: 664
26. Bresnahan GF, Roberts R, Shell WE, Ross JJr, Sobel BE (1974) Deleterious effects due to hemorrhage after myocardial reperfusion. Am J Cardiol 33: 82

# Mechanical balloon catheter recanalization combined with intracoronary lysis and PTCA

R. ERBEL, T. POP, K.J. HENRICHS, K. VON OLSHAUSEN,
T. MEINERTZ, H.J. RUPPRECHT, R. ZAHN, C. STEUERNAGEL,
F. BECK, and J. MEYER

**Summary**

In 127 patients with acute transmural myocardial infarction combined intravenous (iv) and intracoronary (ic) thrombolysis therapy with streptokinase was started. In still occluded vessels a mechanical recanalization was performed with 3 F recanalization catheters (group I, n = 64) or 4 F Grüntzig balloon catheters (group II, n = 63). After reperfusion streptokinase was administered superselectively. After the control coronary angiography angioplasty was performed only in group II. Both groups demonstrated no difference in relation to sex, age, infarct location, CPK levels and time between onset of symptoms and start of treatment. Reperfusion rate in group I was 59/64 patients (92%) and in group II 56/63 patients (89%). PTCA was attempted in 55/56 patients in group II with a success rate of 65% and reocclusion rate of 4%. Reocclusion occurred in 10/59 patients in group I (17%). In group II reocclusion was found in 9/55 patients (16%). By PTCA coronary stenosis in group II could be reduced from $82.6 \pm 6\%$ to $46.9 \pm 30.5\%$, $p<0.001$. Reocclusion was found in 3/36 (8%) of patients with successful and in 6/17 (35%) patients with unsuccessful PTCA, $p \pm 0.01$. Only in group II with PTCA improvement of regional and global left ventricular function was observed in patients with anterior myocardial infarction.

*Conclusion*

By combined medical and mechanical recanalization, reperfusion rate can be increased providing the possibility of full revascularization by PTCA with improvement of regional wall motion and reduction of reocclusion rate.

Restoration of coronary blood flow as soon as possible seems to be the aim of therapy in acute myocardial infarction. Intravenous (iv) and intracoronary (ic) application [1–10] – of streptokinase, urokinase, [11, 12] acylated streptokinase-plasminogen complex (BRL 26921) [13] and tissue plasminogen activators [14] can be used for thrombolysis therapy. A combination of ic and iv routes of application already seems to be effective in increasing the rate of open vessels at the time of the first coronary angiogram [16].

Based on our experience of recanalization of totally occluded coronary artery in the chronic stage of coronary artery disease [17, 18] we combined thrombolysis therapy with mechanical recanalization of occluded coronary arteries and percutaneous transluminal coronary angioplasty (PTCA) for residual stenosis.

## Methods

### Patients

The study was performed in 127 consecutive patients who were admitted to the emergency ward of the medical clinic within 6 h after onset of symptoms of acute myocardial infarction. Diagnosis was based on (1) acute chest pain lasting for more than 30 minutes, (2) persistent ST segment elevation of more than 0.3 mV in leads V1-V6 or 0.2 mV in leads I–III, aVL or aVF. Informed consent was obtained either from the patient or, in the case of cardiogenic shock, from relatives. Exclusion criteria were: (1) resuscitation, (2) history of streptokinase allergy, (3) previous cerebro-vascular accident, (4) surgery in the preceding 10 days, (5) history of acute peptic ulcer, and (6) history of bleeding problems.

### Treatment regimen

All patients received a premedication of 5,000 U heparin, 250 mg prednisolon, 3 mg/h nitroglycerine, and 1 g acetyl salicylate. 250,000 U streptokinase were infused iv prior to heart catheterization within 20 min.

Coronary angiography was performed in a random fashion via a 7 F catheter (group I) or 9 F guide catheter (group II). Coronary angiography was followed by injection of a 50,000 U bolus dose of streptokinase dissolved in saline solution, followed by a continuous regulated infusion of streptokinase in saline at a rate of 4,000 U/min through the coronary catheter until a total dose of 200,000 U was reached. Thus, patients received a total dose of 250,000 U streptokinase both ic and iv, total dose 500,000 U.

During streptolysis therapy, 3 F recanalization catheters (Schneider Medintag, Zürich, Switzerland) in group I or 4 F Gruentzig balloon catheters (Schneider Medintag, Zürich, Switzerland) in group II were prepared. As soon as possible the catheters were introduced into the occluded coronary artery for mechanical recanalization. During this time, streptokinase application had to be interrupted for 2–4 min. Immediately after the recanalization streptokinase was administered superselectively via the 3F or the 4F catheter. After administration of the total dose of streptokinase, coronary angioplasty was attempted in all except one cases in group II using steerable 3.0 or 3.7 mm balloon catheters.

Before discharge, control left cinventriculography was performed during atrial pacing at a rate corresponding to initial cineventriculography in the acute stage in order to exclude rate-related effects on left ventricular function [21].

*Anticoagulation*

Heparin therapy was started within 5–6 h after lysis, when the initial prolongation of the thrombin time started to decrease [20]. Overlapping phenprocoumon therapy was started and maintained between 15–25%.

*Calculations*

Left ventricular volumes were determined using a disc method, as previously described, with a half automatic computer system (Kontron 200, München, Germany) [22].

For regional wall motion analysis a floating system was used with diastolic long axis as a center point, creating 28 radii. Percentage shortening of the 28 segments was calculated and normal values were established in 30 controls [23].

*Statistics*

All results are given as mean ± standard deviation. Students t test for unpaired and Wilcoxon test for paired data were used, as well as the Chi-squared test: a p value of <0.05 was regarded as significant.

**Results**

Analysis of clinical data demonstrated no significant difference between groups I (n = 64) and II (n = 63) with regard to mean age, sex, infarct location and CPK levels.

A typical example of mechanical recanalization is demonstrated in Figure 1. Initial coronary angiography demonstrated an open vessel in 23/64 patients (36%) in group I and in 12/63 patients (19%) in group II (p<0.01). Mechanical recanalization with 3F catheters was succesful in 27/41 patients (66%) in group I and with 4F balloon catheters it was successful in 26/51 patients (51%) from group II with occluded coronary arteries (Fig. 1). Reperfusion rate in group I measured 59/64 patients (92%) and in group II 56/63 patients (89%). Time between onset of symptoms and treatment are listed in Figure 2.

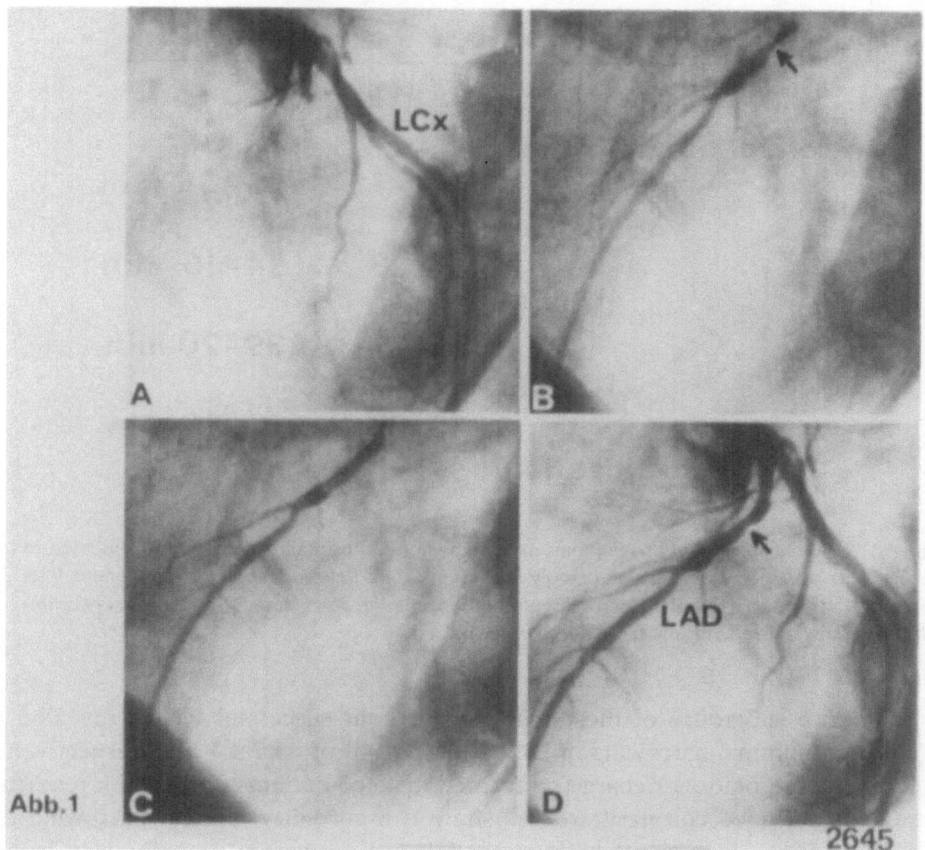

*Figure 1.* A. Occluded left anterior descending coronary artery and opacification of the left circumflex coronary artery (LCx). B. Mechanical recanalization using a balloon catheter of the left anterior descending coronary artery. C. Angioplasty of the coronary luminal narrowing demonstrated in B. D. Control coronary angiogram of the left coronary artery after angioplasty. (From Erbel et al. Cath. and Cardiovasc. Diagn. 11: 361, 1985. Reproduced with permission).

Immediately after thrombolysis, PTCA was performed in 55/56 patients in group II with reopening of the coronary vessel. PTCA was successful in 36/55 patients (65%) and unsuccessful in 15/55 patients (35%) taking an improvement of 20% of coronary luminal narrowing as significant. In 2/55 patients (4%) coronary vessel reocclusion occurred during PTCA.

In group I coronary luminal narrowing measured 94.2 ± 8.6% before and 78 ± 11.9% after recanalization. In 47/64 patients examination before discharge revealed a narrowing of 77.2 ± 14.8%. In group II coronary luminal narrowing measured 96.9 ± 6.6% before and 82.6 ± 6% after medical mechanical recanalization. After PTCA coronary stenosis measured 46.9 ± 30.5%. Dividing pa-

## Medical~Mechanical Recanalisation

|  | Group I | Group II |
|---|---|---|
| onset of symptoms | 156 ± 71 | 153 ± 58 min |
| admission | 18 ± 23 | 14 ± 16 min |
| IV lysis | 39 ± 15 | 39 ± 20 min |
| IC lysis | 13 ± 27 | 14 ± 16 min |
| recanalisation | | |

*Figure 2.* Time between onset of symptoms until admission to hospital, time between admission to hospital and start of intravenous thrombolysis therapy, time between onset of intravenous lysis therapy to intracoronary application of streptokinase, time between start of intracoronary thrombolysis therapy and reperfusion of the coronary artery.

tients into subgroups of those with and without successful PTCA revealed a coronary luminal narrowing of $28.0 \pm 16.3\%$ and of $84.7 \pm 7.6\%$, respectively. Examination before discharge performed in 43/63 patients (79%) with reperfusion of occluded coronary arteries showed a coronary luminal narrowing of $52.5 \pm 34.0\%$. In patients with successful and unsuccessful angioplasty mean values of coronary luminal narrowing remained nearly constant at $29.8 \pm 4\%$ and $87.2 \pm 12\%$, respectively.

During hospital stay reocclusion occurred in 10/59 patients in group I (17%) and in 9/55 patients in group II (16%) (Figs. 3 and 4). After thrombolysis therapy coronary luminal narrowing in group I measured $76.5 \pm 12.8\%$ in patients without and $87.9 \pm 15.8\%$ in patients with reocclusion ($p<0.05$). When patients in group II were divided into those with and without successful PTCA, reocclusion was found in 3/36 patients (8%) and 6/17 patients (35%), coronary luminal narrowing was $33 \pm 20\%$ and $85 \pm 6.8\%$, respectively ($p\pm0.001$). Follow-up during 6 months is illustrated in Figures 5 and 6.

Left ventricular function: Comparison of left ventricular volumes and ejection fraction is demonstrated for patients in group I and II in Figures 7 and 8 divided in those with infarct times 210 min. In patients with inferior myocardial infarction no significant difference of volumes and ejection fraction were found in group I and II.

With regard to regional wall motion a significant improvement was found in group II with anterior myocardial infarction, not demonstrated in group I. In

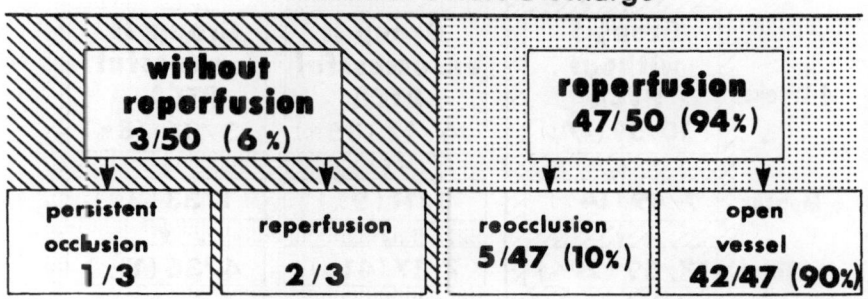

*Figure 3.* Follow-up during hospital stay of group I without PTCA. Included were 50/64 patients where coronary angiography could be performed before discharge. Reocclusion and reperfusion rate is indicated.

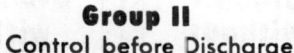

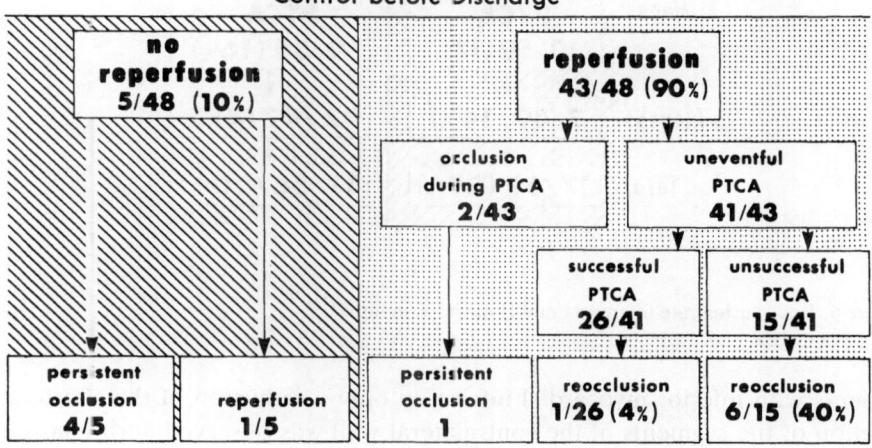

*Figure 4.* Follow-up of group II with percutaneous transluminal coronary angioplasty (PTCA). Included were 48/63 patients with control coronary angiography before discharge. Reocclusion rate is indicated.

## Reocclusion

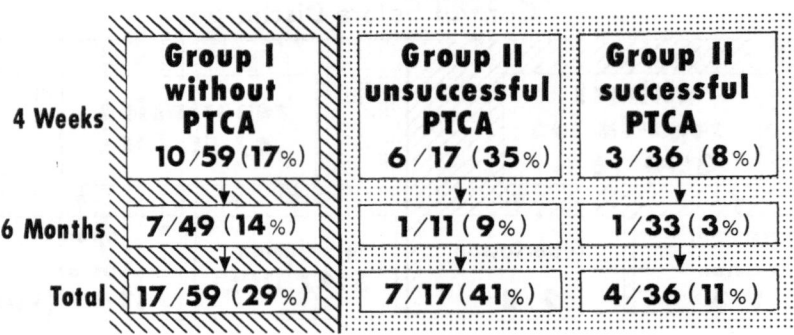

*Figure 5.* Reocclusion rate in group I and group II divided in successful and unsuccessful PTCA during 6 months follow-up time. Included are in both groups patients with reperfusion (group I 59/64, group II 56/63 patients). In group II PTCA was not tried in 1 patient, 2 demonstrated reocclusion during the acute PTCA, follow-up in 56 patients.

## Reocclusion

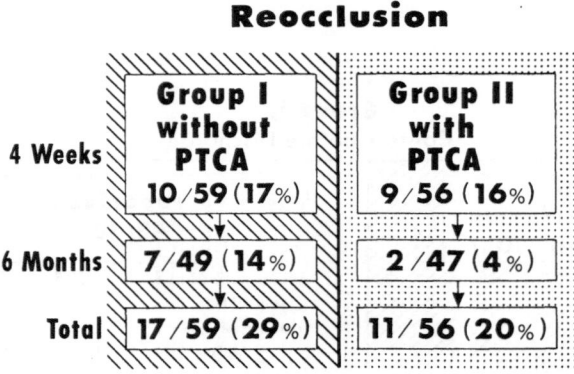

*Figure 6.* Reocclusion rate in group I and II during 6 months.

patients with inferior myocardial infarction only a reduction of the shortening fraction of the segments of the contralateral wall was observed during hospital stay.

During hospital stay 9/64 patients (14%) in group I and 5/63 patients (8%) in group II suffered a cardiac death. In addition, in group II 3 cases of acute respiratory distress syndrome and one case of subarachnoidal bleeding were observed.

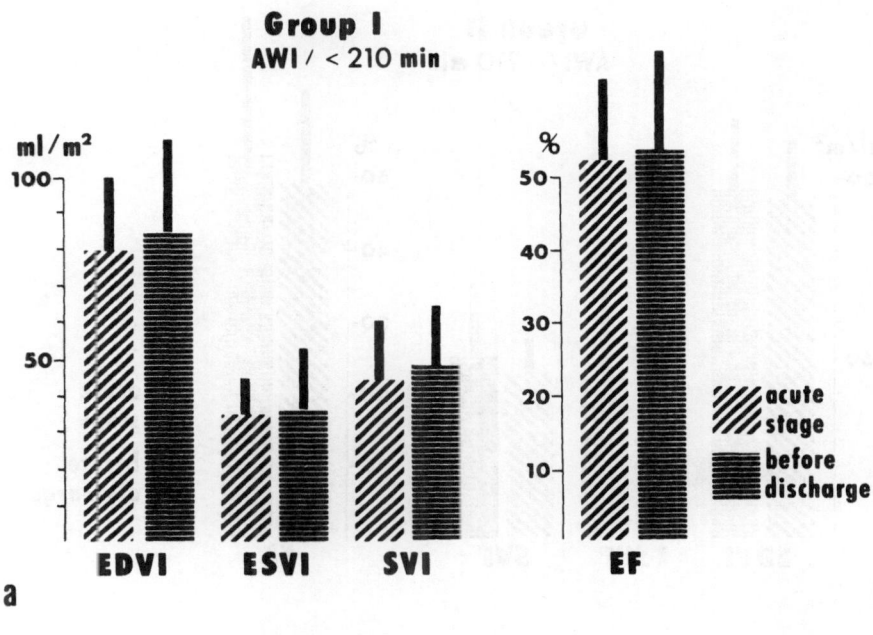

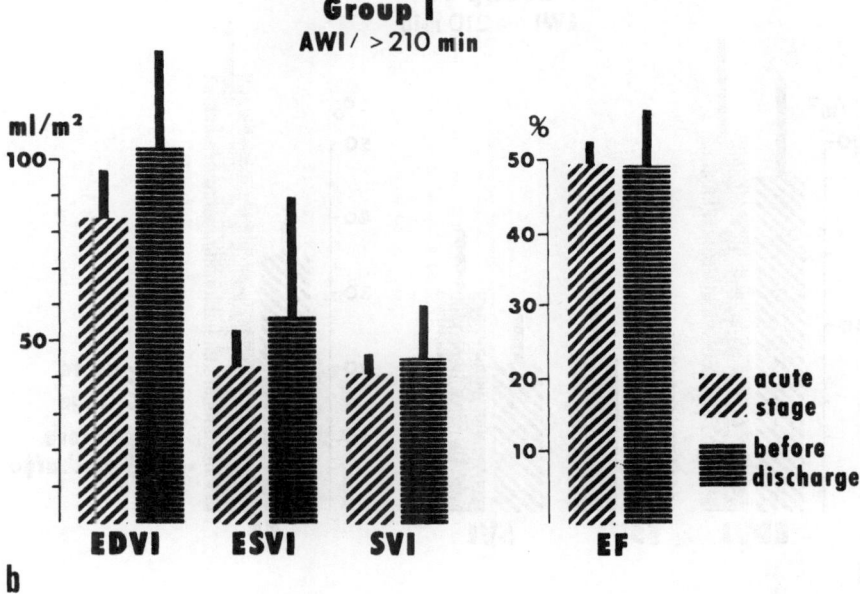

*Figure 7 a/b.* Changes of enddiastolic and endsystclic volume index (EDVI/ESVI), stroke volume index (SVI) and ejection fraction EF) in patients with anterior myocardial infarction in group I with infarct times less than 210 min (time between onset of symptoms and reperfusion) and more than 210 min.

374

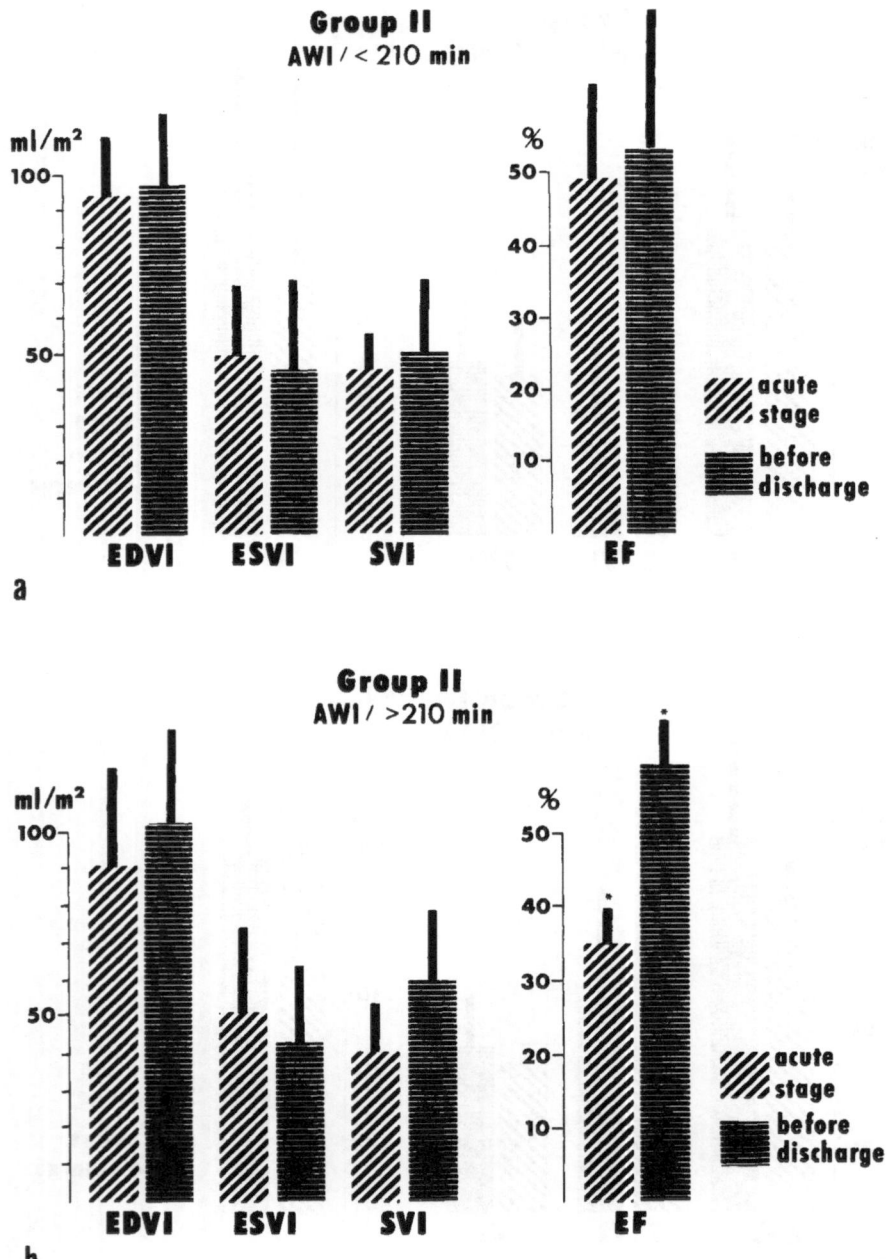

*Figure 8 a/b.* Changes of enddiastolic and endsystolic volume index (EDVI/ESVI), stroke volume index (SVI) and ejection fraction (EF) in patients with anterior myocardial infarction in group II with infarct times less than 210 min (time between onset of symptoms and reperfusion) and more than 210 min.

## Discussion

Rapid restoration of coronary blood flow as soon as possible is the aim of therapy in acute myocardial infarction. Thrombolysis can be achieved by iv and ic administration of streptokinase, urokinase as well as tissue type plasminogen activator [1–16]. Many authors have attempted to reopen occluded vessels mechanically using both guide wires and catheters [1, 24]. Rutsch et al [15] attempted a mechanical recanalization by guide wires in 22% with a success rate of 41%. Our previous studies demonstrated that mechanical recanalization can be performed by 3 F recanalization or 4 F angioplasty catheters in acute myocardial infarction [25]. By combination of thrombolytic therapy with the mechanical approach recanalization rate could be increased up to 88% without coronary perforation, as observed in previous studies in 4% using guide wires [15]. Also other authors reported high reperfusion rates using balloon catheters [19, 26].

By combination of iv and ic thrombolysis therapy of open vessels could be increased up to 35%, according to other authors [16]. In studies with ic thrombolysis therapy, however, only 15% of open coronary vessels were found [10, 27].

In our study recanalization with 3F and 4F balloon catheters was achieved within 15 minutes. This time is shorter than the time reported for ic thrombolysis therapy alone with time intervals of from $23 \pm 12$ min [24] up to $36 \pm 8$ min [29].

Reocclusion during hospital stay occurred in 17% of patients with successful reperfusion in group I and in 16% in group II. Other authors also reported a reocclusion rate of 17% [30] and 18% [24]. Serruys et al [30] reported reocclusion rate of 7/42 (17%) after attempted thrombolysis and of 1/18 (5.5%) after additional PTCA. Coronary stenoses were significantly higher in our patients of group I with reocclusion compared to those without reocclusion. These results are in accordance to those of Schwartz and Kübler, [16] reporting reocclusion rates of 8% in those with coronary luminal narrowing <70% and 26% in those with >70%. PTCA could reduce coronary luminal narrowing in our patients significantly. Reocclusion rate was found to be only 8% in patients with successful PTCA, 35% in those with unsuccessful PTCA because of high grade residual stenosis.

Reocclusion during hospital stay is of course also dependent on continuous full heparinization [10]. In 2/3 cases of successful PTCA and reocclusion an intermittent normalization of thrombin time was observed. One other factor is the persistence of coronary thrombus because in these cases the rethrombosis rate is high, reaching 30% in our study. Prolonged streptokinase infusion should be taken into account in cases of persistent thrombus.

The first cineventriculogram was performed after restoration of coronary blood flow. This means, however, that possible changes of left ventricular function before and after recanalization were not detected. However, these changes seem to be only slight, as previous reports have pointed out [31].

In patients with anterior myocardial infarction and long infarct times a significant increase of left ventricular ejection fraction was found in group II during hospital-phase, whereas it remained constant in group I.

Changes of left ventricular volumes in patients with inferior myocardial infarction were small. Also previous reports described only minor changes of ejection fraction after thrombolysis therapy [8, 33]. The mean ejection fraction was higher in inferior than in anterior myocardial infarction [32].

Regional wall motion improved significantly in patients with anterior myocardial infarction and PTCA, whereas in the group without PTCA regional wall motion was almost unchanged. Increased wall motion of the contralateral wall decreased during the hospital stay. Corresponding to the improvement of global left ventricular function regional wall motion improved in patients from group II and in those with long infarct times significantly, whereas in group I no significant change was found, except for the contralateral wall.

For patients with inferior myocardial infarction observed changes were only slight. In most patients a decrease of wall motion of the contralateral wall was observed combined with a slight decrease of global left ventricular ejection fraction.

In patients admitted to hospital within 4 h after onset of symptoms, hospital mortality was found to be 22% [35]. In control groups the mortality rate of 19% was found for patients with anterior and of 4.8% for patients with inferior myocardial infarction in a conventionally treated group [27]. High mortality rates are reported particularly in patients without reperfusion [9, 18]. Previous not controlled studies reported mortality rates of between 7 and 10% [9, 10, 16, 27]. Rentrop et al [36] found a mortality rate of 13% in patients treated with nitroglycerine, 20% in those treated with streptokinase and 22% in those treated with streptokinase and nitroglycerine. In our study cardiac mortality was 14% in group I, whereas in group II the cardiac mortality rate was 8%.

### Clinical implications

This randomized study demonstrates that by combined medical-mechanical recanalization either with 3F recanalization or 4F balloon catheters reperfusion rate of 90% can be reached in patients with acute myocardial infarction. Immediate elimination of underlying flow-limiting coronary stenosis by PTCA improves global left ventricular function and regional wall motion in anterior myocardial infarction. Reocclusion and reinfarction rate was reduced from 17% to 8%.

### Acknowledgement

We thank Priv. Doz. Dr. Grün, St. Vinzenz, Prof. Dr. Baum, Hildegardis Hospital, Mainz, Prof. Dr. Abel, St. Josef, Prof. Dr. v. Egidy, Dr. Horst Schmidt

Hospital, Wiesenbaden, and Prof. Dr. v. Mengden, Hospital Rüsselsheim, for their good cooperation. We also thank Mrs. Meurer for her graphical, Mrs. Larbi for her photographical work, Mrs. Pahlen and Mrs. Müller for their assistance in preparing the manuscript. Supported by Deutsche Lebensversicherungs-Gesellschaft e.G., Bonn.

## References

1. Neuhaus KL, Köstering H, Tebbe U, Sauer G, Kreuzer H (1981) Intravenöse Kurzzeitstreptokinase-Therapie beim frischen Myokardinfarkt. Z Kardiol 70: 791
2. Schröder R, Biamino G, v. Leitner ER, Linderer Th, Heitz J, Vöhringer HF, Wegschneider K, Andresen D, Arntz HR, Brüggemann Th, Grassot A, Lichey J, Oeff M, Prokein E, Schäfer JH (1982) Systemische Thrombolyse mit Streptokinase-Kurzzeitinfusion bei akutem Myokardinfarkt. Z Kardiol 71: 709
3. Spann JF, Sherry S, Blase A, Carabello BA, Mann RH, McConn WD, Gault JH, Gentzler RD, Rosenberg KM, Maurer AH, Denenberg BS, Warner HF, Rubin RN, Malmud LS, Comerota A (1982) High-dose, brief intravenous streptokinase early in acute myocardial infarction. Am Heart J 104: 939
4. Rogers WJ, Mantle JA, Hood W, Baxley WA, Whitlow PL, Reeves RC, Soto B (1983) Prospective randomized trial of intravenous and intracoronary streptokinase in acute myocardial infarction. Circulation 68: 1051
5. Alderman EL, Jutzky KR, Berte LE, Miller RG, Friedman GP, Gregor WP, Eliastan M (1984) Randomized comparison of intravenous versus intracoronary streptokinase for myocardial infarction. Am J Cardiol 54: 14
6. Anderson JL, Marshall JM, Askins JC, Lutz JR, Sorensen SS, Menlove RL, Yanowitz FG, Hagan AD (1984) A randomized trial of intravenous and intracoronary streptokinase in patients with acute myocardial infarction. Circulation 70: 606
7. Ganz W, Geft J, Shah PK, Lew AS, Rodriguez L, Weiss T, Maddahi J, Berman DS, Charuzi Y, Swan HJC (1984) Intravenous streptokinase in evolving acute myocardial infarction. Am J Cardiol 53: 1209
8. Rentrop P, Blanke H, Karsch R, Kaiser H, Köstering H, Leitz K (1982) Selective intracoronary thrombolysis in acute myocardial infarction and unstable angina pectoris. Circulation 63: 307
9. Mathey DG, Kuck KH, Tilsner V, Krebber HJ, Bleifeld W (1981) Nonsurgical coronary artery recanalization in acute transmural myocardial infarction. Circulation 63: 489
10. Merx W, Dörr R, Rentrop P, Blanke H, Karsch KR, Mathey DG, Kremer P, Rutsch W, Schmutzler H (1981) Evaluation of effectiveness of intracoronary streptokinase infusion in acute infarction: Postprocedure management and hospital course in 204 patients. Am Heart J 102: 1181
11. Tennant ST, Dixon J, Venable TH C, Page HL, Roach A, Kaiser AB, Fredericksen R, Tacoque L, Kaplan Pl, Bahn NS, Anderson EE, Wooten E, Jennings S, Breinig J, Campbell WB (1983) Intracoronary thrombolysis in patients with acute myocardial infarction: comparison of the efficacy of urokinase with streptokinase. Circulation 69: 756
12. Ibba GV, Terrosu P, Franceschino V, Contini GM, Sannia L, Frau G (1982) Short-time high-dose of intravenous urokinase in the treatment of acute myocardial infarction. Eur Heart J 5: (Suppl 1) (abstr)
13. Kasper W, Erbel R, Meinertz T, Drexler M, Rückel A, Pop T, Prellwitz W, Meyer J (1984) Intracoronary thrombolysis with a new acylated streptokinase-plasminogen complex (BRL 26921) in patients with acute myocardial infarction. J Am Coll Cardiol 4: 357
14. Gold HK, Fallon JT, Yasuda T, Leihbach RC, Khow BA, Newell JB, Guerrero, Vislosky FM,

Hoying CF, Grossbard E, Collen D (1984) Coronary thrombolysis with recombinant human tissue-type plasminogen activator: a prospective randomized, placebocontrolled trial. Circulation 70: 1012

15. Rutsch W, Schartl M, Mathey D, Kuck K, Dörr R, Rentrop P, Blanke H, Karsch K (1982) Perkutane, transluminale koronare Rekanalisation: Methodik, Ergebnisse und Komplikationen, Z Kardiol 71: 7

16. Schwarz F, Hofmann M, Schuler G, v. Olshausen K, Zimmermann R, Kübler W (1984) Thrombolysis in acute myocardial infarction: Effect of intravenous followed by intracoronary streptokinase application on estimates of infarct size. Am J Cardiol 53: 1505

17. Schreiner G, Erbel R, Pop T, Meyer et al (1984) Mechanische Rekanalisation von totalen Koronararterienverschlüssen (PTCA). Z Kardiol 73 (Suppl 1) 34, (abstr.)

18. Erbel R, Meinertz T, Wessler I, Meyer J, Seybold-Epting W (1984) Recanalization of occluded left main coronary artery in unstable angina pectoris. Am J Cardiol 53: 1725–1727

19. Uebis R, v. Essen R, Merx W, Schmidt WG, Emons HP, Effert S (1984) Combined medical and mechanical recanalization versus superselective streptokinase alone: reperfusion and time of occlusion. Circulation 70, II: 329

20. Pfeiffer C, Erbel R, Prellwitz W, Meyer J (1984) Antithrombin III levels and starting time for heparin application after streptokinase therapy. Eur Heart J 5 (Suppl 1) 52

21. Erbel R, Schweizer P, Krebs W, Langen HJ, Meyer J, Effert S (1984) Effects of heart rate changes on left ventricular volume and ejection fraction. Am J Cardiol 53: 590–597

22. Erbel R, Krebs W, Henn G, Schweizer P, Richter HA, Meyer J, Effert S (1982) Comparison of single plane und biplane volume determination by two-dimensional echocardiography: A study in asymmetric model hearts. Eur Heart J 3: 469–480

23. Clas W, Henkel B, Erbel R, Schreiner G, Kopp H, Brennecke R, Meyer J (1984) Computergestützte Analyse regionaler Wandbewegungsstörungen bei transluminaler Angioplastie. Biomed Technik 29, Ergänzungsband 73

24. Timmis GC, Gangadharan V, Hauser AM, Ramos RG, Westveer DC, Gordon S (1982) Intracoronary streptokinase in clinical practise. Am Heart J 104: 925–938

25. Erbel R, Pop T, Meinertz T, Kasper W, Schreiner G, Henkel B, Pfeiffer C, Meyer J (1985) Combined medical and mechanical recanalization in acute myocardial infarction. Cath and Cardiovasc Diagn 11: 361

26. Hartzler Go, Rutherford BD, McConahay DR (1984) Percutaneous transluminal coronary angioplasty: Application for acute myocardial infarction. Am J Cardiol 53: 117C–121C

27. Kennedy JW, Ritchie JL, Davis B, Fritz JK (1983) Western Washington randomized trial of intracoronary streptokinase in acute myocardial infarction. New Engl J Med 309: 1477–1482

28. Terrosu P, Ibba G, Contini GM, Franceschino V (1984) Angiographic features of the coronary arteries during intracoronary thrombolysis. Br Heart J 52: 154–63

29. Reduto L, Smalling R, Freund GC, Gould KL (1981) Intracoronary infusion of streptokinase in patients with acute myocardial infarction: Effects of reperfusion on left ventricular performance. Am J Cardiol 48: 403–409

30. Serruys PW, Wijns W, Van den Brand M, Ribeiro V, Fioretti P, Simoons ML, Kooijmon CJ, Reiber JH, Hugenholtz P (1983) Is transluminal coronary angioplasty mandatory after successful thrombolysis. Quantitative coronary angiography study. Br Heart J 50: 257–265

31. Erbel R, Pop T, Meinertz T (1984) Analysis of left ventricular function before and immediately after recanalization in acute myocardial infarction. Eur Heart J 5: Suppl 1–221, (Abstr.)

32. Taylor GJ, Mikell FL, Moses HW, Dore JT, Batchelder JE, Thull A, Hansen S, Wellons HA (1984) Intravenous versus intracoronary streptokinase therapy for acute myocardial infarction in community hospitals. Am J Cardiol 54: 256–260

33. Ritchie JL, Davis B, Williams DL, Caldwell J, Kennedy JW (1984) Global and regional left ventricular function and tomographic radionuclide perfusion: The Western Washington intracoronary streptokinase in myocardial infarction trial. Circulation 70: 867–875

34. Yasuno M, Saito Y, Ishida M, Suzuki K, Endos, Takahashi M (1984) Effect of percutaneous transluminal coronary angioplasty: Intracoronary thrombolysis with urokinase in acute myocardial infarction. Am J Cardiol 53: 1217

35. Meyer J, Erbel R, Rupprecht HJ, v. Essen R, Merx W, Effert S (1981) Relation between admission time, haemodynamic measurements, and prognosis in acute myocardial infarction. Br Heart J 46: 647–656

36. Rentrop P, Feit F, Blanke H, Stecy P, Schneider R, Rey M, Horowitz S, Goldman M, Karsch K, Meilman H, Cohen M, Siegel S, Sanger J, Slater J, Gorlin R, Fox A, Fagerstrom R, Calhoun F (1984) Effects of intracoronary streptokinase and intracoronary nitroglycerin infusion on coronary angiographic patterns and mortality in patients with acute myocardial infarction. New Engl J Med 311: 1457–1463

# Early coronary bypass or coronary angioplasty after successful reperfusion in acute myocardial infarction

P.G. HUGENHOLTZ, P.W. SERRUYS, P.J. DE FEYTER, M. VAN DEN BRAND, H.J. SURYAPRANATA, M. HAALEBOS and E. BOS

## Introduction

The point of no return and the beginning of irreversible necrosis becomes evident somewhere between 5 and 30 minutes after the occlusion of a major nutrient artery to the human myocardium. Depending on the subsequent duration of complete obstruction and the time of reperfusion, the pre-existing load on the ventricle (mainly the product of afterload and heart rate) as well as the extent of available collaterals, the size of the infarction distal to the site of obstruction will vary from a minor lesion via major dyskinetic area to 'sudden death'.

Jennings et al [1] have, in animal studies, quoted specific times for the onset of irreversibility. Depending on the preceeding load, Schaper [2] has confirmed that such irreversibility may occur within 20 minutes in the example of the small rodent, such as the rat, when arterial bloodflow is reduced to below 85% of control, whereas in the guinea pig, an animal supplied with an extensive collateral network, many hours of complete obstruction will not lead to infarction. The human infarction, like that in the pig, occurs somewhere inbetween, so that the period during which areas of severe ischemia may still be returned to normal function is now currently considered to be as long as 4 hours after onset of symptoms. It is now also generally accepted that the interruption of blood-flow in human coronary artery disease, at least in the early hours, is in more than 85% caused by an obstructing thrombus while in the remainder spasm with incomplete thrombus may be the cause. The demonstration therefore of rapid dissolution of the intracoronary thrombus by selective infusion of thrombolytic substances in that coronary artery, first demonstrated in 1960 by Boucek and Hurphy [3], and followed by the clinical introduction of this practice in 1979 by Rentrop et al [4] has galvanized the cardiovascular world in an unprecedented manner. Has it now really become possible to avoid infarction? In fact, a review of the recent literature leaves no doubt that intracoronary and intravenous administration of streptokinase [5, 6, 7] or tissue plaminogen activator [8], can re-establish blood-flow through the acutely occluded coronary artery in approximately 80% of all cases and that acute mortality can be reduced drastically [6].

As clinical experience in acute infarction has grown in the last few years, it has also become evident that the underlying atherosclerotic lesion in the coronary artery was often more severe than suspected beforehand [9, 20]. In other words, although recanalisation was demonstrated, the flow through remaining obstruction often was sufficiently slow and incomplete, that re-infarction became a dreaded complication, the more so since it usually carries a high mortality. Re-occlusion rates reported to vary between 10 and 35%, will negate much of the earlier improvement. More complete restoration of 'normal' bloodflow would therefore seem advisable as is conventional in surgical circles. In 1981 Matthey et al [11] reported that the reinfarction rate could be reduced from 20 to 4% by early referral to coronary artery bypass grafting (CABG). Soon after, Meyer et al [12] claimed the same for early percutaneous transluminal angioplasty (PTCA). Earlier de Wood et al [13] had shown the benefits in terms of improved ventricular function and reduced short and long-term mortality, when complete surgical revascularization was achieved within 6 hours after the onset of symptoms. Eighty-nine percent of those operated upon with acute infarction survived 10 years or more versus 63% in those operated after those 6 hours. This has led to a series of investigation, most of which are still in progress, which are aimed at immediate, or at least early, complete revascularisation. From the above, it would certainly make sense to optimize any reperfusion effort once the decision to recanalize a patient with acute myocardial infarction has been taken. In the present overview the experience will be detailed which has been collected in the Thoraxcenter in Rotterdam over the past 4 years with early 'permanent' re-canalisation, whether by PTCA or by CABG after succesful thrombolysis.

## Methods and results

Currently the final follow up is in progress of a randomised prospective trial in which 533 patients with acute myocardial infarction with 4 hours or less between onset of symptoms and admission to the catheterization laboratory have been enrolled [6]. Inasmuch as this trial is in the process of being published by the Netherlands Interuniversitary Cardiological Institute only the subset of data, seen at the Thoraxcenter in Rotterdam will be alluded to here. Details regarding the patient population, the inclusion and exclusion criteria, the protocol which was followed, the therapies which have been administered and the follow-up and ultimate evaluation procedures have been published elsewhere [14].

From the patients, admitted into the trial up to January 1, 1984, 152 patients had been assigned to intracoronary administration of streptokinase, whilst the patients, who had been randomized during the year 1984 have received, in addition, intravenous streptokinase upon entry into the hospital or emergency ward. Among those randomised to intracoronary or intracoronary plus intravenous streptokinase thrombolysis was achieved in 85%. Improved left ventricular function was demonstrated to be between 6 and 7% of the ejection fraction. Early (≤2 week) mortality in 14 patients was 5,3%, while among those assigned to conventional therapy in the coronary care unit there were 30 deaths, 11.3%. On an intention to treat principle, the difference between these two groups is statistically significant. More important, however, is that among those patients assigned to I.C. streptokinase therapy, there were 16 individuals who refused to participate in the study. Among these, there were 4 early deaths, for a mortality of 25%. Of the 22 in whom thrombolysis was unsuccessful, there were 6 deaths, (27%) versus 6 deaths among the 60 with successful lysis (10%). In the group with lysis and PTCA (27 individuals) only 1 late death took place (4%). Also, among the patients assigned to streptokinase, there were 27 in whom the vessel was found to be patent. None of these died in the following twelve months, although there was one re-infarction. Even more interesting, however, is the fate of all patients (randomized and nonrandomized) in whom the operator in Rotterdam decided to proceed with a percutaneous transluminal angioplasty (Figs. 1 and 2). Among the 40 patients in whom this procedure was carried out, either immediately or soon after lysis, because of persistent signs of obstruction or signs of ischemia, there have been thus far only two late deaths. Accordingly, when one groups all 27 individuals in whom the infarct related vessel became spontaneously patent or remained patent (possible temporary spasm having been the cause of temporary obstruction or spontaneous lysis) with the 40 in whom the vessel, was properly dilated after thrombolysis so that the residual obstruction was 30% or less, the death rate is very low at ≤1%. In contrast, among the refusers and in those in whom the vessel could not be re-opened, a total of 38 individuals, there were 10 deaths, for a mortality of 26%.

As is evident from Figure 1, the need for CABG in the year following lysis is twice as high in the group where reperfusion after streptokinase initially was considered satisfactory, in comparison to those cases where the operator decided to proceed early with PTCA. The outcome of CABG is detailed in Figures 2 and 3. It is again quite clear that mortality after thrombolysis is drastically reduced after CABG is carried out. A similar effect is seen relative to reinfarction. In the conventionally treated group, the need for late CABG failed to influence mortality although it again favourably altered the outcome in terms of reinfarction. When one regards the entire group of CABG patients (47 out of the 221 seen at the Thoraxcenter within the randomized study), it again becomes evident that mortality is low in the group assigned to thrombolysis and lowest in those who had prior PTCA. Since CABG was sequential to and not compared with either thrombolysis or PTCA, a definite conclusion as to the superiority of one above the other cannot be drawn.

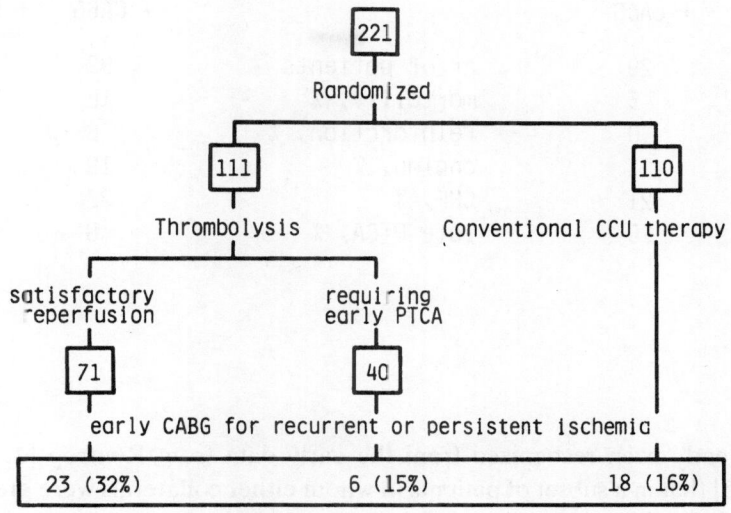

*Figure 1.*

## ONE YEAR CLINICAL FOLLOW-UP OF 221 PATIENTS ENROLLED IN A RANDOMIZED TRIAL OF THROMBOLYSIS (TR) vs CONVENTIONAL TREATMENT (CT)

|              | TR+PTCA N = 40 | TR N = 71 | CT N = 110 |
|--------------|------|-----|-----|
| - Mortality  | 5%   | 14% | 16% |
| - Reinfarction | 12% | 14% | 7% |
| - PTCA/re PTCA | 5% | 3% | 6% |
| - CABG       | 15%  | 32% | 16% |
| - AP         | 12%  | 20% | 19% |

*Figure 2.*

## ONE YEAR FOLLOW-UP WITH AND WITHOUT CABG

| 111, THROMBOLYSIS | | | 110, CONVENTIONAL R$_\downarrow$ | |
|---|---|---|---|---|
| - CABG | + CABG | | - CABG | + CABG |
| 82 | 29 | nr of patients | 92 | 18 |
| 13 | 3 | mortality, % | 16 | 17 |
| 18 | 0 | reinfarction, % | 8 | 0 |
| 18 | 11 | angina, % | 19 | 27 |
| 11 | 21 | CHF, % | 22 | 9 |
| 44 | 10 | late PTCA, % | 8 | 0 |

*Figure 3.*

## Discussion

It had already been recognized from the early data from Rentrop [4, 5] and Blanke [15] that in a subset of patients in whom either collaterals were present at the time of complete obstruction, or in whom reperfusion was achieved within the first few hours after the onset of symptoms, the clinical improvement as well as the augmentation in ejection fraction were highest. Similar data have been reported by others [10, 16]. These data however were all from series in whom selection bias could have played a major role. Schwartz et al [17] compared in an open parallel study, 55 patients pretreated with intravenous streptokinase followed by intracoronary streptokinase, with 46 who received the latter only and demonstrated better outcome with the combined therapy.

The data from the randomized Netherlands trial [6, 14] confirm this and in addition, are supported by further analysis from the Western Washington Trial [7]. All concur that the death rate is most reduced in that subset of patients in whom the degree to which reperfusion is achieved is optimal. Since the recent publication by Davies et al [18] that the origin of the thrombus in the coronary artery is often a fissure in a plaque, the significance of the underlying atherosclerotic lesion has gained importance. Furthermore, now that acute angiography in acute myocardial infarction has become a possibility and is regularly practised, the assessment of residual coronary artery disease after dissolution of the acute thrombus has become of major significance [19].

Today, it would therefore seem rather naive to assume that simple reperfusion, whether by the intravenous or the intracoronary route could in all cases suffice to re-establish adequate blood flow. Rather, it has to be anticipated, that if early optimal reperfusion is to be achieved in all patients in whom there is the suspicion of significant residual obstruction, they should be submitted to early coronary angiography to determine their optimal further treatment.

De Feyter et al [20] performed PTCA as an emergency in 60 patients with unstable angina pectoris, when these patients had proven to be refractory to treatment with maximally tolerated dosis of betablockers, $Ca^{++}$ antagonists and intravenous nitroglycerin for 24 to 36 hours. In this group of interesting patients, of whom Cowley et al [21] have suggested that thrombus may be present in well over 50% of cases, the initial PTCA success rate was 93%. There were also no deaths related to the procedure, although re-occlusion occurred in 4. In these latter patients, immediate CABG alleviated symptoms, although a myocardial infarction could not be avoided. Fifty-five patients were followed for at least 6 months and while there was only 1 death, it was even more significant that progression to complete myocardial infarction was seen in none of the others. Only 13% had recurrent angina pectoris and the one year re-stenosis rate was 28% (13 out of 46) in whom routine repeat angiography was obtained. Furthermore, improved cardiac functional status was demonstrated by an almost normal capacity to bicycle exercise testing and a complete absence of ischemia on thallium isotope studies during exercise in 80%. These authors concluded that in selected patients emergency PTCA had a major place in therapeutic options, when maximal pharmacological efforts fail. Inasmuch as the syndrome of unstable angina pectoris is extremely close to that of impending or early myocardial infarction, these data are highly relevant for what can be expected if PTCA were to be systematically employed in all patients with residual stenosis of more than 50% after successful reperfusion by thrombolytic agents.

In a recent series in Victoria (B.C. Canada) patients, admitted within 2 hours after onset of symptoms, have been treated by primary PTCA, followed, where needed, by thrombolytic therapy. In the first 20 patients so handled, there was not a single death. Keon, [12a] in an overview of early surgical reperfusion of acute myocardial infarction in Canada, concludes that the vast majority of myocardial infarctions are uncomplicated and hence do not need emergency revascularisation. Nevertheless he and his crew participate in a controlled, randomized trial in which patients with acute myocardial infarction are operated. Within hours after the onset of symptoms. Initial analysis of these data would indicate a very much better outcome of those treated with early reperfusion, thus confirming the earlier data by de Wood et al [13] who reported a beneficial effect of early surgical reperfusion, provided it was carried out within the first 6 hours after onset of symptoms, with a 10 year survival of 89%.

The data from our streptokinase trial do not, as yet, permit a final decision regarding which procedure must be considered optimal subsequent treatment, PTCA or CABG. However, a number of observations can be made, which are relevant in this regard. Although surgical standby is required for PTCA, the effort in terms of personnel, time and expense is considerably less then for the 24 hours standby of a fully staffed operating room for CABG. On the other hand, while many acute significant obstructions can be reached with the dilating balloon, certainly not all obstructions can be treated by PTCA. Then there will be instances where the team of cardiac surgeon and cardiologist will jointly decide that surgery is the better overall solution because of extensive multivessel disease, the need for additional surgery or other operational cicumstances.

Ultimately multiple, pragmatic arguments depend on the local circumstances and the merits of the individual case. Therefore the decision to choose between CABG or PTCA for further reperfusion effort, will be subjective. It will be very difficult, if not impossible therefore to carry out a randomised study of this aspect. When mortality and morbidity figures remain as low as they are now, a statistically scientific decision is unlikely to be arrived at. Clinical decision making should suffice here and should favor PTCA over CABG, where possible (Figures 1–4). Laffel and Braunwald [22] in their extensive article develop a new strategy for the treatment of acute myocardial infarction which is remarkable similar to the thoughts and data expressed above. Their last comment is 'what is the best design for a large scale randomized trial of thrombolytic therapy in acute myocardial infarction?' While we would agree that this question must ultimately be answered, we would now plead, as we have done in the abstract with Feinstein [23]: 'Whether we like it or not, most of our future decisions about medical practice, health care and scientific knowledge will have to be made without evidence from randomized trials. To acknowledge this reality, requires no loss of reference, allegiance or respect for the primary goal of randomized trials as a "gold standard", in scientific research'. To understand which therapy after thrombolysis is better, PTCA or CABG we suggest that to study the causeeffect relationships between thrombus, plaque fissure, spasm, obstruction, reperfusion and salvage in acute coronary artery disease, we need at present carefully conducted observational epidemiological research rather than large scale randomized trials with its many subgroups, which will defy sensible interpretation of this new therapeutic strategy.

For these and many other arguments not to be detailed here, it would seem advisable for those centers and healthsystems where intravenous and intracoronary thrombolytic agents can be given, to limit this therapy to those in whom reperfusion efforts can be begun within the first 4 hours after onset of symptoms. In these same individuals at the suspicion of residual ischemia or significant obstruction, an angiogram should be carried out within 4–12 hours so as to decide the optimal fashion in which that given patient should be treated further. This can be PTCA or CABG, preceded by or followed by further thrombolytic or anticoagulant therapy.

There is no doubt however, that all evidence today point towards the need for early and complete restoration of blood flow. If this can be achieved by whatever combination of methods and medicines, the goal of reducing mortality of myocardial infarction to 1% or less, lies just ahead of us. Who could ever have believed that a decade ago!

387

CABG AFTER RANDOMIZED I.C. THROMBOLYSE: ONE YEAR CLINICAL FOLLOW-UP.

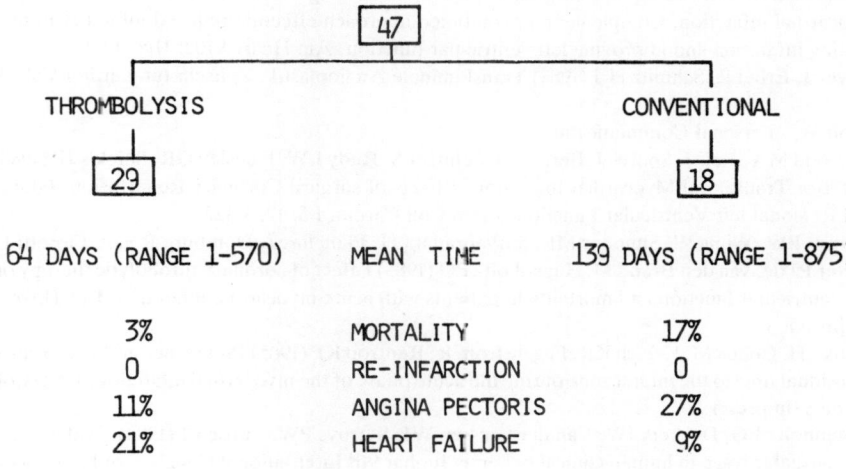

64 DAYS (RANGE 1-570)   MEAN TIME   139 DAYS (RANGE 1-875)

| | | |
|---|---|---|
| 3% | MORTALITY | 17% |
| 0 | RE-INFARCTION | 0 |
| 11% | ANGINA PECTORIS | 27% |
| 21% | HEART FAILURE | 9% |

*Figure 4.*

# References

1. Jennings RB, Gante CE, Reimer KA (1975) Ischemic Tissue Injury. Am J Pathol 81: 179–198
2. Schaper W (1983) Natural defense mechanisms to ischemia. Eur Heart J 4 (Suppl D) 73–78
3. Boucek RJ, Murphy WP Jr (1960) Segmental perfusion of the coronary arteries with fibrinolysis in man following acute myocardial infarction. Am J Cardiol 6: 525–533
4. Rentrop KP, Blanke H, Kostering K, Karsch KR (1979) Acute myocardial infarction: Inracoronary application of nitroglycerin and streptokinase in combination with transluminal recanalization. Clin Cardiol 5: 354
5. Rentrop KP, Feit F, Blanke H et al (1984) Effects of intracoronary streptokinase and intracoronary nitroglycerin infusion on coronary angiographic patterns in patients with acute myocardial infarction. New Engl J Med 311: 1457–1463
6. Simons ML, Serruys PW, van den Brand M, Res J, Verheugt, FWA, Krauss XH, Remme WJ, Bar F, de Zwaan F, Vermeer F, Lubsen J (1985) Improved survival after early thrombolysis in acute myocardial infarction. Submitted to the Lancet
7. Kennedy JW, Ritchie JL, Davis KB, Fritz JK (1983) Western Washington Trial of Intracoronary Streptokinase in Acute Myocardial Infarction. New Engl J Med 309: 1477–1482
8. Verstraete M, Bernard R, Bory M, Brower RW, Collen D, Bono DP de, Erbel R, Huhmann W, Lennane RJ, Lubsen J, Matthey D, Meyer J, Michels JR, Rutsch W, Schartl M, Schmidt W, Uebis R, Essen R van (1985) Randomized trial of intravenous recombinant tissue type plasminogen activator versus intravenous streptokinase in acute myocardial infarction. Lancet 1: 842–847
9. Swan HJC (1982) Thrombolysis in acute myocardial infarction treatment of the underlying coronary artery disease. Circulation 66: 914–916

388

10. Hugenholtz PG, Rentrop P (1983) Thrombolytic therapy for acute myocardial infarction Qio Vadis. A review of the recent literature. Eur Heart J 3: 395–403

11. Mathey DG, Rodewald G, Rentrop KP et al (1981) Intracoronary streptokinase thrombolytic recanalization and subsequent surgical bypass or remaining atherosclerotic stenosis in acute myocardial infarction: Complementary combined approach effecting reduced infarct size, preventing infarction and improving left ventricular function. Am Heart J 102: 1194–1201

12. Meyer J, Erbel R, Schmitz H-J (1984) Transluminale Angioplastik. Zeitschr für Kardiol Vol 73: 73

12a. Keon WJ. Personal Communication

13. de Wood MA, Heit J, Spores J, Berg Jr G, Selinger S, Rudy LW, Hensley GR, Shields JP (1983) Anterior Transmural Myocardial Infarction: Effects of surgical Coronary Reperfusion. Global and Regional left Ventricular Function. J Am Coll Cardiol I 5: 1223–1234

14. Serruys PW, Wijns W, Simoons ML, Suryapranata H, Planellas J, Domburg R van, Floretti P, Feyter PJ de, van den Brand M, Hugenholtz PG (1985) Effect of coronary throbolytic therapy on left ventricular function and mortality in patients with acute myocardial infarction. Eur Heart J (in press)

15. Blanke H, Cohen M, Karsch KR, Fagenstrom R, Rentrop KP (1985) Prevalence and significance of residual flow to the infarct zone during the acute phase of the myocardial infarction. J Am Coll Cardiol (in press)

16. Hugenholtz PG, Deckers JW, Van der Giessen WJ, Serruys PW, Lubsen J (1984) Evidence for myocardial salvage in human clinical ischemia Iuphar 9th International Congress of Pharmacology, London Proceedings. Mac Millan Press Ltd 257–268

17. Schwartz F, Hoffmann M, Schuler et al (1984) Thrombolysis in acute myocardial infarction: Effect of intravenous followed by intracoronary streptokinase application on estimates of infarct size. Am J Cardiol 53: 1505–1510

18. Davies GJ, Chierchia S, Maseri A (1984) Prevention of myocardial infarction by very early treatment with intracoronary streptokinase. New Engl J Med 311: 1488–1492

19. Serruys PW, Wijns W, van den Brand M, Ribeiro V, Fioretti P, Simoons ML, Kooymans G, Reiber JHC, Hugenholtz PG (1983) Is transluminal coronary angioplasty mandatory after successful thrombolysis? Br Heart J 50: 257–265

20. De Feyter PJ, Serruys PW, v.d. Brand M, Balakumaran K, Mochtar B, Arnold AER, Hugenholtz PG (1985) Emergency coronary angioplasty in refractory unstable angina: immediate and follow up results. New Engl J Med (submitted)

21. Cowley MJ, Hastillo A, Vetrovec GW, Fisher LM, Garrett R, Hess ML (1983) Fibrinolytic effects of intracoronary streptokinase administration in patients with acute myocardial infarction and coronary insufficiency. Circulation 67: 1031–1038

22. Laffel GL, Braunwald E (1984) Thrombolytic therapy. A new strategy for the treatment of acute myocardial infarction. New Engl J Med 311: 710–717 and 770–776

23. Feinstein AR (1984) Current problems and future challenges in randomized clinical trials. Circulation 70: 767–774

# Immediate and late results of thrombolysis on infarct size, left ventricular function and survival after successful reperfusion

W. BLEIFELD, D.G.MATHEY and J. SCHOFER

## Summary

The aim of coronary reperfusion by thrombolysis in acute myocardial infarction (AMI) is the improvement of left ventricular function and of survival as a result of the reduction of infarct size. Although most of data presented in the literature are from non-randomized trials the following conclusions seem to be justified:

1. The immediate results in terms of reopening rate, decrease of infarct size, improvement of regional wall motion in the infarct area and early (hospital) mortality depend on
   a) the time delay between AMI and the application of the thrombolytic agent, which is linked to
   b) the reperfusion rate (successful reopening),
   c) the size of the occluded vessel, which determines in combination with the degree of collateralization the initial infarct size and – at least partially – the initial hemodynamic state,
   d) the age.
2. Among these, the time up to reperfusion is the single factor to be influenced by therapy. In 80% of the patients, successfully treated within 2.0 hours, the initial infarct size was reduced and regional wall motion improved.
3. After achieving a favourable immediate result for the longterm course it is of major importance to maintain a sufficient antegrade coronary flow by avoiding reocclusion. Whether aortocoronary bypass-surgery, percutaneous coronary angioplasty, alterations in the dosage and/or duration of the thrombolytic compound or some type of effective anticoagulation or a combination of these measures will be the follow-up therapy of choice has to be clarified by further investigations.

Coronary reperfusion by thrombolysis in acute myocardial infarction (AMI) has become a widely used method for the early reestablishment of coronary flow to the infarcted area [1–5]. This therapeutic intervention is directed to the improvement of left ventricular function and the decrease of mortality by salvaging jeopardized, ischemic myocardium. It is based on the fact that the impairment of left ventricular function, the severity of ventricular arrhythmias, sudden cardiac death and thus mortality are related to the size of acute myocardial infarction [6–8].

With regard to the effect of acute thrombolysis on left ventricular function, at the present time there are only 6 studies with more or less reasonable numbers of patients, from which only two were randomized [9] (Table 9). While the study from Anderson [12] revealed a positive result of coronary reperfusion, khaja and co-workers [11] observed no improvement in ejection fraction and regional wall motion. The other not randomized studies showed an improvement in ejection fraction and in regional wall motion compared to the control group, which was in the study from Sheehan et al [16] in the order of 40% of all patients.

Even the two randomized studies need cautious interpretation, mainly for methodologic reasons: In khaja's study, left ventricular angiograms were compared immediately after reperfusion with the state before lysis. From animal experiments it is, however, wellknown that impaired wall motion following coronary occlusion and reperfusion needs up to 1 to 2 weeks for complete improvement [17]. Thus, it is not astonishing that there was no improvement in their study. The same holds true for the comparison of the values of the ejection fraction (radionuclide ventriculography) taken from the 12th with those at the 2nd day after thrombolysis for two reasons: First, the ejection fraction is by

| Investigator | No. | Rando-mized | Method | Parameter | Results Thrombolysis | Controls |
|---|---|---|---|---|---|---|
| Khaja et al. (1983) | 40 | + | Cine-Angio | EF, reg. wall movement | no change | no change |
| | | | Nuclear-Ventr. | EF | no change | no change |
| Anderson et al. (1983) | 50 | + | Nuclear-Ventr. | EF | + 3.9 % | – 3.0 % |
| | | | Echo | Reg. wall movement | | no change |
| Rentrop et al. | 55 | ∅ | Cine-Angio | EF | + 4.0 % | – 3.0 % |
| | | | | Reg. wall movem. (score) | | no change |
| Gould et al. (1983) | 136 | ∅ | Nuclear-Ventr. | EF | + 7.0 % | + 1.0 % |
| Schwarz et al. (1982) | 27 | ∅ | Cine-Angio | EF | CK<1000 +8.0% / CK>1000 +0.5% | – 4.4 % |
| | | | | Reg. EF | +14.0% / +2.0% | – 6.0 % |
| Sheehan et al. | 52 | ∅ | Cine-Angio | EF | no change | no change |
| | | | | Reg. wall movement | ↑↑ in 40 % | no change |

Table 1. Global and regional myocardial function following intracoronary thrombolysis.

means a parameter to evaluate the alterations of wall motion in a process, affecting only one segment of the left ventricle, where the non-affected segment resp. the contralateral part of the ventricle could hypercontract, thus outbalacing the decreased wall motion in the infarcted area [18]. Second, it is not justified to use the value of the 2nd day as a control value, since at that time already a particular improvement of contraction could have been occured.

One of the positive result from Anderson's study has also to be regarded with caution, since he used a score obtained from echocardiography, a method still under debate in terms of sufficient resolution for this particular purpose.

The other studies have all drawbacks of the lack of randomization. In addition, several of these studies rely only on ejection fraction, which in our own experience revealed no change for the whole group of successful reperfused patients 6 weeks after successful lysis compared to the angiogram at admission. In contrast, in the same patients regional wall motion as evaluated by the centerline method [16] was improved in 40%, irrespective, whether they had early aortocoronary bypass operation or not, while the unsuccessful treated patients showed no improvement and about 30% of these exhibited an impairment of the wall motion in the infarcted area (Table 3). From these data at least a trend for an improvement of left ventricular function resulting from the reduction of infarct size can be taken and a decrease in mortality should be expected. In Table 2 six representative studies are listed. They show uniformely a reduction of mortality in successful intracoronary reperfused patients during the hospital phase [11, 12, 19, 20, 21, 22]. The longest randomized trial revealed with 3.7% in the streptokinase group a

| Investigator | No. | Rando-mized | Controls (n =) | % Mortality Thrombolysis | Controls |
|---|---|---|---|---|---|
| Kennedy et al. (1983) | 250 | + | 116 | 3.7<br>(AWI) 7.9<br>(PWI) 0 | 11.2<br>18.9<br>4.8 |
| | | | | 3.7 | 14.7 |
| Khaja et al. | 40 | + | 20 | 1/20 | 2/20 |
| | | | | 0/19 | 2/18 |
| Anderson et al. (1983) | 50 | + | 26 | 1/24 | 4/26 |
| Merx et al. (1981) | 204 | Ø | 37<br>unsuccessful lysis | 5.4 | 24.0 |
| Weinstein et al. (1983) | 224 | Ø | 77<br>standard therapy | 4.5 | 14.6 |
| Kennedy et al. (1983) | 527 | Ø | 148<br>unsuccessful lysis | 3.7 | 10.8 |

*Table 2.* Mortality of intracoronary thrombolysis in acute myocardial infarction from several randomized and non-randomized studies.

significantly lower mortality than in the control group (14.7%), which was still present after 1 year (22). Although, containing smaller numbers in the two other randomized studies from Khaja [9] and Anderson [10], a decrease in mortality in the treated patients compared to the controls, was observed.

Which other factors in addition to a successful reperfusion of a coronary artery could be important for infarct size, left ventricular function and accordingly mortality?

Among the different parameters as the site of acute occlusion, the coronary anatomy, and the age of a patient, the time up to reperfusion has the highest priority for two reasons: First, AMI is a dynamic process resulting within 6 hours to death of 40–60% of the cells in the infarcted area, while the necrosis in the residual cells develop within 24 hours [24]; second, the time delay from the acute occlusion up to therapy is – to our present knowledge – the only variable and thus the single factor to be influenced in the clinical setting of an AMI. This can be seen from a study by Mathey et al [25] with urokinase 2 millions units as bolus applicated immediately after diagnosing the acute infarction (Table 4). The application of urokinase as a bolus has the advantage over i.v. streptokinase or intracoronary streptokinase that the delay between the occlusion and the reperfusion can be shortened for about one half to one hour. The maximal CPK in unsuccessful treated patients was with almost 2000 U/I markedly higher than those with an immediate reperfusion with urokinase (800 U/I) and in contrast to those patients, who needed more time up to the reperfusion, because urokinase was unsuccessful and the reperfusion was achieved by intracoronary streptokinase and/or percutaneous transluminal coronary angioplasty (PTCA). In all subgroups there was no difference between the acute state and the control values of left ventricular ejection fraction after about 2 weeks. In contrast, regional wall motion – evaluated by the centerline method – was only improved in the group

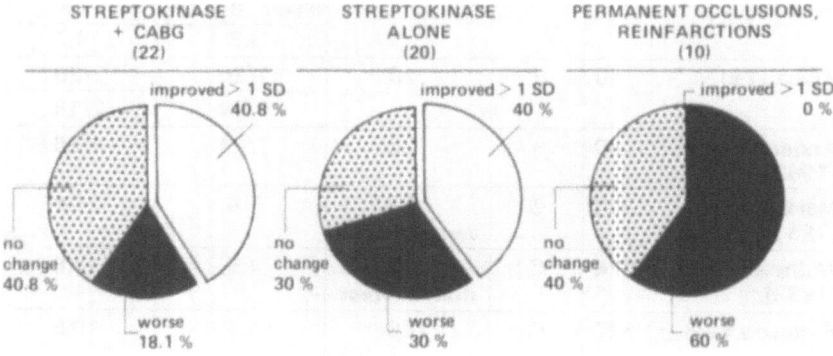

*Table 3.* Alteration of regional myocardial wall motion (size of the hypokinetic segment) at the control state (6 weeks) compared to the angiogram immediately after thrombolysis in patients treated by intracoronary streptokinase. ACVB = coronary artery bypass graft.

with immediate successful reperfusion, which could be obtained within 3ʰ in 70%.

The importance of time is even more demonstrated, when the time up to the application of urokinase was seperated into a 2 hours interval (group I) vs. a 2 to 4 hours interval (group II) (Table 5): Not only the reperfusion rate declined after the longer interval from 70 to 50%, but also the maximal CPK increased to 1000 U/I in the mean (group II) compared to 580 U/I (group I) and the impairment of regional wall motion increased from $-1.2$ (group I) to $-1.8$ standard devia-

| Subgroups | No | Max. CPK U/I | LV eject. fraction acute | control | Reg. wall motion acute | control |
|---|---|---|---|---|---|---|
| All patients 1. | 100 | 1266 | 54 ± 19 | 50 ± 23 | − 2.3 | − 2.0 |
| Rep. with Urokinase 2. | 60 | 802 | 55 ± 10 | 53 ± 11 | − 2.2 | − 1.5 |
| 2. + i.c. Strept/ PTCA | 20 | 1848 | 51 ± 11 | 47 ± 9 | − 2.8 | − 2.6 |
| No reperfusion | 20 | 1973 | 48 ± 8 | 47 ± 12 | − 2.9 | − 2.4 |

*Table 4.* Infarct size (max. CPK), global and regional wall motion after 2.0 millions urokinase i.v. as a bolus.

| | < 2 hours | 2 − 4 hours |
|---|---|---|
| No of patients | 24 | 26 |
| Reperfusion rate (%) | 70.8 | 50 |
| Max. CPK (U/I) | 576 ± 521 | 986 ± 802 |
| Reg. wall motion in infarct area (SD/segment) | −1.2 ± 1.4 | −1.8 ± 1.2 |

*Table 5.* Regional wall motion was evaluated by the centerline method and is given as a standard deviation per segment.

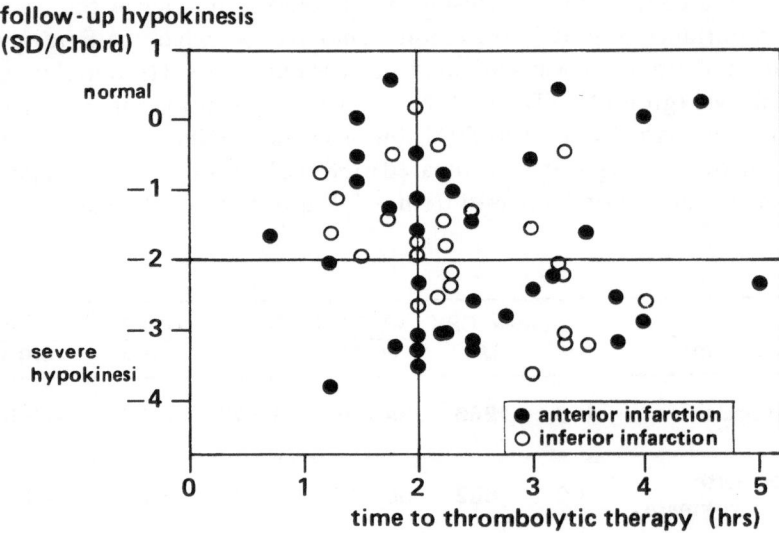

*Figure 1.* Follow-up hypokinesis vs. time to thrombolytic therapy: most of the patients successfully reperfused within 2 hours showed only a slight hypokinesis or normal regional wall motion, while 60% of those recanalized after 2 h had a severe hypokinesis as a result of the infarction.

tions (group II). In Figure 1 time to treatment is plotted against the alteration of regional wall motion at the time of control angiography, 80% of the patients, successfully reperfused within 2.0 hours showed a regional wall motion in the normal range, while this was the case in only 40% of those patients, reperfused within 2.0 to 4.0 hours.

Out of a number of additional clinical and acute angiography variables from the Western Washington Trial [26] comparing intracoronary streptokinase and standard therapy it was reported that the 6 months prognosis after acute myocardial infarction is definitely dependent on the size of the hypokinetic segment (involvement of more than 40% of the circumference of the left ventricle), a moribund clinical state at the time of admission, the age of above 70 years, unsuccessful reperfusion and the absence of collaterals (Table 6). With these parameters a high risk group could be identified with a 6-months mortality of 56% compared to patients with successful reperfusion, with collaterals, lower age, good hemodynamic state and a smaller infarction, who had to face a 6-months-mortality of 4%.

Controversial results have been presented with regard to the effect of mechanical measures as PTCA or aortocoronary bypass surgery (ACBS) to warrant the success of the reperfusion on the clinical follow-up (mortality, recurrent myocardial infarction). In the randomized cooperative Netherlands Study [27] there was no difference in 3 months and 10 months mortality in the intracoronary streptokinase group compared to the untreated controls. ACBS and PTCA did not affect the longterm mortality.

However, the study from v. Essen et al [28] (Table 7) resulted in a 1 month mortality rate of 14% in unsuccessful treated patients with intracoronary strep-

---

i.c. streptokinase : n = 116
standard therapy : n = 91

① Hypo-segment

② Moribund status at cath. time

③ Age

④ Lack of reperfusion

⑤ Absence of collaterals

Low risk group: 6 m. mortality: 4%
High risk group: 6 m. mortality: 56%

---

*Table 6.* 6 months after acute myocardial infarction based on clinical and angiographic data.

| | A ± SD / years | 30 days | 1 year |
|---|---|---|---|
| convent. therapy (n = 204) | 57 ± 12 (21 − 83) | 7.9 % | 21.2 % |
| PTCA (n = 129) | 56 ± 10 (34 − 76) | 3.1 % | 9.3 % |
| early ACB-Op. (n = 78) | 56 ± 7 (39 − 76) | 2.6 % | 6.4 % |
| no success (n = 50) | 54 ± 9 (34 − 79) | 14.0 % | 20.0 % |

*Table 7.* 1 month and 1 year mortality in patients with AMI treated by intracoronary thrombolysis. Upper panel shows the successful groups, lower panel the group without success.

tokinase compared to successful treated patients with 7.9%. The mortality was markedly lower, if the residual stenosis was widened by PTCA (3.1% or treated by early aortocoronary bypass surgery (2.6%). The difference in mortality between the unsuccessful treated group (20.1%) and those, who underwent PTCA (8.3%) or ACBS (6.4%) was still present after 1 year, whereas the initially successful reperfused patients followed by conventional therapy had after 1 year the same mortality (21.2%) as the unsuccessful treated group (20.1%). Thus, although this was a non-randomized study, the major clinical importance to warrant a sufficient coronary blood flow by outruling the effect of the residual stenosis after successful coronary thrombolysis may be suggested.

Age has been claimed to be of clinical relevance for the mortality [26]. As to be seen from Table 8 [28] in 55 patients above 70 years the mortality was with 29% resp. 37% high after 1 year, irrespective of successful or unsuccessful reperfusion. However, when coronary flow to the infarcted segment after successful thrombolysis was maintained either by PTCA or aortocoronary bypass operation, mortality in this small group of 14 patients was markedly diminished.

In conclusion, from the presently available data the short and longterm results in thrombolytic therapy of an acute myocardial infarction depend mainly on the following parameters (Table 9): For the short-term course the first parameter is a successful reperfusion, which has to be achieved, at the best within 2.0 hours. For that purpose the immediate application of thrombolytic agents after AMI is necessary, which is not only accompanied by a higher percentage of successful reperfusion, but also a higher likelihood to decrease infarct size. Moreover, it is clear that time is the only variable and thus the single factor to be influenced by therapeutic measures. Additional determinants are the size of the hypokinetic segment, which depends on the size of the affected infarct vessel and the presence

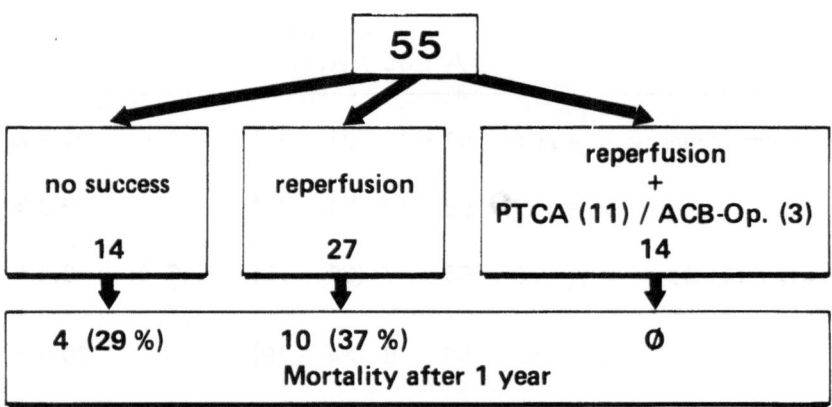

*Table 8.* Reperfusion rate and mortality after intracoronary thrombolysis in AMI in elderly patients (more than 70 years).

Short - and Long Term Results in Thrombolytic Therapy of AMI
Depent on

| SHORT TERM | LONG TERM |
|---|---|
| ● Reperfusion | = |
| ● Time  (< 2.5 h) | = |
| ● Hypok. segment (init. inf. size) (hemod. status) | = |
| ● Age  (< 70 years) | = |
| ● Collaterals | = |
|  | ● Prevention of early reocclusion<br>　a.  Anticoagulation<br>　b.  Early Bypass Op./PTCA |
|  | ● Preservation of ischemia/reinfarction<br>　a.  PTCA  (?)<br>　b.  Aortocoronary Bypass Op. (?) |

Table 9. Parameters, which determine the short and long-term results in the thrombolytic therapy of AMI.

of collaterals, both marking the initial area of jeopardized myocardium or the initially infarct size and, accordingly, the hemodynamic state. This is clearly obvious, if an infarction caused by a thrombosis of the left main coronary artery is regarded. In addition mortality is higher in elderly persons.

If the thrombolytic therapy was successful, for the longterm course it is of major importance to prevent the re-occlusion. The different therapeutic measures, as an effective anticoagulation, early PTCA (29) or aortocoronary bypass-surgery, are still discussed and need further investigations.

## Acknowledgement

With support of the Dr. Werner Otto Foundation, Hamburg, West Germany.

## References

1. Chazov EL, Mateeva LS, Mazaev AV, Sargin KE, Sadoskaya GV, Ruda MY (1975) Intracoronary administration of fibrinolysin in acute myocardial infarction. Terapevticheskii Arkhiv 8: 19
2. Rentrop P, Blanke H, Wiegand V, Karsch KR (1979) Wiedereröffnung verschlossener Kranzgefäße im akuten Infarkt mit Hilfe von Kathetern (transluminale Rekanalisation). Deutsch Med Wsch 104: 1401

398

3.  Mathey DG, Kuck KH, Tilsner V, Krebber HJ, Bleifeld W (1981) Non-surgical coronary artery recanalization in acute transmural myocardial infarction. Circulation 63: 489
4.  Ganz W, Buchbinder N, Marcus H, Mondkar A, Maddahi J, Charuzi Y, O'Connor L, Shell W, Fishbein MC, Kass R, Miyamoto A, Swan HJ (1981); Am Heart J 101: 4
5.  Schröder R (1983) Systemic versus intracoronary streptokinase infusion in the treatment of acute myocardial infarction JACC 1: 1254
6.  Bleifeld W, Mathey DG, Hanrath P, Buss H, Effert S (1977) Infarct size estimated from serial CK in relation to left ventricular hemodynamics. Circulation 55: 303
7.  Sobel BE, Bresnahan B, Shell WE, Yoder RD (1972) Estimation of infarct size and its relation to prognosis. Circulation 46: 640
8.  Bleifeld W (1984) Medical therapy in the acute phase of myocardial infarction. In: Perspectives in Cardiology. Eds.: Sobel BE, Julian DG, Hugenholtz PG, Current Medical Literature Ltd p 84
9.  Mathey DG, Schofer J, Bleifeld W (1984) Intrakoronare Thrombolyse – eine bereits gesicherte Therapie des akuten Herzinfarktes? Dtsch Med Wschr 109: 678
10. Geltman EM, Ehsani AA, Campbell ML, Schechtman K, Robert R, Sobel BE (1979) The influence of location and extent of myocardial infarction on long-term ventricular dysrhythmia and mortality. Circulation 60: 805
11. Khaja F, Walton JA jr, Brymer JF, Lo E, Osterberger L, O'Neill WW, Colfer HT, Weiss R, Lee T, Kurian Th, Goldberg A, Pitt B (1983) Intracoronary fibrinolytic therapy in acute myocardial infarction. Report of a prospective randomized trial. N Engl J Med 308: 1305
12. Anderson JL, Marshall HW, Bray BE, Lutz JR, Frederich PR, Yanowitz FG, Datz LF, Klausner St C, Hagan AD (1983) A randomized trial of intracoronary streptokinase in the treatment of acute myocardial infarction. N Engl J Med 308: 1312
13. Rentrop P, Blanke PH, Karsch KR, Rutsch W, Schartl M, Merx W, Dörr R, Mathey DG, Kuck KH (1981) Changes in left ventricular function after intracoronary streptokinase infusion in clinically evolving myocardial infarction. Am Heart J 102: 1188
14. Smalling RW, Fueuler F, Matthews MW, Freund BL, Hicks ChH, Reduto LA, Walker WE, Sterling RP, Gould GL (1983) Sustained improvement in left ventricular function and mortality by intracoronary streptokinase administration during evolving myocardial infarction. Circulation 68: 131
15. Schwarz F, Schuler G, Katus H, Mehmel HC, v. Ohlshausen K, Kübler W (1982) Intracoronary thrombolysis in acute myocardial infarction. Correlation among serum enzyme, scintigraphic and hemodynamic findings. Am J Cardiol 50: 32
16. Sheehan HF, Mathey DG, Schofer J, Krebber HJ, Dodge HT (1983) Effects of interventions in salvaging left ventricular function in acute myocardial infarction. A study of intracoronary streptokinase. Am J Cardiol 52: 431
17. Baughamm KL, Maroko PR, Vatner SF (1981) Effects of coronary artery reperfusion on myocardial infarct size and survival in conscious dogs. Circulation 63: 317
18. Mathey DG, Sheehan FH, Schofer J, Bleifeld W, Dodge HT (1982) Left ventricular function following intracoronary thrombolysis in acute myocardial infarction. Circulation 66: 335
19. Kennedy JW, Ritchie JL, Davis KB, Fritz JK (1983) Western Washington randomized trial of intracoronary streptokinase in acute myocardial infarction. N Engl J Med 309: 1477
20. Merx W, Dörr P, Rentrop P, Blanke H, Karsch KR, Mathey DG, Kremer P, Rutsch W, Schmutzler H (1981) Evaluation of the effectiveness of intracoronary streptokinase infusion in acute myocardial infarction. Postprocedure management and hospital course on 204 patients. Am Heart J 102: 1181
21. Weinstein J (1983) The international registry to support approval of intracoronary streptokinase thrombolysis in the treatment of myocardial infarction. Assessment of safety and efficacy. Circulation 68: Suppl I, 61
22. Kennedy JW (1983) Intracoronary streptokinase in acute MI. Report from the Society for Cardiac Angiography Registry Circulation 68: III, 121

23. Kennedy JW, Ritchie JL, Davis KB, Fritz JK (1983) Western Washington trial of intracoronary steptokinase in acute myocardial infarction. N Engl J Med 309: 1477
24. Reimer KA, Lowe JE, Rasmussen MM, Jennings RB (1977) The wave-front phenomen of ischemic cell death. I. Myocardial infarct size vs. duration of coronary occlusion in dogs. Circulation 56: 786
25. Mathey DG, Sheehan FH, Schofer J, Dodge HT (in Press) Time from onset of symptoms to thrombolytic therapy: a major determinant of myocardial salvage in patients with acute transmural infarction. Am J Cardiol (in press)
26. Stadius ML, Maynard C, Sheehan FH, Davis K, Fritz JK, Ritchie JL, Kennedy JW (1984) Six months prognosis after acute MI based on clinical and acute angiographic variables from the Western Washington Intracoronary Streptokinase Trial (WWIST). Circulation 70: II, 257
27. Simoons ML, v. Brand M, Serruys PW, Verheugt FW, Res J, Bär F, de Zwaan C, van Hoogenhuyze, Krauss XH, Wijns W, de Feyter P, Lubsen P, van Domburg R (1984) Clinical follow-up after recanalization in acute myocardial infarction. Circulation 70: II, 256
28. v. Essen R, Uebis R, Schmidt W, Dörr K, Merx W, Meyer J, Effert S, Schweizer P, Erbel R, Bardos P, Minale C, Messmer BJ (1985) Dtsch med Wschr 110: 570
29. Erbel R. Meyer J (1985) Mechanical ballon catheter recanalization combined with intracoronary lysis and PTCA. In: Dordrecht, the Netherlands: M. Nijhoff Publishers, Invasive Cardiovascular Therapy. Recent advances and future developments. Hilger HH, Hombach V, Rashkind WJ (Eds)

# V. Cardiac Arrythmias

# History of pacemaker therapy

S. EFFERT and M. SIGMUND

The occupation with the history of one's field is commonly regarded as a clear sign of old age.

In general the past cannot serve as a model for the future, but may be we can learn from what has gone before. Pacemaker-therapy appears to prove this hypothesis. During the thirties impulse generators capable of producing impulses necessary for pacing were certainly available. But even there was obviously no clinican sufficiently familiar with the work being done in related disciplines to know to the publication by the american physiologist Albert S. Hyman entitled: 'Resuscitation of the stopped heart by intracardial therapy' [13].

Hyman had shown that the electrical methods had previously failed because most investigators attempted to reactivate the heart by neurogenic exitation. When electric current was applied directly to the heart it was done by placing the entire organ in the electric circuit; the result was that the heart was unable to maintain its normal cycle. With the application of strong currents the factors discovered in electrocution were seen to be present.

Hyman used a clinical needle through which an electrical impulse was applied. In having two electrodes so close together that only a small pass way is involved in the electric circuit established by the heart muscle, an irritable point is produced. This point becomes the focus from which an excitation wave that follows the normal physiological conditions may spread over the heart muscle.

The apparatus Hyman used consisted of a spring motor activated electro-magnet generating a current which was instantaneously available at any time, at any place, and under all circumstances. The impulses were delivered at a constant rate that could be varied from 30 to 120 beats per minute.

Experimental animal studies had shown that the arrested heart immediately responded to the artificial pacemaker and rapidly returned to automatic activity after this response had restored some of the normal circulatory balance. Hyman writes: 'When correctly used the artificial pacemaker may prove to be of inestimable value in the restoration of those patients now succumbing to cardiac arrest; used together with other established live-saving procedures it may well be included in every physicians armamentarium against the final struggle with death'.

The paper was published in the Archives of Internal Medicine in October 1932. The first communication of a successful external electrical stimulation was given not before 1952 by Zoll from Boston. Two large electrodes applied to the chest wall delivered the impulses to the heart [24].

In 1954 Rosenbaum and Hanssen were the first to use electrodes put closer to the heart through a troicar in emergency situations [18].

Dittmar, Friese, and Nusser successfully applied this method to two patients first time in Germany in 1955 [3].

The first report of a successful postoperative stimulation in a patient with AV-block using epicardial or mycardial electrodes respectively was published by Weirich, Gott, and Lillehei in 1957 [23].

In 1958 Elmquist and Senning implanted the first fully implantable pacemaker with bipolar myocardial electrodes [8]. According to Greatbatch, Senning's device was not clinically successful. It worked only for three hours and then failed. A replacement worked for 8 days whereafter the patient lived without stimulation for another 3 years [11, 19, 20].

In 1960 Chardack, Gage, and Greatbatch started with the successful technique of permanent electrical stimulation using myocardial electrodes [2] (Fig. 1). Despite the fact that many problems remained to be solved pacemaker-therapy became a routine procedure.

The necessety of thoracotomy in the mostly elderly patients when myocardial electrodes were employed initated research to find alternatives.

In 1959 Furman and Schwedel were the first to refer to the possibility of transvenous electrode positioning also for permanent electrostimulation [10]. However, the merit of introducing this method into common clinical practice must go to the swede Lagergren in 1963 [14].

But I would like to mention the Suttgart internist Rienmüller, who reported in the 'Medizinische Welt' in 1957 for the first time on transvenous intracardial stimulations [17]. However, he thought more of anaesthesia problems due to asystole rather than of its possibilities in atrioventricular block. Nevertheless, he described a suitable catheter-technique similar to the one used today and built an impulse generator with technical support from Siemens.

So, the procedure commonly applied today with transvenous electrodes and pacemaker implantation into one of the two upper thoracical quadrants was already fully developed in 1963.

The following steps deal with improvements of catheters and impulse generators. The stiff and compared to now very large bipolar catheter carried a high risk of ventricular perforation (Fig. 2). The development of thinner and highly flexible electrodes which could be fixed to the ventricular wall in different ways ensued.

However, the technical advancement of generators to more longevity and

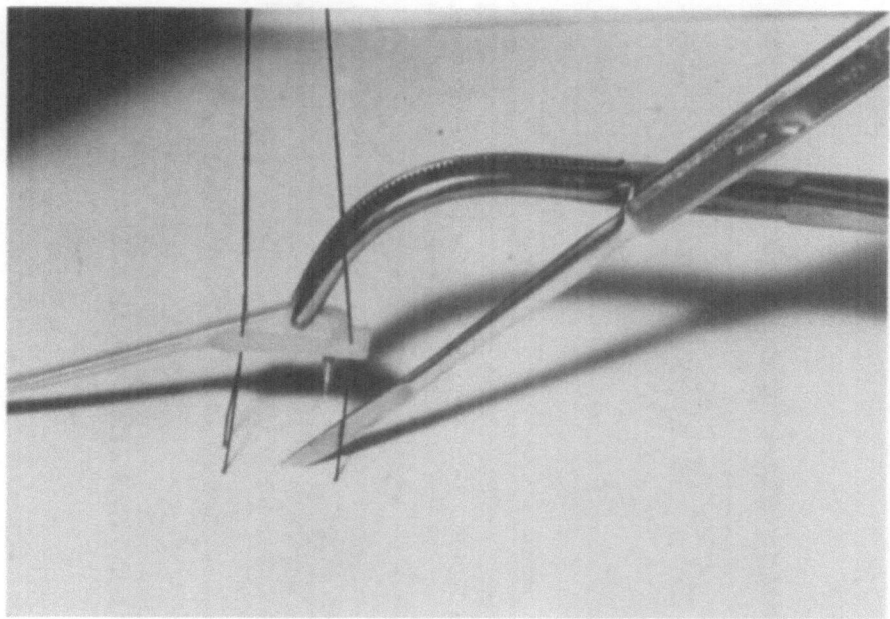

*Figure 1.* Principle of fixation of myocardial electrodes accoring to Chardack.

reliability met more difficulties than initially expected. In 1959 one of the pioneers of pacemaker-therapy, Greatbatch, predicted a five-year-pacemaker [12]. However, even by 1970 the life of the average pacemaker was only two years. 'The warm moist environment of the human body proved a far more hostile environment than outer space or the bottom of the sea.'

The life of mercury-batteries lay between several months and two to three years. Alternative solutions proposed were for example: an externally rechargable accumulator (Leatham) or transcutaneous energy transmission from a transmitter to a receiver. The nickel-cadmium-accumulators of 1958 were abandoned from 1960 in favor of mercury-zinc-batteries.

1970 isotope-pacemakers were introduced to the market and implanted. However, this development is also a thing of the past.

Up to now, the lithium-battery, used since 1972 supplanted all other developments. Its advantages are the high density of stored energy, the low internal losses due to self-discharge, the lack of gas production, and the absence of short circuits caused by reaction products.

The great capacity increases the longevity of the device; the pacemakers have become small and light. Battery and electronics are hermetically sealed.

The reliability could be considerably improved since programmable pacemaker with semi-conductor techniques were introduced. Pacemaker runaway – a feared complication of the older devices – no longer arises.

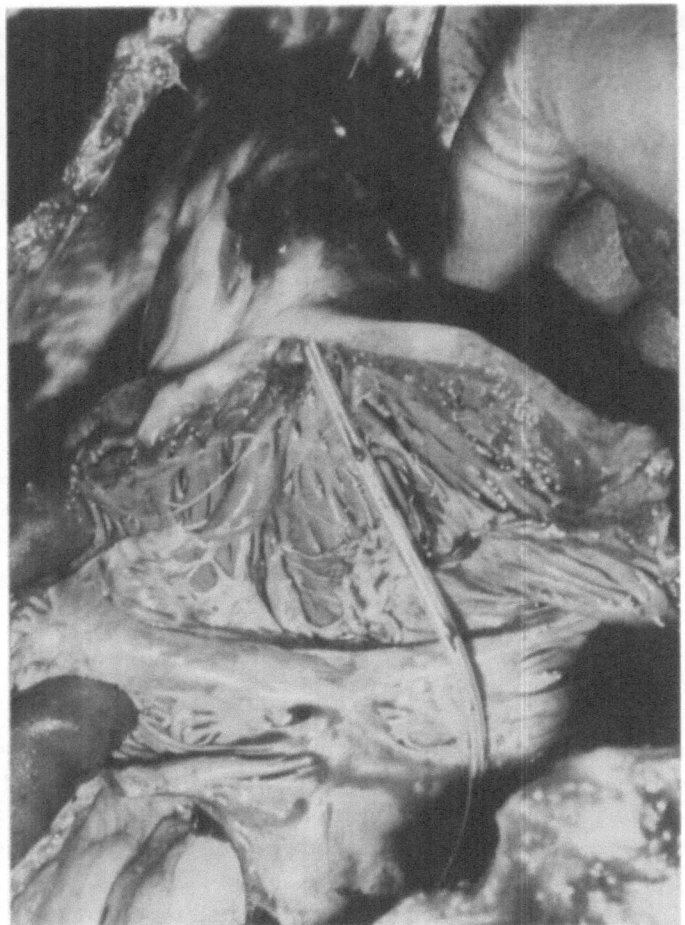

*Figure 2.* Perforation of a bipolar stiff catheter for permanent transvenous electrical stimulation.

Complications like perforation of the pacemaker through the pocket site are very rare nowadays.

The first pacemaker implantation I personally witnessed on October 6, 1961 was the first to be performed in West-Germany [5]. Sykosch implanted a Chardack-Greatbatch-pacemaker that I had brought to Düsseldorf from a visit to the United States. The patient was an 18 year old man with traumatic AV-block. Before implantation external pacing with myocardial and pericardial electrodes and transvenous stimulation had been repeatedly unsuccessful. The patient is still alive today.

There ist no doubt that a synchronous pacing carries a risk of inducing tachyarrhythmias up to ventricular fibrillation if spontaneous electrical activity is present as well. Of course, the problem was soon recognized. Several groups tried to find

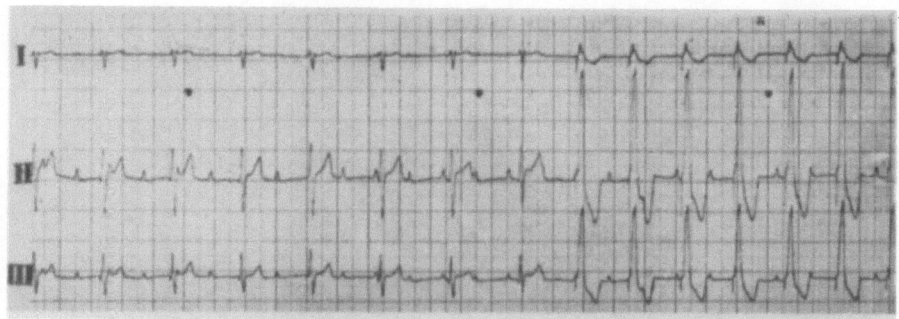

*Figure 3.* Function of a demand-pacemaker in a canine model. Ventricular rate decreases continously due to artificial complete atrioventricular block. At the end of the registration onset of pacemaker action.

a solution. We ourselves tested in 1962 what is now called a VVI-pacemaker developed by Zacouto from Paris [22] (Fig. 3). Both circuits – stimulating and sensing part – were still separated, the electronics were very complex, but the demand-mode worked well. However, the technique was soon appreciably improved with sensing and stimulating parts being combined in one device. The problem posed by the so-called pacemaker-syndrome was soon recognized as well. In 1963 our group together with Bostroem and Kreuzer could demonstrate the typical behavior of ventricular and atrial pressures in a simple ventricular demand-pacemaker (VOO) and a dual chamber sequential pacemaker (VAT-mode) [1].

Figure 4 shows the development from the first pacemaker with two transistors, built by Elmquist to modern device with 50.000 to 100.000 integrated semiconductor circuits. One of the first 'physiological pacemaker systems' – atrial synchronous ventricular pacing – was realized by Nathan and coworkers at the beginning of the sixties [15].

Our group operatively applied atrial electrodes for the first time in 1967 in two patients with sick-sinus-syndrome in order to pace in the AOO-mode [7]. But the transvenous technique of electrode implementation, used for the first time by Porstmann with an electrode with flexible tips developed by Schaldach [16], was also successful in these patients.

The further developments belong to the present, not to the past: first implantation of a DDD-pacemaker by Funke in 1978 [9], possibilities of frequency adaption to physiological needs by measuring pH-value, oxygen partial pressure, temperature, respiratory frequency, QT-time, stroke volume and stimulus threshold; the growing use of dual chamber systems, the introduction of the pacemaker code by Smyth and the systematic follow-up of patients with pacemakers.

At the moment the situation in West-Germany according to the figures of the

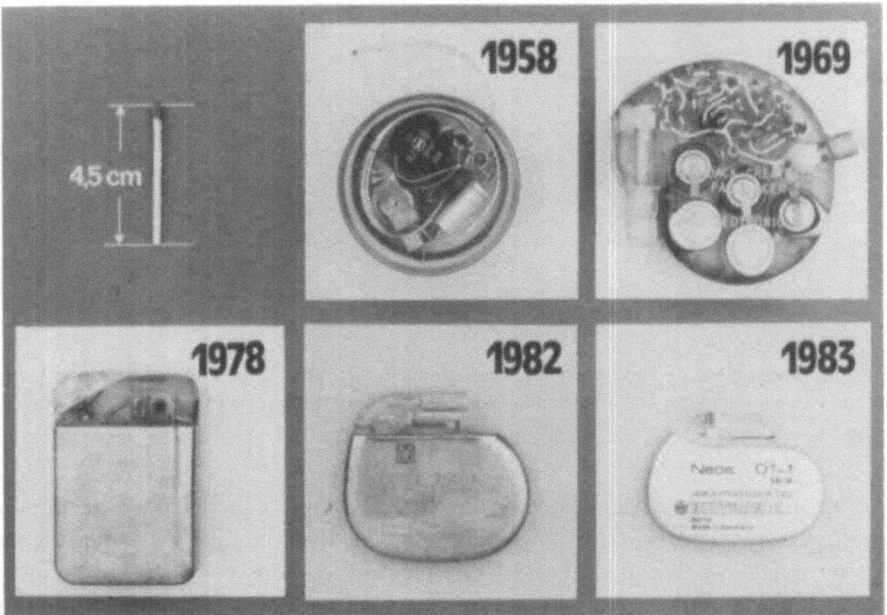

*Figure 4.* Development of pacemakers from 1958 (first pacemaker by Elmquist and Senning) until 1983.

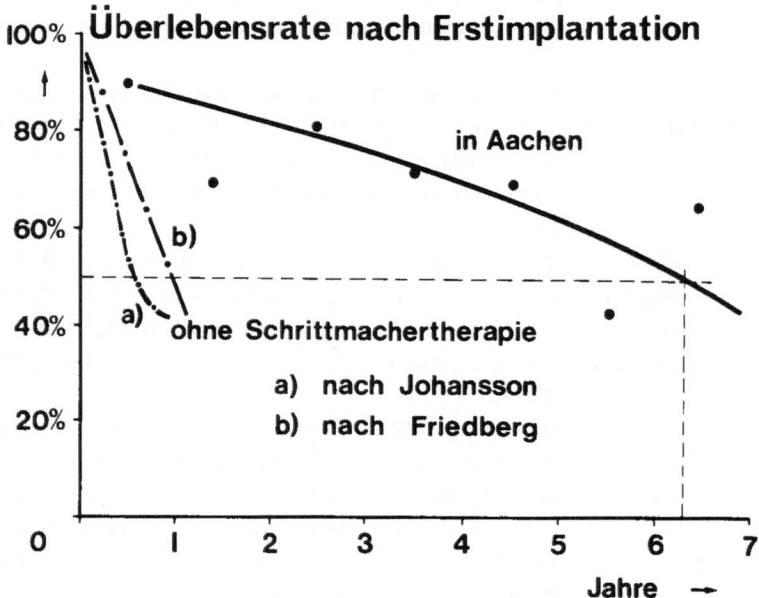

*Figure 5.* Survival rate following the first Adams-Stokes-attack. The respective survival rates before and after availability of pacemaker therapy are compared.

central register for pacemakers in Giessen is as follows: 148.000 patients lived with a pacemaker in 1983; 632 clinics implanted pacemakers. The number of first implantations was 32.000 in 1983, exchange operations were carried out 9.500. Seventeen firms offered 153 different types of pacemaking systems.

It is interesting that many of the implanting clinics have not yet responded to technical progress. 93 percent of the patients still received VVI-systems in 1984.

It is not necessary to mention here that pacemaker-therapy has been one of the milestones of medicine during the past 25 years. The patients do not only live longer they live a life worth living (see Fig. 5).

## References

1. Bostroem B, Effert S, Kreuzer H, Sykosch J (1964) Zur Hämodynamik bei permanenter Stimulierung des Herzens mit implantierbaren elektrischen Schrittmachern. Reanimation et organes artificiels 1: 69–75
2. Chardack WM, Gage AA, Greatbach W (1960) A transistorized self-contained implantable pacemaker for the long-term correction of complete heart block. Surgery 48: 643
3. Dittmar HA, Friese G, Nusser E (1956) Über die Behandlung des Kammerstillstandes beim Morgagni-Adams-Stokes'schen Symptomenkomplex mit einem elektrischen Schrittmacher. Z Kreisl Forsch 45: 416
4. Effert S, Bisping HJ, Irnich W Clinical requirements for pacemaker therapy. In: Schaldach M, Furman S (1975) Advances in pacemaker technology. Springer 3–10
5. Effert S, Greuel H, Grosse-Brockhoff F, Sykosch J (1962) Die Therapie mit elektrischen Schrittmachern beim Adams-Stokes-Syndrom. Dtsch med Wschr 87: 473–479
6. Effert S, Irnich W (1974) 15 Jahre Herzschrittmachertherapie. Dtsch med Wschr 99: 1146
7. Effert S, Meyer J, Petersen H, Reifferscheid M (1968) Elektrische Stimulation bei bedrohlichen tachykarden Arrhythmieformen. Verh Dtsch Ges Kreislaufforsch 34. Tagung: 424–427
8. Elmquist R, Senning A (1960) Implantable pacemaker for the heart. In: Smyth CN: Medical Electronics London 253
9. Funke H, Herpers L (1978) Electrographic findings in patients treated with optimized sequential stimulation. Abstr 1st Europ Symp Cardiac Pacing London 43–44
10. Furman S, Schwedel JB (1959) Use of an intracardiac pacemaker in the control of heart block. New Engl J Med 261: 943
11. Greatbatch W (1984) Implantable pacemakers, a twenty five year journey. IEEF Engineering in Medicine and Biology Magazine 121: 24–26
12. Greatbatch W, Chardack W (1959) A transistorized implantable pacemaker for the longterm correction of the complete atrioventricular block. Proc. New Engl Research and Engineering Meeting 1: 8
13. Hyman AS (1932) Resuscitation of the stopped heart by intracardial therapy. Arch Intern Med 50: 283
14. Lagergren H, Johansson L (1963) Intracardiac stimulation for complete heart block. Acta Chir Scand 125: 562
15. Nathan DA, Center S, Wu IY, Keller W (1963) An implantable synchronous pacemaker for the longterm correction of complete heart block. Amer J Cardiol 11: 362
16. Porstmann W, Witte J, Dressler L, Schaldach M, Vogel J, Warnke H (1972) P-wave synchronous pacing using anchored atrial electrode implanted without thoracotomy. Amer J Cardiol 30: 74–76
17. Rienmüller J (1957) Praktische Erfahrungen in der Prophylaxe des akuten Herzstillstandes. Medizinische Welt 1659–1662

18. Rosenbaum J, Hansen DK (1954) Simple cardiac pacemaker and defibrillator. J Amer med Ass 155: 1151
19. Senning A (1964) Problems in the use of pacemakers. J Cardiovasc Surg 5: 651
20. Senning A (1959) In discussion. J Thorac Cardiovasc Surg 38: 639
21. Siddons H, Sowton E (1967) Cardiac pacemakers. CC Thomas, Springfield
22. Sykosch J, Effert S, Pulver KG, Zacouto F (1963) Zur Therapie mit elektrischen Schrittmachern. Ein implantierbarer, induktiv ausschaltbarer elektrischer Schrittmacher. Elektromedizin 8: 139–142
23. Weirich WL, Paneth M, Gott VL, Lillehei CW (1958) Control of complete heart block by use of an artificial pacemaker and a myocardial electrode. Circulat Res 6: 410
24. Zoll PM (1952) Resuscitation of the heart in ventricular standstill by external electric stimulation. New Engl J Med 247: 768

# Present status and future needs of pacemaker technology

K. STEINBACH and G. JOSKOWICZ

## Introduction

The progress in microelectronics and the development of Lithium powered batteries really have pushed the pacemaker technology to such a level that the question arises which further development may improve the therapeutic facilities for the patient with brady- or tachyarrhythmias or if improvements serve only to satisfy the electronic play instinct of physicians dealing with pacing.

A pacemaker system consists of:

- battery
- one or more sensors
- controller-processor
- one or more stimulus delivery systems

and communicates bidirectionally with the outside world (Fig. 1).

## 1. Batteries

### 1.1. Reliability

The reliability of pacemaker batteries during the last five years with exception for a few models was adequate. Lithium iodine as energy source has solved the problem of internal discharge and has avoided the non predictable depletion, common in Hg-Zn batteries in the Sixties and early Seventies.

The longevity of the battery amounts between 5 and 15 years and is influenced less by battery variation than by other variables. EOL criteria for the different pacing models are well defined and allow timing of the explantation procedure without any risk for the patient. The reliability and longevity of pacemaker batteries is clearly demonstrated by the decrease of the number of replacements in relation to the number of first implants per year (Fig. 2) [1, 2].

412

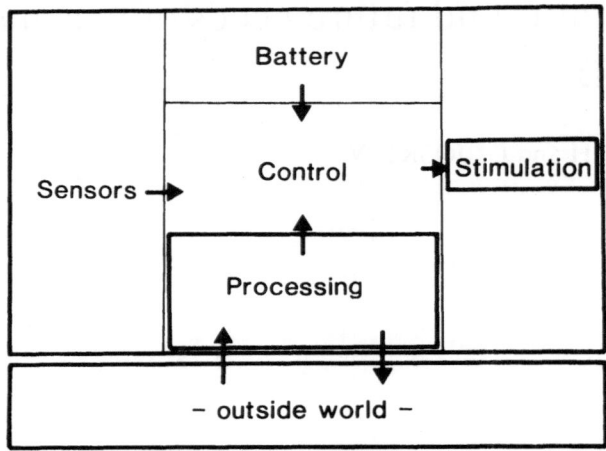

*Figure 1.* Scheme of an implantable pacemaker.

## 1.2. Longevity

The longevity of a battery does not depend on the capacity of the batteries which is in a range of 1.5–3.5 Ah but mainly on the output, pacing mode and pacing rate in programmable units as well as the spontaneous rate of the patient. As an example a pacemaker draws around 6–8 $\mu$A in stand by mode in contrast to 15–40 $\mu$A during active stimulation. Thus, in a dual chamber pacing system the energy drain during stimulation is 10 times higher than in sensing mode. Longevity is also influenced by the energy drain depending on the impedance in the electrode circuit in a range between 600 and 900 $\Omega$. Decrease of the impedance in the electrode circuit and increase of internal impedance of the batteries decrease the longevity up to 50% of the predicted time. In comparison to the theortic battery capacity, the other variables have a higher influence on the longevity. Provided they are well programmed a pacemaker system today offers a function time, long enough that the average patient will not require further replacement [3].

Looking back in the history in 1973 for the first energy controlled pacemaker a safety margine curve was calculated using constant voltage and variable pulse width (Fig. 3). Setting the energy safety margin to 50% instead of 100% over the threshold an increase of longevity by 100% was achieved [4, 5, 6]. Today we are just on the verge of continuous monitoring systems for the stimulation response which will allow on one hand an optimal set up of the output parameters and on the other hand the reduction of safety margin to 10–15% over the threshold. The individual rate set up using simple statistical parameters like counts of sensed or induced QRS-complexes through external or internal Holter monitoring allow to gauge the expected useful life of the system.

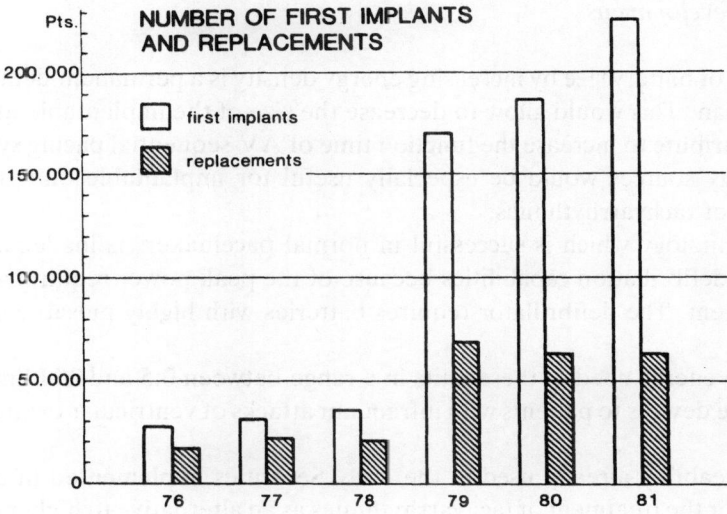

*Figure 2.* Ratio of first implants and replacements; 1976–1978 figures for Europe; 1979–1981 figures for five continents.

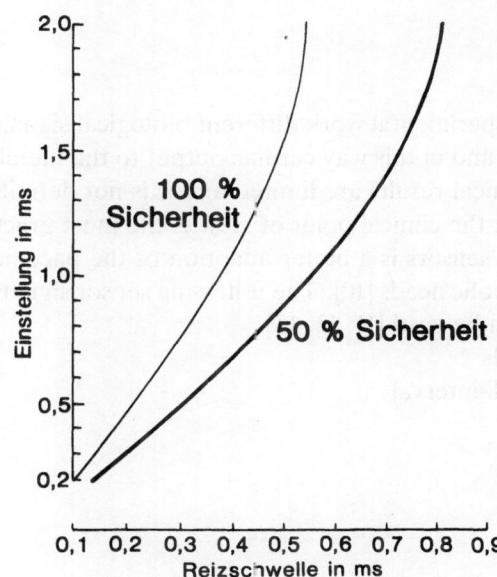

*Figure 3.* 50% and 100% safety margin expressed in duration (ms) of the stimulus.

## 1.3. New developments

Reduction of battery size by increasing energy density is a permanent demand by the physician. This would allow to decrease the size of the implantable unit and would contribute to increase the function time of AV-sequential pacing systems. New energy sources would be especially useful for implantable units for the treatment of tachyarrhythmias.

The technology which is successful in normal pacemakers is inadequate for units with defibrillation capabilities because of the peak power requirements of such a system. The defibrillator requires batteries with highly pulsatile current drains.

Also the energy need of these units in a range between 0.5 and 25 J limits the use of these devices to patients with infrequent attacks of ventricular tachycardia/fibrillation.

Rechargeability already used in the early Seventies implemented in devices designed for the treatment of tachyarrhythmias as an alternative to higher energy density could increase the function time of the batteries. However, the dependence on an external charger, the size of an adequate recharging circuit and the need for reliable monitoring of the capacity leaves this possibility as a very remote one [7, 8, 9].

## 2. Sensors

Since 10 years in experimental work different biological signals have been tested to adapt heart rate and in this way cardiac output to the metabolic demands. At the present the clinical results are limited and it is not definitely decided which sensor system from the clinical point of view is the most practical.

The goal of new sensors is a better adaption of the pacemaker to the hemodynamic and metabolic needs [10]. The following sensor signals for triggering the pacemaker rate can be used [11, 12, 13].
a) Electrical signals
   P-Wave and QT-interval
b) Biological
   pH
   temperature
   $O_2$
   respiration
c) Mechanical
   vibration
d) Volume indices
   stroke volume
   preload dimension
e) Impedance amplitude

About 50% of patients receiving permanent pacemakers have significant chronotropic incompetence. This precludes an appropriate increase of ventricular rate during exercise using P-wave sensing. Shortening of the QT-interval as trigger mechanism depends on serum catecholamin concentration. The rather small experience with implantable units already demonstrates the applicability under clinical conditions [14, 15].

Motion of the pacemaker during physical activity sensed by a piezo-quartz uses a rather simple technical device. Special filters are necessary to differentiate pacemaker motion during physical activity and passive motion of the patient e.g. during car driving [16].

Impedance amplitude maybe a useful adjunct to the analysis of rate and QRS-morphology for automatic detection of ventricular tachycardias. Impedance amplitude decreases up till 30% during ventricular tachycardia. This decrease depends on changes of the ventricular volume.

It has been demonstrated that all the above mentioned parameters are influenced by physical activity. From the technical point of view 3 requirements have to be fulfilled:

I.    Stability
      a) Same action in response to the same trigger
      b) Resistant to noise from system or random sources
      c) no drifts caused by ageing
II.   Practicability
      Use of one electrode, simple insertion technique
III.  Serviceability
      A feed back mechanism should be included in the system accessible from outside to check the behaviour of each element of the loop.

Not only new sensors but also improvement of processing of the ECG-signal e.g. differentiation of antegrade and retrograde depolarization of the atrium can be accomplished by converting the analogue signal in a derived form describing maxima and minima. Amplitude, slew rate, initial deflection and overall polarity could be used as criteria for discrimination (Fig. 4).

Pacemakers using two sensors – one for atrial activity and one for metabolic changes – would be able to check if the increase of atrial rate is appropriate. If this is not the case the rate could be adjusted according to the metabolic needs. The concept of two sensors in the pacemaker also has advantages in the treatment of tachyarrhythmias by improvement of detection and classification of the tachycardia.

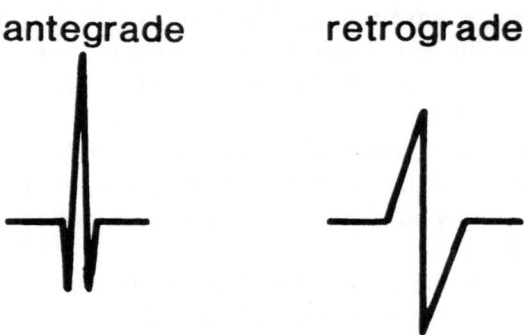

*Figure 4.* Characteristics of an antegrade and retrograde atrial depolarisation.

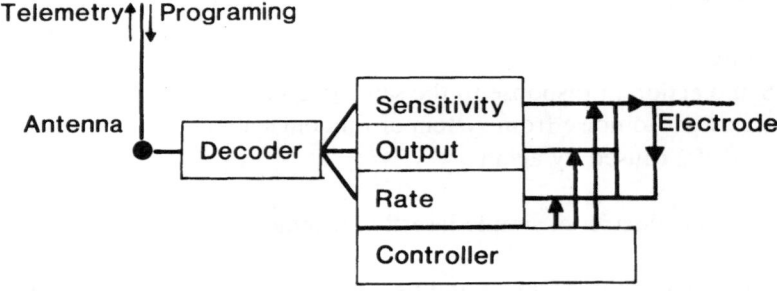

*Figure 5.* Technical principle of a controller.

## 3. Controller – processor

In hardware based pacemakers the so-called controller provides the timing and the characteristics of the stimulus. The specifications of the controller cannot be changed. The system is variable in the sense that the programmable parameters registered in the unit can be changed from outside (Fig. 5).

The controller in the simplest case is a counter which times the next stimulus (Fig. 6). It is an engine which activates sequences through predetermined states. Reprogramming changes the whole sequences e.g. DDD to DVI. but the system will never change the sequence of states through an automatic decision. We can implement through a state machine any pacemaker system.

In a software based pacemaker the relatively inflexible controller is replaced by a processor unit. This processor communicates with a registry (Fig. 7).

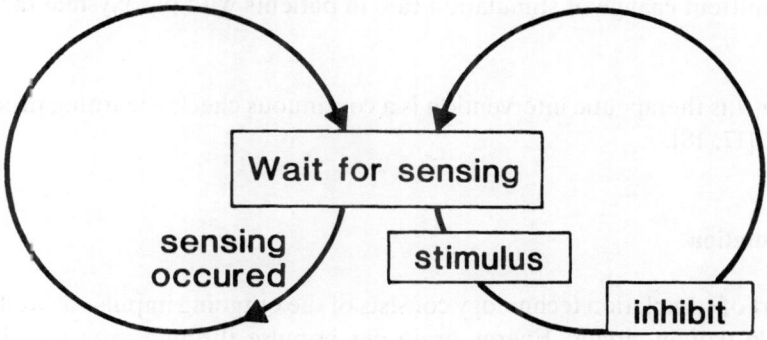

*Figure 6.* Scheme of a hardware based pacemaker.

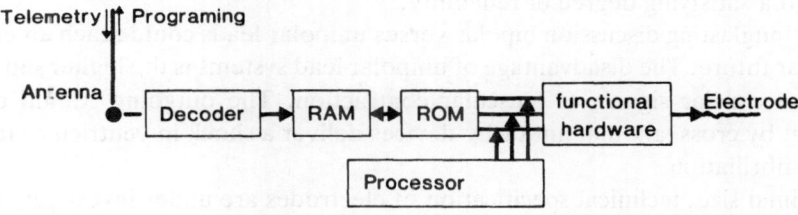

*Figure 7.* Scheme of a software based pacemaker.

In ROM (read only memory) data which cannot be changed are stored. The task of RAM is to store patient related data and diagnostic information. The orchestra of registry, processor and hardware conducted by an appropriate software provide a versatile pacemaker system. The advantage of the software system is obvious. This allows not only total reprogramming of the unit but has also learning capabilities from the outside:

I.  A new operation mode could be introduced in the unit by down loading a new program.
II. Self learning especially for treatment of tachycardias.
    The most effective termination method could be recognized by the system from past experience with different trials.

Examples for clinical application:

1. The behaviour of spontaneous heart rhythm can be continuously evaluated.
2. Adaption of stimulation rate to the spontaneous rate of the patient.
3. Detection of circadian rhythm.

4. Intermittent change of stimulation rate in patients with paroxysmal tachycardias.

Base for this therapeutic intervention is a continuous check – learning process of the unit [17, 18].

## 4. Stimulation

This part of stimulation technology consists of the outgoing impulse as well as the electrode patient circuit. Energy drain per impulse through programming the output according to the individual threshold has been reduced in programmable units leading to increase of function time. The electro-chemical properties of the electrode, the resistance in the circuit as the diameter of the electrodes have reached a satisfying degree of reliability.

The longlasting discussion bipolar versus unipolar leads could reach an end in the near future. The disadvantage of unipolar lead systems is the higher sensivity to extra cardiac signals as muscular contraction. The outgoing stimuli could prevent by cross talk that antitachy-devices deliver a shock in ventricular tachycardia/fibrillation.

Optimal size, technical specification of electrodes are under investigation for treatment of tachyarrhythmias [19]. From the technical point of view the goal should be to reduce the energy need by using multiple electrodes and sequences of shocks with lower energy [20].

## 5. Outside world

A software based pacemaker with a suitable software can be used as an implantable electrophysiological laboratory. This is of course extremely interesting for the clinician. An equipment with these capiabilities could replace Holter monitoring in pacemaker patients for continuous rhythm analysis. Based on the result of the rhythm analysis the antiarrhythmic treatment could be guided by these equipments. In case of the occurrence of ventricular arrhythmia pacing rate could be adapted automatically and simultaneously injection of an antiarrhythmic drug stored in an implantable injector could be initiated by the pacemaker.

Both, the hardware as well as the software pacemaker, comunicate with the outside world via an antenna system. This system transmits the commands generated by the programmer. The decoded signals in a hardware based pacemaker are fed in the different memories for amplitude, pulse duration etc. In software based pacemakers they are fed in RAM. At the present time each pacemaker model uses a different interface. It would be necessary especially for the more complex software pacemakers that they are accessible with the same

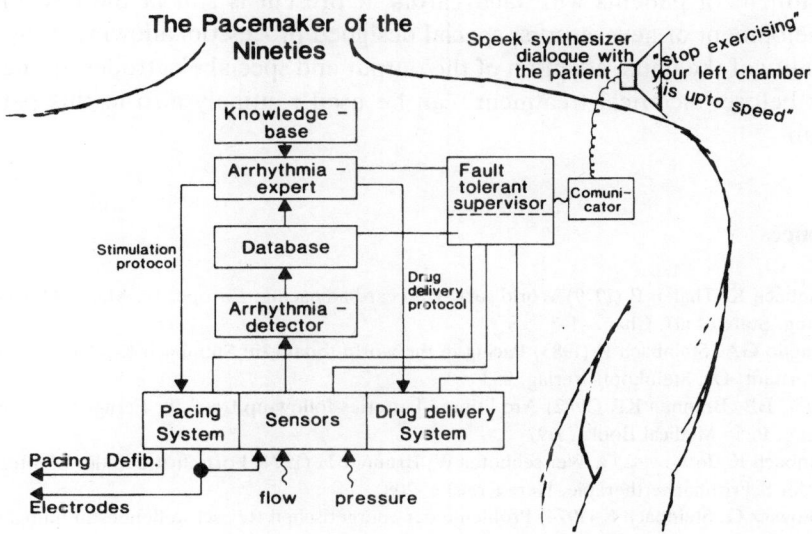

*Figure 8.* The implantable versatile stimulator/defibrillator of the Nineties.

external unit and especially with the same language. This is the prerequesite that in the future an external 'expert' which communicates with the memory of the pacemaker could automatically check the patient's parameter and adapt e.g. in case of increase of the threshold the output to the individual need.

### View into the future

The pacemaker of 1990 is demonstrated in Figure 8. This unit combines capabilities for treatment of brady- as well as tachyarrhythmias. The data base included in this system stores patient related data as behaviour of spontaneous rhythm, arrhythmias etc. The arrhythmia expert is able to decide on the therapeutical intervention as change of pacing rate, pacing mode and additional pharmacological treatment. The fault tolerant supervisor has to control and if necessary to correct the different parts of the system. From the technical point of view it is possible to produce an external unit with these capabilities.

### Summary

1. Improvement of therapeutic facilities for patients with bradycardia can be expected by introducing software based pacemaker with capabilities for continuous monitoring of physiological and pacing related data.

420

2. Treatment of patients with tachycardia at present is still at the beginning. Development of new sensors, special designed processors allowing programmability of the units, adaption of the output and special electrodes are necessary before 'electrical treatment' can be used routinely also in this patient group.

## References

1. Steinbach K, Thalen B (1979) World survey on cardiac pacing: Europe. In: Meere C. Cardiac pacing. State of art. Chap. 41–3
2. Feruglio GA, Steinbach K (1983) Pacing in the world today. In: Steinbach K. Cardiac pacing. Darmstadt: Dr. Steinkopff Verlag, 953
3. Owens BB, Brennen KR (1982) Are lithium batteries follow-up free? In: Feruglio G. Cardiac pacing. Picin Medical Books, 1197
4. Steinbach K, Joskowicz G, Weissenhofer W, Brunner H (1974) Fortschritte in der Meßtechnik bei der Schrittmachertherapie. Herz/Kreisl 6: 208
5. Joskowicz G, Steinbach K (1974) Probleme der energetischen Reizschwellenbestimmungen bei Schrittmacherpatienten. Intensivmedizin 11: 338
6. Joskowicz G, Steinbach K, Domanig E Jr (1975) Practical application of a power controlled pacemaker. ESAOI, 74
7. Frohner K, Kaltenbrunner W, Podczeck A, Steinbach K (1985) Transvenöse low-energy Karioversion bei ventrikulären Tachykardien. Zeitsch f Kardiologie 74: 3–97
8. Mirowski M, Reid PR, Mower MM, Watkins L, Gott VL, Schauble JF, Langer A, Heilman MS, Kolenik SA, Fischell RE, Weisgeldt ML (1980) Termination of malignant ventricular arrhythmias with an implanted automatic defibrillator in human beings. N Engl J Med 303: 322
9. Zipes DP, Prystowsky EN, Brown JW, Miles WM, Heer JJ (1984) Implantable transvenous cardioverter. JACC 3: 553
10. Humen DP, Kostuk WJ, Klein GJ (1985) Activity-sensing, rate-responsive pacing: improvement in myocardial performance with exercise. PACE 8: 52
11. Laczkovics A (1984) The central venous blood temperature as a guide for rate control in pacemaker therapy. PACE 7: 822
12. Rossi P, Plicchi G, Canducci G, et al (1983) Respiratory rate as a determinant of optimal pacing rate. PACE 6: 502
13. Wirtzfeld A, Heinze R, Liess HD, et al (1983) An active optical sensor for monitoring mixed venous oxygen-saturation for an implantable rate-regulating pacing system. PACE 6: 494
14. Donaldson RM, Rickards AF (1983) Towards multisensor pacing. Am Heart J 6: 1454
15. Rickards AF, Norman H (1981) Relation between QT-interval and heart rate. New design of physiologically adaptive cardiac pacemaker. Br Heart J 45: 56
16. Ryden L, Snedgard P, Kruse I, Anderson K (1984) Rate responsive pacing by means of activity sensing. Stimucoeur 3: 181
17. Rothman MT, Pumphrey CW, Skehan JD, Johnston K (1984) Recognition and termination of tachycardia in the right ventricle using an 'intellegent' implanted pacemaker. PACE 7: 463
18. Zipes DP, Prystowsky EN, Miles WM, Heger JJ (1984) Electrical therapy for cardiac tachyarrhythmias: Future directions. PACE 7: 606
19. Winkle RAS, Stinson EB, Bach SM, Echt DS, Oyer P, Armstrong K (1984) Measurement of cardioversion/defibrillation thresholds in man by a truncated exponential wave-form and an apical patch-superior vena cava spring electrode configuration. Circ 69: 766
20. Heilman MS, Langer A, Mower MM, Mirowski M (1975) Analysis of four implantable electrode systems for automatic defibrillator. Circ 52: II–194

# Treatment of bradycardias by physiological pacing

A. WIRTZFELD, G. SCHMIDT and K. STANGL

With the increasing tendency to implant pacemakers not only for life threatening bradycardias but also for improving cardiodynamics with the objective in mind to more effectively treat a failing heart or just to improve the workind capacity in patients with bradycardia, it became soon apparent that classical VVI pacing is unable to truely optimize circulatory performance. Experience has shown that with ventricular pacing augmentation of cardiac output takes place only initially but is not maintained on a long-term basis [1, 53], exercise capacity remains markedly reduced [23, 68, 69], there is only an unsatisfactory influence on the degree and course of heart failure [10, 20, 21, 38, 54, 68] and in an occasional patient cardiac function may even deteriorate as compared to the situation prior to pacing [2, 4, 76, 80]. As it was felt that the disappointing hemodynamic effect of fixed rate ventricular stimulation was at least partly due to the 'unphysiologic' mode of pacing provided by those systems which fail to restore AV synchrony and to increase heart rate with changing metabolic requirements, so called physiological pacemakers were developed. These pacing systems either maintain AV-synchrony and/or reestablish some way to adapt pacing rate (Table 1). This survey delineates the hemodynamic situation of the paced heart with special reference to the role of AV relationship and rate control, describes the clinical experience with physiologic pacing and provides some ideas leading to present and future developments for rate adaptive pacing systems.

## Pathophysiologic fundamentals of physiological pacing

Many clinical studies performed on patients with physiologic pacemakers suffer from the drawback that the data do not allow a definit analysis as to the relative importance of AV synchrony and rate control for the hemodynamic benefit provided by these systems. Often 'physiological pacing' is simply equated with systems which restore normal AV relationship irrespective whether stimulating rate is controlled or not. This is quite illogical indeed as improvement in exercise hemodynamics has only been demonstrated with those pacemakers which increase pacing rate. It appears very important to us trying to seperately consider and to individually analyse both aspects of physiological pacing, namely AV synchrony and rate responsiveness.

## Significance of AV synchrony

### Role of atrial function for ventricular performance
In spite of the fact that the active role the atrium plays in normal cardiac function has been known for long time, the significance of a physiologic AV relationship in the paced heart has been little appreciated in clinical cardiology until recently. In the healthy heart beating in sinus rhythm, atrial contraction at the end of diastole acts as a booster pump to enhance ventricular filling and – even more important – to produce the adequate degree of ventricular myocardial fibre stretch (preload) necessary for maximal ventricular contraction. Thus proper atrial contraction guarantees a high enddiastolic pressure for optimal ventricular performance without the need for high atrial (and pulmonary capillary) pressure throughout diastole. Loss of atrial function leads to a fall in enddiastolic ventricular pressure with insufficient fibre stretch resulting in a fall in stroke volume. To maintain LVEDP (preload) and ventricular contractility, mean atrial and venous capillary pressures will rise with a concomitant risk for pulmonary congestion. It has also been suggested that the lack of an atrial contraction prior to ventricular systole prevents the normal presystolic closure of the AV valves and that the delayed closure caused by ventricular contraction may produce some AV valve regurgitation [3, 57].

### Atrial contribution to ventricular stroke volume
The effect of atrial contribution to ventricular stroke volume of the paced heart has been extensively studied in the experimental animal [33, 55, 57, 71] and in man [32, 34, 61, 74, 70, 83]. It could be shown that not only AV synchronization as

*Table 1.* Physiological pacing systems.

| Pacing mode | AV-Synchrony | Rate-adaptation |
|---|---|---|
| AAI | + | − |
| DVI | + | − |
| VAT/VDD | + | + |
| DDD | + | + |
| Rate-responsive VVI | − | + |
| Rate-responsive AAI | + | + |

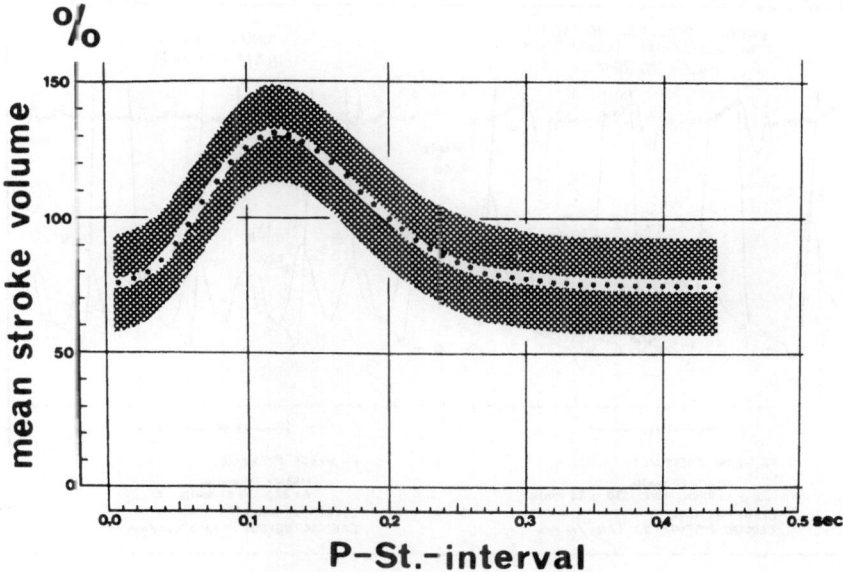

%

*Figure 1.* Dependency of stroke volume (average = 100%) on R-to-pacemaker stimulus interval in 12 patients paced asynchronously for complete AV-block [43].

such was important but also the optimal timing of atrial contraction during the diastolic period. Measuring stroke volume beat by beat by means of impedance cardiography in patients with ventricular pacemakers implanted for complete AV block, Knapp et al [43] observed a maximal stroke volume at a P-to-pacemaker induced R wave interval of 130 ms (Fig. 1). Others found optimal AV intervals between 50 and 250 ms with marked interindividual variations [37, 77]. Furthermore it was shown that an optimal AV interval was even more critical with increasing heart rates [17, 61]; the significance of this observation, however, is debatable as these studies were performed at rest with the heart rate being artificially increased just by pacing (see below).

*Retrograde atrial conduction*
Hemodynamically, the most deleterious event associated with ventricular pacing is the temporal coincidence of atrial and ventricular contractions. In the case of AV dissociation with randomly placed P waves this will occur only occasionally, but it will be present permanently if retrograde ventriculo-atrial conduction occurs. In this situation, the atria contract against the closed AV valves causing retrograde blood flow to the pulmonary and systemic veins (cannon waves) and a marked rise in venous pressures [40, 55]. As it takes some time for the blood to flow back into the atria, atrial pressures are initially low in early diastole and ventricular filling may be severely compromized. The hemodynamic situation is

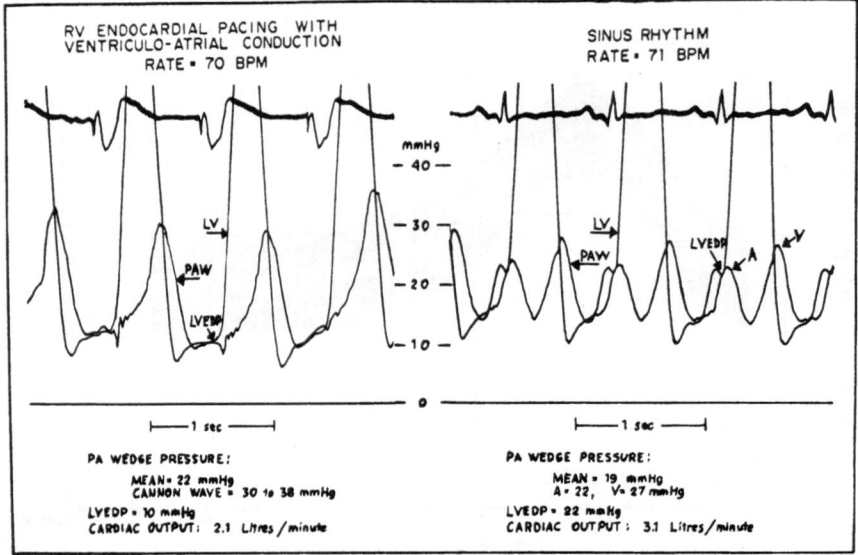

*Figure 2.* Registration of LV and PC wedge pressures during ventricular pacing with retrograde atrial activation (left) and during sinus rhythm (right). Note that during ventricular pacing, LV enddiastolic pressure and consequently cardiac output are low, inspite of the elevated wedge pressure (mean 22 mm Hg) caused by the high cannon waves of 30 to 38 mm Hg. During sinus rhythm wedge pressure is lower but LVEDP is significantly higher being equal to the a-wave in the wedge tracing; this better LV preload leads to an augmentation in cardiac output by 48% [40].

comparable to a patient with mitral stenosis: left atrial and PC wedge pressures are markedly elevated while LV enddiastolic pressure remains low (Fig. 2).

### AV synchrony and myocardial failure

A very important physiologic variable determining the significance of AV-synchrony in an individual patient represents the intrinsic performance of the left ventricle. While initially proper AV synchronization was thought to play a more important role in maintaining cardiac output in the failing than in the normal heart [7], it became evident that the reverse is true [32, 34]. Greenberg et al [34] showed that patients with left ventricular dysfunction and PC wedge pressures over 20 mm of mercury failed to derive any significant benefit from AV synchrony, but that at normal pressures atrial pacing resulted in a 20 to 50% greater stroke volume as compared to ventricular pacing. In a well-devised experiment, the authors altered left ventricular preload by volume expansion (rapid fluid infusion) followed by the application of a venodilating agent (ISDN) and compared the stroke volumes during ventricular and atrial pacing. As seen in Figure 3 both modes of pacing are hemodynamically equal in terms of cardiac output when LV filling pressure is elevated, but atrial pacing is clearly advantageous at low

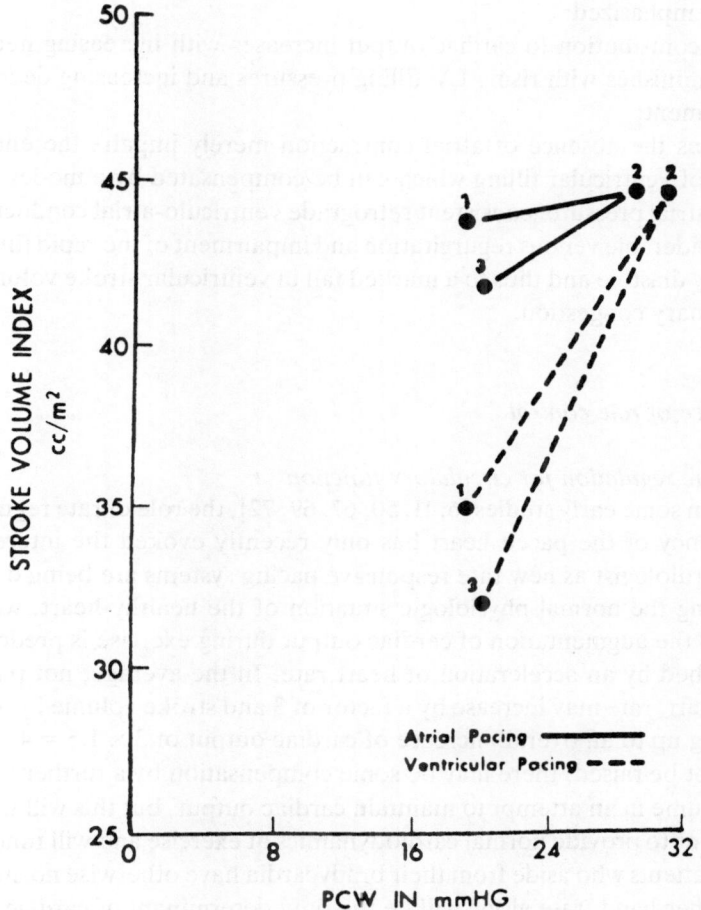

*Figure 3.* Influence of LV filling (PC wedge) pressure on atrial contribution to stroke volume. Measurements were done: 1) at baseline, 2) after volume infusion, and 3) after sublingual ISDN [34].

pressure levels. The reason why atrial contribution to ventricular stroke volume becomes insignificant in the failing heart is that, due to the elevation of overall left atrial pressure, the ventricle will be maximally filled early in diastole and does not require the booster pump of the atrium. Besides, in subjects with impaired LV function, the Starling curve is flat and there would be hardly any augmentation in stroke volume with further rises in filling pressure. Finally, abnormal atrial function (atrial myocardial failure) may also contribute to the observed reduction in atrial efficiency in patients with heart failure [34, 52].

## Conclusion

Summarizing the role of AV-synchrony for the paced heart the following points are to be emphasized:

1) Atrial contribution to cardiac output increases with increasing heart reates and diminishes with rising LV filling pressures and increasing degree of LV impairment;

2) Whereas the absence of atrial contraction merely impairs the enddiastolic phase of ventricular filling which can be compensated by a moderate rise in mean atrial pressure, consistent retrograde ventriculo-atrial conduction leads to considerable venous regurgitation and impairment of the rapid filling phase in early diastole and thus to a marked fall in ventricular stroke volume and to pulmonary congestion.

## Significance of rate control

### Role of rate regulation for circulatory function

Apart from some early studies [6, 11, 50, 67, 69, 72], the role of rate regulation for the efficiency of the paced heart has only recently evoked the interest of the clinical cardiologist as new rate responsive pacing systems are being developed. Considering the normal physiologic situation of the healthy heart, we have to recall that the augmentation of cardiac output during exercise is predominantly accomplished by an acceleration of heart rate. In the average, not particularly trained heart, rate may increase by a factor of 3 and stroke volume by a factor of 1.5, adding up to an overall increase of cardiac output of $3 \times 1.5 = 4.5$. If heart rate cannot be raised, there may be some compensation by a further increase in stroke volume in an attempt to maintain cardiac output, but this will usually not be sufficient to provide normal cardiodynamics at exercise and will function only in those patients who aside from their bradycardia have otherwise normal hearts. On the other hand, rate alone will be the only determinant of cardiac output in those patients who present with a fixed stroke volume due to LV dysfunction [50].

### Relationship of heart rate and cardiac output

In animal experiments it could be shown that in the normal heart cardiac output remains rather constant over a wide range of paced rates but that in hearts with reduced cardiac function rate may become critical and there may be an optimal rate with a maximal cardiac output [7]. Similarly also in man quite different rate/output relationships may be encountered [72]. As demonstrated in Figure 4, patients without myocardial disease tend to show a flat rate/output curve while those with depressed cardiac function demonstrate an obvious optimal rate as evidenced by a peaked curve with cardiac output falling off on either side of a distinct maximum or present slopes showing a continuous rise in output with increasing heart rates up to relatively high levels. These rate/output relationships were obtained during periods of rest; hemodynamically more significant, however, will be the pacing rate during exercise.

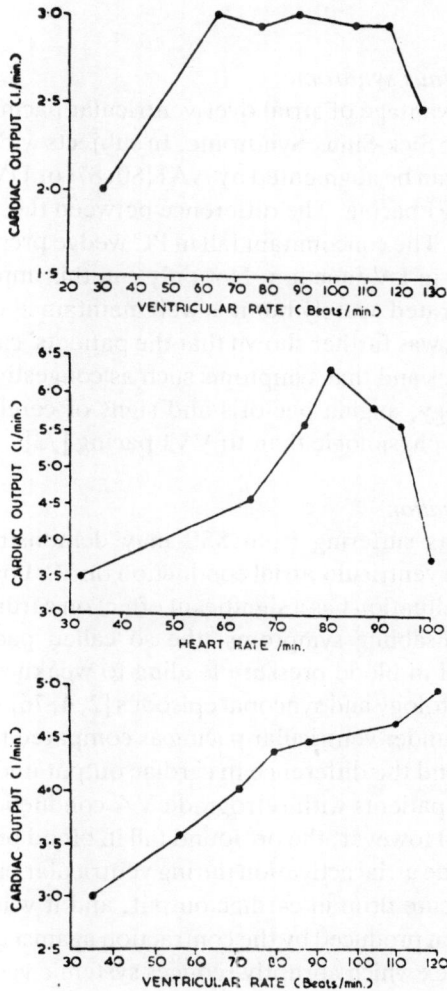

*Figure 4.* Relationship of cardiac output and heart rate at rest in individual patients paced for AV block. a) 'flat' type of rate-output curve; b) 'peaked' type of rate-output curve; c) rate-output curve showing a continuous rise in cardiac output with increasing pacing rates [72].

## Clinical experience with physiological pacemakers

In the clinical setting the role of proper AV sequencing can best be studied in patients with AAI and DVI pacemakers and the effect of rate regulation in those provided with atrial independent rate responsive pacing systems. In atrial triggered units both principles of physiological pacing are realized.

## AAI and DVI pacing

*Atrial pacing in sick sinus syndrome*

The hemodynamic advantage of atrial over ventricular pacing is quite evident in patients suffering from Sick-Sinus-Syndrome. In subjects with sinus bradycardia, cardiac output at rest can be augmented by AAI [80, 87] or DVI [19, 37, 49, 61, 73, 74] but not only by VVI pacing. The difference between these two pacing modes amounts to 20 to 30%. The concomitant fall in PC wedge pressure [74] indicates a definite improvement in LV function. Not only can this improvement in hemodynamics be demonstrated acutely but it is well maintained on a long term basis [39, 75, 83] (Fig. 5). It was further shown that the patients' cardiac symptomatology markedly improves and that symptoms such as congestive heart failure, low output symptomatology, angina pectoris and signs of cerebral dysfunction respond much better to physiologic than to VVI pacing [73].

*Retrograde atrial activation*

40 to 90% of patients suffering from SSS may demonstrate intermittent or permanent retrograde ventriculo-atrial conduction on VVI pacing [30, 31, 56, 76, 80]. This undesirable situation has a significant effect on cardiac performance and may produce quite disabling symptoms, the so called pacemaker syndrome, characterized by a fall in blood pressure leading to weakness, lightheadedness, low output symptomatology and syncopal episodes [2, 4, 76]. Cardiac output falls by 12 to 20% [80, 87] under ventricular pacing as compared to the unpaced heart (sinus bradycardia), and the difference in cardiac output under AAI in comparison to VVI pacing in patients with retrograde VA conduction amounts to 30 to 50% [30, 80] (Fig. 6). However, the profound fall in blood pressure seen in some patients with retrograde atrial activation during ventricular pacing can only partly be explained by an acute drop in cardiac output, and it was suggested that the sudden atrial distension produced by the contraction against the closed AV valves activates an atrial reflex which abruptly reduces systemic vascular resistance [2].

*Development of atrial fibrillation*

A potential limitation of AAI and DVI pacing is the development of atrial fibrillation. The incidence of post-VVI atrial fibrillation may be 7 to 20% [73]. In our opinion, the brady-tachy syndrome with intermittent atrial tachyarrhythmias, however, does not exclude the use of atrial pacing since the ineffective pacemaker discharge during the tachycardic episodes is of no consequence, and on termination of the arrhythmia the pacemaker will take over and prevent prolonged asystole or bradycardia as effectively as a ventricular pacer would do. Atrial pacing may even reduce the incidence of atrial tachyarrhythmias as these frequently develop as an escape rhythm in patients with slow action [83]. In a study comparing the effect of atrial and ventricular pacing on the control of atrial arrhythmias in patients presenting with brady-tachy syndrome it could be shown

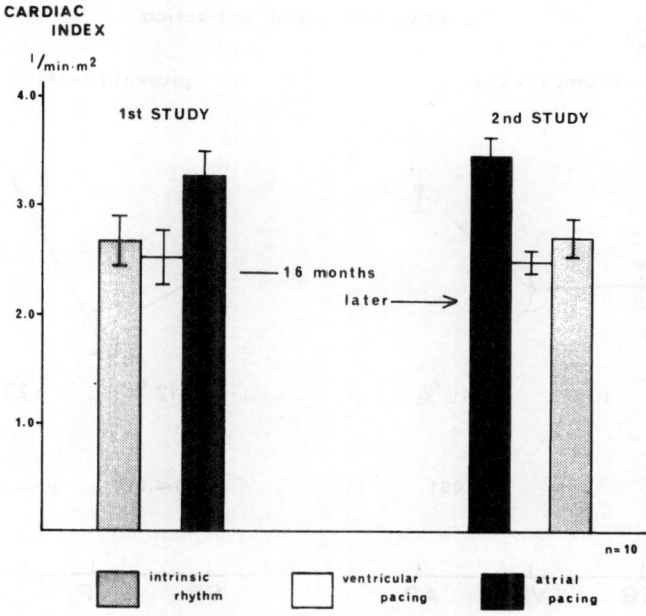

*Figure 5.* Long-term benefit of atrial pacing: Cardiac index during intrinsic rhythm (sinus bradycardia), ventricular pacing and atrial pacing in 10 patients with sick sinus syndrome. Comparison of the hemodynamic situation prior to (left) and 16 months after the implantation of an AAI pacemaker [83].

that in 83% of the patients provided with AAI units tachycardic episodes disappeared, whereas in the VVI group effective suppression was accomplished in only 31% [12].

### Clinical implications
Summarizing the clinical implications from the experience with physiologic pacing in patients with SSS it can be stated that atrial demand or in the case of additional significant AV conduction disturbance bifocal pacing should be employed whenever the objective of pacemaker treatment includes an improvement of hemodynamics. In patients demonstrating retrograde VA conduction on ventricular pacing, physiological pacing becomes mandatory. The major limitation of AAI and DVI pacing modes, however, remains the lack of rate responsiveness of the units available today.

### VAT-(VDD) and DDD pacing

### Exercise hemodynamics
The only rate responsive pacing systems available until recently were atrial

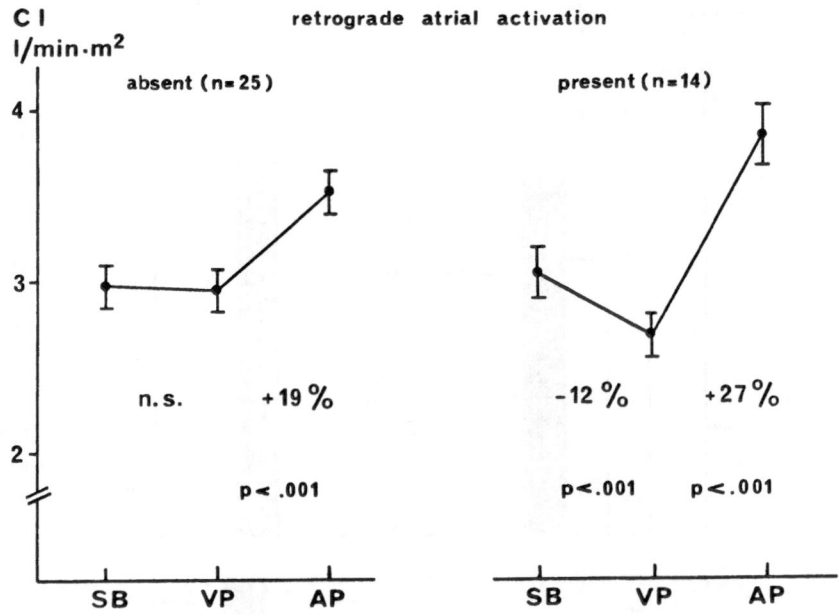

*Figure 6.* Cardiac index during sinus bradycardia (SB), ventricular (VP) and atrial (AP) pacing in patients without (left) and those with (right) retrograde atrial activation during ventricular pacing [80].

triggered VAT or VDD (DDD) units. Several groups have studied their effects on exercise hemodynamics in comparison to fixed rate VVI pacing [9, 41, 42, 46, 53, 79, 81]. They described an augmentation in cardiac output between 15 to more than 50% with the physiologic pacing system. This improvement in cardiac function is long-lasting and, unlike the experience with VVI pacing [1, 54]), the hemodynamic benefit can still be demonstrated after many months of continuous pacing [41, 59] or may even further gain with passage of time [25]. Furthermore, an increase in working capacity and exercise tolerance by 24 to 44% [25, 26, 45, 46, 58, 60, 75] and a reduction in heart size [46] occurs with atrial triggered pacing systems. Finally in a randomized controlled trial, Perrins et al [60] demonstrated a significant improvement in the patients' subjective status as symptoms such as shortness of breath, dizziness and palpitations were markedly reduced and the sensation of well-being was much improved during physiological pacing.

*Relative significance of AV synchrony and rate response*
The beneficial effect of atrial triggered ventricular pacing on exercise hemodynamics may be due to the restoration of AV-synchrony, to the rate increase provided by the system or to a combination of both factors. The question arises as to the relative significance of these two aspects of physiological pacing.

The interrelationship of AV-synchrony, rate and exercise hemodynamics was first analyzed in a study published by Karlöf in 1975 [42]. He measured cardiac performance at rest and during moderate exercise in patients paced externally in VVI and VAT modes. In one group of patients, comparing fixed rate pacing at 70/min with atrial triggered pacing, an increase in exercise cardiac output by 20% was found. In another group of patients, cardiac output was measured during VAT pacing and during a second exercise period while on an asynchronous ventricular pacing the rate of which was adjusted upward to equal the maximum rate achieved during the previous VAT period; cardiac output in these patients was only 8% higher on VAT compared to rate-adjusted VVI pacing and there were no differences in stroke volumes.

We studied the issue of the relative importance of atrio-ventricular synchronization and rate control in 11 patients with multiprogrammable DDD units implanted for complete heart block [53]. Cardiac output at rest and during exercise on a bicycle ergometer set to work loads of 25 to 100 Watts was measured during three different modes of pacing: VVI pacing at 70/min; atrial triggered pacing (VDD); VVI pacing at a rate matched to that previously recorded with VDD pacing. The exercise test was performed in one session, and the mode of pacing was changed on each level of work load while the patient continued pedalling (Fig. 7a). As seen in Figure 7b, with the P wave synchronous compared to the rate matched asynchronous system, there was as slight advantage of 7% and 5%, respectively, in cardiac output at the low work loads of 25 and 50 Watts. At the higher work loads of 75 and 100 Watts, however, cardiac output at both pacing modes were identical indicating that the increase in cardiac output achieved with VDD pacing compared to VVI 70/min pacing (+23%) was entirely due to the higher pacing rate.

Further indication for the limited importance of atrioventricular synchronization in rate adjusted pacing has been contributed by studies assessing the exercise capacity during various pacing modes [26, 58]. They showed that the chronotropic response to exercise accounts for most of the improvement in exercise performance seen in patient with atrial-synchronous pacing systems (Fig. 8).

*Dependency of atrial contribution to CO on LV performance*
Asking for the mechanism behind the diminishing importance of atrial contribution to cardiac output with increasing levels of exercise one has to recall that the contribution of atrial sysstole to ventricular stroke volume is dependent on mean atrial pressure (see above). As in patients with impaired myocardial function and reduced ventricular compliance mean atrial pressure will rise with exercise, the ventricle will be filled passively to its optimal preload early in diastole obviating an active atrial contraction. This situation is quite different from a patient at rest in whom heart rate is just raised by pacing; as there will be no increase in atrial pressure, it is not surprising that in this artificial and unphysiologic situation – unlike the patient performing work – proper timing of atrial systole may contrib-

432

## Study design

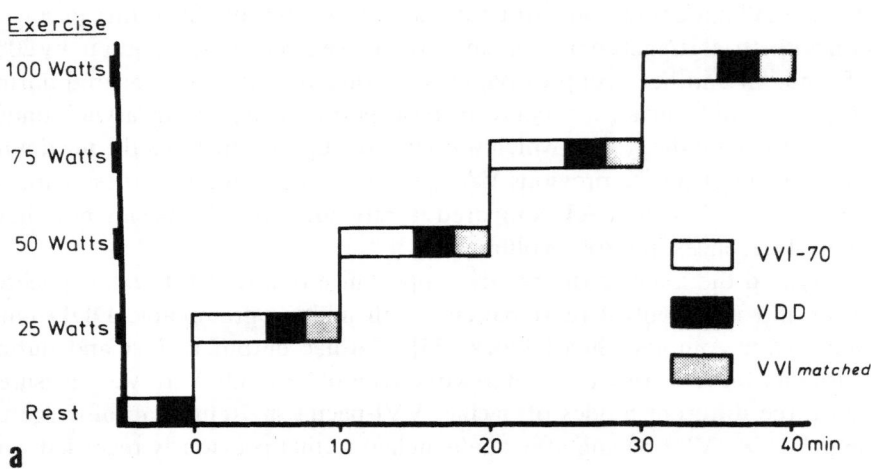

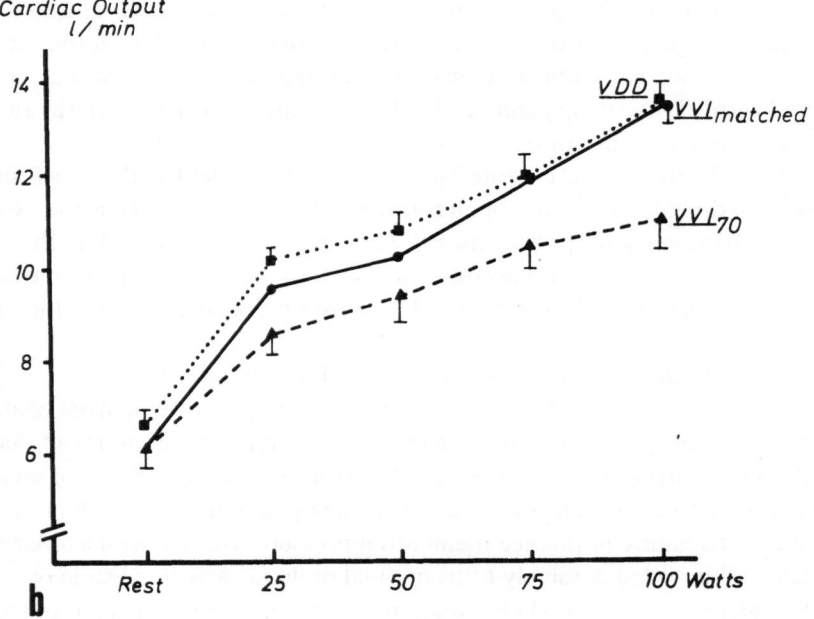

*Figure 7.* Cardiac output at rest and during exercise in 11 patients stimulated at various pacing modes. a) study design; b) results. For details see text.

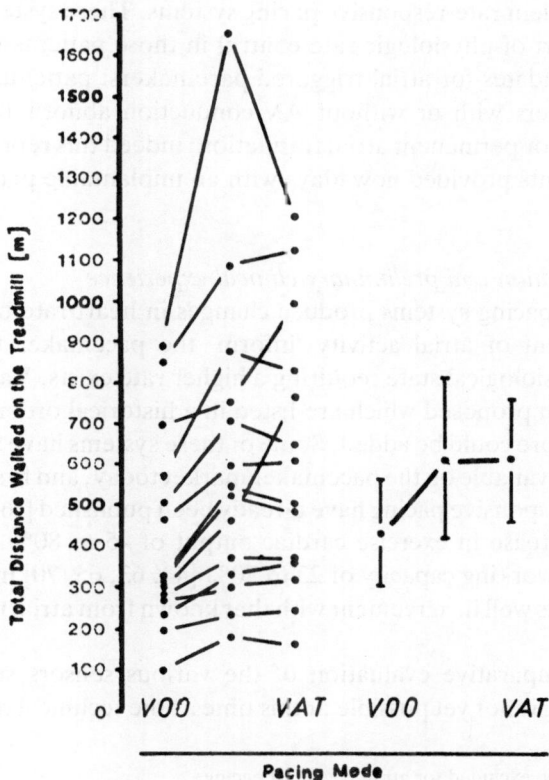

*Figure 8.* Exercise capacity during various pacing modes: VOO 70/min (first line), VAT (third line) and VOO pacing at a rate matched to that reached during VAT pacing (middle line). Left: individual patients; Right: average of the entire group [26].

ute much more to the ventricular stroke volume [17]. On the other hand, one may wonder whether an AV interval which is commonly set to around 150 ms is really optimal for the heart at exercise; the possibility cannot be excluded that a more significant effect of AV-synchrony on cardiac output could have been demonstrated in the studies cited above if a shorter AV interval had been chosen [77]. It might be wise to make the AV interval dependent on heart rate and to automactically shorten it with higher pacing rates [36].

## Atrial-independent rate responsive pacing systems

Since the improvement in exercise performance seen with atrial triggered pacing is predominantly due to the adaptation of heart rate rather than to AV-synchrony, it is to be expected that comparable hemodynamic results can be attained by atrial independent rate-responsive pacing systems. These systems would make possible some sort of physiologic rate control in those patients who have to be excluded as candidates for atrial triggered pacemakers: patients suffering from sinu-atrial disorders with or without AV-conduction abnormalities and those with intermittent or permanent atrial fibrillation; indeed this represents the great majority of patients provided nowadays with an implantable pacemaker (Table 2).

### Principle of operation and preliminary clinical experience

Rate responsive pacing systems produce changes in heart rate by using sensors which independent of atrial activity 'inform' the pacemaker that an altered metabolic or physiological state requiring a higher rate exists. Various biological sensors have been proposed which are listed in a historical order in Table 3 and certainly a few more could be added. Some of these systems have already become a reality and are available on the pacemaker market today, and first reports on the benefits of rate responsive pacing have already been published [16, 44, 63, 65, 70]. The range of increase in exercise cardiac output of 45 to 80% [63, 65] and of improvement in working capacity of 23 to 70% [44, 63, 65, 70] in comparison to fixed rate pacing is well in agreement with that known from atrial triggered pacing systems.

A definite comparative evaluation of the various sensors suitable for rate responsive pacing is not yet possible at this time as the technical development for

*Table 2.* Patients to be excluded for atrial triggered pacing.

| | |
|---|---|
| Sick sinus syndrome | 40% |
| Atrial fibrillation | 20% |
| AV-Block with atrial arrhythmias | 20% |
| | 80% |

*Table 3.* Physiologic sensors proposed for rate responsive pacing.

| Parameter | Year* |
|---|---|
| Respiration rate [28, 39, 64] | 1975 |
| Blood pH [15] | 1977 |
| Blood temperature [78, 47, 35, 27, 3] | 1978 |
| QT-interval [62] | 1981 |
| $O_2$ content of mixed venous blood [82] | 1981 |
| Asynchronous atrial rate [44] | 1982 |
| 'Physical activity' [5] | 1983 |
| Stroke volume [51, 66] | 1984 |
| Right atrial pressure [18] | 1984 |

* first publication in the medical literature.

most of them is still at an early state and clinical experience is either missing or at most quite limited. Such an evaluation has to take into consideration factors such as specificity of the parameter measured, speed of response to exercise, degree of physical work required to evoke a measurable change, reliability and current consumption of the sensor, ease of implantation technique etc.

*Speed of response*
As for the speed of response of a rate responsive pacemaker a definite reaction within 30 to 60 sec. after the onset of exercise should be asked for. In this respect it appears to us that some of the physiologic indicators, especially the QT interval and blood temperature are somewhat slow to pick up exercise. Temperature changes during mild exercise, such as walking, are often very small and insignificant, usually not exceeding levels beyond the physiologic variations seen at rest [48, 86]. Often there is an obvious dip in temperature with changes in body position or at the onset of work and it may take several minutes for the temperature to reach its preexcercise level [86]. This initial drop in core blood temperature can best be explained by an early dilution of right ventricular blood by the colder blood being mobilized from peripheral sources, in particular from the extremities. A special limitation with the QT sensing pacemaker is the fact that this system will be unable to maintain higher pacing rates during prolonged periods of work as it starts to reduce the rate as soon as the QT interval remains constant ('nulling') [62]. Besides, patients with this pacemaker should not be treated with sympatholytic agents because betaadrenergic blockade abolishes the catecholamine induced QT shortening [24]. Interestingly enough, these drugs would also influence the rate response of a temperature regulated pacemaker as the rise in blood temperature induced by exercise is markedly enhanced by betareceptor blockade [14].

*Sensor specificity*
As far as the specificity of a sensor is concerned, we would consider those as being specific which closely – directly or indirectly – reflect cardiac performance and – more precisely – cardiac output. This requirement is ideally met by mixed venous oxygen content [84, 85] and by stroke volume measurements [66] and, because of the interrelationship between minute ventilation and cardiac output, to a lesser extent also by respiratory rate [64], but certainly not by sensors such as body motion [5], QT interval or temperature. We doubt that right atrial pressure [18] could represent a suitable indicator for cardiac performance, because this parameter is not only determined by right ventricular stroke volume and compliance but also by factors such as venous tone (which can be altered acutely, for example by the application of nitroglycerine) or intravascular volume (diuretic therapy!). It is further known that there is but a loose correlation between right atrial and left atrial mean pressures and therefore the information provided by a pressure transducer in the right atrium may be misleading.

An indispensible requirement for a parameter used for rate regulation is that the possibility of inappropriate acceleration of rate in the sense of oscillation of the system is excluded. It appears to us that this might be a special hazard with atrial pressure control because RA pressure may abruptly rise in an ischemic episode: as the ensuing increase in pacing rate would further aggravate ischemia, a vicious cycle could be generated pushing up acutely the driving rate of the pacemaker to its maximal level. Possibly, a similar inappropriate and detrimental acceleration of heart rate may also occur in patients with a respiration controlled pacemaker if hyperventilation due to chest pain and/or ischemia-induced pulmonary congestion develops, or in those patients provided with a QT pacemaker if the QT interval shortens as a consequence of angina induced elevation of circulating catecholamines or due to direct release of norepinephrine from ischemic myocardial cells [88]. Designers of these pacing systems must be aware of this potential danger and try to overcome it by appropriate algorithms, the safety of which can only be documented in the clinical setting.

*Closed feed back loop system for automatic optimization of individual pacing rate*
The ideal system for rate responsive pacing would be one which uses a closed feed back loop for regulating pacing rate. As this can only be realized with a physiologic parameter which reliably reflects cardiac output, only mixed venous oxygen content and stroke volume can be considered as possible physiological variables for such a pacemaker. The idea of this concept is a fully automatic system which at any given moment, at rest as well as during exercise, paces at the lowest rate achieving the highest cardiac output [84, 85]. Unlike the situation with other sensors, no fixed relationship between rate and the physiologic parameter used for its regulation would be required. The advantages of such a system are obvious: there is no need for special assessment of the rate/output relationship in order to define the optimal rate for an individual patient; any change in this relationship occuring with time or with acute pathophysiologic alterations such as ischemia would automatically be taken care of; and finally unnecessarily high pacing rates could be avoided.

*Oxygen content of venous blood for rate regulation*
We have been working on the concept of mixed venous oxygen content as input signal for a rate-responsive pacing system [82, 84–86]. This parameter can be measured continuously by monitoring the oxygen saturation of right ventricular blood; as this can be accomplished opto-electronically by hemoreflectorimetry, the problem of instability and early failure of the sensor inherent to truely chemical sensors is avoided. Mixed venous oxygen saturation could indeed represent the ideal parameter for rate regulation: it starts to decline immediately from the beginning of any degree of work load, is very specific being exclusively determined by cardiac output and peripheral oxygen demand, and meets all requirements for the realization of a closed feed back loop regulation of pacing

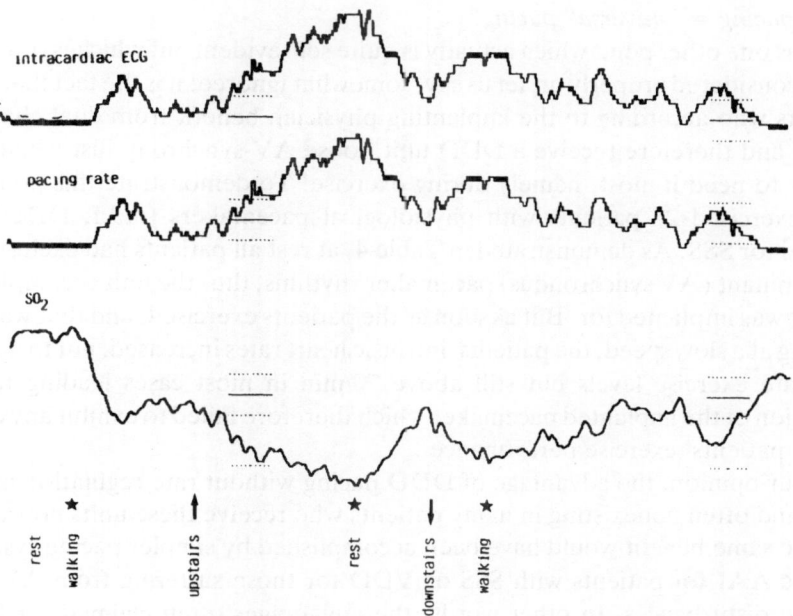

*Figure 9*. Heart rate during various levels of physical activity in a patient with complete heart block stimulated by a VVI pulse generator the rate of which was regulated by central venous oxygen saturation ($SO_2$). Heart rate varies between 65 and 90/min.

rate [84, 85]. Using an appropriate algorith [86], the normal reaction of heart rate to various levels of exercise can be closely matched (Fig. 9).

## Conclusions and further perspectives

### 'Truely physiological' pacemakers

As we have specified in this review, a pacemaker should only be classified as 'truely physiologic' if it takes account of both features of the healthy heart: AV-synchrony and rate responsiveness. For the benefit of cardiodynamics at rest restoring or maintaining normal AV relationship is of some importance, but the main purpose of proper AV sequencing in cardiac pacing is the avoidance of consistently mistimed atrial contractions and thus the prevention of the adverse effects of retrograde VA conduction during ventricular pacing. For the improvement of cardiac function during exercise, however, the ability for increasing pacing rate is essential, no matter whether the regulation of heart rate is accomplished by atrial synchronous or atrial independent pacing systems. The common definition of a 'physiologic' pacemaker as one which restores AV-synchrony neglects the most essential feature of the heart as a blood transporting pump, its variability in rate!

*DDD pacing = 'universal' pacing?*

There is one other point which actually is quite self-evident but which is often not really considered properly or, let us say, somewhat ignored: it is the fact that most patients who according to the implanting physician benefit from dual chamber pacing and therefore receive a DDD unit, loose AV-synchrony just when they appear to need it most, namely during exercise! To demonstrate this point we have exercised 27 patients with physiological pacemakers (AAI, DDD) implanted for SSS. As demonstrated in Table 4, at rest all patients had exclusive or predominant (AV synchronous) pacemaker rhythms, thus the unit accomplished what it was implanted for. But as soon as the patients exercised, and that was just walking at a slow speed, the patients' intrinsic heart rates increased, not to normal adequate exercise levels but still above 70/min in most cases leading to the inhibition of the implanted pacemaker which therefore failed to exhibit any effect on the patients' exercise performance.

In our opinion, the advantage of DDD pacing without rate regulation is very small and often nonexisting in many patients who receive these units nowadays, and the same benefit would have been accomplished by simpler pacing systems, such as AAI for patients with SSS or VDD for those suffering from AV conduction disturbances. In other words, the advantages often claimed for DDD pacemakers, sometimes also connoted 'universal' pacemakers, over simpler systems are greatly exaggerated. What we need are pacemakers which restore AV-synchrony – if possible – but at the same time and even more important adapt pacing rate. It should be clear that one actually cannot achieve permanent AV-synchrony without rate regulation in most cases!

*The future: 'Multisensor pacing' and 'Implantable hemodynamic/metabolic laboratory'?*

We believe that future trend will develop towards what Donaldson and Rickards [22] have called 'multisensor pacing', a dual chamber pacing system which, in addition to sensing atrial activity, also had access to metabolic and/or exercise

*Table 4.* Cardiac rhythm in patients with 'physiological' pacemakers implanted for sinus node dysfunction.

| Rhythm | Rest | Exercise (treadmill 2–4 km/h) |
|---|---|---|
| only PM | 23 | 3 |
| PM + spontaneous rhythm (SB, AV)* | 4 | 3 |
| only spontaneous rhythm | 0 | 21 |
| n = | 27 | 27 |

* SB = Sinusbradycardia, AV = AV rhythyms.

related data, would then truely be able to make logical decisions as to whether atrial rate was appropriate or inappropriate and adjust its pacing function accordingly. Such a pacemaker would no longer be sensitive to the effects of retrograde atrial conduction, ectopic atrial tachycardias, flutter or fibrillation [22]. Finally a multisensor electrode could also provide invaluable hemodynamic and metabolic data which – if transmitted telemetrically – might be of great help for the assessment of the patient's cardiac condition, his exercise capacity, the response to medical therapy etc. Analogous to the concept of the 'implantable electrophysiologic laboratory' [29] it appears well conceivable that in the not too far away future we might have at our disposal a 'hemodynamic and metabolic laboratory' as well.

## References

1. Adolph RJ, Holmes JC, Fukusumi H (1968) Hemodynamic studies in patients with chronically implanted pacemakers. Am Heart J 76: 829
2. Alicandri C, Fouad FM, Tarazi RC et al (1978) Three cases of hypotension and syncope with ventricular pacing: possible role of atrial reflexes. Am J Cardiol 42: 137
3. Alt E, Hirstetter C, Heinz M, Wirtzfeld A (1934) Control of pacemaker rate by central venous blood temperature. Circulation 57: 407
4. Amikam S, Riss E (1979) Untoward hemodynamic consequences of permanent ventricular pacing associated with ventriculo-atrial conduction. In: Meere C (ed): Proceedings of the VIth World Symposium on Cardiac Pacing, Chap. 15–6
5. Anderson K, Humen D, Klein G et al (1983) A rate variable pacemaker which automatically adjusts for physical activity. PACE 3, A–12
6. Astrand I, Landegren J (1965) The effect of varying rate on physical work capacity in patients with complete heart block. Acta Med Scand 177: 657
7. Baller D, Hoeft A, Korb H et al (1981) Basic physiological studies on cardiac pacing with special references to the optimal mode and rate after cardiac surgery. Thorac cardiovasc Surgeon 29: 168
8. Benchimol A, Ellis J, Dimond G (1965) Hemodynamic consequences of atrial and ventricular pacing in patients with normal and abnormal hearts. Am J Med 39: 911
9. Bergbauer M, Sabin G (1983) Hämodynamische Langzeitresultate der bifokalen Schrittmacherstimulation. Dtsch med Wschr 108: 545
10. Bernstein V, Rotem C, Peretz DI (1971) Permanent pacemakers: 8-year follow-up study. Incidence and management of congestive cardiac failure and perforations. Ann Intern Med 74: 361
11. Bevegard S, Johnsson B, Karlöf I et al (1967) Effect of changes in ventricular rate and central pressures at rest and during exercise in patients with artificial pacemakers. Cardiovasc Res 1: 21
12. Boccadamo R, Altamura G, Pistolese M (1982) Antiarrhythmic control of the brady-tachy syndrome by pacing. In: Feruglio G (ed): Cardiac Pacing, p 507, Piccin Medical Books, Padova
13. Brockman SK (1966) Mechanism of the movements of the atrioventricular valves. Am J Cardiol 17: 682
14. Brundin TH (1978) Effects of β-adrenergic receptor blockade on metabolic rate and mixed venous blood temperature during dynamic exercise. Scand J clin Lab Invest 38: 229
15. Cammilli L, Alcidi L, Papeschi G (1977) A new pacemaker autoregulating the rate of pacing in relation to metabolic needs. In: Watanabe Y (ed): Cardiac Pacing, Excerpta Medica, Amsterdam
16. Camilli L, Alcidi L, Shapland E et al (1983) Results, problems and perspectives with the autoregulating pacemaker. PACE 6: 488

17. Carleton RA, Passovoy M, Graettinger JS (1966) The importance of the contribution and timing of left atrial systole. Clin Sci 30: 151

18. Cohen TJ (1984) A theoretical right atrial pressure feedback heart rate control system to restore physiologic control to the rate-limited heart. PACE 7: 671

19. Curtis JJ, Madigan NP, Whiting RB et al (1981) Clinical experience with permanent atrioventricular sequential pacing. Ann Thorac Surg 32: 179

20. Davidson DM, Braak CA, Preston ThA et al (1972) Permanent ventricular pacing. Effect on long-term survival, congestive heart failure and subsequent myocardial infarction and stroke. Ann Intern Med 77: 345

21. Dolder A, Halter J, Nager F (1975) Schrittmacherimplantation bei bradykarder Herzinsuffizienz. Dtsch med Wschr 100: 2070

22. Donaldson RM, Richards AF (1983) Towards multisensor pacing. Am Heart J 106: 1454

23. Eimer HH, Witte J (1974) Zur Leistungsbreite bei Patienten mit festfrequentem Herzschrittmacher unter Berücksichtigung von Hämodynamik, arteriovenöser Sauerstoffdifferenz und Lungenfunktion. Z Kardiol 63: 1099

24. Fananapazir L, Bennett DH, Faragher EB (1983) Contribution of heart rate to QT interval shortening during exercise. Europ Heart J 4: 265

25. Fananapazir L, Srinivas V, Bennett DH (1983) Comparison of resting hemodynamic indices and exercise performance during atrial synchronized and asynchronous pacing. PACE 6: 202

26. Fananapazir L, Bennett DH, Monks Ph (1983) Atrial synchronized pacing: contribution of the chronotropic response to improved exercise performance. PACE 6: 601

27. Fearnot NE, Jolgren DL, Tacker WA et al (1984) Increasing cardiac rate by measurement of right ventricular temperature. PACE 7: 1240

28. Funke HD (1975) Ein Herzschrittmacher mit belastungsabhängiger Frequenzregulation. Biomed. Technik 20: 225

29. Furman S (1984) Foreword: Cardiostim 84. PACE 7: 1099

30. Gamal MIH, vGelder LM (1981) Chronic ventricular pacing with ventriculo-atrial conduction versus atrial pacing in three patients with symptomatic sinus bradycardia. PACE 4: 100

31 Gattenlöhner W, Schneider KW (1973) Schrittmachertherapie und Hämodynamik. Münch med Wschr 115: 2137

32. Gillespie WI, Greene DG, Karatzas NB et al (1967) Effect of atrial systole on right ventricular stroke output in complete heart block. Brit med J I: 75

33. Gilmore J, Sarnoff SJ, Mitchell JH et al (1963) Synchronicity of ventricular contraction: observations comparing haemodynamic effects of atrial and ventricular pacing. Brit Heart J 299

34. Greenberg B, Chatterjee K, Parmley WW et al (1979) The influence of left ventricular filling pressure on atrial contribution to cardiac output. Am Heart J 98: 742

35. Griffin JC, Jutzy KR, Claude JP et al (1983) Central body temperature as a guide to optimal heart rate. PACE 6: 498

36. Günther KR, Duck HJ, Köhler H et al (1981) Ein neues, physiologisch optimiertes Herzschrittmachersystem – ein vorhofgesteuerter, av-delay-kontrollierter Pacemaker. Dt Gesundh.-Wesen 36: 277

37. Hartzler GO, Maloney JD, Curtis JJ et al (1977) Hemodynamic benefits of atrioventricular sequential pacing after cardiac surgery. Am J Cardiol 40: 232

38. Hetzel MR, Ginks WR, Pickersgill AJ et al (1978) Value of pacing in cardiac failure associated with chronic atrioventricular block. Brit Heart J 40: 864

39. Ionescu VL (1980) An 'on demand pacemaker' responsive to respiration rate. PACE 3: 375

40. Johnson AD, Laiken SL, Engler RL (1978) Hemodynamic compromise associated with ventriculoatrial conduction following transvenous pacemaker placement. Am J Med 65: 75

41. Kappenberger L, Gloor HO, Babotai I et al (1982) Hemodynamic effects of atrial synchronization in acute and long-term ventricular pacing. PACE 5: 639

42. Karlöf (1975) Haemodynamic effect of atrial triggered versus fixed rate pacing at rest and during

exercise in complete heart block. Acta med scand 197: 195
43. Knapp K, Gmeiner R, Hammerle P et al (1976) Der Einfluß der Vorhofkontraktion auf das Schlagvolumen bei Schrittmacherstimulation. Z Kardiol 65: 783
44. Knudscn MB, Amundson DC, Mosharrafa M (1982) Hemodynamic demand pacing. In: Barold SS and Mugica J (eds): The third decade of Cardiac Pacing, p 249, Futura, Mount Kisco
45. Kristensson BE, Arnman K, Ryden L (1983) Atrial synchronous ventricular pacing in ischemic heart disease. Europ Heart J 4: 668
46. Kruse I, Arnman K, Conradson TB et al (1982) A comparison of the acute and long-term hemodynamic effects of ventricular inhibited and atrial synchronous ventricular inhibited pacing. Circulation 65: 846
47. Laczkovics A, Simbrunner G, Losert U et al (1982) Temperaturmessungen zur Steuerung der Herzfrequenz in der Schrittmacherchirurgie. Kongreßber Österr Ges Chir 23: 119
48. Laczkovics A (1984) The central venous blood temperature as a guide for rate control in pacemaker therapy. PACE 7: 822
49. Leinbach RC, Chamberlain DA, Kastor JA et al. (1969) A comparison of the hemodynamic effects of ventricular and sequential AV pacing in patients with heart block. Am Heart J 78: 502
50. McGregor M, Klassen GA (1964) Observations on the effect of heart rate on cardiac output in patients with complete heart block at rest and during exercise. Circ Res Suppl II: 215
51. McKay RG, Spears JR, Aroesty JM et al (1984) Instantaneous measurement of left and right ventricular stroke volume and pressure-volume relationship with an impedance catheter. Circulation 69: 703
52. Mitchell JH, Gilmore JP, Sarnoff SJ (1962) The transport function of the atrium. Am J Cardiol 237
53. Munteanu J, Wirtzfeld A, Stangl K et al (1985) Is the hemodynamic benefit of VDD pacing due to AV-synchrony or to rate responsiveness? Proceedings of the IVth Europ Symposium on Cardiac Pacing, Torremolinos
54. Nager F, Bühlmann A, Schaub F (1966) Klinische und hämodynamische Befunde beim totalen Av-Block nach Implantation elektrischer Schrittmacher. Helv med Acta 33: 240
55. Naito M, Dreifus LS, Mardelli TJ et al (1980) Echocardiographic features of atrioventricular and ventriculoatrial conduction. Am J Cardiol 46: 625
56. Nishimura RA, Gersh BJ, Vlietstra RE et al (1982) Hemodynamic and symptomatic consequences of ventricular pacing. PACE 5: 903.
57. Ogawa S, Dreifus L, Shenoy PN et al (1978) Hemodynamic consequences of atrioventricular and ventriculoatrial pacing. PACE 1: 8
58. Pehrsson SK (1983) Influence of heart rate and atrioventricular synchronization on maximal work tolerance in patients treated with arteficial pacemakers. Acta med scand 214: 311
59. Pehrsson SK, Aström H (1983) Left ventricular function after long-term treatment with ventricular inhibited compared to atrial triggered ventricular pacing. Acta med scand 214: 295
60. Perrins EJ, Morley ChA, Chan SL et al (1983) Randomised controlled trial of physiological and ventricular pacing. Brit Heart J 50: 112
61. Reiter MJ, Hindman MC (1982) Hemodynamic effects of acute atrioventricular pacing in patients with left ventricular dysfunction. Am J Cardiol 49: 687
62. Rickards AF, Norman J (1981) Relation between QT interval and heart rate. New design of physiologically adaptive cardiac pacemaker. Brit Heart J 45: 56
63. Rickards AF, Donaldson RM, Thalen HJTh (1983) The use of QT-interval to determine pacing rate: early clinical experience. PACE 6: 346
64. Rossi P, Plicchi G, Canducci G et al (1983) Respiratory rate as a determinant of optimal pacing rate. PACE 6: 502
65. Rossi P, Aina F, Rognoni G et al (1984) Increasing cardiac rate by tracking the respiratory rate. PACE 7: 1246
66. Salo RW, Pederson BD, Olive AL et al (1984) Continuous ventricular volume assessment for

442

diagnosis and pacemaker control. PACE 7: 1267

67. Samet Ph, Bernstein WH, Medow A et al (1964) Effect of alteration in ventricular rate on cardiac output in complete heart block. Am J Cardiol 14: 477
68. Schmid P, Klein WW, Harpf H et al (1979) Körperliche Belastbarkeit von Herzschrittmacherträgern. Z Kardiol 68: 763
69. Segel N, Hudson WA, Harris P et al (1964) The circulation effects of electrically induced changes in ventricular rate at rest and during exercise in complete heart block. J Clin Invest 43: 1541
70. Shapland JE, MacCarter D, Knudson M (1983) Physiological benefits of rate responsiveness. PACE 6: 329
71. Skinner NS, Mitchell J, Wallace AG et al (1963) Hemodynamic effects of altering the time of atrial systole. Am J Physiol 205: 499
72. Sowton E (1964) Haemodynamic studies in patients with artificial pacemakers. Brit Heart J 26: 737
73. Stone JM, Bhakta RD, Lutgen J (1982) Dual chamber sequential pacing in the management of sinus node dysfunction: advantages over single-chamber pacing. Am Heart J 104: 1319
74. Sutton R, Citron P (1979) Electrophysiological and haemodynamic basis for application of new pacemaker technology in sick sinus syndrome and atrioventricular block. Brit Heart J 41: 600
75. Sutton R, Perrins EJ, Morley C et al (1983) Sustained improvement in exercise tolerance following physiological cardiac pacing. Europ Heart J 4: 781
76. Van Mechelen R, Hagemeijer F, De Boer H et al (1983) Atrioventricular and ventriculo-atrial conduction in patients with symptomatic sinus node dysfunction. PACE 6: 13
77. Von Bibra H, Busch U, Wirtzfeld A (1984) Hemodynamic effects of short AV-intervals in DDD pacemaker patients. Circulation 70, Suppl II: 408
78. Weisswange A, Csapo G, Perach W (1978) Frequenzsteuerung von Schrittmachern durch Bluttemperatur. Verh Dtsch Ges Kreislaufforsch 44: 152
79. Westerman KW (1972) Hämodynamische Untersuchungen bei Schrittmacherträgern während AV-Block, starrfrequenter und vorhofgesteuerter Stimulation. Intensivmed 9: 360
80. Wirtzfeld A, Himmler FCh, Präuer HW et al (1979) Atrial and ventricular pacing in patients with the sick sinus syndrome. In: s Ref 4, Chap. 15–5
81. Wirtzfeld A, Himmler FCh, Blömer H (1981) Klinische Gesichtspunkte der Schrittmachertherapie bradykarder Herzrhythmusstörungen. Verh Dtsch Ges Kreislaufforsch 47: 98
82. Wirtzfeld A, Goedel-Meinen L, Bock T et al (1981) Central venous oxygen saturation for the control of automatic rate-responsive pacing. Circulation 64, Suppl IV: 299
83. Wirtzfeld A, Himmler FCh, Klein G et al (1982) Atrial pacing in patient with sick sinus syndrome: acute and long-term hemodynamic effects. In: s Ref 11, p 651
84. Wirtzfeld A, Goedel-Meinen L, Bock Th et al (1982) Central venous oxygen saturation for the control of automatic rate-responsive pacing. PACE 5: 829
85. Wirtzfeld A, Stangl K, Heinze R et al (1983) Mixed venous oxygen saturation for rate control of an implantable pacing system. In: Steinbach K (ed): Cardiac Pacing, p 271, Steinkopff, Darmstadt
86. Wirtzfeld A, Heinze R, Stangl K et al (1984) Regulation of pacing rate by variations of mixed venous oxygen saturation. PACE 7: 1257
87. Witte J, Dressler L, Schröder G (1979) 10 years of experience with permanent atrial electrodes. In: s Ref 4, Chap 16–1
88. Wollenberger A, Shahab L (1965) Anoxia-induced release of noradrenaline from the isolated perfused heart. Nature 207: 88

# Treatment of recurrent supraventricular tachycardias by antitachycardia pacemakers

A.W. NATHAN*

## Introduction

Patients with paroxysmal, atrial or junctional tachycardias represent a common clinical problem. Most regular sustained arrhythmias are reentrant in nature, and may be treated pharmacologically, by ablative techniques (including both catheter-based and surgical methods) or by pacing. Drugs may be ineffective, or cause side effects including proarrhythmias, adverse haemodynamic effects, and both minor and major systemic adverse effects. They may also be inconvenient to take, and many patients dislike taking drugs on a long-term basis. Catheter techniques are in their infancy and may involve the production of complete heart block with the necessity of bradycardia support pacing. Surgical techniques require thoracotomy and usually cardiopulmonary bypass. Antitachycardia pacing represents an alternative method of treatment as implantation is a minor surgical procedure, usually performed under local anaesthesia.

The ideal antitachycardia pacemaker would prevent the initiation of pathological tachycardia. If a pathological tachycardia did occur it would recognise and distinguish its pathological nature. It would automatically attempt to terminate it and if initially unsuccessful would alter its parameters and try again. It would not precipitate unwanted arrhythmias nor cause haemodynamic depression and would be fully versatile, being able to treat all types of tachycardia. Such a pacemaker does not, of course, exist at present but steady progress is being made towards all these goals.

## Prevention of tachycardia

The earliest work on antitachycardia pacing concentrated on prevention, either by increasing the heart rate [1] or by modifying the activation sequence [2].

* Supported by the Britisch Heart Foundation.

Increasing the heart rate by pacing is rarely useful, but modifying the activation sequence by dual site pacing has been proposed as a major option [3, 4]. If the atria and ventricles are paced using an appropriate AV delay, a sensed atrial depolarisation is followed by a ventricular paced beat and collision may occur in one or both limbs of a reentrant circuit, thereby preventing a sustained arrhythmia (Fig. 1). There are however problems with this theoretically attractive concept. A short AV delay is usually necessary and this may be haemodynamically deleterious and uncomfortable for the patient. Electrodes may have to be placed close to the limbs of the circuit to ensure sufficiently early penetration, and if atrial refractoriness is less than the upper rate limit of the pacemaker, an early atrial premature beat capable of initiating tachycardia will not be followed by ventricular pacing, thereby risking tachycardia induction. Furthermore, arrhythmias induced by ventricular stimulation will not be prevented by the present generation of devices, which cannot follow a premature ventricular depolarisation by atrial pacing.

**Termination of tachycardia**

Pacemakers have proved more useful for tachycardia termination than prevention. In any reentrant circuit the circulating impulse is followed by a zone of refractory tissue which is followed by non-refractory tissue, the excitable gap. If an impulse can be generated at the right time from the right site the excitable gap can be entered and collision will take place within the circuit, terminating tachycardia (Fig. 2).

This was first demonstrated by Moe et al in 1963 [5], who described termination of an experimental intra AV nodal tachycardia in a canine model. Although paired pulse pacing had been used to control heart rate in arrhythmias by Chardack et al [6], Haft et al [7] are accredited with the first report of terminating an arrhythmia in man using pacing techniques, when they described the use of rapid atrial pacing to terminate atrial flutter. In the same year, Durrer et al [8] described the use of premature beats(extrastimuli) for the same purpose. In 1968, Ryan et al [9] described the first use of a permanent device for tachycardia termination, using a demand pacemaker together with a magnet to convert the pacemaker to fixed rate for termination of a junctional tachycardia using the underdrive principle. Many developments have occurred since then, with specific antitachycardia devices being devised.

*Tachycardia detection and distinction*

The early tachycardia reversion pacemakers relied on patient recognition of tachycardia, with manual activation of pacing using an external device (magnet,

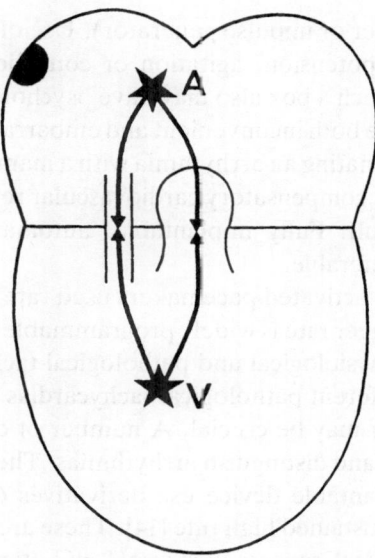

*Figure 1.* Dual site pacing in a patient with the Wolff-Parkinson-White syndrome. The atrial sensed or paced depolarisation (A) and the ventricular paced impulse (V) penetrate into the accessory pathway and AV node, colliding with each other and thus preventing arrhythmia induction.

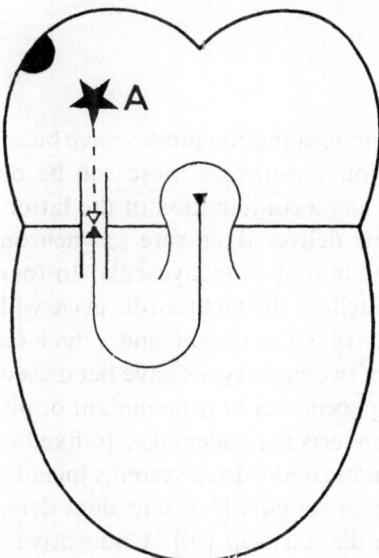

*Figure 2.* This diagram represents orthodromic reentrant tachycardia in a patient with an AV accessory pathway – the circulating wavefront is marked with closed arrows. An atrial paced beat (A) enters the excitable gap (indicated by the open arrowhead) and collides with the oncoming wavefront in the accessory pathway causing tachycardia termination.

radiofrequency transmitter or impulse generator). Use of these external devices can prove difficult if hypotension, agitation or confusion are induced by the tachycardia. The use of such a box also may have psychological disadvantages as external activators may be both inconvenient and embarrassing to patients. Delay always occurs when terminating an arrhythmia with a manual system and this may allow the development of compensatory cardiovascular reflexes which may make termination more difficult. Fully implantable, automatically activated pacemakers are therefore preferable.

The first automatically activated pacemakers used rate alone to trigger pacing [10–13]. Although the trigger rate is widely programmable on some devices, there is an overlap between physiological and pathological tachycardia rates in many patients. In addition, different pathological tachycardias may occur and distinction of one from another may be crucial. A number of different methods have been suggested to detect and distinguish arrhythmias. The only methods actually implemented in an implantable device use derivatives of rate such as sudden onset, rate stability and sustained high rate [14]. These are all useful but certainly not foolproof. 'Physiological' sensors such as pH, $pO_2$, temperature and QT may help to distinguish sinus from pathological tachycardias, but do not aid distinction of different pathological arrhythmias. However, electrographic activation sequence analysis using multiple electrodes or electrogram morphological analysis [15] are likely to prove more valuable.

*Termination modes*

A large number of different termination modes have been described for tachycardia reversion. For descriptive purposes these can be divided into underdrive, extrastimulus, overdrive and a combination of the latter two.

Underdrive pacemakers deliver fixed rate (asynchronous) pacing during tachycardia at a rate less than that of tachycardia. In theory, therefore, a single stimulus is delivered throughout the tachycardia cycle which may, if it happens to be correctly timed, penetrate the circuit and effect tachycardia termination. Permanent pacemakers of two main types have been used for underdrive pacing. A conventional demand pacemaker may be patient or physician activated by the use of a magnet which converts the pacemaker to fixed rate [9], or an automatic unit may be used. Automatic underdrive systems include the upside down pacemaker without bradycardia support [11], and dual-demand pacemakers which have additional bradycardia back-up [10]. Underdrive pacemakers should, in theory, deliver a series of single stimuli that occur throughout the tachycardia cycle. However, if tachycardia and pacing rates are harmonically related or if tachycardia is reset by paced beats and synchronised to the pacing rate, the tachycardia termination window may be missed. Stimulation may occur in the vulnerable period and unwanted and possibly more dangerous arrhythmias may be initiated. In addition, a single stimulus may be insufficient to penetrate the tachycardia circuit and may fail to terminate the tachycardia, even if the best practical electrode position is chosen [16].

In order to refine the underdrive technique and provide an adaptive system that was unlikely to cause haemodynamic deterioration or unwanted arrhythmias, Spurrell introduced the scanning extrastimulus pacemaker in 1975 [17]. The tachycardia cycle is systematically scanned with one or two extrastimuli until tachycardia termination is achieved. Initially an external pacemaker connected to exteriorised permanent electrodes was used [17], but Critelli et al [18] then introduced an external stimulator controlling, and communicating with an implanted receiver using a radiofrequency link. More recently a fully implantable automatic system has been used [13]. Electrode position may be critical as theoretically the electrode should be positioned 'on circuit'. This is frequently not possible, particularly in patients with left sided accessory pathways. Although coronary sinus pacing may be used in such patients, pacing thresholds tend to be high and sensing is complicated by the complexity of the coronary sinus electrogram.

Overdrive pacemakers allow capture of progressively more tissue until the tachycardia focus or circuit is penetrated, entrained and disrupted. It is a very effective form of tachycardia reversion [16], but very rapid rates may be necessary which can lead to the induction of more dangerous arrhythmias [19], or may cause haemodynamic embarrassment.

The earliest pacemakers of this type were radiofrequency systems, which consisted of an implantable inductive coil and electrode together with an external transmitter which is either patient or physician operated [20, 21]. Similar units that require two-way communication for confirmation of tachycardia have been described, and fully implantable automatic units have been used more recently [11, 12]. Early implantable burst pacemakers were non-adaptive, but newer models have adaptive capabilities [14].

There is a close relationship between a number of different factors when considering tachycardia termination. These include the coupling interval (rate) of pacing stimuli, the number of stimuli used, the site of stimulation and the energy used. Other factors include the presence or absence of drugs such as digoxin, and associated cardiac pathologies such as ischaemic heart disease. There is a delicate balance between terminating an arrhythmia and provoking an unwanted arrhythmia. In order to minimise the risks of closely coupled stimuli, which may fall in the vulnerable period and initiate unwanted arrhythmias, and to maximise the chances of terminating an arrhythmia, a limited burst may be optimal. Any intervention must be adaptive and many different kinds of scans have been described. Algorithms used have included constant rate bursts [22], constant rate bursts with scanning initial [23] or final intervals [24], as well as decremental [25] or incremental cycle length bursts. Scans may be decremental, incremental or a combination of both in a searching pattern [26, 27]. There is some advantage in favour of simplicity and the author has described a method, the concertina mode [22], in which a small number of stimuli are used (usually four to eight) with all pacing intervals being equal including the initial coupling interval. If tachycardia is not terminated, all intervals decrement by a similar amount (usually 5 to 10 ms) until termination is achieved. A clear relationship has been shown between the maximum coupling interval effective in terminating tachycardia and the number of stimuli delivered – prescription of more stimuli allows the use of longer pacing intervals [25].

**Patient assessment**

Careful assessment is necessary to determine which patients are suitable for antitachycardia pacing. Factors to note from the history include the occurrence of symptoms such as syncope at the onset of tachycardia, which probably will not be prevented by pacing. Attacks that are extremely frequent may be a contraindication to tachycardia reversion pacing, as may be attacks of a very short duration. The patients preference for a pacemaker is also important.

Electrocardiographic tracings from spontaneous attacks are useful to carefully delineate spontaneous arrhythmias. Twenty-four hour ambulatory electrocardiograms are essential for a number of reasons, including the disclosure of previously unsuspected arrhythmias and the documentation of changes in sinus rate. A maximal exercise electrocardiogram is also mandatory, in order to determine the maximum sinus rate. Other cardiac investigation such as echocardiography, nuclear angiography or invasive angiographic studies may be necessary in selected patients.

A full electrophysiological study must be performed to determine the mechanism and origin of induced arrhythmias. The risk from the arrhythmia substrate must also be determined. For example, those with the Wolff-Parkinson-White syndrome with an accessory pathway capable of rapid anterograde conduction, will not be protected from rapid ventricular rates in association with atrial fibrillation by a pacemaker, and indeed pacing may precipitate this arrhythmia. The suitability of different modes of pacing must be determined from a number of different atrial sites. In the past ventricular stimulation has been used in a number of patients suffering from supraventricular arrhythmias, but because of the risks of inducing ventricular arrhythmias, including ventricular fibrillation, this is not currently recommended. The chosen mode of pacing must be assessed frequently, preferably using an external form of the intended device. Any other requirements, for example bradycardia support, should also be assessed. Following the initial electrophysiological study the efficacy and safety of pacing must be assessed on at least two further occasions with temporary electrodes positioned in the sites chosen for permanent use. Once again an external version of the implantable device should be used where possible and a large number of terminations performed with the patient lying, sitting, standing and undergoing mild exercise, as physiological alterations cause large changes in the termination window. In some patients it may be decided that some form of additional antiarrhythmic drug therapy is necessary and this should be tested prior to implantation of the permanent device. Finally, those patients suffering from arrhythmias on a daily frequency can have ambulatory studies performed with an external device whilst in hospital.

The implantation of such a pacemaker is simple and is similar to the implantation of a conventional bradycardia demand pacemaker. It is usually performed using local anaesthesia, using conventional tined or active fixation electrodes. Virtually all systems are bipolar because of the importance of artefact-free sensing [28]. Routine electrode measurements are performed including the threshold, impedance, endocardial potential and electrogram, all in sinus rhythm. The measurements should then be repeated during tachycardia with emphasis on the sensing values as these may be dramatically different from those in sinus rhythm, particularly if the atrial electrogram is conducted retrogradely during tachycardia. Tachycardia terminating characteristics should be checked quickly with the permanent lead in its final site. The pacemaker should then be implanted and the wound closed. Correct pacing and sensing functions should be confirmed and the device programmed to the appropriate settings. However, the precise set-up of the pacemaker should be left for a day or two until the patient is more comfortable and the electrode has settled. Post-implant studies include verifying optimal termination and trigger settings, and establishing the safety of the device. Tachycardia must be initiated, preferably using the pacemaker for non-invasive stimulation if possible, and termination must be verified in a variety of physiological states. Ambulatory and exercise electrocardiography are essential, as is full patient education.

## Conclusions

There are many indications for permanent antitachycardia pacing. These include arrhythmias that are refractory to previous medical or surgical treatment, but also as an alternative to such treatment in women wishing to become pregnant who do not wish to be exposed to the teratogenic risk of drugs; patients with poor ventricular function, which may be further impaired by antiarrhythmic agents, and in whom surgical therapy may carry a prohibitive risk; and patients with side effects from otherwise effective treatment. Pacing may also emerge as a treatment of first choice in many others.

There are of course contraindications to antitachycardia pacing. These include extremely frequent arrhythmias unless preventative pacing is used; early auto-degeneration of tachycardia; easily inducible atrial fibrillation ($\pm$ flutter); the Wolff-Parkinson-White syndrome especially with a short refractory period and tachycardias responding only to ventricular pacing.

With advances in technology providing both flexibility and the possibility of using more complex and effective recognition and termination algorithms and with the encouraging clinical experience gained so far, antitachycardia pacing promises to be a major therapeutic option for significant numbers of patients with a wide range of tachyarrhythmias.

## References

1. Sowton E, Leatham A, Carson P (1964) The suppression of arrhythmias by artificial pacemaking. Lancet (II) 1098–100
2. Coumel P, Cabrol C, Fabiato A, Gourgon R, Slama R (1967) Tachycardie permanente par rythme reciproque. I. – Preuves du diagnostic par stimulation auriculaire et ventriculaire. Arch Mal Coeur 60: 1830–64
3. Spurrell RAJ, Sowton E (1976) Pacing techniques in the management of supraventricular tachycardias: part 2. An implanted atrial synchronous pacemaker with a short atrioventricular delay for the prevention of paroxysmal supraventricular tachycardias. J Electrocardiol 9: 89–96
4. Davies DW, Bucknall CA, Curry PVL (1984) Prophylactic antitachycardia pacemaker: permanent pre-excitation. Br Heart J 51: 104
5. Moe GK, Cohen W, Vick RL (1963) Experimentally induced paroxysmal A-V nodal tachycardia in the dog: a 'case report'. Am Heart J 65: 87–92
6. Chardack WM, Gage AA, Dean DC (1964) Slowing of the heart by paired pulse pacemaking. Am J Cardiol 14: 374–84
7. Haft JI, Kosowsky BD, Lau SH, Stein E, Damato AN (1967) Termination of atrial flutter by rapid electrical pacing of the atrium. Am J Cardiol 20: 239–44
8. Durrer D, Schoo L, Schuilenburg RM, Wellens HJJ (1967) The role of premature beats in the initiation and the termination of supraventricular tachycardia in the Wolff-Parkinson-White syndrome. Circulation 36: 644–62
9. Ryan GF, Easley RM, Zaroff LI, Goldstein S (1968) Paradoxical use of a demand pacemaker in treatment of supraventricular tachycardia due to the Wolff-Parkinson-White syndrome: observation on termination of reciprocal rhythm. Circulation 38: 1037–43
10. Krikler D, Curry P, Buffet J (1976) Dual-demand pacing for reciprocating atrioventricular tachycardia. Br Med J 1: 1114–6
11. Fisher JD, Furman S (1978) Automatic termination of tachycardia by an implanted 'upside down' demand pacemaker. Clin Res 26: 231A
12. Griffin JC, Mason JW, Calfee RV (1980) Clinical use of an implantable automatic tachycardia-terminating pacemaker. Am Heart J 100: 1093–6
13. Nathan AW, Camm AJ, Bexton RS, Hellestrand KJ, Spurrell RAJ (1982) Initial experience with a fully implantable, programmable, scanning, extrastimulus pacemaker for tachycardia termination. Clin Cardiol 5: 22–6
14. Nathan AW, Davies DW, Sweeney MB, Camm AJ (1985) Initial clinical experience with a new software based tachycardia reversion pacemaker. PACE 8: 301
15. Davies DW, Wainwright R, Tooley M, Lloyd D, Nathan A, Spurrell R, Camm AJ (1985) Electrogram gradient detection: a new method of tachycardia recognition. PACE 8: 290
16. Ward DE, Camm AJ, Spurrell RAJ (1979) The response of regular re-entrant supraventricular tachycardia to right heart stimulation. PACE 2: 586–95
17. Spurrell RAJ (1975) Artificial cardiac pacemakers. In: DM Krikler and JF Goodwin (eds): Cardiac arrhythmias: the modern electrophysiological approach, London, WB Saunders, pp 238–58

18. Critelli G, Grassi G, Chiariello M, Perticone F, Adinolfi L, Condorelli M (1979) Automatic 'scanning' by radiofrequency in the longterm electrical treatment of arrhythmias. PACE 2: 289–96

19. Fisher JD, Mehra R, Furman S (1978) Termination of ventricular tachycardia with bursts of rapid ventricular pacing. Am J Cardiol 41: 94–102

20. Iwa T, Abe H, Sugiki K, Wada J (1970) Treatment of supraventricular tachycardia with inductive radiofrequency atrial stimulation. Progress in Medicine 74: 372–4

21. Fruehan CT, Meyer JA, Klie JH, Johnson LW, Obeid AI, Smulyan H, Eich RH (1974) Refractory paroxysmal supraventricular tachycardia: treatment with patient controlled permanent radio frequency atrial pacemaker. Am Heart J 87: 229–37

22. Nathan A, Hellestrand K, Bexton R, Nappholz T, Spurrell R, Camm J (1982) Clinical evaluation of an adaptive tachycardia intervention pacemaker with automatic cycle length adjustment. PACE 5: 201–7

23. Spurrell RAJ, Nathan AW, Camm AJ (1984) Clinical experience with implantable tachycardia reversion pacemakers. PACE 7: 1296–1300

24. Gardner MJ, Waxman HL, Buxton AE, Cain ME, Josephson ME (1982) Termination of ventricular tachycardia: evaluation of a new pacing method. Am J Cardiol 50: 1338–45

25. Nathan AW, Spurrell RAJ, Camm AJ (1984) Steps towards the development of a safe and effective tachycardia termination pacemaker. Eur Heart J 5: 993–1003

26. Sowton E (1984) Clinical results with the Tachylog antitachycardia pacemaker. PACE 7: 1313–7

27. Vallin H, Hard af Segerstad C, Insulander P, Echag O, Lagergren H (1983) Centrifugal geometrical scanning – an alternative concept in pacemaker treatment of tachycardias. PACE 6: A–141

28. Hauser RG (1982) Bipolar leads for cardiac pacing in the 1980s: a reappraisal provoked by skeletal muscle interference. PACE 5: 34–7

# Surgery for supraventricular tachyarrhythmias

A.J. CAMM

**Summary**

Surgical techniques may be applied to the treatment of supraventricular tachycardias by excluding the tachycardia mechanism from the rest of the heart or by destroying the focus or reentrant pathway which generates the tachycardia. Cryosurgery and direct dissection are the most common methods. Most accessory pathways responsible for Wolff-Parkinson-White syndrome may be destroyed by croyablation from the epicardial surface of the heart, thus obviating the need for open heart surgery. However, septal accessory pathways, the His bundle and most atrial tachycardia foci have usually required an endocardial approach. Although the surgical destruction of the His bundle has been superceded by modern catheter-based techniques new operations designed to modify rather than destroy AV conduction have recently be described. These offer substantial advantages over the crude division of the normal AV conduction pathway. Thus surgery offers an opportunity of curing an arrhythmia and short term results support this possibility. The long term results of surgery, particularly cryosurgery and dissection around the region of the AV node are not yet known and some caution must be applied when considering surgery for those who have not yet exhausted other better understood forms of therapy.

## Introduction

Supraventricular tachycardias arise above the level of the His bundle and conduct to the ventricles through the His bundle or through an accessory AV pathway. For the purpose of this paper supraventricular tachycardia also includes the common form of reciprocating tachycardia associated with the Wolff-Parkinson-White atrioventricular reentrant tachycardia. Thus there are four major varieties of supraventricular tachycardia: atrial fibrillation/flutter, atrial tachycardia, intra AV nodal tachycardia and atrioventricular tachycardia for which surgical therapy may be advised.

## Indications for surgery

Other strategies for the treatment of supraventricular tachycardia include medical management and the use of implantable pacemaker devices. Because of the essential risk associated with cardiac surgery this therapeutic modality is confined to those who cannot or will not be managed by the other techniques. The general indication is drug inefficacy or intolerance in patients with arrhythmias unsuitable for control with pacemakers. Not surprisingly many patients would prefer a surgical 'cure' to pharmaceutical or electronic suppression.

However, it is not yet certain that surgery produces a definite cure. Often another problem is substituted intentionally (for example, creation of AV block) or develops as a late complication (for example sinus node dysfunction or atrial tachyarrhythmias following atrial surgery). However, there is a general optimism about the longterm success of surgery for the management of supraventricular arrhythmias and follow-up results confirm the therapeutic value. The realisation that the risks of surgery are relatively small but that the dangers and distress from some supraventricular arrhythmias are high and that successful surgery can almost be guaranteed has led to liberal indications in some centres. Others argue that because the natural history of supraventricular tachycardia is variable, the prognosis is generally good, and the long term outcome of surgery is uncertain, even the small risk of surgery is not justified. However a life threatening accessory pathway unresponsive to medical management is a definite indication for surgery, but patient preference and physician enthusiasm are still uncertain reasons for a surgical approach to supraventricular arrhythmias.

## Theoretical basis for surgery

Supraventricular tachycardias may arise from a 'point source' and conduct through the atrial myocardium, the His bundle or an accessory AV connection to reach the ventricles. Such a focus of tachycardia may be surgically excised or ablated. Alternatively the essential conduction pathway(s) between the focus and the ventricles may be interrupted thus preventing the expression of the supraventricular tachycardia at ventricular level. Some tachycardias for example atrioventricular tachycardias associated with Wolff-Parkinson-White syndrome involve circus movement over a large, so called 'macro' reentrant circuit. In such cases tachycardia may be entirely prevented by dividing an obligatory conduction pathway within that circuit. For example, in the Wolff-Parkinson-White syndrome atrioventricular reentry may be rendered impossible by dividing the AV node/His bundle or preferably by destruction of the accessory connection.

454

## Surgical ablation techniques

The surgeon may select a variety of instruments to divide or destroy cardiac tissue. Four such techniques which have been applied to the division of accessory pathways. Dissection by hook and knive are described elsewhere in the symposium by Gallagher. Cryoablation has now been used for more than six years for the destruction of conduction pathways and ablation of cardiac tissue. The main advantage of the technique is that cooling to zero degrees centigrade produces reversible conduction block and cooling to lower temperatures creates permanent block. Thus transient cooling to freezing point may be used as a 'mapping technique' to seek out the most suitable point at which to destroy tissue by freezing. The other advantages of cryosurgery are indicated in Table 1.

Although both liquid nitrogen and nitrous oxide cryosurgical systems have been used, the nitrous oxide system (e.g. Spembley UK Limited, Newbury Road, Andover, England and Frigitronics Inc, Shelter, CT, USA) has been most used. In this system gaseous nitrous oxide is allowed to expand into a small chamber at the tip of the cryoprobe. The expansion results in cooling because of the Joule-Thompson effect. The flow of gas is controlled by a regulating valve and larger flows result in the cooling of a larger mass of tissue. The mass of frozen tissue is also proportional to the size of the cryoprobe. With the Spembley system and a cryoprobe of 4.5 mm tip diameter an iceball of 9 mm can be produced. The Frigitronics device produces an iceball 25 mm in diameter with a probe size of 14 mm diameter. With nitrous oxide a temperature of $-60$ degrees centigrade can be achieved.

Of the techniques available for destruction of cardiac tissue the endocardial approaches require full cardiopulmonary bypass and cardiotomy. Dissection

*Table 1.*

Advantages of cryoablation.

1. Reversible conduction block may be achieved by cooling to just below 0 degrees centrigrade.
2. Permanent conduction block may be achieved by cooling to $-60$ degrees centigrade for 2 minutes.
3. Fibrous tissue is not damaged.
4. Haemostasis is not necessary.
5. The cryolesion is histologically and electropysiologically discrete.
6. The cryolesion is not arrhythmogenic.

Disadventages of cryoablation

1. Usually cardiopulmonary bypass is required.
2. Epicardial coronary vessels may be damaged.
3. A focus deep in the myocardium is not readily assessible to cryoablation.

necessitates cardioplegia or fibrillatory arrest. Endocardial cryosurgery can be performed on the beating heart with immediate electrocardiographic confirmation of accessory pathway destruction. Epicardial cryosurgery can also be performed with the beating heart without the need to open the heart. Epicardial d.c. shock is a new method which can be performed on the beating heart without resort to cardiopulmonary bypass and without the need for any dissection. This is further described in the symposium by Gallagher.

**Specific surgical procedures**

*a) His bundle cryoablation*

This operation is used for these purposes: to isolate a supraventricular arrhythmia from the ventricles, to interrupt a reentrant circuit which includes the AV node or to ablate a tachycardia arising from within the AV node or His bundle. In 1967 Gianelli and colleagues first reported the intentional division of the human AV conduction system. They used a ligature around the AV node by 'blind' insertion of sutures in the region of the AV node in a patient with atrioventricular tachycardia due to WPW syndrome. Sealy and others (1977) developed an operation which involved severing the AV conduction system at the junction of the AV node and His bundle by dissection of the atrial septum from the right fibrous tissues trigone. The technique of cryoablating the AV node/His bundle was reported by Klein et al (1979). The position of the His bundle is determined electrographically and confirmed by 'cryo' mapping. Usually several destructive lesions are then made in this region. The cryosurgical technique appears to be slightly better than direct dissection but to a large extent open heart division of the AV conduction system has been superceded by the catheter fulguration technique. Table 2 shows comparative results of direct dissection, cryoablation and

*Table 2.*

| Method | Patient | Complete AV block | Modified AV block | No AV block | Mortality |
|---|---|---|---|---|---|
| Direct dissection (Sealy) | 11 | 9 (82%) | – | 2 (18%) | – |
| Direct dissection (SBH) | 10 | 7 (70%) | – | 3 (30%) | – |
| Cryoablation (German & SBH) | 51 | 44 (86%) | 2 (4%) | 5 (10%) | 3 (7%) |
| Fulguration (German & SBH) | 48 | 39 (81%) | 9 (19%) | 5 (10%) | 0 |

Data derived from 3 sources:
Sealy = American Journal of Surgery 145, 711, 1983.
German et al = Circulation 70, II–412, 1984.
SBH = St. Bartholomew's Hospital Series.

fulguration. Cryoablation which is an open chest, open heart procedure, has a definite risk associated with the operation. All these techniques are of similar efficacy (70–86%). The new non-operative catheter based ablation technique, known as fulguration, appears to be the superior technique for AV node/His bundle ablation. However, the long term results are not known.

## b) Endocardial cryoablation of accessory pathways

A variety of techniques have been used to interrupt accessory pathway conduction. The technique of direct dissection with knife and hook devised by Sealy and Gallagher (1981) has been particularly successful. Cryoablation from the endocardial surface has also been used. This technique requires the institution of cardiopulmonary bypass and localisation of the accessory pathway by electrographic mapping techniques. The atrial electrogram around the appropriate AV valve ring is recorded and timed during orthodromic atrioventricular re-entrant tachycardia. In this arrhythmia retrograde conduction from ventricle to atrium occurs over the accessory pathway and the earliest atrial activation therefore indicates the atrial insertion of the accessory pathway. Cryomapping is then performed and provided that the tachycardia is terminated, retrograde conduction through the accessory pathway is prevented and preexcitation in response to atrial pacing disappears, that part of the AV annulus is frozen to −60 degrees centigrade for 2 minutes. Adjacent areas are similarly treated. The results from St. Bartholomew's Hospital (Table 3) indicate that whilst free wall pathways may be relatively easily destroyed by this technique connections situated in the septum are more difficult to destroy. Because major epicardial vessels lie in the AV groove there is some concern about the possible damage to these arteries by closely applied cryosurgery.

*Table 3.* Endocardial cryolesions in WPW Syndrome (St. Bartholomew's Hospital).

| Position of accessory pathway | Complete ablation | Modified conduction | No change | Total |
|---|---|---|---|---|
| Left free wall | 41 (95%) | 0 | 2 (5%) | 43 |
| Right free wall | 7 (100%) | 0 | 0 | 7 |
| Anteroseptal | 1 (25%) | 3 (75%) | 0 | 4 |
| Posteroseptal | 0 | 4 (100%) | 0 | 4 |
| Total | 49 (85%) | 7 (12%) | 2 (3%) | 58 |

## c) Epicardial cryoablation of accessory pathways

In their report of the cryosurgical ablation of accessory pathways responsible for incessant AV junctional tachycardia Camm, Ward and Spurrell (1980) record that they were able to destroy accessory pathway conduction by epicardial application of the cryoprobe in the posterior left AV groove. This technique has been considerably improved by Guiraudon and colleagues (1985) who, because of concern about the cryosurgical effect on major epicardial coronary arteries, dissect the vessels away from the AV sulcus before applying cryotherapy over the supposed region of atrial/ventricular preexcitation. They have used this technique in eighty cases (Table 4) with a remarkable degree of success. They account for their single failure by the observation that right free wall pathways seem to be located predominantly on the endocardial surface. Although cardiopulmonary bypass has been employed in most of these patients a small proportion have been successfully treated without its use. A similarly excellent success has been recently reported by Page and his colleagues (1985).

## d) Other surgical techniques for the management of supraventricular tachycardia

There is a growing number of reports of the surgical exision, cryoablation or exclusion of foci of reentrant and automatic atrial tachycardia. Tachycardias arising from both the left and the right atria have been successfully treated with surgical techniques (Gillette et al 1980; Sealy and Seaber, 1980; Wyndham et al 1980; Anderson et al 1982; Josephson et al 1982; Ott et al 1985). Occasionally an atrial reentrant circuit, such as that supporting typical atrial flutter, has been permanently interrupted by an atrial incision. When tachycardias arise in the left atrium or are caused predominantly by a left atrial pathology, for example atrial fibrillation due to mitral valve disease, the left atrium can be electrically isolated from the atrial septum and right atrium by an excision extending from the coronary sulcus posteriorly to the fibrous trigone anteriorly. In their description of this operation Williams and colleagues (1980) point out that any conducting

*Table 4.* Epicardial cryoablation for WPW syndrome.

|  | Total | Success |
|---|---|---|
| left free wall | 53 | 53 (100%) |
| right free wall | 6 | 5 (83%) |
| posterior septal | 13 | 13 (100%) |
| anterior septal | 8 | 8 (100%) |
| Total | 80 | 79 (99%) |

from Guiraudon 1985 – personal communication.

fibres at the extremes of the incision must be destroyed, for example by cryoablation.

There have been several attempts to prevent reentry in and around the AV node without impairing anterograde AV conduction during sinus rhythm. Holman et al (1984) and Cox (1985) have used discrete cryoablation along the borders of the triangle of Koch to modify AV conduction in such a way as to prevent AV nodal re-entry or to impair conduction of rapid supraventricular tachycardias without affecting the conduction of sinus beats. Guarnieri et al (1984) have operated on eight patients with atypical (long R-P') junctional reciprocating tachycardia. In seven of the eight cases dissection of the postero-septal region resulted in ablation of the retrograde limb of the circuit which was presumed to be a postero-septal AV connection operating with decremental characteristics and only in the ventriculo atrial direction. Recently Johnson et al (1984) have introduced a new operation for typical intra AV nodal re-entrant tachycardia. Basically this consists of dissecting the tissue overlying the His bundle away from its inferior attachments. This surgery has resulted in abolition of the re entrant tachycardia but no impairment of anterograde conduction including the duality of AH conduction. Initial results are very promising but long term follow up is needed before recommending this form of surgery more widely.

**Conclusion**

When supraventricular tachycardia proves refractory to medical therapy and unsuitable for electrotherapy a surgical treatment should be considered. There is a wide range of operations designed to excise, ablate, interrupt or exclude the tachycardia focus or mechanism. Apart from the immediate risks of surgery, which are small in this otherwise healthy group of patients, the results are usually excellent. Cryosurgical techniques have been successfully applied to the destruction of tachycardia foci and to the ablation of the His bundle and accessory connections, particularly in the free wall. Deeply located pathways may often require a direct dissection technique or a combination of dissection and cryosurgery.

The therapeutic option of His bundle division is the least attractive form of surgery because an artificial ventricular (or dual chamber) pacemaker is necessary to support the ventricular rate and because His bundle destruction can be very easily produced by the technique of catheter ablation or 'fulguration'. However, surgery to AV nodal region offers the possibility of selective destruction of those structures responsible for tachycardia without impairing normal AV conduction. This new development in the surgical approach to supraventricular tachycardia offers a considerable advantage.

# References

Anderson KP, Stinson EB, Mason JW (1982) Surgical exclusion of focal paroxysmal atrial tachycardia. Am J Cardiol 49: 869

Camm AJ, Ward DE, Spurrell RA (1980) Cryothermal mapping and cryoablation of refractory cardiac arrhythmias. Circulation 62: 67

Cox JL (1985) Status of surgery for cardiac arrhythmias. Circulation 71: 413

Gillette PC, Garson A, Kugler JD, Cooley DA, Zinner A, McNamara DG (1980) Surgical treatment of supraventricular tachycardia in infants and children. Am J Cardiol 46: 281

Giannelli S, Ayres SM, Gomprecht RF, Conklin EF, Kennedy RJ (1967) Therapeutic surgical division of the human conduction system. JAMA 199: 3

Guarnieri T, Sealy WC, Kasell JH, German LD, Gallagher JJ (1984) The nonpharmacologic management of the permanent form of junctional reciprocating tachycardia. Therapy and Prevention – Arrhythmia 69: 2

Guiraudon G, Klein G, Sharma A, Jones D (1985) Surgical correction of the Wolff-Parkinson-White syndrome in the closed heart using cryosurgery: Further observations and long-term follow-up. PACE 8: 304

Holman WL, Ikeshita M, Lease JG, Ferguson TB, Lofland GK, Cox JL (1984) Alteration of antegrade atrioventricular conduction by cryoablation of peri-atrioventricular nodal tissue. Implications for the surgical treatment of atrioventricular nodal reentry tachycardia. J Thorac Cardiovasc Surg 88: 67

Johnson DC, Ross DL, Denniss AR, Uther JB (1984) A new operation for 'AV nodal' tachycardia: Abolition of tachycardia with preservation of normal AV conduction. Circulation 70: part II–99

Josephon ME, Spear JF, Harken AH, Horowitz LN, Dorio RJ (1982) Surgical excision of automatic atrial tachycardia: Autonomic and electrophysiologic correlates. Prog in Cardiol 1076

Klein GJ, Harrison L, Ideker RF, Smith WM, Kasell J, Wallace AG, Gallagher JJ (1979) Reaction of the myocardium to cryosurgery: Electrophysiology and arrhythmogenic potential. Circulation 59: 364

Ott DA, Gillette PC, Garson A, Cooley DA, Reul GJ, McNamara DG (1985) Surgical management of refractory supraventricular tachycardia in infants and children. Am Coll Cardiol 5: 124

Page PL, Shenasa M, Cardinal R, Cossette R, Nadeau R (1985) Closed heart surgical interruption of accessory pathways in the Wolff-Parkinson-White syndrome. PACE 8: 313

Sealy WC, Anderson RW, Gallagher JJ (1977) Surgical treatment of supraventricular tachyarrhythmias. J Thorac & Cardiothorac Surg 73: 511

Sealy WC, Gallagher JJ (1981) Surgical treatment of left free wall accessory pathways of atrioventricular conduction of the Kent type. J Thorac Cardiovasc Surg 81: 698

Sealy WC, Seaber AV (1980) Surgical isolation of the atrial septum from the atria. Identification of an atrial septal pacemaker. J Thorac Cardiovasc Surg 80: 742

Williams MJ, Ungerleider RM, Lofland GK, Cox JL (1980) New technique for the treatment of supraventricular arrhythmias. Thorac Cardiovasc Surg 80: 73

Wyndham CRC, Arnsdorf MF, Levitsky S, Smith TC, Dhingra RC, Denes P, Rosen KM (1980) Successful surgical excision of focal paroxysmal atrial tachycardia. Circulation 62: 1365

# Ablation techniques for accessory pathways in the Wolff-Parkinson-White syndrome

J.J. GALLAGHER, J.G. SELLE, W.C. SEALY, J.M. FEDOR, R.H. SVENSON, and S.H. ZIMMERN

## Introduction

The first successful interruption of an accessory pathway in a patient suffering from the Wolff-Parkinson-White (WPW) syndrome [1–6] was performed on a fisherman from the coast of North Carolina on May 28, 1968 [7–8]. Sustained reciprocating tachycardia refractory to medical therapy had resulted in the development of congestive heart failure and the patient was offered the opportunity to undergo surgical correction. Epicardial mapping demonstrated the earliest point of ventricular activation at the right lateral base of the heart [7]. Using a external dissection of the atrioventricular groove in this region, Dr. Will C. Sealy successfully divided the pathway. The patient's electrocardiogram returned to normal and his recurrent supraventricular tachycardia ceased. Over the ensuing years a variety of modifications have been introduced into the procedure originally described [7–38]. In this communication, these modifications will be reviewed with emphasis on current results.

## Anatomic aspects of preexcitation surgery

A variety of mechanisms have been advanced to explain the presence (or persistence) of anomalous A-V connections in the human heart. Truex [39] and Lune [40] have proposed that anomalous bundles pass through gaps or holes in the annulus fibrosus. Morphologic and clinical observations, however, cannot support this theory in its entirety. We know for example that an anomalous fiber can pass from atrium to ventricle anywhere from a superficial epicardial location to one closely adjacent to an intact annulus fibrosus. This raises the possibility that a gene mediated step may be responsible for regression of anomalous fibers rather than the postulated mechnical disruption of these fibers as a result of the developing annulus fibrosus. The detailed nature of the anatomic studies required to adequately define an accessory pathway explains to some extent the paucity of information about such fibers [41, 42]. Literally hundreds of sections are required to locate these fibers which range in width from 0.1–7.0 mm (average 1.3 mm) [40]. Multiple pathways can be anticipated in up to 10% of patients with no associated cardiac abnormalities, while the incidence increases to over 50% in patients with associated Ebstein's malformation of the tricuspid valve. The above anatomical features must be taken into account in the development of ablative techniques. Accessory pathways are invisible to the naked eye and cannot be seen or palpated by the operating surgeon. Their localization depends largely on the information provided by preoperative and intraoperative endocardial and epicardial activation studies. In general, an attempt is made to localize both the ventricular and atrial insertions of the accessory pathways. Recently it has become evident that the use of operating loupes by the surgeon permits visualization of microscopic strains coursing in through the atrioventricular groove in some cases [21]. Nevertheless, the presence or absence of this visual identification should not be used to primarily direct the surgical intervention. Furthermore it should be emphasized that activation studies can only define the location of the accessory pathway along the atrioventricular groove but cannot as yet reliably define the exact depth in which the pathway crosses.

## Classification of accessory pathways

Accessory pathways can be located at any site along the right or left atrioventricular junction as well as the septal area. For descriptive purposes, it is useful to classify accessory pathways as right freewall (RFW), left freewall (LFW), anterior septal (AS), and posterior septal (PS) (Figs. 1A and 1B). The atrium and ventricle are adjacent to each other but separated by the annulus fibrosus and epicardial fat around the entire circumference of both the tricuspid and mitral orifices except where the left atrium is attached to the aortic ring. In the region of aortomitral continuity, there is no portion of the left ventricle in immediate contact with the left atrium; no accessory pathways would be expected in this region and surgical experience confirms this. In a recent review [41] we found that the distribution of accessory pathways was as follows: left freewall – 46%; posterior septal – 26%; right freewall – 18%; and anterior septal – 10%. The distribution was not different in medically vs. surgically treated patients. The anatomy of the posterior septal area is the most complex and will be pursued in greater detail below.

## Intermediate septal accessory pathways (para-hisian pathways): proposal of a new subgroup

As noted above septal pathways have traditionally been subdivided into anterior

462

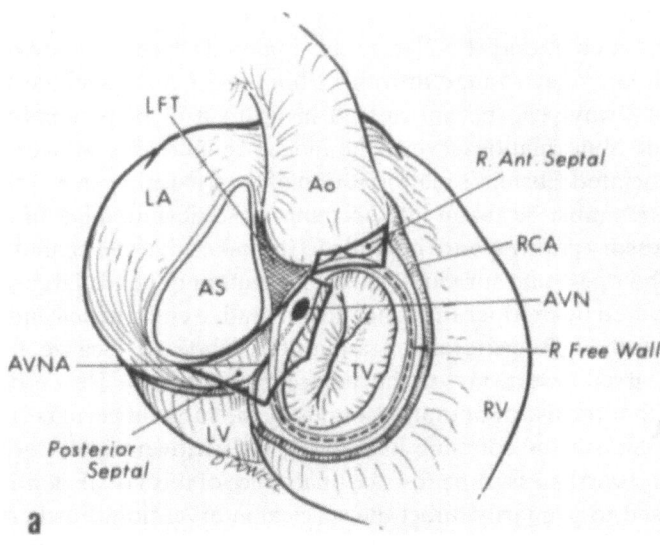

*Figure 1.* Classification of accessory atrioventricular pathways. *Panel A.* Accessory pathway locations are schematically shown, viewed from the right side of the heart. Right freewall accessory pathways traverse the right atrioventricular groove in relationship to the portion of the tricuspid annulus indicated by the dotted line. The location of right anterior septal pathways as well posterior septal pathways is also indicated. RCA = right coronary artery; AVN = AV node; RV = right ventricle; TV = tricuspid valve; LV = left ventricle; AVNA = AV nodal artery; AS = atrial septum; LA = equals left atrium; LFT = left fibrous trigone; AO = aorta.

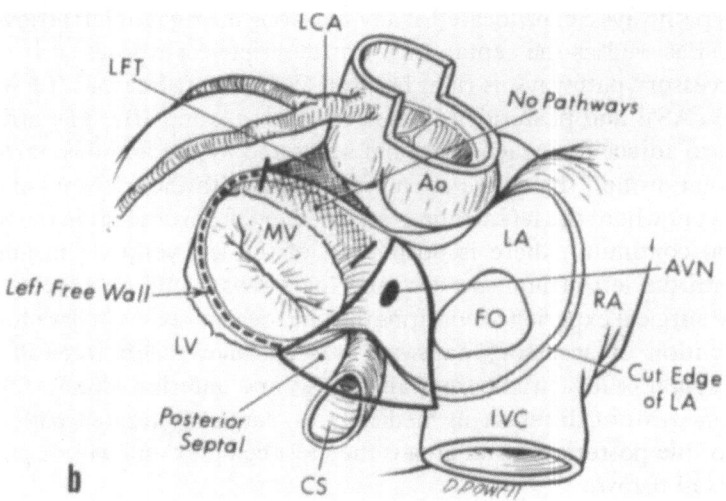

*Figure 1.* Classification of accessory atrioventricular pathways. *Panel B.* Accessory pathway location viewed from the left side of the heart. Left freewall accessory AV pathways traverse the left AV groove in relation to the portion of the mitral valve annulus indicated by the dotted line. No pathways are thought to be situated in the region where the mitral valve is suspended from the aortic annulus. The location of posterior septal pathways is also indicated. LCA = left coronary artery; FO = fossa ovalis; CS = coronary sinus; MV = mitral valve. Remainder of abbreviations as in Panel A.

septal and posterior septal pathways based on electrocardiographic and electrophysiologic criteria which appeared to have good correlation with intraoperative findings. In reviewing the previously operated cases, however, a subset of septal accessory pathways was identified with *discordant* electrocardiographic and electrophysiologic features. For descriptive purposes these will be referred to as *intermediate* septal accessory pathways.

*Anterior septal* pathways generally manifest initially positive forces of preexcitation (initial forces of the Delta wave) in leads I, II, AVL (and at times also AVF) as well as $V_1$ (where there is a rS morphology). The earliest area of retrograde atrial activation is typically found in the anterior portion of the interatrial septum or in the anteromedial right atrium. Intraoperative mapping has shown that earliest ventricular activation occurs at the base of the anterior right ventricle anywhere from the mid anterior wall over to the infundibulum. In contrast, *posterior septal* pathways generally manifest positive initial forces of preexcitation in I and AVL but negative forces in leads II, III and AVF. The initial forces are usually isoelectric in $V_1$ but an abrupt transition is seen with almost exclusive positivity observed by $V_2$. During reciporcating tachycardia, earliest retrograde atrial activation is typically demonstrated just inside the orifice of the coronary sinus. Intraoperatively, ventricular preexcitation is usually demonstrated on the posterior base of the heart in the region of the crux.

Review of a large number of patients who had undergone both electrophysiologic study as well as intraoperative mapping revealed a subset in whom the pathway appeared to be a right anterior septal by electrocardiographic criteria because they had positive initial forces of preexcitation in limb leads I and II as well as $V_1$ (with a rS morphology in $V_1$) On the other hand, the earliest area of retrograde atrial activation during reciprocating tachycardia was situated in the orifice of the coronary sinus. Intraoperative mapping in this subset of patients suggested that the positivity of the initial forces of preexcitation in lead II was due to simultaneous breakthrough of anterior and posterior wavefronts on the epicardium due to preexcitation of the mid portion of the summit of the ventricular septum. These patients were found to have a higher risk of surgical failure and development of heart block. In several of these patients it was demonstrated by 'cryothermal mapping' that cooling of the region of the His bundle to 0 degrees centigrade resulted in simultaneous block of conduction over both the accessory pathway and the normal AV node His bundle. These observations in concert suggested that there is a subset of accessory pathways which run near-contiguously with the His bundle and which are properly termed 'para-Hisian'. Recognition of this subset of patients may allow one to select out patients who are at higher risks for surgical failure and/or induction of heart block in the course of surgical interruption of their accessory pathway.

**Techniques to divide accessory pathways**

Current attempts to interrupt accessory pathways can be subdivided into open-chest (surgical) and closed-chest (catheter ablation) procedures. The open-chest surgical procedures can be further subdivided into open-heart and closed-heart techniques.

*Open-chest open-heart technique: Sealy*

The surgical principles involved in endocardial dissection of accessory pathways derive from the anatomic features noted above, complimented by empiric observations made during surgery of over 300 WPW patients. The accessory pathway, as mentioned earlier, can be located anywhere from the annulus fibrosus to the epicardium (Fig. 2). Historically the first accessory pathway was divided using an *external* approach but it readily became apparent that a safer, more thorough dissection could be accomplished by a *endocardial* approach.

A great deal of modifications and improvements have been introduced over the years by Drs. Will Sealy, Jim Cox [30] and Jay Selle [28]. Essentially all dissections are now performed during cardioplegic arrest of the heart. Each of the four anatomic areas where accessory pathways can occur in the Wolff-Parkinson-White syndrome are defined by specific boundaries. The accessory pathway courses from atrium through a portion of this bounded space to insert on the ventricle. A thorough and meticulous plane of dissection must be established at the site of ventricular insertion in the region of the pathway. The dissection is usefully guided by the use of 2.5 power optical loupes.

The surgical approach to *left freewall* A-V pathways is begun with entry made through an incision in the posterior interatrial groove. Deep hypothermia is used. The incision is begun just above the mitral annulus and is extended anteriorly to the left fibrous trigone and posteriorly to the junction of the freewall and the septum. The dissection is then extended from the region of the mitral valve annulus all the way to the epicardial reflection. The latter is the most important structure to visualize along the entire length of the supra-annular incision. A sharp and blunt dissection using a nerve hook is used immediately at the level of the mitral annulus to interrupt any accessory pathway which might cross the A-V groove contiguous with the annulus itself. The integrity of the epicardium itself is usually preserved for purposes of hemostasis. Occasionally a small portion of the atrial side of the incision is undermined to facilitate a closure of the edges without risking injury to the coronary artery.

Surgical approach to *right freewall* pathways is similar. On the right side, however, endocardial mapping is also used in addition to epicardial mapping to obtain a more detailed localization. Because hemostasis does not constitute such a problem with closure on the right side, a complete through-and-through dissec-

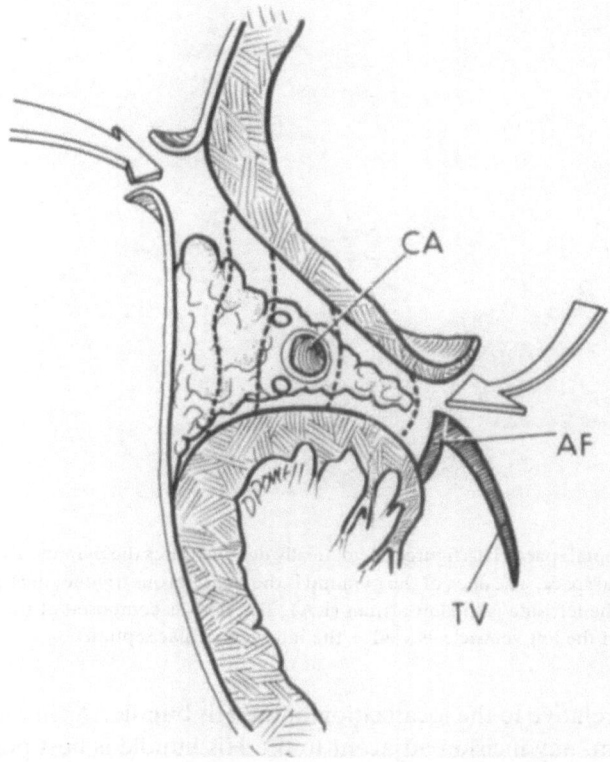

*Figure 2*. Potential locations of accessory pathways. This figure schematically shows a cross section of the right atrioventricular groove with the variety of accessory pathway locations which have been empirically confirmed by clinical studies. The accessory pathways are shown as dotted lines and can occur anywhere from the epicardium to the endocardial aspect of the atrioventricular groove. The large arrows indicate potential external and internal dissections which would be required to disrupt the accessory pathway in its course from atrium to ventricle.

tion of the A-V groove is sometimes resorted to especially when the tricuspid annulus is not well developed.

The *septal* region is divided into anterior and posterior regions. The term septum in this instance is utilized loosely since it is obvious that the true atrioventricular septum is a very tiny area confined to the region of the right fibrous trigone and membranous septum. Nonetheless, the emphasis on the 'septal' localization is justified since this is a more difficult area to work in and injury to the normal conduction tissues may result either from direct trauma or indirectly from traction on the neighboring tissues.

The *anterior septal* space is bounded by the membranous portion of the interatrial septum posteriorly, the right anterior freewall anteriorly, and extends from the tricuspid valve annulus to the epicardial reflection. Endocardial mapping in this area is particularly useful to define the precise location of the

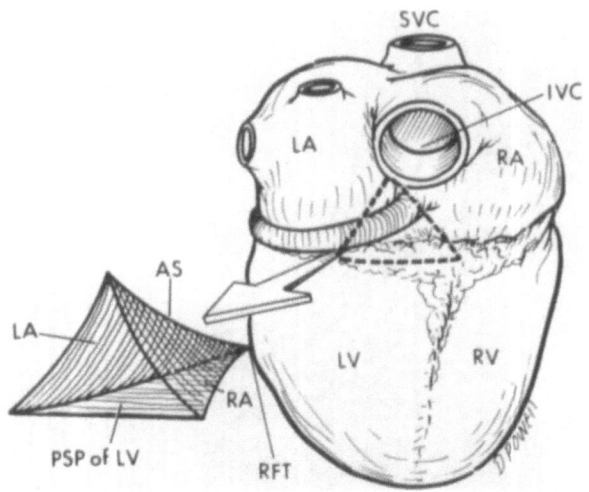

*Figure 3.* The posterior septal space. This figure schematically demonstrates the pyramidal configuration of the posterior septal space. The apex of the pyramid is the right fibrous trigone; the right side is the right atrium (RA); the left side is the left atrium (LA). The floor is composed of the posterior superior process (PSP) of the left ventricle as well as the interventricular septum.

accessory pathway relative to the localization of the His bundle. As in the case of the posterior septum, any incision adjacent to the His bundle is best performed with the heart beating and with continual monitoring of the His bundle to ensure that damage to the A-V node His bundle does not occur; the remainder of the dissection can be carried out with cardioplegia. In cases where excessive motion of the heart would cause dissection in this manner to be hazardous, the localization of the His bundle is clearly defined by mapping and marked, with dissection proceeding later under the protection of cardioplegic arrest.

The greatest modifications of technique have occurred in the surgical approach to the *posterior septal* accessory pathways (Fig. 3). The space which overlies the crux of the heart can be best compared to a toppled pyramid. The pyramidal space through which posterior septal accessory pathways cross is bounded anteriorly by the insertion of the atrial extension of the membranous septum into the right fibrous trigone and posteriorly by the epicardium overlying the crux of the heart. The floor of this space is made up of the interventricular septum and the posterior superior process of the left ventricle. The lateral walls of the space are formed by the diverging walls of the right and left atria respectively. Again, endocardial mapping during ventricular pacing or reciprocating tachycardia is used to define not only the location of the His bundle but also the area of earliest retrograde atrial activation. An incision is begun approximately 1 cm posterior to the region of the recorded His bundle and entry is thus made into the posterior pyramidal space (Fig. 4). The anterior extent of the incision is not allowed to proceed

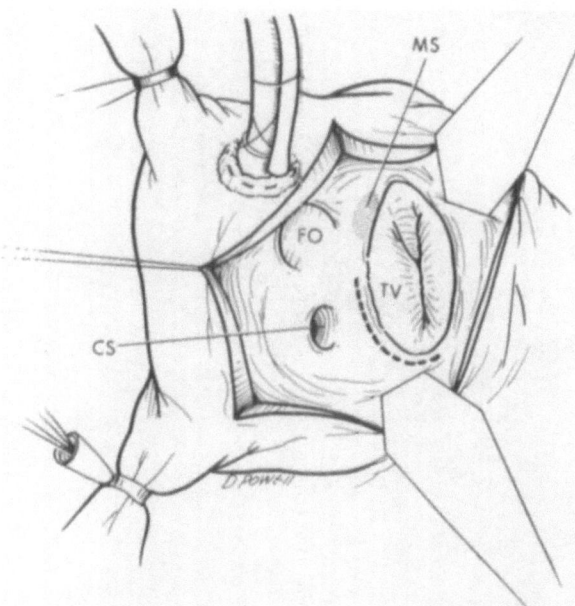

*Figure 4.* The endocardial approach for dissection of posterior septal accessory pathways. The right atrium is schematically shown opened after an atriotomy while on cardiopulmonary bypass. The dotted line indicates the initial incision which is made just above the tricuspid annulus. The incision is initiated posterior to the membranous septum after first locating the region of the His bundle and is extended onto the right freewall to facilitate exposure (see text for discussion).

beyond the convergence of the right and left atrium anteriorly [30] to minimize any damage to the His bundle. Traction on the atrial septum as well as dissection above the level of the annulus is avoided in order to protect the integrity of the A-V node. The endocardial incision is extended posteriorly well on the right posterior freewall to facilitate exposure. Historically, this dissection has been the most difficult of all because the need for good exposure in this difficult small area must be balanced against the risk of potential damage to the A-V node His bundle. The mitral annulus must be carefully identified and thoroughly cleaned. The left corner of the pyramidal space is the most difficult of all to expose and has long been suspected as the trouble spot where previous failures occurred. The epicardial reflection of the ventricle is identified on the right side and followed across the mid-line until the posterior superior process of the left ventricle is encountered. External examination of the heart at this point should verify that the dissection plane has extended over to the beginning of the left ventricular freewall (Fig. 5). When adequate exposure cannot be obtained, alternative possibilities include either cryosurgery of the left corner of the parietal space (with possible risk to the coronary artery) or performing a left atriotomy to complete the dissection with a left supra-annular incision.

468

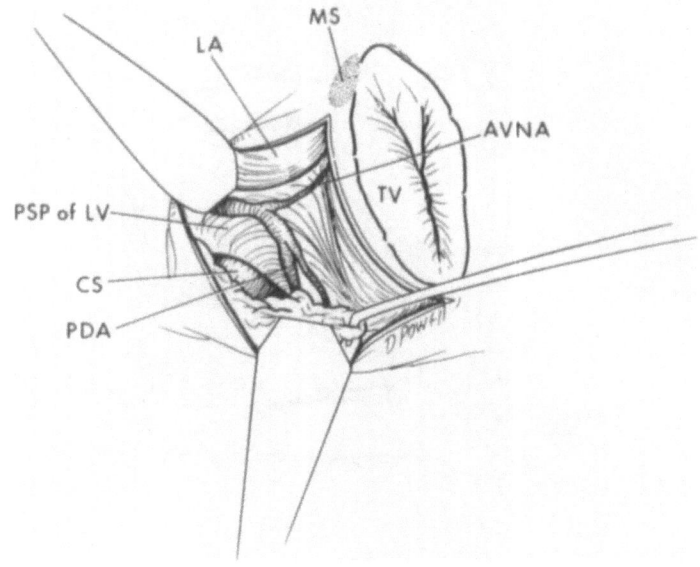

*Figure 5.* Surgical dissection of the posterior pyramidal space (see text for discussion). MS = membranous septum; AVNA = AV nodal artery; TV = tricuspid valve; PDA = posterior descending artery; CS = coronary sinus; PSPLV = posterior superior process of the left ventricle (see text for discussion).

In our earlier series at Duke University Medical Center (May 1968 – January 1983), three surgeons – Drs. Will Sealy, James Cox, and James Lowe – operated on a total of 267 patients who had 304 accessory pathways (15% multiple pathways). Successful interruption of accessory pathways was as follows: 52/53 right freewall (98%), 134/143 left freewall (94%), 66/81 posterior septal (81%), and 23/27 anterior septal (85%). Sixteen of the *posterior* septal pathway patients developed heart block (20%) while only one of the *anterior* septal pathway patients developed heart block (0.04%). The overall mortality was 4%; reoperation was required in 15%. The last 118 consecutive patients in this series was separately reported recently [30] to emphasize the improved results which have been obtained with the procedure described above. Thus the success rate for division of accessory pathways rose from an overall of 85% to 99.3%, there was a decrease in reoperation rate from 15% to 0% and a decrease in the incidence of permanent heart block from 10.5% to 0.8%. The mortality again was 5% for the entire series but only one death occurred following elective operation in the *absence* of associated abnormality (0.85%).

In July of 1983, a new series was initiated at the Sanger Clinic by the authors. From July 1983 through January 1986, 77 additional patients underwent surgical treatment of 93 accessory pathways (2 patients had 3 accessory pathways and 12 patients had 2 accessory pathways). In contrast to previously reported analyses, the *intermediate* septal accessory pathway classification was utilized (Table 1). Successful interruption of the accessory pathway was achieved in all but 2 patients, both with septal accessory pathways. The first (patient #45) had a right freewall and a posterior septal accessory pathway; the right freewall was successfully divided at surgery but the posterior septal pathway returned and was later ablated by the transvenous catheter electrode technique to be discussed in a subsequent section. The second patient (#44) had a para-Hisian pathway (intermediate septal pathway) that remained blocked only when conduction in the His bundle was also obtunded; he is currently scheduled to undergo deliberate transvenous His bundle ablation. Three patients were felt to fall into the intermediate septal pathway group. Two of these had their accessory pathways successfully divided but in the process acquired either complete heart block or persistent second degree block. The third patient is the failure noted above (patient #44) who is scheduled to undergo deliberate His bundle ablation. There was one death (#12) encountered in a patient with a posterior septal pathway who died of congestive cardiomyopathy thought to be related to ligation of an excessive number of veins draining into the coronary sinus; this is now avoided.

*Open-chest closed-heart technique: Guiraudon*

Recently, Guiraudon proposed an epicardial approach for ablation of accessory atrioventricular pathways which does not require cold cardioplegic cardiac arrest. Using this technique, ablation is carried out on a beating heart with or without the assistance of normothermic cardiopulmonary bypass [26, 43]. The rationale for this approach is based on the pathological evidence that the vast majority of the accessory pathways course within the atrioventricular groove rather than in the subendocardium and therefore are accessible from the epicardial approach. The epicardial approach involves dissection and mobilization of the atrioventricular fat pad with exposure of the atrioventricular junction and is followed by cryoablation of the atrioventricular junction. This approach has now been applied to left

*Table 1.* Results of surgical treatment of 77 patients with W-P-W syndrome; Sanger Clinic, July 1983– February 1986.

| Pathway location | Successful division | Heart block |
| --- | --- | --- |
| Left freewall | 49/49 | 0 |
| Right free wall | 15/15 | 0 |
| Anterior septal | 2/2 | 0 |
| Intermediate septal | 2/3 | 2 |
| Posterior septal | 23/24 | 0 |

* Later ablated by catheter electrode technique.

and right freewall pathways as well as posterior septal accessory pathways; anterior septal pathways generally require an *open* heart approach to the septum. Guiraudon recently reported his experience [43] in a total of 105 consecutive patients with 74 left ventricular freewall pathways [24], posterior septal pathways, and 11 right ventricular freewall pathways operated on between July 1982 and September 1985. Three patients had multiple accessory pathways. All but one pathway was successfully ablated with no mortality and no incident of heart block. One pathway was modified. Four patients, however, required a second operation for recurrence of pathway conduction within the first few weeks and one patient required a third operation.

Certain unique pitfalls and potential limitations were encountered. The surgical approach to the *anterior* left atrioventricular groove in the region of the left atrial appendage was particularly complex because of the absence of a good plane of dissection. Dissection in the left atrioventricular groove had to be particularly delicate and meticulous in order to avoid circumflex coronary arteries (which were intramural in 14 patients), and to avoid puncture (5 patients) or tearing (2 patients) of the left atrium, which might result in air embolism. Pathways adjacent to the left fibrous trigone as well as right anterior septal pathways did not appear accessible by this surgical approach. Extensive external dissection of the atrioventricular groove was obviously required in every case with division of coronary veins carried out when these impaired adequate exposure of the atrioventricular groove. Although this theoretically might predispose patients to bleeding complications, only 2 patients apparently required reoperation because of excessive bleeding. It is useful to point out that the mean age of the patients in this series was 32.8 years. It remains to be seen whether in a larger series, the more elderly patient may prove more susceptible to bleeding complications because of friable tissues. Potential advantages of the epicardial approach include the ability to continually monitor preexcitation during dissection and to avoid cardioplegia and aortic cross-clamping. The absence of postoperative atrial fibrillation in Guiraudon's series to date may be due to the absence of atriotomies using this approach.

*Open-chest closed-heart technique: Bockeria*

Bockeria [34] in the Sovjet Union recently reported a new open-chest procedure for surgical treatment of W-P-W syndrome which avoids aortic cross-clamping and cardioplegia. After opening the chest and performing epicardial mapping, cardiopulmonary bypass was used to empty the heart. Specially fabricated electrodes which conformed to specific regions of the atrioventricular groove were used to apply external epicardial shocks of 200 joules, resulting in lesions approximately 12 mm$^2$ in diameter. No dissection of the atrioventricular groove was performed. Twenty-five patients with freewall accessory pathways were reported successfully treated by this approach although it was emphasized that the long-term sequelae to the coronary arteries in the atrioventricular grooves is presently unknown. No septal pathways were attempted.

### Closed-chest catheter ablation of accessory pathways

The availability of catheter techniques to localize and record from sites of cardiac rhythm disturbances naturally led to attempts to deliver energy through the same catheters in order to ablate or modify the responsible cardiac tissues. A number of animal studies previously indicated the feasibility of transvenous catheter ablation of the A-V junction. In 1982, Gallagher [44] and Scheinman [45] reported successful therapeutic induction of heart block in man utilizing discharges of high voltage D-C current through catheter electrodes positioned in the region of the His bundle. The technique has subsequently been extended to ablation of atrial foci, accessory pathways and ventricular foci.

Catheter electrodes can be used to localize the atrial insertion of most accessory pathways which conduct retrogradely. A limited amount of experimental data supports the feasibility of catheter ablation of accessory pathways. Thus Brodman and Fisher [35] reported *bipolar* discharges of 35–250 joules across adjacent poles of a catheter electrode introduced into the coronary sinus of man. *Acutely, burns of the coronary sinus with ecchymosis and edema in the adjacent left atrial and left ventricular wall were noted. Two dogs received 240 joules with perforation and tamponade occurring in one of these.* Chronic lesions were characterized by fibrosis, occlusion of the coronary sinus and occasional intimal hyperplasia of the circumflex coronary artery. It is difficult to extrapolate these canine studies to man because of marked differences in size and compliance of the heart and particularly of the coronary sinus, not to mention the obvious differences in thoracic impedance.

Application of this technique world wide had been somewhat limited [36–38]. A number of theoretical problems will limit the widespread application of this technique to ablation of accessory pathways in man. Little if any success has been encountered during application to right freewall and left freewall accessory pathways, and at present only posterior septal pathways appear suitable for ablation by this approach [36–38]. The topography of the right atrioventricular groove makes catheter placement difficult. In the left atrioventricular groove, the coronary sinus tapers in its diameter as it extends laterally making perforation a distinct risk in this location; furthermore the coronary sinus descends onto the ventricle and is at some distance from the atrioventricular goove in its more lateral course.

Septal accessory pathways appear to be the most favorable substrate for this technique. Such pathways are generally located close to the orifice of the coronary sinus where a stable catheter position can be maintained. The proximal

472

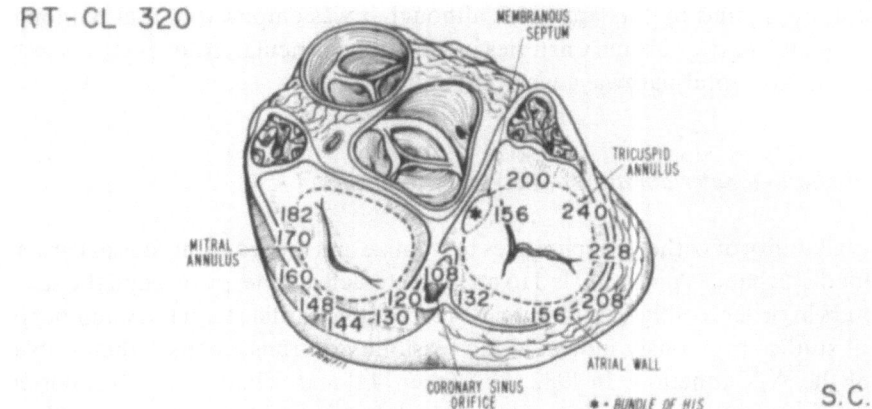

RT-CL 320

*Figure 6.* Retrograde sequence of atrial activation resulting from a posterior septal accessory pathway successfully ablated by transvenous catheter electrode shock. The heart is shown schematically in cross section at the level of the atrioventricular groove. The ventriculoatrial intervals recorded by catheter electrode technique during sustained reciprocating tachycardia are shown. The earliest area of retrograde atrial activation was 108 msec. and was situated in the orifice of the coronary sinus. Cases such as this are ideal for consideration for transvenous catheter electrode ablation. In this case, delivery of a single 200 joule unipolar shock to the catheter electrode situated just at the orifice of the coronary sinus ablated the posterior septal accessory pathway, leaving intact normal conduction in the AV node His bundle.

coronary sinus has a large diameter to absorb the pressure transient or so called barotrauma which occurs, probably minimizing the possibility of perforation or rupture. Potential risks, however, include damage to the circumflex artery either acutely or chonically (ie spasm [46], intimal lesion leading to stenosis), thrombosis or perforation of the coronary sinus, and damage to the AV node in the adjacent atrial septum. There is still a great deal of controversy concerning the mechanism of therapeutic injury of the accessory pathway. The actual ablation may result from electrogenic forces, local thermal effects, or result from the high pressures generated locally by the shock. The role of 'barotrauma' has been especially suggested by the experimental studies of Coltorti and co-workers [47]. The best results appear to be obtained when the shock is delivered in a unipolar fashion to an electrode reaching the orifice of the coronary sinus with the indifferent electrode placed on the chest wall. Energy levels of 200 joules or less appear suitable, with perforation perhaps more likely with higher energies. The procedure has been applied in at least 40 patients worldwide, with approximately 75% success in the posterior septal group. At least 2 instances of tamponade have been reported. In our own experience with 4 cases of posterior septal pathways, successful ablation was achieved in 3/4. Two of these patients had previously undergone unsuccessful surgery (one from our series, one referred), and were successfully ablated with two 400 joule shocks. In the two unoperated cases, energy was limited to 200 joules: one succeeded (Fig. 6). In the failed case, a small area of ecchymosis was noted on the *superior* aspect of the coronary sinus orifice at surgery.

It should be emphasized that this technique remains investigational. Coronary angiography is mandatory prior to attempting the procedure to establish the location of the coronary artery relative to the catheter electrode; late films can also demonstrate the size of the coronary sinus in the location where the delivery of shock is proposed. Administration of calcium channel blockers are probably advisable to avoid potential coronary artery spasm. Finally in all cases, the surgical team with cardiopulmonary bypass facility should be on standby during the procedure.

## Conclusion

Extensive modifications of surgical techniques has resulted in the ability to divide accessory pathway in essentially every case. In the absence of associated abnormalities, mortality is minimal and comparable to elective closure of congenital atrial septal defects. Heart block is extremely uncommon and it now appears possible to identify the subset of septal accessory pathways which may at higher risk for surgical failure and/or the creation of heart block. Compared with the prospect of life-long dependence on cardiac medications with the attendant side effects and risks of arrhythmia recurrence, surgical interruption of accessory pathways appears to offer not only a reasonable alternative therapy but perhaps the most desirable of all. Excellent results have been achieved despite the variety of different surgical approaches utilized. Larger series with long-term followup will be required before the safety and efficacy of catheter electrode ablation of posterior septal pathways can fully assessed.

## References

1. Gallagher JJ, Gilbert M, Svenson RH, Sealy WC, Kasell J, Wallace AG (1975) Wolff-Parkinson-White syndrome. The problem, evaluation, and surgical correction. Circulation 51: 767–785
2. Gallagher JJ, Pritchett ELC, Benditt DG, Tonkin AM, Campbell RWF, Dugan FA, Bashore TM, Tower A, Wallace AG (1977) New catheter techniques for analysis of the sequence of retrograde atrial activation in man. Eur J Cardio 6: 1014
3. Gallagher JJ, Pritchett ELC, Sealy WC, Kasell J, Wallace AG (1978) The preexcitation syndromes Progress in Cardiovascular Diseases 20: 285–327
4. Gallagher JJ, Kasell J, Sealy WC, Pritchett ELC, Wallace AG (1978) Epicardial mapping in the Wolff-Parkinson-White syndrome. Circulation 57: 854–866
5. Gallagher JJ, Sealy WC, Kasell J (1979) Intraoperative mapping studies in the Wolff-Parkinson-White syndrome. PACE 2: 523–537
6. Prystowsky EN, Miles WM, Heger JJ, Zipes DP (1984) Preexcitation syndromes. Mechanisms and management. Med Clin N Am 68: 831–893
7. Cobb FR, Blumenschein SD, Sealy WC, Boineau JP, Wagner GS, Wallace AG (1968) Successful

surgical interruption of the bundle of Kent in a patient with Wolff-Parkinson-White syndrome. Circulation 38: 1018–1029

8. Sealy WC, Gattler BG, Blumenschein SD, Cobb FR (1969) Surgical Treatment of Wolff-Parkinson-White syndrome. Ann Thorac Surg 8: 1–11

9. Svenson RH, Gallagher JJ, Sealy WC, Wallace AG (1974) An electrophysiologic approach to the surgical treatment of the Wolff-Parkinson-White syndrome. Report of two cases utilizing catheter recording and epicardial mapping techniques. Circulation 49: 799–804

10. Sealy WC, Wallace AJ, Ramming KP, Gallagher JJ, Svenson RH (1974) An improved operation for the definitive treatment of the Wolff-Parkinson-White syndrome. Ann Thorac Surg 18: 107–113

11. Sealy WC, Wallace AG (1974) Surgical treatment of Wolff-Parkinson-White syndrome. J Thorac Cardiovasc Surg 68: 757–770

12. Wallace AG, Sealy WC, Gallagher JJ, Svenson RH, Strauss HC, Kasell J (1974) Surgical correction of anomalous left ventricular preexcitation: Wolff-Parkinson-White (Type A). Circulation 49: 206–212

13. Sealy WC, Gallagher JJ, Pritchett ELC, Wallace AG (1978) Surgical treatment of tachyarrhythmias in patients with both an Ebstein anomaly and a Kent bundle. J Thorac Cardiovasc Surg 75: 847–853

14. Gallagher JJ, Sealy WC, Anderson RW, Kasell J, Millar Roger, Campbell RWF, Harrison L, Pritchett ELC, Wallace AG (1977) Cryosurgical ablation of accessory atrioventricular connections. A method for correction of the preexcitation syndrome. Circulation 55: 471–479

15. Sealy WC, Gallagher JJ, Pritchett ELC (1978) The surgical anatomy of Kent bundles based on electrophysiologic mapping and surgical exploration. J Thorac Cardiovasc Surg 76: 804–815

16. Iwa T, Kawasuji M, Misaki T, Takaaki I, Magara T (1980) Localization and interruption of accessory conduction pathway in the Wolff-Parkinson-White syndrome. J Thorac Cardiovasc Surg 80: 271–279

17. Sealy WC, Gallagher JJ (1980) The surgical approach to the septal area of the heart based on experiences with 45 patients with Kent bundles. J Thorac Cardiovasc Surg 79: 542–551

18. Sealy WC, Gallagher JJ (1981) Surgical problems with multiple accessory pathways of atrioventricular conduction. J Thorac Cardiovasc Surg 81: 707–712

19. Sealy WC, Gallagher JJ (1981) Surgical treatment of left free wall accessory pathways of atrioventricular conduction of the Kent type. J Thorac Cardiovasc Surg 81: 698–706

20. Sealy WC, Mikat EM (1983) Anatomical problems with identification and interruption of posterior septal Kent bundles. Ann Thorac Surg 36: 584–595

21. Brodman R, Fisher J, Mitsudo S, Kim SG, Matos J (1982) Kent pathways visualized in situ and removed at operation. Brief Reports 1457–1458

22. Holmes DR, Osborn MJ, Gersh B, Maloney JD, Danielson GK (1982) The Wolff-Parkinson-White syndrome – A surgical approach. Mayo Clin Proc 57: 345–350

23. Sealy WC (1983) The evolution of the surgical methods for interruption of right free wall Kent bundles. Ann Thorac Surg 36: 29–36

24. Sealy WC (1983) Kent bundles in the anterior septal space. Ann Thorac Surg 36: 180–186

25. Sealy WC (1984) The Wolff-Parkinson-White syndrome and the beginnings of direct arrhythmias surgery. Ann Thorac Surg 38: 176–180

26. Guiraudon GM, Klein GJ, Gulamhusein S, Jones DL, Yee R, Perkins DG, Jarvis E (1984) Surgical repair of Wolff-Parkinson-White syndrome: a new closed-heart technique. Ann Thorac Surg 37: 67–71

27. Sealy WC (1984) A review of the surgical treatment of cardiac arrhythmias. Clin Prog in Pacing and Electrophysiol 2: 120–138

28. Selle JG (1984) Temporary division of the superior vena cava for exceptional mitral valve exposure. J Thorac Cardiovasc Surg 88: 302–304

29. Ott DA, Garson A, Cooley DA, McNamara DG (1985) Definitive operation for refractory

cardiac tachyarrhythmias in children. J Thorac Cardiovasc Surg 90: 681–689

30. Cox JL, Gallagher JJ, Cain ME (1985) Experience with 118 consecutive patients undergoing operation for the Wolff-Parkinson-White syndrome. J Thorac Cardiovasc Surg 90: 490–501

31. Bredikis J, Bukauskas F, Zebrauskas R, Sakalauskas J, Loschilov V, Nevsky V, Bredikis A, Liakas R (1985) Cryosurgical ablation of right parietal and septal accessory atrioventricular connections without the use of extracorporeal circulation. J Thorac Cardiovas Surg 90: 206–211

32. Bredikis J, Bredikis A (1985) Cryosurgical ablation of left parietal wall accessory atrioventricular connections through the coronary sinus without the use of extracorporeal circulation. J Thorac Cardiovasc Surg 90: 199–205

33. Gallagher JJ, Sealy WC, Cox JL, German LD, Kasell JH, Bardy GH, Packer DL (1984) The results of surgery for preexcitation due to accessory atrioventricular pathways in 267 consecutive cases. In: Tachycardias; Mechanisms, Diagnosis, Treatment. Josephson Mark, and Wellens Hein, Eds. Publ. by Lea and Febiger. Chapter 11: 259–269

34. Bockeria L (1985) Epicardial electric shock ablation of accessory pathways in preexcitation syndrome. Proceedings of the International Symposium on Fulguration and Laser in Cardiac Arrhythmias, Paris, France. Ed. by Fontaine G, April 12–13. In preparation.

35. Brodman R, Fisher J (1983) Evaluation of a catheter technique for ablation of accessory pathways near the coronary sinus using a canine model. Circulation 67: 923–929

36. Morady F, Scheinman MM, Winston SA, DiCarlo LA, Davis JC, Griffin JC, Ruder M, Abbott JA, Eldar M (1985) Efficacy and safety of transcatheter ablation of posteroseptal accessory pathways. Circulation 72: 170–177

37. Ward DE, Camm AJ (1985) Treatment of tachycardias associated with the Wolff-Parkinson-White syndrome by transvenous electrical ablation of accessory pathways. Br Heart J 53: 64–68

38. Critelli G, Gallagher JJ, Perticone F, Monda V, Scherillo M, Condorelli M (1985) Transvenous catheter ablation of the accessory atrioventricular pathway in the permanent form of junctional reciprocating tachycardia. Am J Cardiol 55: 1639–1642

39. Truex RC, Bishof JK, Downing DF (1960) Accessory atrioventricular muscle bundles. II. Cardiac conduction system in a human specimen with Wolff-Parkinson-White syndrome. Anat Rec 137: 417

40. Lunel AAV (1972) Significance of annulus fibrosus of heart in relation to AV conduction and ventricular activation in cases of Wolff-Parkinson-White syndrome. Br Heart J 34: 1263

41. Gallagher JJ, Sealy WC, Cox JL, Kasell JH, German LD (1983) Part XI: Updating of Wolff-Parkinson-White syndrome. Anatomic substrates of the Wolff-Parkinson-White syndrome. In: Frontiers of Cardiac Electrophysiology, Rosenbaum MB, and Elizari MB, eds., Published by Martinus Nijhoff. pp. 689–701

42. Sealy WC, Pritchett ELC, Kasell JH, Gallagher JJ (1979) Surgical treatment of Wolff-Parkinson-White syndrome. In: Update I: The Heart. Willis Hurst J, ed. New York: McGraw-Hill, pp 275–289

43. Guiraudon GM, Klein GJ, Sharma AD, Mitstein S, McLellan DG: Closed-heart technique for Wolff-Parkinson-White syndrome: further experience and potential limitations. Ann Thor Surg in press

44. Gallagher JJ, Svenson RH, Kasell JH et al (1982) Catheter technique for closed-chest ablation of the atrioventricular conduction system. A therapeutic alternative for the treatment of refractory supraventricular tachycardia. NE J Med 306: 194

45. Scheinman MM, Morady F, Hess DS, Gonzales R (1982) Catheter-induced ablation of the atrioventricular junction to control refractory supraventricular arrhythmias. JAMA 248: 851

46. Hartzler GO, Giorgi LV, Diehl AM, Hamaker WR (1985) Right coronary spasm complicating electrode catheter ablation of a right lateral accessory pathway. JACC 6: 250–253

47. Coltorti F, Bardy GH, Reichenbach D, Greene HL, Thomas R, Breazeale DG, Ivey TD (1985) Unipolar vs bipolar catheter shocks at the coronary sinus orifice. Circulation 72: 1557

# His bundle ablation in refractory supra-ventricular tachycardia: a report of the Percutaneous Cardiac Mapping and Ablation Registry

G.T. EVANS-BELL, M.M. SCHEINMAN, and the Executive Committee of the Percutaneous Cardiac Mapping and Ablation Registry*

## Introduction

Direct surgical interruption of the His bundle is an accepted technique for the management of patients with drug or pacemaker resistant supraventricular tachycardia. Since the initial animal studies using closed-chest approaches to induce atrioventricular (A-V) block, catheter ablation of the A-V junction has supplanted surgical interruption of the His bundle as the preferred technique for management of these difficult patients. This chapter will describe the development of catheter ablation techniques, the actual ablation procedure, provide a summary of the data collected by the Percutaneous Cardiac Mapping and Ablation Registry (PCMAR), review the literature on catheter ablation of the A-V junction and look at future developments in the field.

## Preliminary studies

Open or closed-chest techniques for induction of A-V block in both experimental and clinical settings have included injection of caustic material [1–5], electro- or cryo-coagulation of the A-V junction [6–12], and various surgical techniques involving direct transection of the His bundle [13–15], production of septal infarction [16] and direct mechanical crushing [17–18]. Among these techniques, cryoablation has the ability to most precisely control the extent of injury, albeit necessitating a thoracotomy [12].

In 1976, Beazell et al [19], described a technique for the production of A-V

* The Executive Committee of the Percutaneous Cardiac Mapping and Ablation Registry: David Benditt, M.D., Kevin Browne, M.D., Nabil El-Sherif, M.D., John Fisher, M.D., Guy Fontaine, M.D., Larry German, M.D., Geoffrey Hartzler, M.D., Mark Josephson, M.D., Fred Morady, M.D., Jeremy Ruskin, M.D., Melvin Scheinman, M.D., Fons Timmermans, M.D., and Douglas Zipes, M.D., Mr. David Mai, Secretary.

block in dogs using a closed-chest electrosurgical approach with delivery of pulsed energy via an insulated transseptal needle.

In 1981, Gonzalez et al [20], using a modification of Beazell's technique, produced chronic stable A-V block in nine of ten dogs which persisted for the duration of the three month follow-up period. Synchronized shocks of 35 joules were delivered to the region of the A-V junction. Five dogs responded to a single shock and two to four shocks were necessary in the remaining dogs. One dog died in ventricular fibrillation as a result of improper QRS synchronization with the shock. The other dogs appeared healthy, had a stable heart rate and did not require cardiac pacing during this time. The A-V block persisted during exercise and atropine administration. Gross post-mortem examination revealed neither evidence of myocardial or valvular scars, nor perforation of the septum. Histologic evidence of necrosis and fatty infiltration of the approaches to the A-V node, the A-V node itself and the His bundle were found in the four dogs studied. Bardy et al [21] confirmed these findings in a later study in dogs using shocks of 280 joules and also noted discrete scars at the base of the leaflet of the tricuspid valve. In all their animals, complete A-V block was refractory to isoproterenol and atropine administration. Total amounts of tissue destroyed compared favorably with results of cryoablation methods. Thus, a suitable closed-chest animal model demonstrated that the technique of catheter ablation of the A-V junction could produce stable chronic third degree A-V block with acceptable amounts of tissue loss.

**Initial human experience with closed-chest catheter ablation**

The first report of closed-chest catheter-induced A-V block in man occurred in 1979, when Vedel et al [22] reported a patient who fortuitously developed A-V block. A DC shock was inadvertently delivered through an intracardiac catheter which was in contact with the paddle electrodes being used to treat ventricular tachycardia induced during an electrophysiologic study. The first patient to undergo therapeutic catheter ablation occurred in April 1981 at the University of California San Francisco Medical Center.

Three years later, Gallagher et al [23], and Scheinman et al [24] reported their results in a total of 15 patients undergoing catheter ablation of the A-V junction for control of refractory supraventricular tachycardia (SVT). Single or multiple shocks ranging from 25 to 500j were effective in producing chronic third degree A-V block in the patients. A-V conduction with RBBB pattern resumed in one patient at six weeks, one patient had first and second degree A-V block, and three patients had intra-His-bundle conduction delay. CPK-MB ranged from zero to 121 IU (mean $26 \pm 31$). Technetium Tc 99m pyrophosphate scan was positive in two of fourteen patients. No evidence of procedure-induced arrhythmias or valvular dysfunction occurred. One patient died suddenly five and one-half weeks after the procedure.

## Technique of catheter ablation

All patients undergo standard electrophysiological studies prior to ablation. After obtaining informed, written consent, the patients are taken to the catheterization laboratory, where a temporary pacing catheter is inserted percutaneously through a subclavian or femoral vein and positioned in the right ventricular apex. A standard tripolar His-bundle catheter or quadripolar catheter (USCI) is introduced via the right femoral vein and positioned across the tricuspid valve to record a His-bundle deflection. Filtered unipolar recordings are obtained, and the electrode which demonstrates the largest His bundle deflection is connected to the cathodal output of a standard defibrillator. Another patch electrode is firmly positioned over the left scapula and connected as the anode. Patients are anesthetized with intravenous short-acting barbituates in preparation for the shock. The defibrillator is charged and DC shocks synchronized to the QRS complex are delivered through the electrode showing the largest unipolar His bundle deflection. After delivery of the shock, demand ventricular pacing is initiated via the previously inserted catheter. The patients are observed in the laboratory and transferred to the coronary care unit. Creatine phosphokinase determinations, technetium Tc 99m pyrophosphate scans and ambulatory electrocardiographic monitor (Holter) tracings are obtained. After 48 to 72 hours of stable chronic third degree A-V block, a permanent transvenous pacemaker is inserted into the apex of the right ventricle. Patients are followed with Holter recordings and stress testing, as well as with standard checks of pacemaker function.

## Development of the registry

Shortly after the initial reports of closed chest catheter ablation of the A-V junction desxribed above, a voluntary international organization, the Percutaneous Cardiac Mapping and Ablation Registry, was developed to collect and collate data on catheter ablation techniques. An Executive Committee was formed, under the chairmanship of Melvin M. Scheinman M.D., and Douglas Zipes, M.D., to coordinate the data and disseminate the information about these new techniques. There are presently sixty-three reporting centers, forty in the United States, and twenty-three representing thirteen foreign countries. An initial report of the Registry has been published [25].

## Registry patient characteristics

Two hundred and nine cases of attempted A-V junction ablation have been reported to the Registry over the past two years. Females and males are almost equally distributed, 53% and 47%, respectively, with an average age of 55 ± 17 years, (range from nine to eighty-four years of age). Table 1 summarizes the characteristics of the registry patients.

The most common indication for catheter ablation was atrial fibrillation or flutter with a rapid ventricular response (61%). This was followed by A-V node re-entrant tachycardias (20%), orthodromic A-V tachycardia utilizing an accessory pathway (13%), atrial tachycardia resulting from interatrial reentry or ectopic atrial tachycardia (11%), the permanent form of junctional reciprocating tachycardia (3%), and nonparoxysmal sinus or junctional ectopic tachycardia (4%).

Forty-five percent (45%) of patients had no organic heart disease. The remainder had diagnoses of coronary heart disease (17%), cardiomyopathy (15%), valvular heart disease (10%), hypertensive heart disease (4%), cor pulmonale (4%), and other heart disease in 5%.

All patients but one had failed at least one antiarrhythmic drug trial, with the mean number of failed drug categories equal to 3.5 ± 1.5. This underestimates the actual number of drugs used, since multiple trials of a variety of beta blockers, type I antiarrhythmic drugs, calcium channel blockers, and other experimental drugs were all coded under a general classification for the drugs.

Digitalis preparations and the type I antiarrhythmics were the most common drugs failed, 83% and 81%, respectively. This was followed by beta blockers in 78% and calcium channel blockers in 77%. Forty-seven percent (47%) proved intolerant of or failed amiodarone, while 21% failed other experimental antiarrhythmics. Eight percent of patients had failed therapy with an antitachycardia pacemaker.

*Table 1.* Clinical findings in patients with drug and/or pacemaker resistant supraventricular tachycardia.

| Heart disease (type/% of patients) | Arrhythmia (type/% of patients) | Symptoms (type/% of patients) | Prior treatment (type/% of patients) |
|---|---|---|---|
| No organic disease/45 | Atrial fibrillation/flutter/61 | Palpitations/60 | Digitalis/83 |
| Coronary artery disease/17 | Atrioventricular nodereentry/20 | Dizziness/38 | Type 1/81 |
| Cardiomyopathy/15 | | Dyspnea/38 | B-Blockers/78 |
| Valvular heart disease/10 | Accessory pathway/13 | Syncope/29 | Calcium-channel blockers/77 |
| Cor pulmonale/4 | Atrial tachycardia/11 | Chest pain/21 | Amiodarone/47 |
| Hypertensive cardiovascular disease/4 | Permanent JRT/3 | Fatigue/16 | Other experimental drugs/21 |
| Other/5 | Other/4 | Angina/9 | Antitachycardia pacemaker/8 |
| | | Other/4 | |

The percentages total more than 100% since more than one parameter may have been present in a given patient. JRT = junctional reciprocating tachycardia.

The most common symptom was palpitations (60% of patients), followed by both dizziness (pre-syncope) and dyspnea in 38% of patients. Twenty-eight (28%) had frank syncopal episodes. Other symptoms included chest pain (21%), fatigue (916%), angina (9%) and rare episodes of hypotension and diaphoresis (4%).

A USCI catheter (no. 6 or 7 F) was used in 92% of attempted ablations, while the remainder included a specially designed hemiquadripolar electrode catheter (3%), a Josephson quadripolar electrode catheter (3%), and other catheter types (3%). The distal electrode was used in 92% of cases, a more proximal electrode in 9%, and a bipolar arrangement in 2%.

## Results of the procedure

A wide variety of protocols for number, sequencing, and energy level of DC shocks was used for the ablation attempts. Approximately two thirds of patients received single or double shocks of 200, 300, or 400 joules. There was no significant difference in the amount of energy delivered or number of shocks used in patients in whom third degree A-V block did or did not develop. The relationship between the number of shocks and the development of permanent third-degree A-V block is shown in Figure 1. Figure 2 depicts the cumulative (delivered) energy in patients with and without development of chronic third-degree A-V block after attempted catheter ablation. Ninety percent of patients had third degree A-V block induced by up to 800 joules delivered energy, and eighty-three percent of patients had third degree A-V block induced by either one or two shocks.

In forty-five patients in the Registry in whom unipolar His bundle amplitude was recorded, a His deflection of greater than or equal to 0.15 mV was predictive of successful production of third-degree A-V block. (P = 0.02) The size of the atrial deflection greater than or equal to 0.15 mV was predictive of success (P = 0.04), but data was available for analysis in only twenty-seven patients.

In the one hundred sixteen patients in whom it was performed, the mean maximal level of creatine kinase was $316 \pm 641$ IU, while in the ninety patients in whom CK-MB levels were determined the mean maximal level was $31 \pm 31$ IU. There was no correlation between the peak CK-MB fraction and the total amount of delivered energy. In the one hundred and twenty-two patients in whom data were available, the mean rate of the escape pacemaker was $45 \pm 15$ beats per minute.

## Short term complications of the procedure

Arrhythmias related to the attempted ablation included ventricular fibrillation

```
                    THIRD DEGREE A-V BLOCK

     NUMBER OF        NUMBER OF
      SHOCKS          OBSERVATIONS
        1                63        **********************************
        2                56        *****************************
        3                16        ********
        4                 6        ***
        5                 3        **


                   NO THIRD DEGREE A-V BLOCK

     NUMBER OF        NUMBER OF
      SHOCKS          OBSERVATIONS
        1                16        ****************
        2                24        ************************
        3                10        **********
        4                 7        *******
        5                 5        *****
```

*Figure 1*. Number of shocks delivered and number of patients for those who developed complete A-V block (top figure) compared to those in whom A-V conduction returned.

```
                    THIRD DEGREE A-V BLOCK

    CUMULATIVE
     ENERGY          NUMBER OF
    (JOULES)         OBSERVATIONS
        0                 1        *
       200               30        ****************************
       400               47        ***********************************************
       600               27        ***************************
       800               25        *************************
      1000                6        ******
      1200                1        *
      1400                1        *
      1600                3        ***
      1800                2        **
      2000                1        *


                   NO THIRD DEGREE A-V BLOCK

    CUMULATIVE
     ENERGY          NUMBER OF
    (JOULES)         OBSERVATIONS
        0                 1        *
       200                6        ******
       400               10        **********
       600               18        ******************
       800               12        ************
      1000                5        *****
      1200                0
      1400                1        *
      1600                4        ****
      1800                3        ***
      2000                2        **
```

*Figure 2*. Cumulative energy delivered and number of patients for those who achieved complete A-V block (top figure) compared to those in whom A-V conduction returned.

482

(two patients) which was converted with external shock, two cases of non-sustained ventricular tachycardia, and one case each of A-V junctional tachycardia, enhanced His rhythm, and transient premature ventricular complexes. Later arrhythmias occurring within the hospitalization period encompassing the ablation attempt included one case of ventricular tachycardia with syncope in a patient with a prior history of myocardial infarction and another of torsades de pointes on the evening of the procedure in a patient taking amiodarone.

Pericardial tamponade requiring surgical drainage occurred in one patient, hypotension lasting from ten minutes to seventy-two hours and necessitating dopamine therapy occurred in four patients, one patient developed a hemothorax, four patients had either staph sepsis, bacteremia, or fever of unknown origin and one patient had unspecified chest pain. The patient with gram negative sepsis died of complications of the sepsis six weeks later. This patient was thought to be immunodeficient.

**Follow-up data**

The two hundred and nine patients were followed for a mean of 7.9 ± 7.2 months (one month to three years). These data are summarized in Figure 3. One hundred forty-four patients (70%) achieved chronic stable third-degree A-V block and were taking no antiarrhythmic drugs for symptom control, seventeen patients (8%) had resumption of A-V conduction but were asymptomatic from arrhythmias and required no antiarrhythmic drug therapy, while another twenty-six patients (13%) had resumption of A-V conduction and had their arrhythmias controlled with previously unsuccessful drugs. In nineteen patients (9%) the procedure was clearly unsuccessful, with resumption of conduction and symptoms refractory to drug therapy. Six of these latter patients underwent cardiac electrosurgery for direct interruption of the His bundle.

**Mortality statistics**

Fourteen patients (7%) died during the follow-up period. Sudden death occurred in five patients at from three weeks to five months following the procedure. Underlying heart disease was present in all five patients and included cardiomyopathy in three, endocardial fibrosis in one and coronary heart disease with a postmyocardial infarction aneurysm in one. One patient who died with ventricular tachycardia had experienced this arrhythmia prior to the ablation procedure.

Five patients had cardiac deaths, four died in refractory congestive heart failure, which was present prior to ablation, from one to eight months after the ablation and one died over one year later after surgery for interruption of an accessory pathway. Four noncardiac deaths occurred, two from respiratory

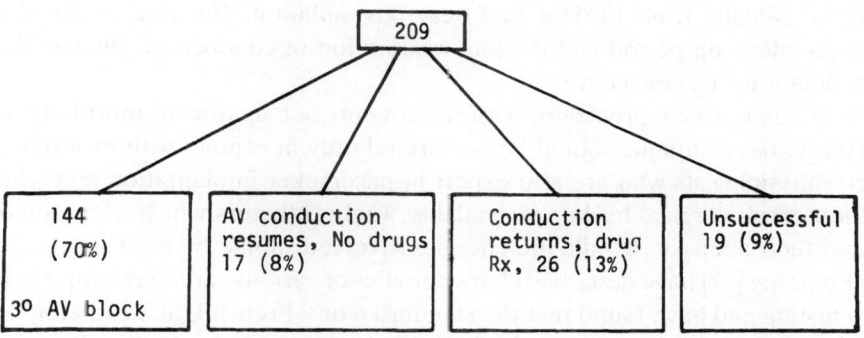

*Figure 3.* Follow-up summary for 209 patients who underwent attempted catheter ablation of the A-V junction. Third-degree A-V block was achieved in 144 (70%) while A-V conduction was sufficiently modified in 17 (8%) so that drug therapy was no longer needed. In 26 patients (13%), the arrhythmia became unresponsive to previously unsuccessful drugs, while in 19 patients (9%), the procedure proved unsuccessful.

failure at two and ten months after the ablation, one from a cerebrovascular accident at six months, and the patient with gram negative sepsis described above.

**Pacemaker problems**

Pacemaker problems were reported in ten patients (5%). These included pacemaker failure in two patients with syncope in one of these, myopotential sensing with syncope in one, diaphramatic pacing in two, and pacemaker erosion in one. In six patients rate or mode changes occurred, including pacemaker-mediated tachycardia, symptoms necessitating rate adjustment and pacemaker tracking of atrial tachycardia or fibrillation in two patients each.

**Discussion**

The Registry has attempted to collect data which will allow for meaningful analysis of the safety and efficacy of catheter ablation techniques for management of patients with refractory SVT.

The available data suggest that catheter ablation is successful in producing chronic third-degree A-V block in seventy percent of patients. In the patients who had an unsuccessful outcome, A-V conduction returned in most cases within the hospitalization encompassing the attempted ablation procedure(s) (mean $29 \pm 39$ hours). Return of A-V conduction resumed later than one week in seven patients, ranging from 10 days to 1 year post-ablation. Because of the short average follow-up period and the late resumption of conduction, further long-term data must be collected.

Since this is a new procedure with infrequent, but significant morbidity and mortality, the technique should be performed only in centers with experienced electrophysiologists who are also expert in pacemaker implantation and where cardiothoracic surgical backup is available. Only catheters which have demonstrated their ability to handle the energies involved should be used. Fisher [26] and Fontaine [27] have described characteristics of various catheters subjected to vitro testing and have found that the standard 6 or 7 French USCI catheter 'old-technology' could tolerate maximal defibrillator output with no gross disruption and minor pitting of the electrode surface. This type of catheter was used in 92% of Registry ablation attempts with no reports of frank catheter disruption. In the data available, all catheters were reported as intact though pitted.

## Immediate complications

Of arrhythmic complications immediately related to the shock, two patients with ventricular fibrillation were successfully defibrillated. This complication has been reported as a result of QRS synchronized external countershock in other patient populations [28–30]. The two episodes of non-sustained ventricular tachycardia were transient. The exact cause of the one case of cardiac tamponade is still unclear. The patient had production of third-degree A-V block, suggesting that the ablation catheter was positioned properly and did not discharge into the atrial free wall. A 'roughness' at the apex of the right ventricle was reported by the surgeon (J. Fisher: personal communication). Perforation of the temporary right ventricular pacing catheter or catheter whip damaging the right atrium cannot be excluded.

## Later complications

Depression of myocardial function has been reported after both external and internal shock to the ventricle. In three patients, transient hypotension responded to dopamine. In one elderly patient with cardiomyopathy due to coxsackie viral myocarditis, the shock induced hypotension lasting three days and necessitating dopamine. This patient had a peak CPK value of 181 with a peak CK-MB of 18 IU, with production of chronic third-degree A-V block. Whether this prolonged hypotension was due to further insult to a compromised myocardium or to loss of A-V synchrony attending the A-V block is unclear.

There was no connection between the peak energy delivered and the maximal CK-MB release. In addition, successful outcome was inversely correlated with peak cumulative energy, since more shocks were required if A-V block did not occur.

Gallagher [23] has emphasized the importance of the size of both the His and atrial deflections as predictors of successful production of third-degree A-V block after catheter ablation. In the forty-five Registry patients with data available for analysis, a unipolar His amplitude $\geq$0.15 mV was significantly correlated with production of third-degree A-V block. Similar results were obtained relative to the size of the atrial deflection. These results tend to support the hypothesis that catheter position is critically important to successful outcome.

In comparing mortality statistics from catheter ablation with that of surgical His bundle ablation, the data are hampered because of a lack of a concurrent surgical series. The sudden death rate for the Registry during the follow-up period was 2.5%. Prior surgical data for cryoablation of the A-V junction have shown a 5% to 10% operative mortality for this procedure [11–12]. Approximately one-half of all registry patients (45%) had no organic heart disease and no cardiac deaths were reported from this group. On the other hand, all patients with sudden death (2%) or other cardiac death (2%) had significant prior cardiac pathology ranging from post myocardial infarction aneurysm to various types of cardiomyopathy. The causes of the sudden deaths were not known, but do not appear related to pacemaker failure [31]. All prior patients had pre-existing conditions as noted above which predispose to sudden death. Enhanced ventricular arrhythmogenesis as a result of the ablation procedure cannot be definitely excluded as a cause for these patients' demise.

Further reports of catheter ablation have shown results very similar to the Registry experience [32–38]. McComb et al [39] have recently reported results of interruption or modification of A-V conduction using successive shocks at low energy settings. This is promising area for future study, since in approximately 20% of Registry patients, A-V conduction resumed but patients were now controlled either without antiarrhythmic therapy or with previously unsuccessful drugs. Such modification of conduction might also obviate the need for permanent pacemaker implantation.

Recent developments in laser technology have made this method of energy delivery attractive as an alternative to electrical coagulation [40–42]. It is hoped that the ability to more precisely localize the area to be destroyed by the laser-catheter combination might be an advance over electrode catheter techniques. This technology is still in its infancy, however.

In summary, catheter ablation of the A-V junction has been shown in cases thus far reported to be an effective (91%) means of arrhythmia management in patients with drug or pacemaker-resistant supraventricular tachycardia. It must be considered a 'tactic of last resort' [43–44] because of the small but definite risk of sudden death, direct complications related to the catheter technique itself and induction of a pacemaker-dependent state. Nevertheless, it compares favorably with open-chest methods, not only in lower mortality, but in hospital costs and

486

attendant morbidity [45]. Future trends to develop effective means of modifying A-V conduction without producing chronic third-degree A-V block should add an exciting new chapter to arrhythmia management.

## Acknowledgements

We thank Mr. David Mai and Mansfield Scientific Corporation for support of the Registry and Ms. Marjorie Glines for expert secretarial assistance.

## References

1. Fisher VJ, Lee RJ, Christianson CC, Kavaler F (1966) Production of chronic atrioventricular block in dogs without thoracotomy. J Appl Physiol 21: 1119–21
2. Steiner C, Kovalik ATW (1968) A simple technique for production of chronic complete heart block in dogs. J Appl Physiol 25: 631–2
3. Turina MI, Babotai I, Wegmann W (1968) Production of chronic atrioventricular block in dogs without thoracotomy. Cardiovasc Res 2: 389–93
4. Babotai I, Brownlee R (1971) Experimental atrioventricular block without thoracotomy: a new instrument. Cardiovasc Res 5: 416–8
5. Randall DS, Westerhof N, Van den Bos GC, Sipkema P (1981) Production of chronic heart block in closed-chest dogs: an improved technique. Am J Physiol 241 (Heart Circ Physiol 10): H279–82
6. Wieberdink J (1966) Experimental production of permanent heart block (total or bundle branch block) without circulatory arrest for extracorporeal circulation. Thorax 21: 401–4
7. Pruett JK, Woods EF (1967) Technique for experimental complete heart block. J Appl Physiol 22: 830–1
8. Edmonds LH Jr, Ellison RG, Grews TL (1969) Surgically induced atrioventricular block as treatment for recurrent atrial tachycardia in Wolff-Parkinson-White syndrome. Circulation 39 & 40 (Suppl I) I-105-11
9. Dunaway MC, King SB Jr, Hatcher CR Jr, Logue RB (1972) Disabling supraventricular tachycardia of Wolff-Parkinson-White syndrome (type A) controlled by surgical A-V block and a demand pacemaker after epicardial mapping studies. Circulation 45: 522–8
10. Harrison L, Gallagher JJ, Kasell J, Anderson RH, Mikat E, Hackel DB, Wallace AG (1977) Cryosurgical ablation of the A-V node-His bundle: a new method for producing A-V block. Circulation 55: 463-70
11. Klein GJ, Sealy WC, Pritchett ELC, Harrison L, Hackel DB, Davis D, Kasell J, Wallace AG, Gallagher JJ (1980) Cryosurgical ablation of the atrioventricular node-His bundle: Long-term follow-up and properties of the junctional pacemaker. Circulation 61: 8–15
12. Ohkawa S-I, Hackel DB, Mikat EM, Gallagher JJ, Cox JL, Scaly WC (1982) Anatomic effects of cryoablation of the atrioventricular conduction system. Circulation 65: 1155–62
13. Starzl TE, Gaertner RA (1955) Chronic heart block in dogs: a method for producing experimental heart failure. Circulation 12: 259–70
14. Giannelli S Jr, Ayres SM, Gromprecht RF, Conklin EF, Kennedy RJ (1967) Therapeutic surgical division of the human conduction system. JAMA 199: 155–60
15. Cole JS, Wills RE, Winterscheid LC, Reichenbach DD, Blackmon JR (1970) The Wolff-Parkinson-White syndrome: problems in evaluation and surgical therapy. Circulation 42: 111–21
16. Hashiba K, Katayama T, Takahashi A, et al (1965) Atrio-ventricular block produced by ligation of septal arteries in the dog. Jpn Heart J 6: 256–67

17. Erlanger J, Blackman JR (1910) Further studies on the physiology of heart-block in mammals: chronic auriculo-ventricular heart-block in the dog. Heart 1: 177–229
18. Meakins J (1913) Experimental heart-block with atrio-ventricular rhythm. Heart 5: 281–6
19. Beazell J, Tan K, Criley J, Schulman J (1976) The electrosurgical production of heart block without thoracotomy. Clin Res 24: 137A. Abstract
20. Gonzalez R, Scheinman MM, Margaretten W, Rubinstein M (1981) Closed-chest electrode catheter technique for His bundle ablation in dogs. Am J Physiol 241 (Heart Circ Physiol 10): H283–7
21. Bardy GH, Ideker RE, Kasell J, Worley SJ, Smith WM, German LD, Gallagher JJ (1983) Transvenous ablation of the atrioventricular conduction system in dogs: electrophysiologic and histologic observations. Am J Cardiol 51: 1775–82
22. Vedel J, Frank R, Fontaine G, Fournial JF, Grosgogeat Y (1979) Bloc auriculo-ventriruclaire intra-hisien définitif induit au cours d'une exploration endoventriculaire droite. Arch Mal Coeur 72: 107–12
23. Gallagher JJ, Svenson RH, Kasell JH, German LD, Bardy GH, Brougton A, Critelli G (1982) Catheter technique for closed-chest ablation of the atrioventricular conduction system. NEJM 306: 194–200
24. Scheinman MM, Morady F, Hess DS, Gonzalez R (1982) Catheter-induced ablation of the atrioventricular junction to control refractory supraventricular arrhythmias. JAMA 248: 851–5
25. Scheinman MM, Evans-Bell T, and the Executive Committee of the Percutaneous Cardiac Mapping and Ablation Registry (1984) Catheter ablation of the atrioventricular junction: a report of the percutaneous mapping and ablation registry. Circulation 70: 1024–9
26. Fisher JD, Brodman R, Johnston DR, Waspe LE, Kim SG, Matos JA, Scivin G (1984) Nonsurgical electrical ablation of tachycardias: importance of prior in vitro testing of catheter leads. Pace 7: 74–81
27. Fontaine G, Cansell A, Lechat P, Frank R, Tonet JL, Grosgogeat Y (1984) Endocavitary electric shock. Problems related to equipment. Arch Mal Coeur 77: 1307–14
28. Killip T (1963) Synchronized DC precardial shock for arrhythmias. Safe new technique to establish normal rhythm may be utilized on an elective or an emergency basis. JAMA 186: 1–7
29. Rabbinc MD, Likoff W, Dreifus LS (1964) Complications and limitations of direct-current countershock. JAMA 190: 417–20
30. Ross EM (1964) Cardioversion causing ventricular fibrillation. Arch Int Med 114: 811–4
31. Broughton A, Gallagher JJ, German LD, Guarnieri T, Trantham JL (1983) Escape rhythm properties following His ablation by the catheter technique. J Am Coll Cardiol 1 (2): 653. Abstract
32. Trantham JL, Gallagher JJ, German LD, Broughton A, Guarnieri T, Kasell J (1983) Effects of energy delivery via a His bundle catheter during closed chest ablation of the atrioventricular conduction system. J Clin Invest 72: 1563–74
33. Gillette PC, Garson A Jr, Porter CJ, Ott D, McVey P, Zinner A, Blair H (1983) Junctional automatic ectopic tachycardia: New proposed treatment by transcatheter His bundle ablation. Am Heart J 106: 619–23
34. Critelli G, Perticone F, Coltorti F, Monda V, Gallagher J (1983) Closed chest modification of atrioventricular conduction system in man for treatment of refractory supraventricular tachycardia. Br Heart J 49: 544–9
35. Wood DL, Hammill SC, Holmes DR Jr, Osborn MJ, Gersh BJ (1983) Catheter ablation of the atrioventricular conduction system in patients with supraventricular tachycardia. Mayo Clin Proc 58: 791–5
36. Manz M, Steinbeck G, Luderitz B (1983) His-Bündel-Ablation: Eine neue Methode zur Behandlung bedrohlicher Supraventrikulärer Herzrhythmusstörungen. Internist 24: 95–8
37. Pop T, Henkel B, Kasper W, Meinertz T, Rückel A, Treese N, Schuster CJ, Pfeiffer C, Meyer J (1984) Erfolgreiche Transvenose elektrische Ablation des A-V Überleitungssystems beim thera-

pierfraktären Vorhofflattern. Z Cardiol 73: 120–4

38. Nathan AW, Bennett DH, Ward DE, Bexton RS, Camm AJ (1984) Catheter ablation of atrioventricular conduction. Lancet 1: 1280–4

39. McComb JM, McGovern BA, Garan H, Ruskin JN (1985) Modification of atrioventricular conduction using low energy transcatheter shocks. J Am Coll Cardiol 5: 454. Abstract

40. Narula OS, Bharati S, Chan MC, Embi AA, Lev M (1984) Laser micro transection of the His bundle: a pervenous catheter technique. J Am Coll Cardiol 3: 537. Abstract

41. Lee Bi, Fletcher RD, Cohen AI, Cutler DJ, Del Negro AA, Singh SN (1984) Transcatheter endocardial ablation – a comparison of laser photoablation and electrode shock ablation. J Am Coll Cardiol 3: 536. Abstract

42. Narula OS, Boveja BK, Cohen DM, Tarjan PP (1985) Laser catheter induced A-V nodal (AVN) delays and block: acute and chronic studies. Circulation. Suppl II: 99. Abstract

43. Surawicz B (1982) A tactic of last resort. NEJM 306: 234–6

44. Rosen KM, Dhingra RC, Wyndham CRC (1980) Trading arrhythmia for atrioventricular block. Circulation 61: 16–7

45. German LD, Pressley J, Smith MS, O'Callaghan WG, Ellenbogen KA (1984) Comparison of cryoablation of the atrioventricular node versus catheter ablation of the His bundle. Circulation 70: II-412. Abstract

# Dynamic overdrive pacing for the suppression of ventricular ectopic activity: long-term application using implantable pacemakers

U.J. WINTER, D.W. BEHRENBECK, M. HÖHER, TH. BRILL, H. EBELING, HJ. HIRCHE, and H.H. HILGER

## Introduction

Overdrive pacing is a commonly used method for terminating tachycardias [2]. Furthermore, overdrive suppression of repetitive Purkinje fibre activity is a well known electrophysiological phenomenon. The so far discussed working mechanisms are shown in Table 1. Dynamic overdrive pacing (DO), which means an overdrive stimulation with varying rate, was incorporated in the DPG 1 (Vitatron) for tachycardia prevention. In order to investigate the reliability of this new pacing mode, we first induced complex ventricular extrasystoles (VES) and ventricular tachycardia by bipolar, epicardial direct current (DC) application in 5 pig hearts (20 to 30 kg) in situ during neuroleptanalgesia (method: 24). During

*Table 1.* So far discussed working mechanisms of overdrive pacing on the cellular level.

| Authors [1] | Year | Discussed mechanism [1] |
|---|---|---|
| Han et al | 1966 | Increase in heart rate leads to an increase of the fibrillation threshold and to better synchronization of repolarization. |
| Vassalle et al | 1967 | Increase of heart rate leads to an increase of $[K^+]$ in the coronary sinus. |
| Ten Eick et al | 1968 | Increase in heart rate induces a higher threshold for the triggering of conducted potentials in the Purkinje fibres. |
| Krellenstein et al | 1969 | Increase in heart rate influences the extracellular electrolytes. |
| Carpentier et al | 1971 | A higher heart rate causes a $Na^+$-Efflux in the Purkinje fibres which leads to a higher RMP. This causes a delay in the diastolic depolarization. |
| Janse et al | 1971 | Higher heart rate in local ischemia leads to lower fibrillation threshold and desynchronization of repolarization process. |
| Lüderitz | 1983 | High heart rate shortens the duration of diastole and reduces the probability of extrasystolies. |
| Camm et al | 1983 | Increased heart rate leads to a reduction of coordinated impulse propagation of arrhythmias by increasing the depolarization between stimulation site and ectopic impulse generating tissue. |

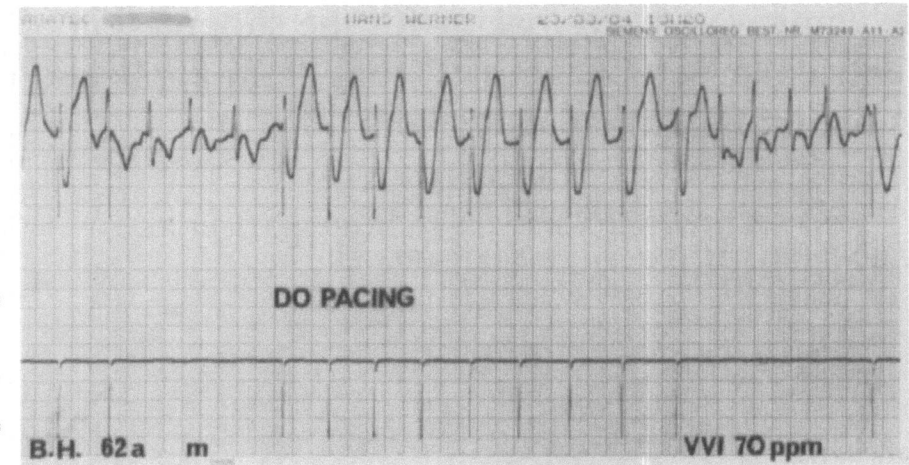

*Figure 1.* Dynamic overdrive pacing in VVI pacemaker (Vitatron DPG 1). The pacemaker-Holter-ECG (Ela Medical Anatec), with the recointed spike in the second channel shows the varying pacing intervals during dynamic overdrive.

ventricular DO pacing, DC-induced complex VES disappeared and tachycardias needed significantly higher current strengths to be induced. In some cases, tachycardias could not be initiated any more.

**Methods**

After these successful animal investigation findings, 10 patients with bradyarrhythmias and VES due to coronary heart disease were treated with the DPG 1 pacemaker (VVI) and a Helifix lead (Vitatron). Since 7/10 patients had VES of Lown ≥II° in spite of being treated with 1 to 3 antiarrhythmic drugs (in case of VES ≥Lown III°) the DPG's dynamic overdrive pacing mode was switched on. Its antiectopic effect was investigated by 24-hour-continuous-Holter-ECG-recordings (Anatec of Ela Medical, Paris) and the pacemaker's premature beat counter. The patients were controlled during a follow-up period of up to 3 years.

**Results**

In 5/10 patients we observed a change to VES of Lown ≥I° and in another 5/10 patients a reduction of ≥80% of the total number of premature beats. In 5/10 patients with low Lown grade and little number of premature beats the reduction of the arrhythmias was not significant (Table 2). During the follow up period no patient showed a recurrence or the first manifestation of ventricular tachycardias.

*Table 2.* Long-term ventricular DO stimulation with a significant VES reduction and a continously high ventricular rate can lead to cardiac decompensation in patients with elevated mean pulmonary artery pressure ($\overline{PAP}$) and decreased cardiac output (60) at rest.

| Myocardial decompensation | VES reduction | DO [ppm] range | CO [l·min⁻¹] (rest) | $\overline{PAP}$ [cm H$_2$O] (rest) |
|---|---|---|---|---|
| Yes | 81% | 70–127 | Reduced* | Increased* |
| n = 3 | 88% | 90–100 | 3.01 | 25 |
| | 83% | 100–120 | 4.08 | 28 |
| No | 0% | 90–100 | 2.42 | 17 |
| n = 7 | 9% | 90–100 | Reduced * | Increased * |
| | 23% | 70–80 | Reduced* | Increased* |
| | 23% | 80–100 | 3.18 | 10 |
| | 47% | 80–90 | (Reduced)* | Normal* |
| | 81% | 70–100 | (Reduced)* | Normal* |
| | 98% | 70–100 | 3.39 | 25 |

* No invasive studies possible, $\overline{PAP}$ and CO were concluded from the clinical examination.

## Disadvantages

3/10 patients revealed a progression of the myocardial insufficiency during long-term DO pacing. This phenomenon was mainly seen in patients with reduced cardiac output and elevated mean pulmonary artery pressure at rest (Table 2). These patients were examined by bicycle stress test (20 to 25 W, supine postion, right heart catheter) during repeated 4 minute periods. During exercise the DO pacing mode led to a 10 to 15% reduction of the stroke volume (as compared with spontaneous rhythm) which was accompagnied by the heart rate increase. In comparison, atrial DO (n = 1) leads to a higher cardiac output due to an increased heart rate and atrio-ventricular synchrony. In all 10 patients the number of stimulations and thus the power consumption was significantly increased.

## Discussion

After the recent success in the field of tachycardia terminating pacing (TTP) by means of endocardial cardioversion and epicardial defibrillation, tachycardia research now returns more to tachycardia preventing pacing (TPP). Different kind of TPP were proposed during the last years.

*Overdrive pacing*

The simplest kind of tachycardia preventing pacing is the use of overdrive suppression. This stimulation technique refers to the effect of higher pacing rates in preventing the occurrence of repetitive arrhythmias or tachycardias (Table 1). Prevention of rapid ventricular arrhythmias (tachycardias, fibrillation) by increasing the stimulation rate up to 80 ppm was first described by Zoll et al 1960 [28]. Klassen et al [11] and Sowton [20] used endocardial electrodes for the pacing. They performed this preventing pacing also in patients without av-block or bradycardia. During the following years, several investigators demonstrated the reliability of overdrive pacing for tachycardia prevention in patients with and without bradycardia (Heiman et al [7]; Lew and March [13]; Hornbaker et al [8]; Zipes et al, 1969, [26]; Beller et al [1]; Moss and Rivers, 1974 [18]). The design of a dynamic overdrive pacing mode (Vitatron DPG 1), combined with programmable upper and lower rate limits, enabled a more flexible application of this pacing technique. The long-term use of dynamic overdrive in the ventricle may lead to myocardial decompensation in patients with reduced left ventricular performance, as demonstrated by our data. These hemodynamic side effects were not observed during long-term atrial DO (Fontaine et al [5]; Winter et al, unreported data, 1985). Suppression of repetitive ventricular arrhythmias can also be achieved by atrial overdrive pacing (Kastor et al [9]; Moss et al [17]; Zipes et al [26]; De Francis et al [4]; Lichstein et al [14]; Sowton et al [21]; Fontaine et al [5]) proposed an atrial DO, in which the ventricular premature beats were sensed by an additional, that means ventricular lead. DO pacing is now also possible with a dual chamber device (Vitatron Quintech DDD). The effectiveness of overdrive pacing for the prevention of arrhythmias during acute myocardial infarction is not yet completely clear. Whereas B. Scherlag (personal communication, 1984) reported that the infarct size can be significantly increased by overdrive pacing in ischemic dog hearts, there are some clinical reports (Meltzer, 1974 [16]; J. Camm, personal communication, 1984; D.W. Behrenbeck, personal communication, 1984) which indicate a significant reduction of premature ventricular beats during overdrive pacing and thus tachycardia prevention.

*Dual site pacing*

Coumel et al [3] paced atria and ventricles simultaneously in order to prevent junctional tachycardias (DOO-Mode). Also other modalities of atrio-ventricular pacing were proposed: VAT-mode (Spurrell and Sowton, 1976 [22]); DVO-DVI-mode (Maloney et al, 1981 [15]; Sung et al, 1980, [23]). Atrio-ventricular pacing as prevention of junctional tachycardias implies a collision of the atrial and ventricular impulses within the reentry circuit. During long-term prevention of junctional tachycardias by means of atrio-ventricular pacing, closely coupled ventricular stimulations (triggered by atrial premature beats) and fast ventricular rates due to atrial tachycardias were observed (Spurrell and Sowton, 1976 [22]; Sung et al, 1980 [23]).

## Continuous high-rate pacing

Continuous high-rate atrial pacing in patients with supraventricular tachycardias may lead to an effective reduction of the ventricular rate due to pacing-induced second degree av-block. If, for example, the stimulation rate to induce av-block has to be 200% of the tachycardia rate, this pacing technique obviously cannot be applied. Since also variations in the autonomic tone influence av-conduction and atrial refractoriness, this technique can only be used on a short-term base [2].

*Paired and coupled stimulation.* Paired and coupled stimulation prolong the refractory period, thus leading to a rate reduction [2]. During ventricular paired or coupled stimulation ventricular tachycardia or fibrillation may occur if the stimulus falls within the vulnerable period [2]. Guize et al (1971, [6]) investigated a so-called orthorythmique pacemaker which adjusted the interval of the coupled extrastimulus to the preceding R-R-interval. If single premature beats occurred the pacemaker stimulated with a time delay Z which was the function of the distance between the previous rate respectively R-R-interval (Y). It was possible to shorten the intervention interval up to 40% of the distance of the last cardiac actions (spontaneous rhythm or premature beats). Recently Kuck et al [12] reported that tachycardias of atrio-ventricular, accessory pathways could be reproducibly induced from the high right atrium with a single premature beat and that the initiation of tachycardia could be prevented from the same position by a introducing a second premature beat. The second extrastimulus prevented tachycardia initiation if it was delivered within the preventive zone (10 ms outside the refractory period of the stimulus, which initiated the tachycardia). Whether or not this stimulation technique is also valid in prevention of ventricular tachycardia initiation is not yet clear. Furthermore the question cannot yet be answered whether or not trains of extrastimuli or subthreshold stimuli can prevent reentry tachycardia induction. Recently, Prystowsky et al [19] achieved myocardial inhibition by using a conditioning bipolar stimulus at intervals, shorter than the effective refractory period. Conditioning stimuli significantly prolonged the ventricular effective refractory period (VERP). This effect was dependent on the current and the impulse duration used. Trains of conditioning stimuli caused an even more pronounced prolongation of the VERP. This kind of preventing pacing is not yet available in implantable pacemakers. Von Leitner et al [24] achieved a tachycardia (rates between 160 and 220 bpm) termination by means of right ventricular, bipolar subthreshold burst pacing (10 to 30 impulses at a rate of 300 per minute; impulse width 2.0 ms; 10 to 20% below the patient's pacing threshold). Whether or not this new stimulation technique is also able to prevent tachycardias is still under investigation.

494

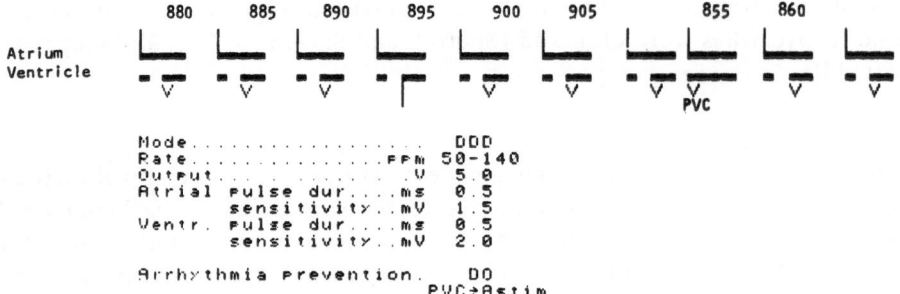

*Figure 2.* Ventricular sensing of a ventricular premature beat leads to the initiation of the atrial dynamic overdrive pacing mode in the Vitatron Quintech DDD.

## Summary

Ventricular DO stimulation can reduce CHD-related, drug-refractory extra-systoles significantly (≥80%) in patients with VES ≥Lown II° and a large quantity of VES. The cardiac output during ventricular DO pacing is not significantly influenced since the lower stroke volume (due to VVI pacing) is balanced by a higher ventricular rate. Pacemaker patients with elevated pulmonary artery pressure at rest due to myocardial insufficiency have to be excluded from long-term ventricular DO pacing. The continuous higher ventricular rate often leads to cardiac decompensation.

## Conclusions

Dynamic overdrive pacing seems to be the technically and clinically simplest way of premature beat reduction and tachycardia initiation inhibition. All so far reported preventing pacing techniques have limited indications and some not neglectable disadvantages. However, the ventricular DO can only be used in patients with normal left ventricular performance. Since most of the premature beats are related to progressing coronary heart disease and cardiomyopathy, patients with normal left ventricular pump function are rarely to be found. Atrial DO has a normal av-conduction as necessary pre-requesite. So, atrial DO in dual chamber pacemakers seems to be the best kind of application (Vitatron Quintech DDD; Fig. 2). Whether or not myocardial inhibition [19], subthreshold burst pacing [24] or other pacing techniques will be applicable in the future in pacemakers, cannot be stated in the moment. Whereas B. Lown propagates that a significant reduction of premature beats also leads to a tachycardia/prevention, this opinion is rejected by M.E. Josephson [8]. In our study, also patients with low Lown grade and little number of premature beats as well as patients with normal and reduced left ventricular performance were included, in order to find out the reliable indications. Future investigations should focus on patients with VES ⩾III°, left ventricular insufficiency and atrial DO in dual chamber devices.

## References

1. Beller BM, Kotler MN, Collens R (1970) The use of ventricular pacing for suppression of ectopic ventricular activity. Am J Cardiol 25: 467
2. Camm J, Ward D (1983) Pacing for tachycardia control. Telectronics Publications
3. Coumel P, Cabrol C, Fabiato A, Gourgon R, Slama R (1967) Tachycardic permanente par rhythme reciproque. Archives des Maladies du Coeur et des Vaisseaux 60: 1830
4. De Francis NA, Giordano RP (1968) Permanent epicardial atrial pacing in the treatment of refractory ventricular tachycardia. Am J Cardiol 22: 742
5. Fontaine G, Frank R, Grosgogeat Y (1984) Value of a software pacemaker in the management of cardiac arrhythmias. Proceedings of the 6th International Congress on Cardiology, Marilleva, p 433–439
6. Guize L, Zacouto F, Lenegre J (1971) Un nouveau stimulateur du coeur: Le pacemaker orthorhythmique. La Presse Médical 79: 2071
7. Heiman DF, Helwig J (1966) Suppression of ventricular arrhythmias by transvenous cardiac pacing. J of the Am Medical Assoc 195: 1150
8. Hornbaker JH, Humphries JO, Ross RS (1969) Permanent pacing in the absence of heart block. An approach to the management of intractable arrhythmias. Circulation 39: 189
9. Josephson ME (1984) Personal communication
10. Kastor JA, De Sanctis RW, Harthorne JW, Schwartz GH (1967) Transvenous atrial pacing in the treatment of refractory ventricular irritability. Annals of Internal Medicine 66: 339
11. Klassen GA, Broadhurst C, Peretz DI, Johnson AL (1963) Cardiac resuscitation in 126 medical patients using external cardiac massage. Lancet 1: 1290
12. Kuck KH, Kunze K-P, Schlüter M, Bleifeld W (1984) Tachycardia prevention by programmed stimulation. Am J Cardiol 54: 550–554
13. Lew HT, March HW (1967) Control of recurrent ventricular fibrillation by transvenous pacing in the absence of heart block. Am Heart J 73: 794
14. Lichtstein E, Chadda K, Fernig S (1972) Atrial pacing in the treatment of refractory ventricular tachycardia associated with hypokalemia. Am J Cardiol 30: 550
15. Maloney JM, Medina VR, Pieretti OH, Portillo B, Maduro C, Berkovits B, Moliero F (1981) Long-term effectiveness of dual-demand sequential pacing for automatic conversion and prevention of refractory reentry supraventricular tachycardias. Cardiology 47: 476
16. Meltzer LE (1975) The significance and treatment of bradycardias associated with acute myocardial infarction. Cardiovascular Clinics 7: 183
17. Moss AJ, Rivers RJ, Griffith LSC, Carmel JA, Millard EB (1968) Transvenous left atrial pacing for the control of recurrent ventricular fibrillation. New Engl J Med 278: 928
18. Moss AJ, Rivers RJ (1974) Termination and inhibition of recurrent tachycardias by implanted pervenous pacemakers. Circulation 50: 942
19. Prystowsky N, Miles WM, Windle JR, Skale BT, Zipes DP. Myocardial inhibition in: Hombach V, Hilger HH, Rashkind WJ: Invasive Cardiovascular Therapy. Martinus Nijhoff Publishers, in press
20. Sowton, E (1964) The use of artificial pacemaking in cardiac resuscitation. Proceedings of the Royal Society of Medicine 57: 368
21. Sowton E, Balcon R, Preston T, Leaver D, Yacoub M (1969) Long-term control of intractable supraventricular tachycardia by ventricular pacing. Brit Heart J 31: 700

22. Spurrell RAJ, Sowton E (1976) Pacing techniques in the management of supraventricular tachycardia. Part 2; J of Electrocardiology 9: 89

23. Sung RJ, Styperek JL, Castellanos A (1980) Complete abolition of the reentrant supraventricular tachycardia zone using a new modality of cardiac pacing with simultaneous atrioventricular stimulation. Am J Cardiol 45: 72

24. Von Leitner E-R, Linderer Th. Subthreshold burst pacing in: Behrenbeck DW, Sowton E, Fontaine G, Winter UJ. Cardiac pacing

25. Winter UJ, Ebeling H, Kebbel U, Hirche Hj (1983) Induction of ventricular arrhythmias and ventricular late potentials by epicardial direct current application in pig hearts in situ: importance of stimulation position. Circulation 68 (Suppl II): 1151

26. Zipes DP, Festoff B, Schaal SF, Cox C, Sealy W, Wallace AG (1968) Treatment of ventricular arrhythmia by permanent atrial pacemaker and cardiac sympathectomy. Annals of Internal Medicine 68: 591

27. Zipes DP, Wallace AG, Sealy W, Floyd WL (1969) Artifical atrial and ventricular pacing in the treatment of arrhythmias. Annals of Internal Medicine 70: 885

28. Zoll PM, Linenthal AJ, Zarsky LRN (1960) Ventricular fibrillation. Treatment and prevention by external electric currents. New Engl J Med 262: 105

# Myocardial inhibition

N. PRYSTOWSKY, J.R. WINDLE, W.M. MILES, F. GILMOUR,
BRIAN T. SKALE and DOUGLAS P. ZIPES

An electrical stimulus that does not completely depolarize myocardium has the ability to interact with a subsequent stimulus that activates myocardium. In 1926 Drury and Love [1] showed in the frog ventricle that a subthreshold electrical stimulus initiated before a threshold stimulus could prevent the threshold stimulus from evoking a recordable ventricular depolarization. Lewis and Drury [2] made similar observations in the dog atrium, and Tamargo et al [3] demonstrated that subthreshold stimuli could inhibit threshold stimuli from activating canine ventricle.

We have been interested in this phenomenon for several years, and have investigated myocardial inhibition in humans at electrophysiologic study as well as in *in vivo* and *in vitro* experiments [4–7]. These observations and potential clinical implications of myocardial inhibition are discussed in this manuscript.

## Clinical studies

In our initial study [4] 16 patients receiving no cardioactive medicines were investigated in the postabsorptive nonsedated state at electrophysiologic study. All patients gave informed written and verbal consent before entering the study. Three to four electrode catheters were inserted percutaneously into the femoral and/or brachial veins and positioned under fluoroscopic guidance to multiple areas of the heart. In all patients ventricular pacing was performed with a quadripolar catheter (USCI) with 10 mm interelectrode distance. The right ventricular catheter for all studies was positioned at the apex. Atrial pacing was performed with a quadripolar catheter with 5 mm interelectrode distance (USCI) that was positioned in the high right atrial area. A second atrial catheter was positioned near the first atrial catheter to record the bipolar atrial electrogram.

**Pacing protocol**

For the inhibition studies in the atrium or ventricle, the following protocol was used. A programmable custom-built stimulator (MECA) was used to pace the heart with rectangular pulses (WPI) delivered through an isolation unit for the basic drive train ($S_1$) and the premature stimulus ($S_2$). The pulse width of $S_1$ and $S_2$ was 2.0 msec and the current used was twice late-diastolic threshold (1.0 to 1.4 mA). A second current output generator (WPI) that delivered 2 msec rectangular stimuli through an isolation transformer was used to introduce the conditioning stimulus ($S_c$). The $S_1$, $S_2$, and $S_c$ stimuli were bipolar and, regardless of whether the distal or proximal bipolar electrode pair on the quadripolar catheter were used for stimulation, the distal pole of the pair was always the cathode and the proximal pole the anode. Ventricular and atrial refractoriness were determined by stimulating the myocardium with a train of eight complexes and after each eight complex a premature stimulus was introduced beginning in late diastole. The $S_1S_2$ interval was shortened progressively until $S_2$ consistently failed to evoke a response. The longest $S_1S_2$ interval that did not result in myocardial depolarization on two consecutive attempts was defined as the effective refractory period of the tissue being tested.

To test for ventricular inhibition, the stimulator delivering the basic train and premature interval was set at a fixed $S_1S_2$ and $S_1S_2$ interval. The $S_1S_2$ interval was 10 to 20 msec longer than the effective refractory period and $S_2$ always produced a ventricular response. Then, with the use of a separate current generator, $S_c$ was introduced beginning 20 msec before the occurrence of $S_2$ and within the duration of the ventricular effective refractory period. The current of $S_c$ always was subthreshold and by itself $S_c$ never produced a ventricular response. As the current of $S_c$ was increased, especially at levels of 6.0 mA or more, $S_c$ was periodically introduced without $S_2$ to ensure that $S_c$ by itself did not result in myocardial depolarization. The current level of $S_c$ was increased in 0.1 to 0.3 mA increments until $S_c$ inhibited ventricular depolarization of $S_2$. At this point, the current level of $S_c$ was kept constant but the $S_c$ stimulus was moved 10 msec earlier than the previous $S_cS_2$ interval. If $S_c$ failed to inhibit $S_2$ then the mA was again increased progressively until $S_c$ inhibited $S_2$. This process was repeated until an $S_cS_2$ interval was obtained at which an $S_c$ of 10 mA no longer inhibited $S_2$. In 11 patients $S_1$, $S_2$, and $S_c$ were initiated at the distal bipolar pair and the proximal bipolar pair was used to record the local electrogram. In nine patients $S_1$ and $S_2$ were initiated at the distal bipolar electrode pair but $S_c$ was introduced at the proximal bipolar pair. For these patients the catheter was positioned so that late-diastolic pacing threshold was similar for the distal and proximal bipolar pair.

For atrial inhibition a protocol similar to that detailed above for ventricular inhibition was used. Five patients underwent this protocol and for all five patients, $S_1$, $S_2$, and $S_c$ were initiated at the distal bipolar pair. A second electrode catheter positioned near the first catheter was used to record atrial potentials because the stimulus artifact often obscured atrial depolarization recorded from the same catheter that delivered the stimulus.

## Ventricular inhibition

Eleven patients underwent ventricular inhibition testing. When the $S_1$, $S_2$, and $S_c$ were applied at the distal bipolar pair all patients demonstrated inhibition in the ventricle. For the entire group the maximum mean $S_cS_2$ interval at which inhibition still occurred at 10 mA or less was 85 msec, with a range of 40 to 150 msec. Figure 1 illustrates analog data from one patient. The $S_1S_2$ interval was 270 msec and this was held constant for the entire study. Figure 1, left demonstrates the maximum current for each $S_cS_2$ interval at which the conditioning stimulus did not inhibit $S_2$, while figure 1, right illustrates the minimum current at which $S_c$ always inhibits $S_2$. As shown, more current is needed for $S_c$ to inhibit $S_2$ as $S_c$ precedes $S_2$ at increasing intervals.

When the current of $S_c$ required to inhibit $S_2$ was plotted as a function of the time at which $S_c$ preceded $S_2$ a curvilinear relationship was noted; the current required for $S_c$ to inhibit $S_2$ varied directly as the $S_cS_2$ interval increased. For the entire group of 11 patients, the maximum mean $S_cS_2$ interval at which $S_c$ still inhibited $S_2$ when currents for $S_c$ were less than 5 mA was 56 msec, with a range of 0 to 110 msec. Therefore, approximately two-thirds of the maximum $S_cS_2$ interval at which $S_c$ still inhibited $S_2$ occurred at current strengths for $S_c$ of 5.0 mA or less.

Three of 9 patients demonstrated inhibition when $S_c$ was introduced at the proximal ventricular pacing pair and $S_1$ and $S_2$ stimuli were applied at the distal pair. In these 3 patients inhibition was compared with $S_c$ initiated at the distal bipolar electrode pair.

The mean maximum $S_cS_2$ inhibition interval with currents of 10 mA or less for $S_c$ was 113 msec (range 90 to 150) with $S_c$ at the distal electrode pair vs 77 msec (range 20 to 130) with $S_c$ at the proximal electrode pair. When $S_c$ was 5.0 mA or less, maximum mean $S_cS_2$ inhibition interval was 83 msec (range 50 to 110) vs 50 msec (range 20 to 90) with $S_c$ at the distal and proximal electrode pair, respectively. Thus, inhibition was much more effective when the $S_c$ was applied nearer to the point at which $S_2$ was delivered. This demonstrated the relatively localized effect of subthreshold stimuli to inhibit subsequent myocardial depolarization.

## Atrial inhibition

Atrial inhibition occurred in all 5 patients tested. The maximum mean $S_cS_2$ interval at which $S_c$ still inhibited $S_2$ was 102 msec, with a range of 80 to 190 msec. The maximum mean $S_cS_2$ interval at which $S_c$ still inhibited $S_2$ with $S_c$ of 5.0 mA or less was 36 msec (range 0 to 50). In other words, a significant portion of inhibition

500

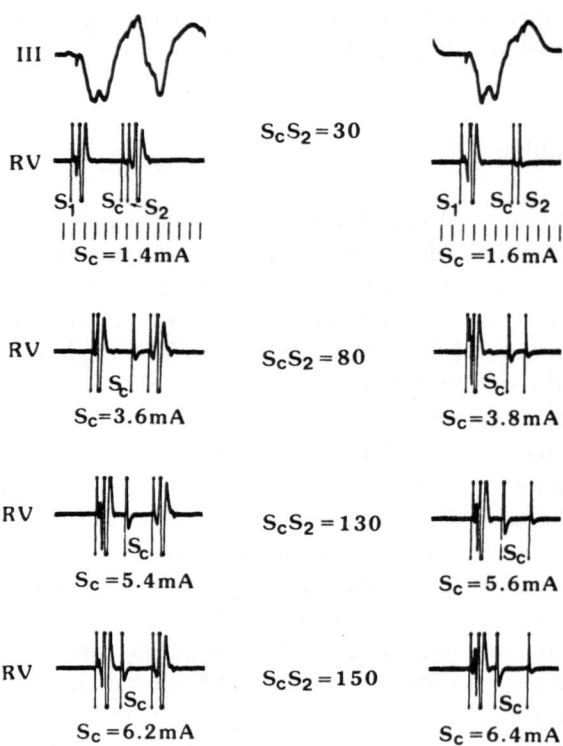

*Figure 1.* Inhibition of human ventricle (patient 5). The $S_1S_2$ interval for this patient was 270 msec. Left, For each $S_cS_2$ interval the highest $S_c$ (mA) at which no inhibition occurred. Right, The lowest $S_c$ (mA) at which $S_2$ was inhibited. As the $S_cS_2$ interval increases the current of $S_c$ needed to inhibit $S_2$ increases. Time line intervals are 50 msec. RV = right ventricle. (Reproduced with permission of the American Heart Association.)

(65%) could be obtained as the milliamperes of $S_c$ exceeded 5.0 mA, in contrast to results for ventricular inhibition.

The results of our initial investigation demonstrated that subthreshold stimuli can prevent subsequent threshold stimuli from depolarizing human atrium and ventricle. We further showed that inhibition was both time and voltage dependent, and is markedly more effective if the inhibitory stimulus is delivered at the same site as the $S_2$. However, further studies were necessary to investigate the mechanism responsible for myocardial inhibition, as well as to evaluate the relationship of heart rate, $S_c$ pulse width, and $S_c$ current intensity or inhibition.

### Effect of $S_c$ on ventricular refractoriness [5, 7]

*Methods*

Thirty-four patients having a variety of arrhythmias were studied in a postabsorptive, nonsedated state. All patients gave informed written and verbal consent before entering the study. The study population included 28 men and 6 women with a mean age of $52 \pm 14$ years. In all patients, ventricular pacing was performed from the right ventricular apex using the distal bipolar pair of a quadripolar catheter (USCI) with ten mm interelectrode distance. Similar to our initial study [4], the basic drive ($S_1$) and premature stimulus ($S_2$) were delivered through the same isolator unit (WPI) and $S_c$ was delivered through a separate current generator (WPI). All stimuli were introduced at the distal bipolar electrode pair. The pulse width of $S_1$ and $S_2$ was 2.0 msec and the current intensity used (1.2–2.0 mA) was twice the late diastolic threshold. The current intensity and pulse width of $S_c$ varied with individual protocols.

Ventricular refractoriness was evaluated by the following protocol. A premature stimulus was introduced after a drive train of 8 complexes. The $S_1S_2$ interval was shortened progressively by 5 msec steps until the ventricular effective refractory period (ERP) (defined as the shortest $S_1S_2$ interval at which $S_2$ always evoked threshold ventricular depolarization) was determined. The ventricular ERP was reconfirmed periodically throughout the study. Next, $S_c$ was introduced after the eight complex of the drive train but before the timing of $S_2$ and the $S_1S_c$ interval was increased by 5 msec intervals until the longest $S_1S_c$ interval was obtained at which $S_c$ always failed to evoke a response. The $S_1S_c$ interval was defined as the time between the onset of $S_1$ and the offset of $S_c$. The $S_c$ was introduced periodically without $S_2$ to insure that $S_c$ by itself did not produce myocardial depolarization.

Following determination of the $S_1S_c$ interval, ventricular pacing was performed using the $S_1S_2$ interval that had defined the ventricular ERP. Then, $S_c$ at the previously defined $S_1$-$S_c$ interval was interpolated between $S_1$ and $S_2$. If $S_c$ prevented $S_2$ from eliciting a ventricular depolarization, noted by the absence of a local ventricular electrogram and scalar ECG QRS complex, the $S_1S_2$ interval was increased progressively by 5 msec increments and testing repeated until $S_2$ produced ventricular depolarization. The change in ventricular ERP was defined as the difference between the control ventricular ERP and the ventricular ERP determined after $S_c$.

*Results*

In 20 patients the effect of $S_c$ on ventricular ERP was evaluated at a constant paced cycle length using $S_c$ with a current intensity of 10.0 mA and a pulse

502

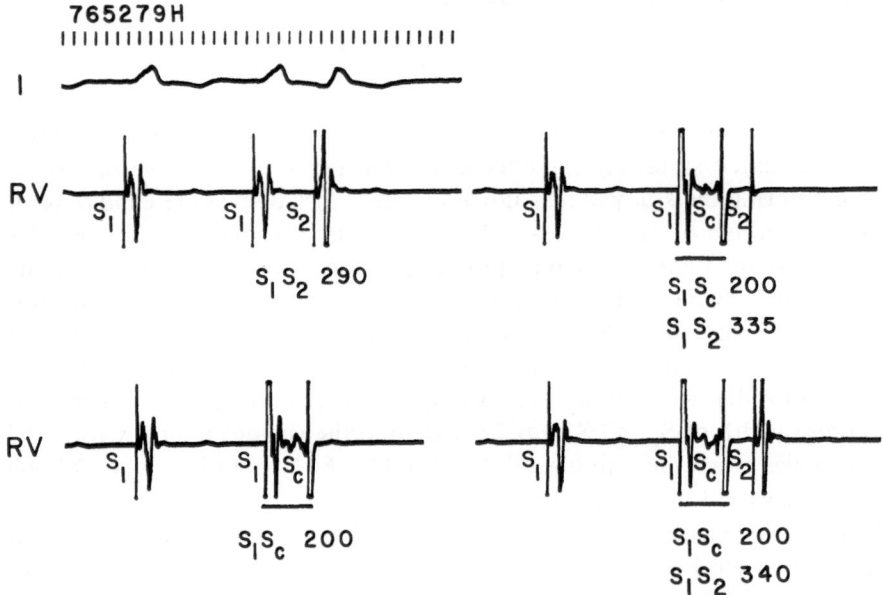

765279H

*Figure 2.* Effect of $S_c$ on ventricular ERP. The ventricular ERP was 290 msec in this patient (upper left). The longest $S_1S_c$ interval that never caused ventricular depolarization was 200 msec (lower left). $S_c$ was introduced between $S_1$ and $S_2$ and inhibition occurred at an $S_1S_2$ interval of 335 msec (upper right). At an $S_1S_2$ interval of 340 msec, ventricular depolarization occurred (lower right).

duration of 2.0 msec. Figure 2 demonstrates the prolongation of ventricular ERP caused by $S_c$. In all 20 patients $S_c$ prolonged ventricular ERP, and the mean increase was 21 msec (255 to 277 msec, p<.001).

The influence of heart rate on the ability of $S_c$ to increase ventricular refractoriness was tested in 6 patients. Refractoriness was determined at pacing cycle lenght 600 and 400 msec with and without introduction of $S_c$ with a current intensity of 10.0 mA and a pulse width of 2.0 msec. The conditioning stimulus prolonged ventricular ERP equally at pacing cycle length 600 msec (259 to 289 msec) and 400 msec (236 to 258 msec).

The effect of $S_c$ pulse duration and current intensity on ventricular ERP prolongation was evaluated in 13 patients. In 7 patients, $S_c$ current intensity was kept constant at 10 mA but $S_c$ pulse duration was either 100, 10, or 2 msec. The $S_1S_c$ interval was established as the longest interval at which $S_c$ of 100 msec pulse duration never caused ventricular depolarization. At $S_c$ pulse durations of 2, 10, and 100 msec ventricular ERP prolonged by $16 \pm 6$, $33 \pm 11$, and $66 \pm 25$ msec respectively. The increase in ventricular ERP was significantly different for each group (p<.01).

In 6 patients, pulse duration was fixed at 100 msec but the $S_c$ current intensity was 2, 5 or 10 mA. The longest $S_1S_c$ interval at which $S_c$ at 10 mA and 100 msec pulse duration always failed to cause ventricular depolarization was determined. At $S_c$ current intensities of 2, 5, and 10 mA ventricular ERP increased $6 \pm 5$, $40 \pm 22$, and $81 \pm 31$ msec respectively, and values were significantly different from each other ($p < .02$).

We concluded from these studies that subthreshold stimuli ($S_c$) significantly increased local ventricular tissue refractoriness in patients. Prolongation of refractoriness by $S_c$ depended on both current intensity and pulse duration of $S_c$, but was independent of the pacing cycle length over the range of physiologic pacing rates tested.

**In vivo canine experiments (6)**

In these studies mongrel dogs anesthetized with intravenous secobarbitol (25 mg/kg) were used. A quadripolar electrode catheter with 10 mm interelectrode spacing was introduced into an internal jugular vein and advanced under fluoroscopic guidance to the right ventricular apex. The method to study ventricular ERP and the effect of $S_c$ on refractoriness was similar to that described earlier for human investigations. One major difference was the adition of testing the effect of trains of subthreshold stimuli on ventricular ERP.

Trains of subthreshold conditioning stimuli (250–500 Hz, stimuli duration 1–2 msec, interstimulus interval 1–2 msec) were introduced after the 15 beat drive train to inhibit $S_2$ in 13 dogs. The initial $S_1$–$S_2$ interval was 10 ms greater than the right ventricular ERP. The train of conditioning stimuli (Frederick Haer stimulator) was delivered using a current generator separate from the generator delivering $S_1$ and $S_2$. The conditioning train, $S_1$, and $S_2$ were all delivered to the same distal bipolar pair on the pacing catheter positioned at the right ventricular apex. The train of conditioning stimuli was initiated 75 ms after the final $S_1$ of each drive train and terminated with delivery of $S_2$. The current of each stimulus within the train of stimuli was constant and was 0.1 mA initially, increasing in increments of 0.05 mA until $S_2$ was inhibited or the conditioning train depolarized the ventricle. After inhibition of $S_2$ occurred, the $S_1$–$S_2$ interval was increased by 10–20 ms and the process was repeated. For inhibition to be present, the following criteria had to be met: 1) the train of conditioning stimuli inhibited propagated ventricular depolarization in response to $S_2$ at the same current three consecutive times, 2) the train of conditioning stimuli when delivered without $S_2$ did not produce propagated ventricular depolarization, 3) $S_2$ delivered without the train of conditioning stimuli depolarized the ventricle, and 4) the train of conditioning stimuli delivered with $S_2$ after completion of the previous events again inhibited $S_2$.

Trains of high frequency stimuli inhibited the response to an $S_2$ delivered during diastole most successfully at a frequency of 333 Hz (stimulus interval 2 ms and stimulus duration 1 ms). The mean right ventricular ERP of the 13 dogs tested with conditioning trains was 162 ms (range 140–180 ms) at a mean pacing cycle length of 302 ms (range 280–350 ms). The mean late diastolic pacing threshold for $S_1$ and $S_2$ was 0.47 mA (range 0.26–0.8 mA). The mean maximal $S_1$–$S_2$ interval at which inhibition of the response to $S_2$ occurred was 321 ms (range 220–600 ms) employing a maximal conditioning train with a mean current of 1.21 mA (range 0.46–1.85 mA). The mean increase in the right ventricular ERP produced by trains of conditioning stimuli was 152 ms (range 70–460 ms). Trains of conditioning stimuli in the current range used in this study did not cause ventricular tachycardia or ventricular fibrillation in any dog.

Three dogs each were tested with conditioning trains before and after either lidocaine administration or autonomic blockade. Neither lidocaine nor autonomic blockade altered the curvilinear response comparing the control with the drug state.

**In vitro experiments [7]**

Two tissue preparations were studied in these investigations, either human ventricular endocardium or canine Purkinje fibers. In 2 studies human ventricular myocardium obtained from the recipient heart at the time of heart transplantation was used. Strips of ventricular endocardium were dissected free and placed in a tissue bath. Histologic examination of the ventricular endocardium demonstrated diffuse interstitial fibrosis consistent with cardiomyopathy in one patient and a healed myocardial infarction in the second patient. In 6 additional studies we used canine Purkinje fibers.

The preparations were stimulated via one of two bipolar Teflon coated electrodes positioned near the ends of the fiber. The distance between the stimulating electrodes was 10 to 20 mm. Microelectrodes were placed within 1 to 2 mm of each stimulating electrode. Transmembrane potentials were recorded with glass microelectrodes filled with 3 molar KCl (DC resistance 10 to 30 M). The electrodes were coupled to silver-silver chloride wires leading to the input stages of a high impedance, capacitance neutralizing amplifier, (WPI Model M 707, or 701). The recordings were displayed on a memory oscilloscope (Tektronix 5115) and photographed with a Polaroid camera (C-59).

Figure 3 shows the effect of $S_c$ on transmembrane action potentials from human ventricle. The bottom tracing represents actual data obtained from 1 experiment, and these data are correlated with the expected electrocardiographic and right ventricular endocardial events schematically depicted in the top and middle tracings respectively. The preparation was paced ($S_1$, $S_2$, and $S_c$) from the left-hand side, and the upper transmembrane action potential (proximal) was recorded near the pacing electrode and the lower action potential (distal) was recorded from a microelectrode situated 1 to 2 cm to the right of the proximal microelectrode (figure 3, bottom tracing). Oscilloscope sweeps were recorded

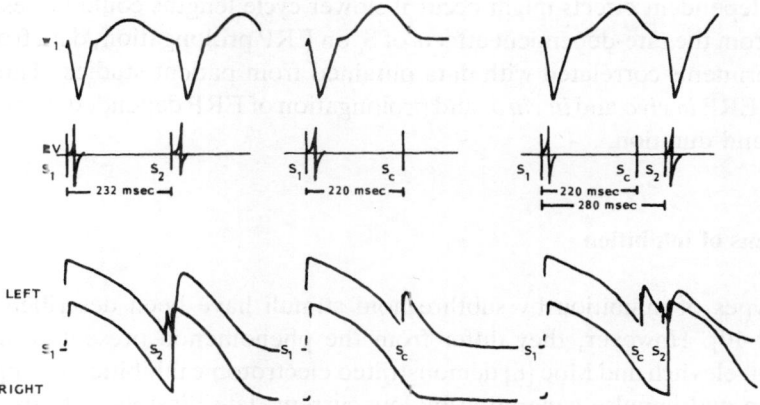

*Figure 3.* Demonstration of *in vitro* efect of $S_c$ on human ventricular ERP. See text for details.

with the last action potential of the drive train ($S_1$), $S_2$, and $S_c$ with the cellular response to $S_c$ shown.

The initial ERP was 232 msec (left panel). The $S_1$–$S_c$ interval was 220 msec (middle panel), and $S_c$ current intensity was 10 mA with a pulse width of 10 msec. Note that $S_c$ produced a local response at the proximal electrode site that did not propagate to the site of the distal electrode recording (middle panel). When the $S_1S_2$ interval was increased to 280 msec a threshold response occurred and it propagated to the distal microelectrode recording site (right panel). Thus, $S_c$ altered the morphology of the action potential and prolonged action potential duration.

For all experiments, $S_c$ of 10 mA intensity and 10 msec duration produced a mean increase in ERP of 43 msec in human ventricle and 99 msec in canine Purkinje fibers. Increasing $S_c$ intensity or duration produced progressively greater increase in ERP. In Purkinje fibers, magnitude of changes in ERP were affected by the pacing cycle tested, and the mean increase in ERP was 67 msec, 99 msec, and 125 msec at cycle length 300, 500 and 1000 msec respectively ($p < .05$). These rate-dependent differences in degree of ERP lengthening were not observed in the studies performed on patients (see earlier).

A number of explanations may account for this discrepancy. First, in patients, shortening of the cycle lengths from 600 to 400 msec resulted in a difference in ERP of only 25 msec. In isolated canine Purkinje fibers, a decrease in pacing cycle lengths yielded greater baseline differences in ERP: 50 msec for 300 vs 500 msec, and 80 msec for 500 vs 1000 msec. Since the effects of $S_c$ depended on the $S_1$–$S_c$ interval, greater changes in the prolongation of ERP by $S_c$ would be predicted by wider ranges in the baseline ERP. Second, these studies compared ventricular myocardium in patients to canine Purkinje fibers *in vitro*. Third, the range of rates tested in patients were limited by the resting sinus cycle length, and it is possible that rate dependent effects might occur if slower cycle lengths could be tested.

Aside from the rate-dependent effects of $S_c$ on ERP prolongation, data from *in vitro* experiments correlated with data obtained from patient studies. Thus, $S_c$ increased ERP *in vivo* and *in vitro*, and prolongation of ERP depended on both $S_c$ intensity and duration.

## Mechanisms of inhibition

Several types of inhibition by subthreshold stimuli have been described previously [8–10]. However, they differ from the phenomenon presented in this study. Antzelevitch and Moe [8] demonstrated electrotonic inhibition of impulse conduction and impulse generation by low current, late diastolic subthreshold stimuli and suggested that inhibition resulted from resetting of the pacemaker current ($I_F$). In our study, $S_c$ was delivered during the plateau or rapid repolarization phase of the action potential and therefore it is unlikely that $S_c$ activated or altered $I_F$. Cranefield and Hoffman [10] demonstrated that spatial inhibition could be produced by colliding wavefronts in branched Purkinje fibers encased in $K^+$ agar. However, our studies were performed in nondepressed myocardium and the subthreshold stimuli in our studies did not propagate.

We demonstrated that subthreshold stimuli delivered during the relative refractory period of the myocardium prolonged ERP by altering the morphology of the action potential and prolonging action potential duration. It is unknown whether this represented reactivation of inward sodium or calcium currents, or whether the cellular response produced by $S_c$ was purely an electrotonic phenomenon. In addition, it is possible that a subthreshold stimulus introduced during the relative refractory period produced a local threshold response that was extinguished upon entering tissue with a longer ERP, thereby rendering the local tissue refractory to a subsequent stimulus. In this regard, Elizari et al [11] demonstrated that a suprathreshold depolarization introduced near the penetrating His bundle failed to propagate into the branching His bundle at short coupling intervals.

## Clinical implications

It is possible that a properly timed and located subthreshold stimulus may prevent or terminate tachycardia by altering the local tissue refractoriness near the tachycardia focus [12, 13]. For example, Ruffy [12] reproducibly terminated ventricular tachycardia using catheter-induced stimuli delivered during the refractory period of the ventricle. This ability to terminate tachycardia was related to the intensity and timing of the subthreshold stimulus. In addition, Von Leitner and coworkers [13] introduced trains of subthreshold stimuli that successfully terminated ventricular tachycardia in six of eight patients. Prolongation of refractoriness could also be arrhythmogenic, however by creating unidirectional block and facilitating the development of reentry. To date, we have produced no arrhythmias in patients who have had prolongation of ventricular refractoriness by $S_c$.

Current approaches to electrical treatment of ventricular arrhythmias involve initiation of therapy (pacing, cardioversion, or defibrillation) *after* the tachycardia becomes manifest [14]. A preferable goal would be to *prevent* electrically the occurrence of ventricular tachycardia or ventricular fibrillation. More research is needed to obtain this goal, but it is not unreasonable to imagine such an electrical device (Fig. 4). In this example, ventricular tachycardia is initiated by a premature ventricular complex (PVC) as noted on the surface ECG ($V_1$) (upper panel). Ventricular tachycardia has been localized to a specific site in the left ventricle (LV) as noted by the early occurrence of LV electrograms in relation to the QRS complex. A patch electrode connected to an implantable generator has been attached to the LV at and around the site of the ventricular tachycardia focus (left diagram). The generator is programmable, and the appropriate timing, intensity, duration, and number of subthreshold stimuli are entered into the generator. The device also may have pacing, cardioversion, and defibrillation capabilities. The device is activated and after each sensed QRS complex delivers the prescribed subthreshold stimulus (i) to 1 or more electrodes in the patch. As demonstrated in the lower panel, subthreshold stimulation prolongs ventricular ERP and *prevents* the PVC from initiating ventricular tachycardia.

The above example is only one of several potential mechanisms by which subthreshold stimulation could prevent induction of ventricular tachycardia. The possibility of electrical prevention of ventricular arrhythmias is exciting and deserving of future investigation.

## Acknowledgement

Supported in part by the Herman C. Krannert Fund, Indianapolis, Indiana; by Grants HL-06308 and HL-07182 from the National Heart, Lung and Blood Institute of the National Institutes of Health, Bethesda, Maryland; and by the Attorney General of Indiana Public Health Trust and by the Toudebush Veterans Administration Medical Center, Indianapolis, Indiana, and by a Grant-in-Aid from the American Heart Association, Indiana Affiliate, Inc., Indianapolis, Indiana.

508

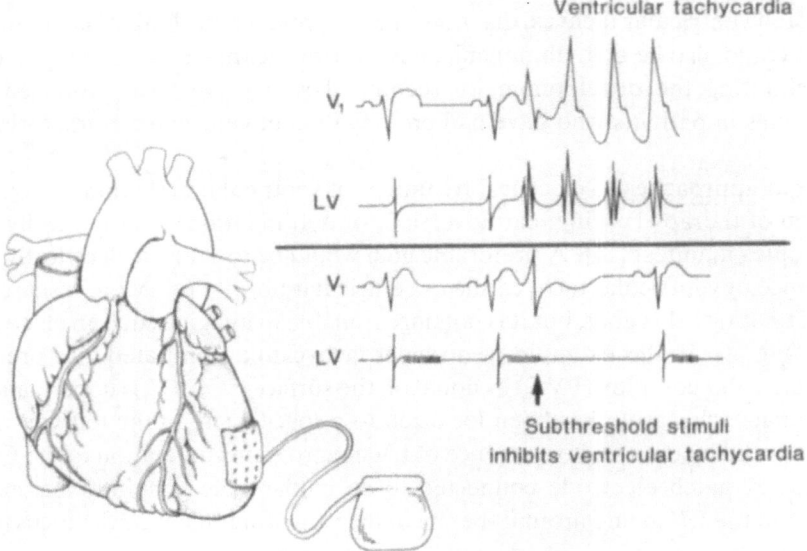

*Figure 4.* Electrical prevention of ventricular tachycardia – A device for the future. See text for details.

## References

1. Drury AN, Love WS (1926) The supposed lengthening of the absolute refractory period of frog's ventricular muscle by veratrine. Heart 13: 77
2. Lewis T, Drury AN (1926) Revised views of the refractory period in relation to drugs reputed to prolong it, and in relation to circus movement. Heart 13: 95
3. Tamargo J, Moe B, Moe GK (1975) Interaction of sequential stimuli applied during the relative refractory period in relation to determination of fibrillation threshold in the canine ventricle. Circ Res 37: 534
4. Prystowsky EN, Zipes DP (1983) Inhibition of the human heart. Circulation 68: 707
5. Windle JR, Miles WM, Zipes DO, Prystowsky EN (1984) Prolongation of human ventricular refractoriness by subthreshold stimuli: Effect of heart rate, pulse width and current strength. (abstr) Circulation 70: II-201
6. Skale BT, Kallok MJ, Prystowsky EN, Gill RM, Zipes DP (in press) Inhibition of premature ventricular extrastimuli by subthreshold conditioning stimuli. J Am Coll Cardiol
7. Windle JR, Prystowsky EN, Zipes DP, Gilmour RF Jr (in press) Inhibition of propagated myocardial excitation by subthreshold stimulation: clinical and cellular correlation. (abstr) PACE
8. Antzelevitch C, Moe GK (1983) Electrotonic inhibition and summation of impulse conduction in mammalian Purkinje fibers. Am J Physiol 245: H42
9. Jalife J, Antzelevitch C (1979) Phase resetting and annihilation of pacemaker activity in cardiac tissue. Science 206: 695
10. Cranefield PF, Hoffman BF (1971) Conduction of the cardiac impulse. II. Summation and inhibition. Circ Res 28: 220

11. Elizari MF, Lazzari JO, Rosenbaum MB (1983) Aberrant ventricular conduction: Electrocardiographic manifestations and mechanisms. In: Rosenbaum MB, Elizari MV (eds) Frontiers of Cardiac Electrophysiology, The Hague: Martinus-Nijhoff,, p 608

12. Ruffy R, Friday KJ, Southworth WF (1983) Termination of ventricular tachycardia by single extrastimulation during the ventricular effective refractory period. Circulation 67: 457

13. Von Leitner ER, Linderer T (1984) Subthreshold burst pacing, a new method of termination of ventricular and supraventricular tachycardia. (abstr) J Am Coll Cardiol 3: 472

14. Zipes DP, Heger JJ, Prystowsky EN (1983) Pacing and transvenous cardioversion to control tachyarrhythmias. In: Zipes DP (ed) Cardiac Arrhythmias, Philadelphia: Cardiology Clinics, PA, W.B. Saunders Co., p 341

# Antitachycardia pacing for treatment of recurrent sustained ventricular tachycardia

J.D. FISHER

## Introduction

Pacing is commonly effective for termination of ventricular tachycardia (VT) in the Electrophysiology Laboratory and elsewhere in a hospital setting, especially when the VT rate is modest [1–6]. Diagnosis is performed by the physician, and acceleration of ventricular fibrillation can be treated promptly with external countershock. A host of different pacing techniques have been developed in the electrophysiology laboratory [1–16]; many of these have been incorporated into increasingly sophisticated implantable units. Widespread use of implantable units continues to be limited, however, by the small number of patients who respond reliably to the same pacing technique [4]. Introduction of increasingly sophisticated diagnostic algorithms for automatic pacers, and incorporation of back-up countershock capability may make implantable units for antitachycardia pacing much more attractive.

## Mechanisms for the success and failure of pacing for termination of VT: [17–19]

It is generally agreed that most VTs are due to a reentrant mechanism. Such arrhythmias can be terminated if bidirectional block in the reentrant circuit can be achieved. Many variables are operative, among them the physical relationship and distance between the pacing site and the reentrant circuit; the 'excitable gap' in the circuit; properties of conductivity and refractoriness in the circuit and the myocardium intervening between the circuit and the pacing site; the possibility of several different pathways from the pacing site to the circuit, or of multiple potential circuits; and the number and timing of pacing stimuli. These interrelationships are complex, variable, and still subject to much speculation, but have been presented in some detail elsewhere [17–19].

## Pacing for termination of VT

*Single capture techniques*

Atrial pacing is occasionally able to produce conduction to the ventricle during VT, but usually only over a small range of the cardiac cycle, and the technique is not a mainstay of anti-VT pacing. Slow, competitive, 'underdrive' pacing results in a random or sometimes harmonic pattern of ventricular stimulation. Although no sophisticated equipment is required, the technique is inherently inefficient, and useful only in slow, well tolerated tachycardias with a broad termination zone. More sophisticated techniques include programmed electrical stimulation (PES) and related scanning techniques which explore the cardiac cycle in an orderly fashion. Based on the observation that the termination zone, when present, begins immediately, following the effective refractory period, trains of ultrarapid stimulation, limited in duration so as to achieve only a single capture, may be effective [11]. Single capture techniques are usually effective only with slow VTs, and are rarely effective on a reproducible or chronic basis. [4–6, 10, 11].

*Multiple capture techniques*

Multiple capture techniques, especially bursts of rapid ventricular pacing (BRVP) are much more effective than single capture techniques. The price of this effectiveness is high, however, in that the risks of acceleration are considerably greater with multi-capture techniques [3–6, 20]. In a study from our institution in patients with well tolerated VT, single capture techniques were able to terminate 57% of 390 episodes, with acceleration in 0.5%; multicapture techniques terminated 94% of 157 episodes, with acceleration in 4.5%.[4].

*Multiple extrastimuli*
Multiple programmed electrical stimuli can be delivered with sophisticated equipment. Beyond two extrastimuli, the risks of acceleration become comparable to those associated with rapid pacing methods.

*Burst pacing*
Bursts of rapid ventricular pacing (BRVP) continue to be the standard against which other methods must be judged. Burst pacing is intrinsically simple, and effective for the majority of VTs. 'Improvement' are directed primarily towards reducing the incidence of acceleration. Both the efficacy and the frustrations associated with single and multicapture techniques have recently been illustrated in a series of 13 figures [19].

In our laboratory, BRVP is usually initiated at a rate perhaps 20 bpm higher than the VT rate, for five to six captures. Another attempt is made at the same rate for eight to ten captures. The pacing rate is then increased in steps of 20–25 bpm, and the process repeated until the VT is terminated or accelerated. When it appears that the VT will not be well tolerated, initial BRVP rates 50 bpm in excess of the VT may be tried initially [3].

With simple equipment, bursts are delivered asynchronously, i.e. the initial stimulus occurs at a random point in the cardiac cycle. There has been some interest in burst pacing with the first stimulus synchronized in some fashion with the cardiac cycle, in the hopes of decreasing the incidence of acceleration. The value of synchronized burst pacing remains to be confirmed.

### BRVP plus PES
The combination of burst pacing plus extrastimuli may be effective in patients where either method alone has proved useless [21]; the method is not without its own risks of acceleration [20].

### Ramp pacing
Pacing with continuously changing stimulus cycle lengths can be imagined graphically as a ramp. We have found the method useful in several variations. [4, 7, 19]. For rapid VTs, i.e. those requiring the most rapid pacing and the most likely to accelerate, burst pacing appears to have a 'jolting' effect. It is our impression that the risks of acceleration are less if the pacing is initiated at a rate similar to that of the tachycardia, gradually ramped up, and after a pause ramped down. Slower VTs may respond well to a 'tune-down' ramp in which pacing is initiated at a rate only modestly above that of the VT, and then very slowly decreased.

### Newer termination techniques

Increased current strength may have a salutory effect [22]. At the other end of the scale, subthreshold single stimuli [23] and subthreshold burst pacing [24] have reportedly been useful in terminating some VTs. Our own experience with these techniques has been disappointing, even when the stimuli are delivered very near to the tachycardia circuit [19]. Pacing at multiple sites may prove useful in VT [25] as well as in AV nodal reentrant tachycardias [26].

### Entrainment

A special form of rapid pacing involving the concept of entrainment has received recent attention [13–16]. First explored in atrial flutter, and then extended to other arrhythmias including VT, Dr. A. Waldo and his colleagues have noticed that during rapid pacing, the ECG often showed morphologies which were fusions between the fully paced and pure tachycardia morphologies. At slower pacing rates, tachycardia morphology predominated, and at faster rates the paced morphology terminates. At any given rate, the degree of fusion is constant except for the last entrained beat. At a critical rate, a purely paced morphology becomes evident, and this is frequently associated with termination of the arrhythmia, due to conduction block. Demonstration of entrainment requires a large excitable gap in the VT circuit, presumably due to a relatively short refractory period. If slow conduction in the antegrade limb is added to relatively short refractory periods, a greater degree of fusion will be evident at slower pacing rates. Analysis of entrainment has led to an increased appreciation of some of the mechanisms involved in tachycardia perpetuation and termination. In addition, the risks of acceleration may be smaller if the minimum possible pacing rate is used; this rate can be inferred from the ECG by examining the morphology of the complexes as pacing rates are increased, and identifying the minimum rate at which entrainment/fusion disappears.

*Prevention of tachycardia*

Recognition of the pattern of extrasystoles likely to result in a tachycardia, and responding with programmable preventive pacing patterns has been used in the orthorhythmic pacemaker and its derivatives to 'abort' incipient arrhythmias [27].

Inhibition of subsequent beats by stimulation during the effective refractory period is being investigated [28] and is detailed in another chapter. Future biologic sensors may be able to detect physiologic changes leading to arrhythmias and provide preventive pacing.

*Hemodynamic improvement without termination of tachycardias*

Occasionally a patient will become 'stuck' in VT, often due to transient causes such as the administration of certain antiarrhythmic drugs. Pacing techniques can be helpful in some such patients, to slow the effective ventricular response, or to achieve a gain in blood pressure and/or cardiac output to tide the patient over until the offending drug has dissipated. Useful techniques include synchronization of the atrial and ventricular depolarizations to maximize ventricular filling (AVT pacing); multi site pacing to create a more satisfactory sequence of ventricular depolarization; and coupled pacing [7]. None of these techniques is useful except in relatively acute situations.

**Implantable anti-VT pacers**

Implantable anti-VT pacers are burdened with a sword of Damocles. Even if tachycardia may be terminated in a majority of instances, any given acceleration could prove fatal. Nevertheless, there has been much progress in the development of antitachycardia pacers.

There are two ways to cope with the possibility of acceleration: 1) a manual antitachycardia pacer can be used, to be activated only when medical support is available and 2) a back-up cardioverter/defibrillator can be incorporated into the unit. Both of these approaches have been used, with the latter undergoing very earnest development at the present time.

Manual units are limited in their application to patients whose tachycardias are well enough tolerated to allow time for access to medical back-up. This can prove a major nuisance to patients, and inhibit them from travelling or otherwise leading normal, active lives. We have observed many patients who are unable to restrain themselves from activating their own devices without adequate back-up. For all of these reasons, manually activated units have not enjoyed widespread use.

Automatic antitachycardia pacemakers must be capable of accurate tachycardia diagnosis, and effective antitachy pacing; at the present time we strongly believe that these units should also incorporate a back-up cardioverter/defibrillator. Early automatic units had simple diagnostic algorithms, usually amounting to a limited selection of rate/duration criteria. Responses to tachycardias in earlier units were typically simple, with the unit continuing to respond until the tachycardia was terminated.

### Newer diagnostic algorithms

Implantable antitachycardia pacemakers now becoming available incorporate several different diagnostic algorithms. These include suddenness of tachycardia onset in order to distinguish pathologic tachycardias from physiologic rate increases [29]; and stability of the tachycardia cycle length in order to avoid pacing irregular rhythms such as atrial fibrillation. Responses to test stimuli may also have diagnostic value [30]. The use of multiple leads within a single or several chambers, can provide diagnostic information on the basis of sequence of depolarization; and electrogram information including morphology, amplitude, and slew rate may also be useful in differentiating between physiologic and pathologic tachycardias [7]. Pacers capable of sensing biologic functions including respiration, pH, $pO_2$, hemoglobin saturation, etc may prove useful.

### Tachycardia responses

Presently available devices offer an array of very flexible antitachycardia responses. In some instances, the pacemaker can be programmed to perform a series of different responses until the tachycardia is terminated. Some units can remember the effective technique, and will automatically use this as the first response if another tachycardia with similar characteristics recurs. Available units are capable of slow competitive pacing, scanning/PES, bursts, ramp pacing, and ultrarapid train stimulation. Bursts can be programmed to be delivered at a preselected cycle length, or in an 'adaptive' mode, in which the cycle length of the burst is programmed as a percentage of the tachycardia cycle length. The timing of the first stimulus of the burst is also individually programmable, and in some units (such as the Intermedics Intertach), the timing of the first beat may also be scanned independently from the delivery of the remaining scan and/or burst, so that responses such as 'scanning adaptive bursts' become possible. A Medtronic device is currently able to provide back-up cardioversion but not defibrillation, nevertheless a step in the right direction. Intec/CPI, the manufacturers of the automatic implantable defibrillator, will soon be incorporating an antitachycardia pacemaker capability for use when appropriate prior to delivering countershock. Many devices, including the Intertach and the Cordis Orthocor II also provide rather sophisticated Holter capability, so that the physician can determine how many episodes of tachycardia have been diagnosed, treated, and which treatments are most effective.

*Non-invasive PES*

Most of the sophisticated antitachy devices described above incorporate provisions for non-invasive PES. Simple manual units, such as the Medtronic 5998 radiofrequency unit, can be used for non invasive PES. Several conventional antibradycardia pacers can also be used for non-invasive PES and temporary burst pacing, either as a standard feature [31], or with special programmers or modules. The ability to perform non-invasive PES allows the physician to follow the stability of the patients' arrhythmias over a number of years, without resort to further invasive procedures.

**Conclusions**

Pacing for recurrent sustained VT has many advantages. Pacing therapy is painless and largely avoids compliance problems and side effects associated with medications. The risks of implantation are much lower that those of open heart surgery. Improved diagnostic algorithms and the flexible antitachycardia pacing responses are leading to increasingly effective antitachycardia pacing. The combination of a sophisticated antitachycardia pacemaker with a back-up defibrillator in a moderately sized and cost effective package is likely to expand markedly the role of implanted pacemakers in patients with recurrent sustained VT.

516

## Acknowledgement

The author gratefully acknowledges the long-term contributions of his present and prior colleagues, including Drs. S. Furman, D. Escher, S. Kim, L. Waspe and J. Matos. The help of many fellows, technicians, and nurses has been great and that of Ms. R. Simak indispensible.

## References

1. Escher DJW, Furman S (1970) Emergency treatment of cardiac arrhythmias. JAMA 214: 2028
2. Wiener I (1980) Pacing techniques in the treatment of tachycardias. Ann Int Med 93: 326
3. Fisher JD, Mehra R, Furman S (1978) Termination of ventricular tachycardia with bursts of rapid ventricular pacing. Amer J Cardiol 41: 94
4. Fisher JD, Kim SG, Matos JA et al: Comparative effectiveness of pacing techniques for termination of well-tolerated sustained ventricular tachycardia. PACE 1083,6: 915
5. Naccarelli GV, Zipes DP, Rahilly TG et al: (1983) Influence of tachycardia cycle length and antiarrhythmia drugs on pacing termination and acceleration of ventricular tachycardia. Amer Heart J 105: 1
6. Roy D, Waxman HL, Buxton AE et al (1982) Termination of ventricular tachycardia: Role of tachycardia cycle length. Amer J Cardiol 50: 1346
7. Fisher JD, Kim SG, Furman S, et al (1982) Role of implantable pacemakers in control of recurrent ventricular tachycardia. Amer J Cardiol 93: 194
8. Critelli G, Grassi G, Chiariello M et al (1979) Automatic 'scanning' by radiofrequency in the long-term electrical treatment of arrhythmias. PACE 2: 289
9. Nathan A, Hellestrand K, Bexton R, et al (1982) Clinical evaluation of an adaptive tachycardia intervention pacemaker with automatic cycle length adjustment. PACE 5: 201
10. Reddy PC, Todd EP, Kuo CS et al (1984) Treatment of ventricular tachycardia using an automatic scanning extrastimulus pacemaker. JACC 3: 225
11. Fisher JD, Ostrow E, Kim SG et al (1983) Ultrarapid single-capture train stimulation for termination of ventricular tachycardia. Amer J Cardiol 51: 1334
12. Spurrell RAJ, Sowton E (1975) Pacing techniques in the management of supra-ventricular tachycardias. J Electrocardiol 8: 287
13. Waldo AL, MacLean WAH, Karp RB et al (1977) Entrainment and interruption of atrial flutter with atrial pacing. Circulation 56: 737
14. Waldo AL, Plumb VJ, MacLean WAH (1983) Transient entrainment and interruption of AV bypass pathway type paroxysmal atrial tachycardia: A model for understanding and identifying reentrant arrhythmias in man. Circulation 67: 73
15. Waldo AL, Henthorn RW, Plumb VJ, et al (1984) Demonstration of the mechanism of transient tachycardia with rapid atrial pacing. JACC 3: 422
16. Anderson KP, Swerdlow CD, Maston JW (1984) Entrainment of ventricular tachycardia. Amer J Cardiol 53: 335
17. Fisher JD, Kim SG, Waspe LE et al (1983) Mechanisms for the success and failure of pacing for termination of ventricular tachycardia: Clinical and hypothetical considerations. PACE 6: 1094
18. Fisher JD, Kim SG, Matos JA et al (1984) Pacing for Tachycardias: Clinical Translations. Zipes D (Ed) Grune and Stratton
19. Fisher J, Kim SG, Matos JA, Waspe LE (1984) Pacing for Ventricular Tachycardia. PACE 7: 1278–1290
20. Jentzer JH, Hoffmann RM (1984) Acceleration of Ventricular Tachycardia by Rapid Overdrive

Pacing Combined with Extrastimuli. PACE 7: 922–924

21. Gardner MJ, Waxman HL, Buxton AE, Cain ME, Josephson ME (1982) Termination of Ventricular Tachycardia. Amer J Cardiol 50: 1338–1345

22. Waxman HL, Cain ME, Greenspan AM, et al (1982) Termination of ventricular tachycardia with ventricular stimulation: Salutary effect of increased current strength. Circulation 65: 800

23. Ruffy R, Friday KJ, Southworth WF (1983) Termination of ventricular tachycardia by single extrastimulation during the ventricular effective refractory period. Circulation 67: 457

24. Von Leitner R, Linderer T (1984) Subthreshold burst pacing: A new method for termination of ventricular and supraventricular tachycardia. JACC 3: 472 (abstract)

25. Mehra R, Gough WB, Zeller R, et al (1984) Dual ventricular stimulation for prevention of reentrant ventricular arrhythmias. JACC 3: 472

26. Sung RJ, Styperek JL, Castellanos A (1980) Complete abolition of the reentrant tachycardia zone using a new modality of cardiac pacing with simultaneous atrioventricular stimulation. Amer J Cardiol 45: 72

27. Zacouto F, Juillard A, Gerbaux A (1982) Letter to the Editor, PACE 5: 781

28. Prystowsky EN, Zipes DP (1983) Inhibition in the human heart. Circulation 68: 707

29. Fisher JD, Goldstein M, Ostrow E, et al (1983) Maximal rate of tachycardia development: Sinus tachycardia with sudden exercise vs spontaneous ventricular tachycardia. PACE 6: 221

30. Munkenbeck FC, Bump TE, Arzbaecher RC (1984) Differentiation of sinus tachycardia from paroxysmal tachycardias using single rate diastolic atrial extrastimuli. JACC 3: 473 (abstract)

31. Fisher JD, Furman S, Kim SG, Matos JA, Waspe LE (1984) DDD/DDT Pacemakers in the Treatment of Ventricular Tachycardia. PACE 7: 173–178

# Clinical application of transvenous cardioversion

J.J. HEGER, E.N. PRYSTOWSKY, W.M. MILES, AND D.P. ZIPES

## Introduction

Transvenous electrical cardioversion refers to the reversion of cardiac arrhythmia by delivery of synchronized electrical shock to the endocardial surface of the heart through a transvenous catheter. The application of a catheter system for transvenous intracardiac cardioversion represents a logical extension of the techniques and concepts of electrical cardioversion and defibrillation. The concept of delivering electrical shocks directly to the heart through a catheter has been advanced by the work of investigative teams lead by Mirowski et al [1, 2]. They demonstrated the feasibility and safety of such an approach with work that has progressed to the development of an implantable defibrillation system. With this background, it was further reasoned that synchronized shocks delivered through a catheter electrode system would successfully cardiovert ventricular tachycardia using very low energies.

Implantable systems for cardioversion and defibrillation offer advantages over other antiarrhythmic treatment modalities. Electrical shock is a highly effective method to terminate a variety of tachyarrhythmas. As such, cardioversion and defibrillation are relatively nonspecific or generic treatments especially as compared to antiarrhythmic drugs. Thus, electrical countershock is widely applicable. Given the large number of patients at risk for recurrent ventricular tachycardia and ventricular fibrillation and the problems of identifying and maintaining effective drug treatment regimens, it is apparent that new directions are needed.

## Animal studies

Initial testing of low energy transvenous cardioversion was performed by Jackman and Zipes in canine model of inducible ventricular tachycardia at three to eight days following myocardial infarction [3]. Cardioversion shocks were delivered through a specially designed catheter. A pair of electrodes at the right ventricular apex served as the cathode and a pair of electrodes at the right atrial superior vena cava junction was the anode. A total of 627 episodes of sustained ventricular tachycardia were tested by the cardioverter system. Cardioversion energies of 1.0 joules or less synchronized to the QRS complex terminated 83 percent of induced sustained ventricular tachycardias that had a cycle length of 200 msec or less. Repetitive ventricular responses were rare and acceleration of ventricular tachycardia or degeneration to ventricular fibrillation never occurred when the delivered shock fell within the initial 80 percent of the QRS interval.

These animal studies indicated that in a model of post-myocardial infarction ventricular tachycardia, transvenous electrical cardioversion using a single catheter was effective and safe. The success rate of cardioversion was high when the ventricular tachycardia cycle length was longer than 200 msec, but success could not be further related to rate or other variables including epicardial activation sequence. Similarly, cardioversion was safer in the slower ventricular tachycardias. Synchronized ventricular shocks that were often unsynchronized to atrial systole could produce atrial arrhythmias. Conversely, electrical cardioversion or atrial fibrillation was demonstrated on several occasions.

**Initial clinical studies**

With the animal studies as a background, initial clinical evaluations in humans were performed. A total of 13 patients entered the initial trial to test the transvenous cardioversion system [4, 5]. Ventricular tachycardia either occurred spontaneously or was induced during electrophysiological study. Ten of 13 patients were successfully cardioverted using up to 2 joules (Fig. 1). Two patients could not complete the testing protocol because hemodynamic deterioration during ventricular tachycardia necessitated immediate transthoracic cardioversion. One patient experienced 311 episodes of sustained ventricular tachycardia over a 12 hour period that were terminated by transvenous cardioversion at energies of 4 to 25 joules using the cardioversion catheter interfaced to a standard defibrillator.

The clinical utility of the internal cardioversion system in acute cardiac care was reported in eight patients hospitalized in a cardiac intensive care unit for recurrent ventricular tachycardia and ventricular fibrillation [6]. Transvenous cardioversion converted ventricular tachycardia in 86 of 99 (87 percent) attempts and ventricular flutter/fibrillation in 7 of 16 (44 percent) attempts.

The safety and efficacy of transvenous cardioversion were then evaluated in a multicenter trial [7]. In total, 72 of 96 patients (75 percent) and 397 of 467 (85 percent) episodes of sustained ventricular tachycardia had successful cardioversions through the catheter lead system. Ventricular tachycardia cycle lengths successfully converted ranged from 170 to 575 msec (mean 375 ms) and those not successfully converted ranged from 180 to 620 msec (mean 318 ms). Cardioversion

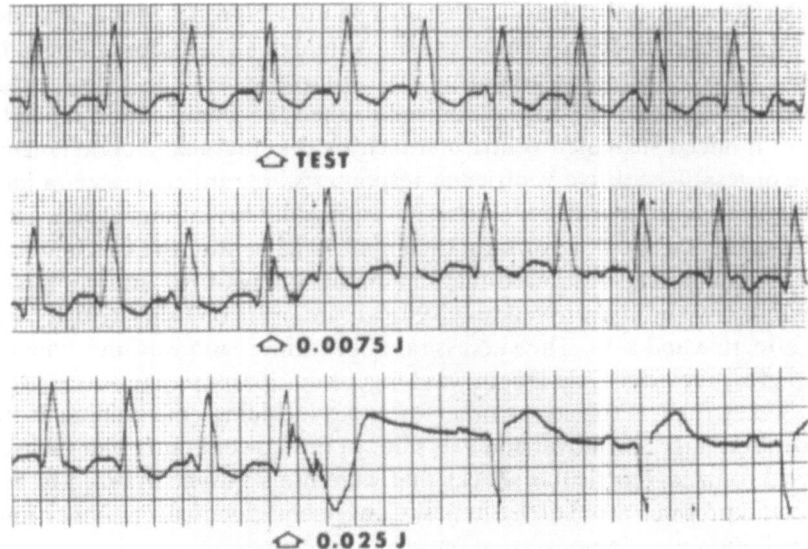

*Figure 1.* ECG records from a patient undergoing successful transvenous cardioversion of spontaneous sustained ventricular tachycardia. Top: A test pulse is delivered to verify timing within the QRS complex. Middle: An energy of 0.0075 joules fails to terminate ventricular tachycardia. Bottom: A 0.025 joule shock terminates ventricular tachycardia.

energy levels were from 0.03 to 28 joules. Further studies of the efficacy and safety of transvenous electrical cardioversion included 52 patients in whom 75 of 111 episodes of spontaneous or induced ventricular tachycardia were terminated by transvenous shocks [8–11]. The mean termination threshold for each patient ranged from 0.67 to 1.47 joules. Acceleration of ventricular tachycardia or precipitation of ventricular fibrillation occurred in from 6 percent to 15 percent of episodes. As with prior reports, ventricular tachycardias successfully converted tended to have slower rates than those in which cardioversion was unsuccessful.

**Permanent implantable cardioverter**

On the basis of the initial successes using temporary transvenous electrical cardioversion, development and implantation of a permanent device was pursued [12]. The automatic cardioversion system consists of three components, the implantable pulse generator, cardioversion lead and external programmer.

*Cardioverter pulse generator*

The pulse generator, Medtronic model 7210, is contained in a titanium case

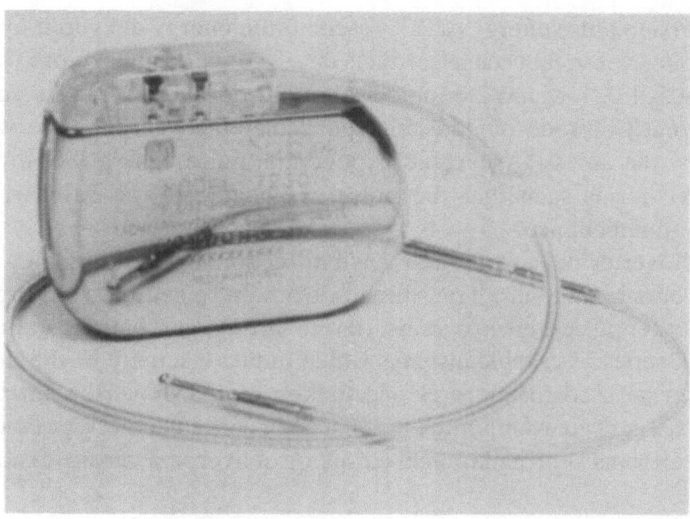

*Figure 2.* The cardioverter pulse generator and cardioversion lead.

measuring 57 × 73 × 19 mm and weighing 95 gm (Fig. 2). Power is supplied by two independent lithium batteries. The unit is designed to detect ventricular tachycardia and deliver pulses of 0.06 to 2.0 joules in synchrony with ventricular depolarization. The tachycardia detection and cardioversion functions may be programmed on or off. The unit also performs ventricular demand pacing, ventricular asynchronous pacing or programmed electrical stimulation independently of the cardioversion features. Pacing parameters of rate, pulse width and sensitivity are programmable. The cardioversion mode has four progammable parameters which include interval change threshold, tachycardia trigger interval, number of intervals to trigger, and cardioversion pulse energy. The first three relate to ventricular tachycardia detection.

The interval change threshold (ICT) uses a criterion of paroxysmal onset of tachycardia. The device continuously monitors ventricular depolarization rate. When an R–R interval decreases from the previous R–R interval by more than the programmed amount, the ICT criterion is satisfied. This parameter helps distinguish the paroxysmal onset of ventricular tachycardia from the more gradual onset of sinus tachycardia. Tachycardia trigger interval (TTI) is a rate detection parameter. The criterion is satisfied if a sensed R–R interval is less than the interval programmed in TTI. Number of intervals to trigger (NIT) delineates the number of consecutive R–R intervals, at rates exceeding TTI, that must be counted for the device to detect ventricular tachycardia.

The tachycardia algorithm employs one of two methods. The first utilizes the TTI and NIT parameters alone with the ICT inactive. The second method uses all three parameters. In this case, the ICT parameter must be met first before the other criteria may begin to be applied.

Cardioversion pulse energy (CPE) refers to the energy delivered by the pulse generator once ventricular tachycardia is detected. CPE may be programmed at 0.06, 0.2, 0.5, 1.0, 1.8, and 2.0 joules. The unit delivers up to five consecutive shocks for each episode of detected ventricular tachycardia. The wave form delivered by the unit is a truncated exponential pulse. The pulses are constant energy wave forms such that the pulse width adjusts for differing levels of cardioversion impedance.

The cardioverter pulse generator has bidirectional radiofrequency telemetry with the programming unit. Transmission from pulse generator to programmer includes marker pulses, electrograms, device settings and battery status. Marker pulses are a series of graphic displays which indicate activity of the device and, thereby, can be used to interpret pacemaker and cardioverter functions. The marker pulses indicate whether the unit paced or sensed in the VVI mode, sensed a depolarization as ventricular tachycardia or delivered a cardioversion pulse.

*Cardioversion lead*

The permanent implantable lead is 9.5 French diameter with four tines at the tip which help secure the lead at the right ventricular apex. The separation between the distal electrode pair and proximal electrode pair may be 100 mm, 125 mm or 150 mm. The variable interelectrode distances accomodate different heart sizes to permit approximation of the proximal electrode pair at the superior vena cava-right atrial junction. The interelectrode spacing for each pair is 5 mm and each electrode has a surface area of $1.25 \, cm^2$. The distal electrode pair is used for bipolar pacing and for sensing ventricular depolarizations. For delivery of shocks, the distal electrodes are coupled to form the cathode with the proximal pair as the anode.

*Cardioverter programmer*

The programmer unit, Medtronic model SP 6000, uses standard line power and provides telemetry communication to the pulse generator through a magnet head placed over the pulse generator. Each function key for programming is color-coded. A digital light display cues all programming functions and indicates whether the programmed parameters have been accepted by the pulse generator. The unit provides a hard copy printout of all pulse generator settings and interfaces with a multichannel recorder to provide marker channel or sensed electrogram outputs.

## Cardioverter implantation protocol

*Preoperative evaluation*

Each patient undergoes extensive preoperative electrophysiological evaluation. At the preoperative electrophysiological study, each patient is receiving the antiarrhythmic regimen expected to be used for long-term treatment. A temporary cardioverter catheter electrode is inserted percutaneously through an arm vein or an interval jugular vein and positioned at the right ventricular apex under fluoroscopic guidance. Using the cardioverter lead as a pacing electrode, programmed electrical stimulation is performed to induce the clinically recurring ventricular tachycardia for that patient. When the induced ventricular tachycardia has stabilized, cardioversion shocks are delivered by an external cardioversion unit. Energy levels similar to those employed by the permanent unit are tested with shocks of increasing intensity until the tachycardia terminates. The cardioversion threshold is defined as the minimal energy required to terminate ventricular tachycardia consistently. To be considered a candidate for implant at this time, cardioversion thresholds must be below 1.7 joules and the shocks may not be associated with more than five repetitive ventricular responses or acceleration or ventricular tachycardia by more than 15 beats per minute. The cardioversion threshold shocks should also be reasonably well tolerated by the patient. To date, approximately 70 percent of patients selected as possible candidates for cardioverter implantation have met these criteria during preoperative testing.

*Operative procedure*

Permanent cardioverter implantations have usually been performed in surgical suites. The technique is nearly identical to that of permanent pacemaker implantation. Usual skin preparation and strict asepsis are employed. Following local anesthesia, the permanent cardioverter lead is introduced into the left cephalic vein and positioned at the right ventricular apex under fluoroscopic guidance. Adequate sensing and pacing parameters are confirmed. Using the permanent lead, ventricular tachycardia is induced by programmed electrical stimulation and cardioversion using the external unit is performed to confirm the performance observed at the preoperative study. Once lead position, pacing, sensing and cardioversion thresholds are adequate, the lead is connected to the implantable cardioverter. The cardioverter pulse generator is positioned in a subcutaneous skin pocket created in the subclaviculan area. By telemetry from the programmer, programmed electrical stimulation is performed through the implanted unit to induce sustained ventricular tachycardia. With the device in the automatic mode, its ability to detect ventricular tachycardia, charge and deliver synchronized cardioversion shocks is then observed (Fig. 3). This sequence is repeated

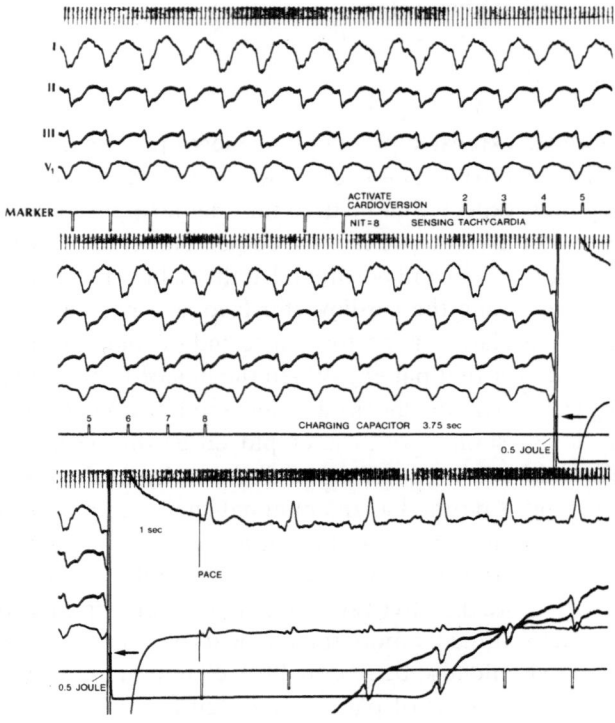

*Figure 3.* Continuous recording illustrating the function of the permanent cardioverter after permanent implantation. Initially, the cardioversion mode is inactivated. After the programmed command to initiate cardioversion, the detected rhythm satisfies the rate criteria for ventricular tachycardia. After 8 sensed beats of VT the capacitor charges and delivers 0.5 joules to terminate the arrhythmia.

several times. The skin incision is then closed and the patient is returned to the coronary intensive care unit.

## Post-operative procedures

Post-operatively, patients are monitored in the coronary intensive care unit for a period of at least three days. The device is maintained in the automatic mode during this period. Because of the risk of acceleration of ventricular tachycardia or precipitation of ventricular fibrillation by a cardioversion shock and since the device at present does not terminate ventricular fibrillation, the tachycardia detection and cardioversion modes are programmed off at the time of hospital discharge. The unit then functions as a ventricular demand pacemaker as described earlier. It is anticipated that if patients develop recurrent ventricular tachycardia during follow-up, their physicians will activate the device so that cardioversion will be done in a setting that has resuscitation and external defibrillation capabilities. Once several cardioversions have been successful and safe in this manner, the unit may be set in the automatic cardioversion mode in selected patients.

For the long-term follow-up protocol, patients are seen after the first month and thereafter at three-month intervals by the investigators. Using the external programmer with the implanted device, ventricular tachycardia is initiated noninvasively. Cardioversion shocks are automatically delivered to terminate the induced ventricular tachycardia. This procedure helps assess the stability of pacing and cardioversion thresholds.

**Clinical experience**

Candidates for consideration of permanent cardioverter implantation must meet several criteria. They must have recurrent episodes of a stable, monomorphic ventricular tachycardia without spontaneous ventricular fibrillation or cardiac arrest other than that associated with acute myocardial infarction. The episodes of ventricular tachycardia must be recognized by the patients and the patients must remain hemodynamically stable for up to several hours such that they can be evaluated by their physicians during an episode of ventricular tachycardia. Patients must have required repeated cardioversions for recurrent ventricular tachycardia over the prior several months despite antiarrhythmic drug trials. It must be judged that the patient is not a candidate for surgical procedures to control the arrhythmia. Finally, patients must give verbal and written informed consent to the procedure and follow-up protocols. The restrictive nature of these indications reflects the developmental nature of the present device and the imperative that patient safety be maximized. Future devices that possess defibrillation capabilities will have much broader applications.

Based on the above considerations for patient entry, the worldwide experience has included 27 permanent cardioverter implantations with the first implant performed in August 1983. Currently, 12 patients have received permanent cardioverter implantations with the present device at Indiana University Hospital. Each has had three or more episodes of ventricular tachycardia converted automatically or by physician-initiated telemetry. One patient has died suddenly. After receiving the device, this patient has five episodes of spontaneous ventricular tachycardia that were converted without incident by physician-activiated programming. The device was then programmed to the automatic mode. Eight episodes of spontaneously occurring ventricular tachycardia were converted automatically. During one episode of ventricular tachycardia, however, cardioversion was followed by atrial fibrillation with a rapid ventricular response that met all criteria for tachycardia detection and initiated attempts at cardioversion. Eventually a cardioversion shock delivered into the ST segment of ventricular tachycardia precipitated ventricular flutter and ventricular fibrillation. The patient was enroute to his local hospital and arrived in time to be successfully resuscitated without sequelae. The unit was reprogrammed to disable the automatic cardioversion mode, but over time and in association with further hemodynamic deterioration, episodes of recurrent sustained ventricular tachycardia became more frequent and the patient insisted on having the automatic mode reprogrammed, fully aware of the potential risk. Several successful cardioversions of ventricular tachycardia followed, but the patient died suddenly at home after experiencing another recurrence of ventricular tachycardia and receiving at least one cardioversion shock. Another patient had several successful cardioversions of ventricular tachycardia during testing, but during follow-up cardioversion shocks during induced ventricular tachycardia accelerated the arrhythmia precluding the use of automatic mode.

## Complications and limitations

In human studies, transvenous shocks have not been associated with diagnostic elevations of myocardial-specific creatine kinase enzymes or with electrocardiographic changes. Post-mortem examination in a patient who had received multiple cardioversion shocks of 2.0 joules or less disclosed endocardial fibrosis and sheath formation associated with the intracavitary lead but no myocardial necrosis attributable to the shocks.

The presence of an intravascular device carries the usual risks associated with pacemaker wire implantation which include infection, cardiac perforation and thrombosis, among others. The main limitations and complications unique to low energy cardioversion relates to the induction of arrhythmia. The shocks are timed to ventricular depolarization and may find the atria in a vulnerable period with resultant precipitation of atrial fibrillation or other atrial tachyarrhythmias. While the induced atrial fibrillation usually terminates spontaneously without sequelae, the events experienced in the patient described earlier deserve attention. A rapid ventricular response to atrial fibrillation may satisfy the tachycardia detection criteria and initiate attempts at cardioversion. It is recommended that the pre-implantation protocol include an evaluation of the response to atrial fibrillation in each patient and that an appropriate drug therapy be given to control the ventricular rate.

The device in its present configuration does not have defibrillation capabilities. Inappropriately timed electrical shocks whether transthoracic or transvenously delivered may accelerate ventricular tachycardia or produce ventricular flutter or ventricular fibrillation. Because of this protocol, the use of the automatic mode in this first generation device has been limited.

Patient tolerance of the delivered cardioversion shock is important since a major aim is to convert sustained ventricular tachycardia in the conscious, unsedated patient. There is great interpatient variability in tolerance to intracardiac cardioversion. Diaphragmatic and intercostal muscle stimulation appears to be the cause of perceived discomfort. In general, shocks of 0.5 joules or less are tolerated satisfactorily. The stated sensations range from a mild 'hiccup' to feeling a strong blow or kick in the chest.

Finally, all devices suffer from a major deficiency in accurate rhythm detection and identification. Similar problems exist for any automatic arrhythmia detection algorithm whether used for ambulatory ECG monitoring or an implantable antitachycardia unit. Clearly, heart rate, paroxysmal onset of tachycardia, tachycardia duration or other parameters employed at present do not provide a completely reliable system. Future devices need better methods to differentiate tachycardias accurately.

**Future developments**

Next generation devices are planned to correct several of the limitations inherent in the first generation unit. The initial emphasis is to examine methods for defibrillation capability. Preliminary studies using two sequential shocks have shown promising results [13, 14].

Efforts to provide reliable cardioversion and defibrillation capabilities will continue with additional focus on more accurate methods for tachycardia detection. It is likely that a device will soon be developed that combines automatic intravenous drug delivery, antitachycardia pacing, synchronized cardioversion and automatic defibrillation in a small, implantable device that will also provide a continuous memory and telemetry of cardiac rhythms.

**Acknowledgement**

Supported in part by the Herman C. Krannert Fund, Indianapolis, Indiana; by Grants HL-06308, and HL-07182 from the National Heart, Lung and Blood Institute of the National Institutes of Health, Bethesda, Maryland; and by the Attorney General of Indiana Public Health Trust and by the Roudebush Veterans Administration Medical Center, Indianapolis, Heart Association, Indiana Affiliate, Inc., Indianapolis, Indiana.

**References**

1. Mirowski M, Mower MM, Gott VL, Brawley RK (1973) Feasibility and effectiveness of low-energy catheter defibrillation in man. Circulation 47: 79–85
2. Mirowski M, Reid PR, Mower MM, Watkins L. Gott VL, Schauble JF, Langer A, Heilman MF,

Kolenik SA, Fischell RE, Weisfeldt ML (1980) Termination of malignant ventricular arrhythmias with an implanted automatic defibrillator in human beings. N Engl J Med 303: 322–324

3. Jackman WM, Zipes DP (1982) Low-energy synchronous cardioversion of ventricular tachycardia using a catheter electrode in a canine model of subacute myocardial infarction. Circulation 66: 187–195

4. Zipes DP, Jackman WM, Heger JJ, Chilson DA, Browne KF, Naccarelli GV, Rahilly GT Jr, Prystowsky EN (1982) Clinical transvenous cardioversion of recurrent life-threatening ventricular tachycardias: Low energy synchronized cardioversion of ventricular tachycardia and termination of ventricular fibrillation in patients using a catheter electrode. Am Heart J 103: 789–94

5. Zipes DP, Prystowsky EN, Browne KF, Chilson DA, Heger JJ (1982) Additional observations on transvenous cardioversion of recurrent ventricular tachycardia. Am Heart J 104: 163–164

6. Yee R, Zipes DP, Gulamhusein S, Kallok MJ, Klein GJ (1982) Low energy countershock using an intravascular catheter in an acute cardiac care setting. Am J Cardiol 50: 1124–1129

7. Kallok MJ, Fischer JD, Fletcher RD, Hartzler GO, Kehoe RF, Klein GJ, Prystowsky EN, Ruffy R, Zipes DP (1983) Intracavitary cardioversion and defibrillation: A multicenter study. (abstr). Circulation 68 (Suppl III): 89

8. Waspe LE, Kim SG, Matos JA, Fischer JD (1983) Role of a catheter lead system for transvenous countershock and pacing during electrophysiologic tests. An assessment of the usefulness of catheter shocks for terminating ventricular tachyarrhythmias. Am J Cardiol 52: 477–484

9. Perelman MS, Rowland E, Krikler DM (1984) Assessment of a prototype implantable cardioverter for ventricular tachycardia. Relations between synchronisation of sensing and origin of the tachycardia. Br Heart J 52: 385–91

10. Nathan AW, Bexton RS, Spurrell RA, Camm AJ (1984) Internal transvenous low energy cardioversion for the treatment of cardiac arrhythmias. Br Heart J 52: 377–84

11. Hombach V, Höpp HW, Behrenbeck DW, Osterspey A, Jansen W, Winter U, Tauchert M, Hilger HH (1984) (Endocardial cardioversion – a new method for treating recurrent ventricular tachycardia.) Dtsch Med Wochenschr 109: 1443–8

12. Zipes DP, Heger JJ, Miles WM, Mahomed Y, Brown JW, Spielman SR, Prystowsky EN (1984) Early experience with an implantable cardioverter. N Engl J Med 311: 485–490

13. Zipes DP, Kallok MJ, Gill RM, Kammerling JM (1984) Efficacy of sequential electrical shocks to terminate ventricular fibrillation in dogs after myocardial infarction. (abstr) Circulation 70: 407

14. Jones DL, Klein GJ, Guiraudon GM, Sharma AD, Bourland JD, Tacker WA, Kallok MJ (1985) Improved internal cardiac defibrillation in man using sequential pulse countershock energy delivery. (abstr) J Am Coll Cardiol 5: 457

# The use of the automatic implantable cardioverter-defibrillator in ventricular tachycardias and fibrillation

M. MIROWSKI, E.P. VELTRI, M. MOWER, P.R. REID and
J.M. JUANTEGUY

## Summary

The automatic implantable cardioverter-defibrillator is an electronic device designed to continuously monitor the heart, identify malignant ventricular tachyarrhythmias, and then to deliver electrical countershock to restore normal heart rhythm. This device is composed of a pulse generator and two defibrillating electrodes, one located in the superior vena cava, the other over the cardiac apex; these electrodes are also used for waveform analysis. A third bipolar right ventricular electrode serves for rate counting and R-wave synchronization. The initial pulse has a 25-joule energy; if the discharge is not effective, the device can deliver up to three additional 30-joule pulses. In presence of ventricular tachycardia, the discharge is R-wave synchronized. To date, the device has been implanted in nearly 600 patients with a follow-up period up to 62 months. The risks and complications associated with this treatment modality were found to be acceptable. Actuarial analysis has demonstrated significant impact on the survival rate of the implantees, with one-year arrhythmic mortality rate reduced to 2% or less. The automatic cardioverter-defibrillator is capable of reliably identifying and correcting potentially lethal ventricular tachyarrhythmias and its use has resulted in a substantial improvement in survival in properly selected high-risk patients.

## Introduction

Sudden cardiac death is a major health problem in the developed countries of the world. In the United States alone, the number of victims is estimated to be approximately 450,000 annually, a casualty rate of one every 50 seconds. Approximately two-thirds of these victims die before reaching the hospital [1]. The available evidence indicates that the mechanism of death is arrhythmic and that the culprits in the vast majority of cases are ventricular tachycardia and/or fibrillation [2, 4]. Approaches used to deal with this problem include the identification of high-risk patients – particularly survivors of sudden cardiac death – patients with histories of recurrent sustained ventricular tachycardia, malignant ventricular arrhythmias in the late phase post-myocardial infarction period, severe left ventricular dysfunction, prolonged QT interval syndrome and/or other primary electrical disturbances of cardiac impulse generation and conduction [5–11]. The work-up for risk stratification involves continuous ambulatory electrocardiographic monitoring, exercise stress testing, invasive and noninvasive assessment of coronary anatomy and left ventricular function, and electrophysiologic evaluation. Within the community, educational programs geared toward comprehensive training in cardiopulmonary resuscitation and advanced life-support systems capable of responding expeditiously to life-threatening situations are being promoted [12].

Extensive research and development of new antiarrhythmic drugs have improved the treatment of malignant ventricular arrhythmias [13], although to date only beta-blockers (in the post-myocardial infarction population) appear to decrease the incidence of sudden cardiac death [14–16]. Even a drug as effective as amiodarone has a 10–20% incidence of failure at one year [17–19]. Also not withstanding, the effectiveness of antiarrhythmic drugs depends upon strict patient compliance in order to maintain protective blood concentration [20, 21]. These drugs, however, are fraught with side effects and may even have proarrhythmic effects in approximately 10% of patients [22, 23]. While acute and chronic drug testing in the electrophysiologic laboratory is rapidly replacing the traditional empirical approach [24–27], successful drug responses are found in only a minority of patients [28].

The management of malignant ventricular arrhythmia has recently been complemented by a number of innovative procedures such as subendocardial resection [29], encircling ventriculotomy [30], and fulguration techniques [31], all aimed at the eradication of arrhythmogenic foci. For optimum results, these procedures require identification of the sites of origin or of the perpetuating pathways of the tachyarrhythmias, as assessed by electrophysiologic study. Many patients, however, have poorly defined morphologic forms of ventricular tachyarrhythmias (pleomorphic ventricular tachycardia or ventricular fibrillation); therefore, the arrhythmias cannot be 'mapped' for definitive localization. Also, despite initially successful surgery, recurrences of arrhythmias are still noted in some 20% of patients and the mortality associated with the procedure itself is approximately 10% [32].

The inability to satisfactorily control ventricular tachyarrhythmias with pharmacologic and surgical means prompted the development of electronic devices – antitachycardia pacemakers, implantable cardioverters, and the implantable cardioverter-defibrillator [33–35]. These devices are being used with increasing frequency to detect and treat ventricular tachyarrhythmias. The main limitation of antitachycardia pacemakers and of implantable cardioverters, however, is the danger that they may accelerate the ventricular tachycardia or even induce ventricular fibrillation. In addition, these modalities are powerless in presence of ventricular fibrillation and they are unable to terminate a significant proportion of ventricular tachycardias. Today, the only implantable electronic device capable of treating the broad spectrum of ventricular tachyarrhythmias is the automatic implantable cardioverter-defibrillator (AICD).

The intent of this paper is to review the status of the ongoing clinical trials of the AICD with particular emphasis on the effect of this therapeutic intervention on the survival rates of implantees and its impact on future directions in the treatment of sudden cardiac death.

## Background

The development of an implantable electronic system with capabilities of recognition and termination of ventricular tachyarrhythmias was prompted by the difficulties in dealing with out-of-hospital cardiac arrests. While trans-thoracic delivery of a sufficiently strong electrical discharge to the heart frequently terminates the arrhythmia, the effectiveness of the countershock and resultant long-term clinical sequelae depend for the most part on the prompt availability of specialized personnel and equipment. The critical factor determining the chances of recovery from hemodynamically compromising sustained ventricular tachycardia and from ventricular fibrillation is the time that elapses between its onset and the delivery of effective countershock. In the absence of cardiopulmonary resuscitation this time usually cannot exceed two minutes which, in the majority of instances, is clearly insufficient for the victim to reach medical facilities or for a specialized rescue team to reach the stricken patient.

The implantable defibrillator*, a self-contained automatic diagnostic and therapeutic system, was initially designed to recognize and treat ventricular fibrillation. In February 1980, after more than a decade of research and preclinical testing, the first such device was implanted in a human being at The Johns Hopkins Hospital in Baltimore. More recently, a new generation of the device with additional cardioverting capabilities was introduced into clinical practice [36]. This implantable automatic cardioverter-defibrillator (AICD) continuously monitors cardiac electrical activity, recognizes the presence of a life-threatening ventricular tachyarrhythmia, and then promptly delivers electrical countershock to restore normal heart rhythm. Thus far, approximately 600 patients suffering from malignant ventricular arrhythmias have undergone implantation of this device.

---

* Developed and manufactured by Intec Systems, Inc., Pittsburgh, Pennsylvania, U.S.A., under the trademark AID.

## Characteristics of the device

### Pulse generator and leads

The AICD (Fig. 1) is composed of a pulse generator and leads. Housed in a titanium can, the pulse generator is hermetically sealed with a laser beam; it weighs 292 grams and occupies a volume of 162 cc. Specifically designed lithium batteries characterized by low resistance and high energy density provide between two and three years of monitoring life or can deliver approximately 100 discharges. The two defibrillating electrodes also serve as sensors. One, the anode, is incorporated into an intravascular catheter which is placed in the superior vena cava near the right atrial junction; the other electrode, the cathode, is a flexible rectangular patch designed for placement over the apex of the heart. A third catheter-lead, containing at its tip two close bipolar electrodes, serves for rate-counting and R-wave synchronization. This lead is usually wedged into the right ventricular apex by way of percutaneous intravascular access, although two epicardial screw-in electrodes may be inserted instead at time of thoracotomy. Also, not infrequently, in order to lower the defibrillation energy requirements, the defibrillating superior vena cava catheter electrode is replaced by another patch-electrode. The epicardial patch electrodes are available in two sizes and are usually placed on the opposite surfaces of the heart.

### Sensing mechanisms

Two sensing channels are used for the recognition of the malignant arrhythmia. One is the rate-detection channel, which utilizes local signals derived from the implanted bipolar right ventricular electrode. Using these signals, the device determines whether the QRS rate exceeds that of the preset rate cut-off value determined by the clinician for the individual patient. The second channel analyzes the morphology of the electrogram as sensed by the transcardiac defibrillating leads to determine whether there is a significant absence of isoelectric potential segments. This analysis is expressed in terms of the probability density function (PDF) of cardiac electrical activity. Since ventricular fibrillation and many ventricular tachycardias are characterized by the virtual absence of isoelectric potential segments, the time spent by the differentiated input electrogram near the baseline is markedly reduced.

While this dual sensing system is incorporated in the great majority of the AICD's, a few investigators prefer a variant of the device with a sensing algorithm that uses the rate channel only. Each of these models has its advantages and limitations. The dual detection scheme is less sensitive to supraventricular tachycardias but may miss certain nonsinusoidal, 'spiky' ventricular tachycardias. The 'rate only' system is able to correctly sense such 'spiky' tachycardias but, on

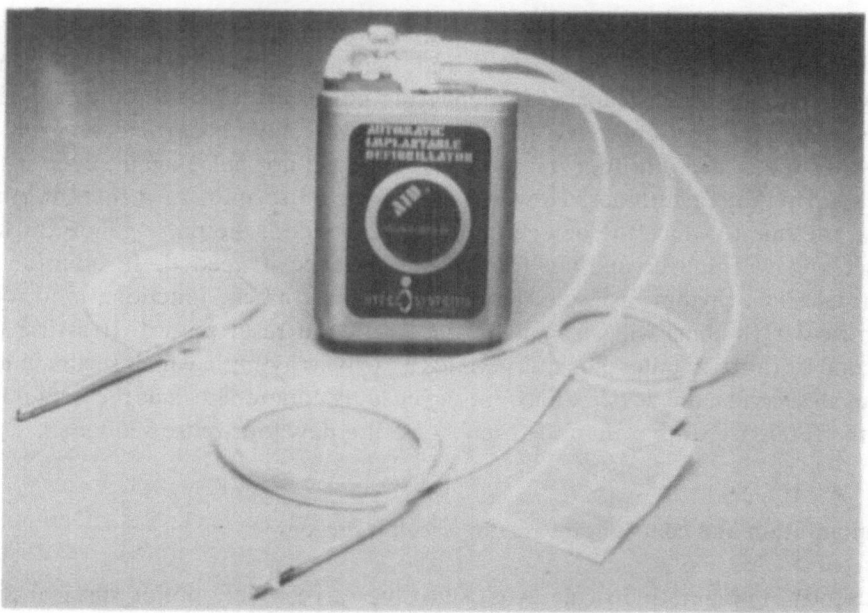

*Figure 1.* The automatic implantable cardioverter-defibrillator with, left to right, its superior vena cava, bipolar right ventricular, and apical patch electrodes. For more details, see text.

the other hand, will also react to supraventricular tachycardias with normal ventricular conduction which are faster than the device's predetermined threshold value. The 'rate only' device may therefore be indicated when a 'spiky' ventricular tachycardia is seen during perioperative testing, and certainly when a nondetection or a delayed detection occurs as a result of such morphology.

## Cardioversion-defibrillating mechanism

Once the rate and morphology criteria – a process which usually requires approximately 5 to 15 seconds – have been satisfied, the AICD makes the diagnosis of a 'treatable' arrhythmia. This initiates the capacitor charging cycle and when the voltage on the capacitors reaches approximately 720 volts, a truncated exponential pulse is delivered to the patient. The total time which elapses between the onset of the arrhythmia and the pulse delivery ranges between 10 and 35 seconds. The strength of the initial pulse is 25 joules and the pulse duration ranges between 3 and 8 milliseconds, as a function of the interelectrode resistance. When the detected arrhythmia is ventricular tachycardia, the cardioverting discharge is synchronized to the R-wave.

If the first discharge is ineffective, second, third, and even fourth countershocks can be delivered after additional individual detection and charging periods of 10 to 35 seconds; their energy is increased to 30 joules. Thus, the complete four-pulse sequence, if required, may last up to two minutes or more. Higher energy devices capable of delivering pulses of up to 40 joules are also available for the patient in whom defibrillating threshold is particularly high.

After the delivery of four pulses, the AICD will not pulse again, even if the tachyarrhythmia continues. However, following 35 seconds of a rhythm other than the one to which the detection circuit responded, the pulse generator will reset and will deliver another four-pulse sequence if needed. In addition to normal sinus rhythm, asystole, bradycardia, heart block, junctional and idio-ventricular rhythms will also satisfy the 35-second reset period. If a first (or second or third) countershock terminates a tachyarrhythmia which recurs in less than 35 seconds, the device will count the ensuing countershock as the next pulse of the sequence, rather than the first shock of a new four-pulse sequence.

**Implantation and concomitant cardiovascular surgery**

Presently, implantation of an AICD involves a relatively major surgical procedure because the placement of the apical patch requires entrance into the thoracic cavity. A number of techniques are available [37–40]. Left lateral thoracotomy is used for patients who have undergone previous thoracic surgery; this approach avoids dissecting through any residual scar tissue. Median sternotomy is used when the patient requires concomitant surgery such as coronary artery bypass grafting, valve replacement, aneurysmectomy, or subendocardial resection. In patients who have not had previous cardiac surgery, minimally invasive procedures via the subxiphoidal and subcostal approaches are used. However, at some centers, thoracotomy is preferred and routinely performed because it provides the best possible exposure for apical patch lead placement or for positioning the two patches sometimes necessary to achieve consistent defibrillation in patients with high energy requirements. Whichever technique is selected, the leads are then tunneled subcutaneously and connected to the pulse generator which is implanted in a paraumbilical pocket.

The implantation of the device involves, in addition to its surgical aspects, an intraoperative electrophysiologic evaluation aimed at selecting the most appropriate device and lead configuration to be used in a particular patient. For this purpose, a number of measurements, including the determination of the energy requirements for defibrillation, must be obtained. An external, non-automatic, cardioverter-defibrillator unit capable of delivering adjustable energy (ranging from one to 40 joules) is connected to the leads during surgery. By introducing low level alternating current (AC) into the heart, the non-automatic unit can then revert programmed stimulation or AC-induced sustained malignant arrhythmias [41]. The 'defibrillation threshold' is the amount of energy necessary to consistently revert these arrhythmias.

The system chosen for implantation is then attached with temporary lead wires to allow continuous recording of rate and transcardiac signals. The malignant arrhythmia is reinduced to ensure that the selected AICD is able to recognize and correct it automatically. The success rate after the first discharge is 90%, and virtually all patients convert after the second discharge. If the chosen system functions successfully, the temporary lead wires are replaced by permanent nylon caps to cover the set screws and the terminals are sealed.

During the final stages of implantation and also in the immediate postoperative period, the device is temporarily deactivated to avoid false triggering when cautery is in use or during rapid supraventricular arrhythmias which occur frequently during the early postoperative period.

At Hopkins, implantation of the AICD is combined, whenever indicated and feasible, with other cardiovascular procedures, especially with antiarrhythmic surgery. In the first 112 patients treated in this institution, 25 underwent subendocardial resection (many with aneurysmectomy and coronary artery bypass grafting), while another 13 patients had coronary artery bypass grafting alone. Approximately 20% of the Hopkins patients who had undergone subendocardial resection suffered recurrences of sustained malignant arrhythmias and thus benefited from the added protection afforded by the AICD that was implanted concomitantly [42]. The recurrences were attributed to either incomplete ablation of the arrhythmogenic mechanism or progression of the underlying disease process.

*Noninvasive function testing*

Techniques for noninvasive communication with the AICD prior to, during, and following implantation have also been developed. Basically, the device can be set in one of two modes, active or inactive. These modes are determined through the use of a magnet, and the status of the device is indicated by coded audio-signals generated by a built-in piezoelectric transducer. A similar technique also provides information about the integrity of the rate channel.

An external analyzer, the AIDCHECK* (Fig. 2), in conjunction with a probe transducer and magnet, is most helpful in indicating the degree of battery depletion, capaciter deformation and cumulative number of pulses delivered by the AICD to the patient.

---

* Developed and manufactured by Intec Systems, Inc., Pittsburgh, Pennsylvania, U.S.A., under the trademark AIDCHECK.

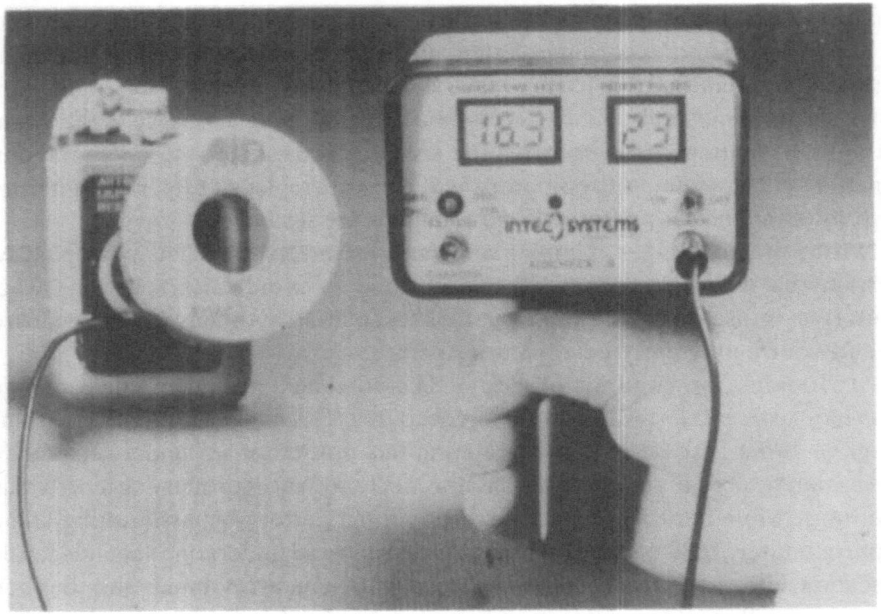

*Figure 2.* The defibrillator analyzer with a magnet and electro-magnetic transducer placed over the automatic defibrillator pulse generator. The digital display on the left indicates the capacitor charging time, while that on the right shows the number of discharges delivered by the device to the patient.

## The clinical program

The clinical evaluation study of the AICD, initially limited to the Johns Hopkins Hospital, soon extended to the Stanford University Hospital and then to additional institutions worldwide. By April 1, 1985, the total number of implantees was 571, with almost 7,000 pulse generator implant-months accumulated. The longest follow-up had been 62 months, and the mean follow-up slightly over 12 months.

The implantee population is comprised of patients who are at a very high risk of sudden cardiac death. Originally, the implantation criteria required that the potential implantees had 1) experienced at least two episodes of cardiac arrest, unassociated with acute myocardial infarction, acid-base or electrolyte abnormality, or drug toxicity and 2) failure of conventional drug therapy as assessed clinically or by programmed electrical stimulation. The current criteria have been somewhat relaxed in that only a single episode of arrhythmic cardiac arrest is required for inclusion into the study. Evidence of incomplete protection of the patients by antiarrhythmic drugs must also be documented. This incomplete protection is indicated by inducible ventricular tachycardia or fibrillation during programmed ventricular stimulation or the inability to suppress complex ventricular ectopy on Holter monitoring or during stress testing. Most of the potential implantees have evidence of severe left ventricular dysfunction; however, none are excluded from consideration for this reason.

The clinical profile of the patients treated with the AICD is quite typical. The great majority are survivors of recurrent cardiac death. They are predominantly male, their mean age is 53 years and the mean ejection fraction is approximately 33%. About 75% of these patients suffer from coronary artery disease and the underlying cardiac disease in the remaining quarter is predominantly non-ischemic, dilated, congestive cardiomyopathy. A few patients with primary electrical disease, long QT interval syndrome, congenital and valvular heart disease are also included. The patients had failed an average four antiarrhythmic drugs and many also had failed aggressive surgical therapy as well.

## Clinical benefits

### In-hospital setting

The clinical experience with the use of the AICD is now based on a follow-up of approximately 600 patients. Initially, the AICD's ability to perform its diagnostic monitoring and therapeutic functions was evaluated within the hospital setting. Numerous spontaeous malignant ventricular arrhythmias were documented in the hospital, and all patients had had similar arrhythmias induced during electrophysiologic studies. Figure 3 depicts induced ventricular fibrillation automatically converted by the device. Virtually all of the spontaneous and the overwhelming majority of the induced rhythms have been properly identified and converted to sinus rhythm by the implanted unit. A single shock was usually effective in terminating the arrhythmia, but occasionally, one or two recyclings were necessary to restore normal heart rhythm. Post-shock bradycardias were rare and transient.

The diagnostic accuracy of the device as determined in the electrophysiology laboratory is 99% for both ventricular tachycardia and ventricular fibrillation. The few instances of non-detection were usually due to lead fracture or malposition, 60-cycle interference, or interaction with a unipolar pacemaker. The average time between the onset of arrhythmia and its termination is 17 seconds. Acceleration of ventricular tachycardia to a faster rhythm or degeneration to fibrillation is occasionally noted, with subsequent successful handling of this problem by AICD recycling. This unique ability sets the AICD apart from other currently available implantable devices such as antitachycardia pacemakers or transvenous cardioverters.

538

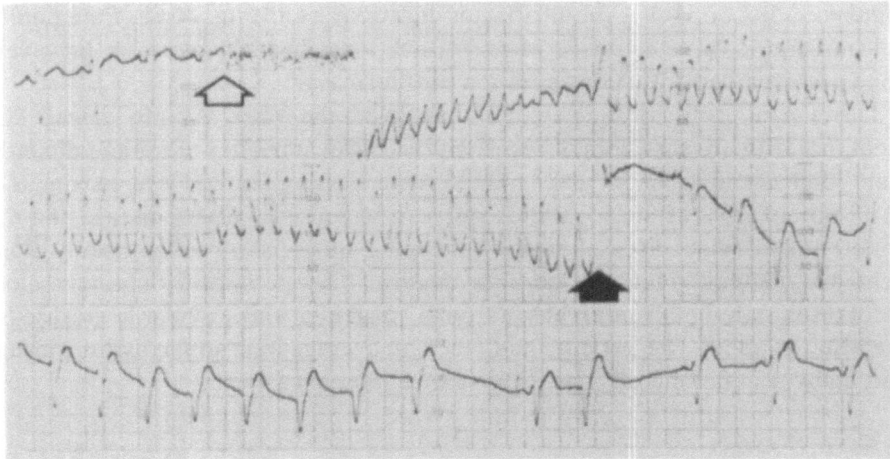

*Figure 3.* Automatic termination of induced ventricular flutter by the AICD. Open arrow: induction of the arrhythmia with low-level alternating current. Closed arrow: intracardiac countershock restores normal sinus rhythm. The strips are continuous.

## Out-of-hospital setting

Following their return to the community, many patients report symptoms indicative of recurrent malignant arrhythmias automatically terminated by their implanted AICD's. Because of the present difficulties in graphically documenting these events, the diagnosis of such out-of-hospital recurrences is frequently based on a characteristic sequence of events reported by the patient, his/her family, or by bystanders. Typically, palpitations and weakness are the initial symptoms, followed by dizziness or syncope and then by prompt evidence of internal discharge consisting of diffuse muscle contraction and immediate recovery accompanied by a feeling of well-being. Figure 4 depicts an out-of hospital episode of sustained ventricular tachycardia successfully converted by the AICD on continuous electrocardiographic recording. On several occasions, the exact nature of an internal discharge reported by the patient was not entirely clear and, in such instances, the remote possibility of a false-positive shock should always be considered.

The countershock itself is usually well-tolerated, even when the patient is in a conscious state. The subjective reactions range from lack of any perceptible sensations to a very painful shock. Most patients describe the event as a moderate blow to the chest resulting in a momentary discomfort.

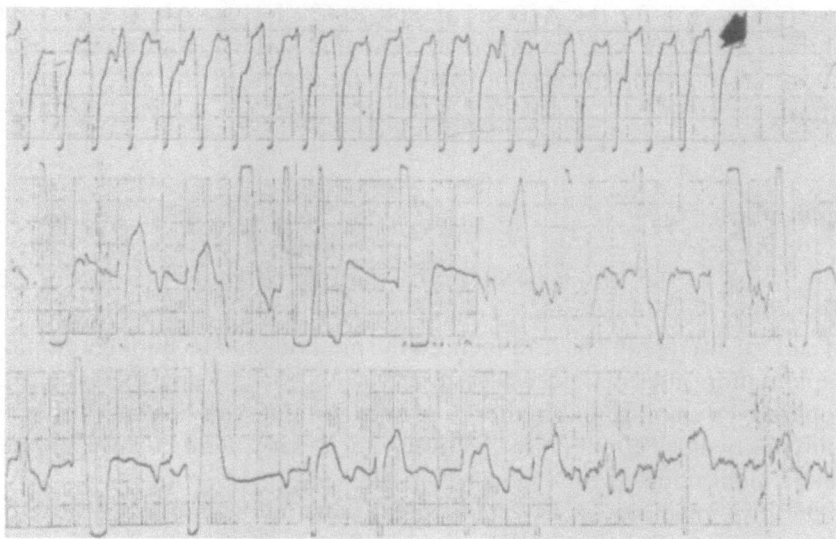

*Figure 4.* Mcnitoring strip recorded in the emergency room during a recurrent episode of hypotensive ventricular tachycardia. At the arrow, the automatic discharge was delivered. After a short period of frequent premature ventricular contractions, the underlying sinus mechanism is seen. (Reproduced with permission from the *American Heart Journal* 103: 147–148, 1982.)

## Effect on mortality

Because patients treated with this device are already at a very high risk of dying from ventricular tachyarrhythmias and given the substantial number of implantees, it is possible to determine the effect of this treatment modality on the survival rate of these patients. The initial information in this regard was derived from the analysis of the first 52 implantees (42 from Hopkins, 10 from Stanford); the great majority of these patients has received the original AID device [36]. The expected one-year mortality without the automatic defibrillator was calculated to be 48% compared to the actual 22.9% one-year mortality in the group. This indicated a 52% decrease in the anticipated incidence of death. The one-year sudden death mortality, assumed to be arrhythmic in origin, was only 8.5%.

More recently, in an attempt to compare the respective effectiveness of the first generation device (AID) to the AICD, 89 patients at Hopkins were divided into two groups according to the model they had received, and their mortality data were analyzed [43]. Patients whose early model was subsequently replaced with the AICD were transferred at that time from the AID group and entered a new into the AICD population. At one year, the mortality due to arrhythmias was 10.6% for the AID group and 2% for the AICD group. The total one-year mortality was 26% for the AID group and 16.6% for the AICD group. These results are consistent with the report by Echt et al [44] who found an arrhythmic one-year mortality of 1.8% in 70 patients treated with the AICD model at Stanford.

## Complications

So far, most of the problems observed during the study period have been satisfactorily resolved; however, a number of potential complications continue to be of clinical interest and have influenced the methods and technology employed.

Implantation involves extensive surgery with general anesthesia and thus, perioperative complications in these very sick patients can be expected to occur despite metriculous attention to electrolyte, acid-base, fluid balance and hemo-dynamic monitoring.

In our own initial series of 112 implantees, there has been one operative death due to perforation of the subclavian vein. Two patients with significant post-operative subcutaneous bleeding required transfusions. There have been two episodes of superior vena cava thrombosis which have resolved with anticoagula-tion therapy. Transient pleuropericardial friction rubs in the early postoperative period are the rule and sterile fluid accumulation in the pulse generator pocket of a few patients have been noted and uneventfully reabsorbed.

Infection, despite aseptic technique and prophylactic antibiotics during im-plantation, has occurred in six patients. In most instances, infection was traced to the pulse generator pocket, although in one case was related to an antecubital cut-down; the origin of infection was unknown in one other case. Though the patients responded fairly well to antibiotics, complete explantation of the system was necessary in two.

Lead dislodgement has been noted in seven patients with repositioning accom-plished without complication in all cases. Lead features, observed early in the study, have been virtually eliminated since the silver tinsel material used for fabrication of the leads was replaced with drawn brazed strands.

False-positive discharges may occur whenever the input signal satisfies the sensing algorithm of the device. In the early stages of the study, the most frequent mechanism was miscounting of the heart rate as sensed by the transcardiac electrodes. Therefore, a separate rate channel was added to the AICD, resulting in reliable determination of the heart rate except in instances of interaction with an implanted unipolar cardiac pacemaker. In the past, interference signals due to lead discontinuity also resulted in unwanted discharges, a problem that was solved by the above mentioned improvements in lead construction.

Spurious discharges may still occur in the presence of particularly rapid supra-ventricular arrhythmias that are faster than the rate threshold of 'rate only' devices. Some of these supraventricular arrhythmias might also satisfy the PDF sensing criteria of the device based on intrinsic intra-ventricular conduction delays or other rate-related morphologic changes, thereby leading to an unwarranted shock. Indeed, prior to discharge from the hospital after implantation, patients are routinely given an exercise stress test in order to evaluate such circumstances. Occasionally, these patients require a beta-blocker to limit the rate of the supraventricular tachycardia. Although still a concern, spurious shocks have never resulted in serious arrhythmias or long-term untoward effects.

Other potential problems involve creating and maintaining the appropriate milieu of patient, cardiac substrate, concurrent antiarrhythmic drug therapy and device – the so-called bio-electric interface [45]. These variables can profoundly affect the device's diagnostic and therapeutic function. More research is needed to evaluate the effects of drugs, electrolytes, and ischemia on the ability to cardiovert or defibrillate a tachyarrhythmia. Drugs, for instance, may either slow the rate of ventricular tachycardia or raise the defibrillating threshold, thereby interfering with the arrhythmia-sensing and terminating functions of the device, respectively.

## Conclusion

The automatic implantable cardioverter-defibrillator is an effective diagnostic-therapeutic system that reliably monitors cardiac electrical activity, recognizes malignant ventricular tachyarrhythmias, and terminates such arrhythmias promptly with effective transcardiac cardioverting or defibrillating countershock. An impressive decrease in arrhythmic mortality suggests its ultimate goal in prevention of a significant number of sudden cardiac deaths may be achievable. This modality represents a promising approach for patients who are at high risk for developing sustained ventricular tachyarrhythmias and in whom other available medical or surgical therapy is not completely effective.

## References

1. Lown B (1979) Sudden cardiac death: the major challenge confronting contemporary cardiology. Am J Cardiol 43: 313–328
2. Nikolic G, Bishop RL, Singh JB (1982) Sudden death recorded during holter monitoring. Circulation 66: 218–225
3. Panidis IP, Morganroth J (1983) Sudden death in hospitalized patients: cardiac rhythm disturbances detected by ambulatory electrocardiographic monitoring. J Am Coll Cardiol 2: 798–805
4. Kempf FC, Josephson ME (1984) Cardiac arrest recorded on ambulatory electrocardiograms. Am J Cardiol 53: 1577–1582
5. Liberthson RR, Nagel EL, Hirschman JC, Nussenfeld SR (1974) Prehospitalized ventricular defibrillation. Prognosis and follow-up course. N Engl J Med 291: 317–321
6. Schaffer WA, Cobb LA (1975) Recurrent ventricular fibrillation and modes of death in survivors of out-of-hospital ventricular fibrillation. New Engl J Med 293: 259–262

7. Swerdlow CD, Winkle RA, Mason JW (1983) Determinants of survival in patients with ventricular tachyarrhythmias. N Engl J Med 308: 1436–42
8. Bigger JT, Weld FM, Rolnitsky LM (1981) Prevalence, characteristics and significance of ventricular tachycardia (three or more complexes) detected with ambulatory electrocardiographic recording in the late hospital phase of acute myocardial infarction (1981) Am J Cardiol 48: 815–823
9. Follansbee WP, Michelson EL, Morganroth J (1980) Nonsustained ventricular tachycardia in ambulatory patients: characteristics and association with sudden cardiac death. Ann Int Med 92: 741–747
10. Moss AJ, Schwartz PJ, Crampton RS, Locati E, Carleen E (1985) The long QT syndrome: a prospective international study. Circulation 71: 17–21
11. Warren JV (1982) Critical issues in the sudden death syndrome. In: Cardiology series, Baylor College of Medicine 5: 6–23
12. Thompson RG, Hallstron AP, Cobb LA (1979) Bystander-initiated cardiopulmonary resuscitation in the management of ventricular fibrillation. Ann Intern Med 90: 737–740
13. Zipes DC, Troup PJ (1978) New antiarrhythmic agents: amiodarone, aprindine, disopyramide, ethmozin, mexiletine, tocainide, verapamil. Am J Cardiol 41: 1005–1024
14. The Norwegian Multicenter Study Group (1981) Timolol-induced reduction in mortality and reinfarction in patients surviving acute myocardial infarction. N Engl J Med 304: 801–807
15. Beta-Blocker Heart Attack Research Group (1981) A randomized trial of propanolol in patients with acute myocardial infarction. I. Mortality results. J Am Med Assoc 247: 1707–1714
16. Hjalmarson A, Elmfeldt D, Herlitz J, et al (1981) Effect on mortality of metroprolol in acute myocardial infarction. A double-blind randomized trial. Lancet 11: 823–827
17. Morady F, Sauve MJ, Malone P, et al (1983) Long-term efficacy and toxicity of high-dose amiodarone therapy for ventricular tachycardia or ventricular fibrillation. Am J Cardiol 52: 975–979
18. Green HL, Graham EL, Werner JA, et al (1983) Toxic and therapeutic effects of amiodarone in the treatment of cardiac arrhythmia. J Am Coll Cardiol 2: 1114–28
19. Peter T, Hamer A, Weiss D, Mandel WJ (1984) Prognosis after sudden cardiac death without associated myocardial infarction: one year follow-up of empiric therapy with amiodarone. Am Heart J 107: 209–213
20. Myerburg RJ, Conde C, Sheps DS, et al (1979) Anti-arrhythmic drug therapy in survivors of prehospital cardiac arrest: comparison of effects on chronic ventricular arrhythmias and recurrent cardiac arrest. Circulation 59: 855–863
21. Vlay SC, Kallman CH, Reid PR (1985) The utility of aprindine blood levels in the management of ventricular arrhythmias. J Am Coll Cardiol 5: 738–743
22. Velebit V, Podrid P, Lown B, Cohen BH, Graboys TB (1992) Aggravation and provocation of ventricular arrhythmias by antiarrhythmic drugs. Circulation 65: 886–894
23. Ruskin JN, McGovern V, Garan H, DiMarco JP, Kelly E (1983) Antiarrhythmic drugs: a possible cause of out-of-hospital cardiac arrest. N Engl J Med 309: 1302–1306
24. Fisher JD, Cohen HL, Mehra R, Altschuler H, Escher DJW, Furman S (1977) Cardiac pacing and pacemaker II. Serial electrophysiologic-pharmacologic testing for control of recurrent tachyarrhythmias. Am Heart J 93: 658–668
25. Mason JW, Winkle RA (1978) Electrode-catheter arrhythmia induction in the selection and assessment of antiarrhythmic drug therapy for recurrent ventricular tachycardia. Circulation 58: 971–985
26. Horowitz LN, Josephson ME, Farshidi A, Spielman SR, Michelson EL, Greenspan AM (1978) Recurrent sustained ventricular tachycardia. 3. Role of the electrophysiologic study in selection of antiarrhythmic regimens. Circulation 58: 986–997
27. Ruskin JN, DiMarco JP, Garan H (1980) Out-of-hospital cardiac arrest. Electrophysiologic observations and selection of long-term antiarrhythmic therapy. N Engl J Med 303: 607–613
28. Waxman HL, Buxton AE, Sadowski LM, Josephson ME (1983) The response to procainamide

during electrophysiologic study for sustained ventricular tachyarrhythmias predicts the response to other medications. Circulation 67: 30–37

29. Josephson ME, Markin AC, Horowitz LN (1979) Endocardial excision. A new surgical technique for the treatment of recurrent ventricular tachycardia. Circulation 60: 1430–9

30. Guiraudon G, Fontaine F, Frank R, Esconde G, Etievent P, Cabrol C (1978) Encircling endocardiol ventriculotomy: a new surgical treatment for life-threatening ventricular tachycardia resistant to medical treatment following myocardial infarction. Ann Thorac Surg 26: 438–444

31. Hartzler GO (1983) Electrode catheter ablation of refractory focal ventricular tachycardia. J Am Coll Cardiol 2: 1107–1113

32. Miller JM, Kienzle MG, Harken AH, Josephson ME (1984) Subendocardial resection for ventricular tachycardia: predictors of surgical success. Circulation 70: 624–631

33. Fischer JD, Kim SG, Furman S, Matos JA (1982) Role of implantable pacemakers in control of recurrent ventricular tachycardia. Am J Cardiol 49: 194–206

34. Zipes D, Heger JJ, Miles WM, et al (1984) Early experience with an implantable cardioverter. N Engl J Med 311: 485–490

35. Mirowski M, Ried PR, Mower MM, et al (1980) Termination of malignant ventricular arrhythmias with an implanted automatic defibrillator in human beings. N Engl J Med 303: 322–324

36. Mirowski M, Reid PR, Winkle RA, et al (1983) Mortality in patients with implanted automatic defibrillators. Ann Int Med 98: 585–588

37. Watkins L Jr, Mirowski M, Mower MM, et al (1981) Automatic defibrillation in man: the initial surgical experience. J Thorac Cardiovasc Surg 82: 492–500

38. Watkins L Jr, Mirowski M, Mower MM, et al (1982) Implantation of the automatic defibrillator: the subxiphoidal approach. Ann Thorac Surg 34: 515–520

39. Lawrie GM, Griffin JC, Wyndham CRC (1984) Epicardial implantation of the automatic implantable defibrillator by left subcostal thoracotomy. PACE 7: 1370–1374

40. Brodman R, Fischer JD, Furman S, et al (1984) Implantation of automatic cardioverter-defibrillators via median sternotomy. PACE 7: 1363–1369

41. Mower MM, Reid PR, Watkins L Jr, Mirowski M (1983) Use of alternating current during diagnostic electrophysiologic studies. Circulation 67: 69–72

42. Platia EV, Reid PR, Watkins L, Mower MM, Mirowski M, Griffith LSC (1984) Endocardial resection combined with automatic cardioverter-defibrillator implantation in patients with malignant ventricular tachycardias: late follow-up. Circulation 70 (Suppl II): II-413

43. Reid PR, Mower MM, Griffith LSC, et al (1984) Comparative effects on mortality of the first and second generation implantable defibrillators. Circulation 70 (Suppl II): II-101

44. Echt DS, Armstrong K, Schmidt P, Oyer P, Stinson EB, Winkle RA (1985) Clinical experience, complications, and survival in 70 patients with the automatic implantable cardioverter/defibrillator. Circulation 71: 289–296

45. Reid PR, Mower MM, Mirowski M (1984) Pathophysiology of ventricular tachyarrhythmias amenable to electric control. PACE 7: 505–513

# Endocardial fulguration in the treatment of resistant chronic ventricular tachycardia*

G. FONTAINE, R. FRANK, J.L. TONET, G. FARENQ
and Y. GROSGOGEAT

## Introduction

Management of chronic ventricular tachycardia (VT) is generally performed by anti-arrhythmic drug therapy. In rare cases anti-tachycardia pacemakers, cardioverters, or implantable defibrillators are considered; antitachycardia surgery by encircling endocardial ventriculotomy or endocardial excision being resorted to as an alternative the purpose of which is to modify the arrhythmogenic substrate in such a way that arrhythmia is no longer possible. In most of the cases however surgery is attempted only when the previous methods prove inadequate.

Endocavitary fulguration (electrode-catheter ablation), is a well-established technique in the treatment of certain supraventricular tachycardias [1–3]. This technique has been recently extended to the management of chronic recurrent VT [4–7]. In this approach the basic principle is to send the electrical energy provided by a conventional external defibrillator to the distal electrode of a catheter positioned at the site of the VT focus. This report concerns our preliminary clinical results in this field.

## Material and methods

### Clinical series

Comprised of 22 cases (18 males, 4 females) our clinical series included subjects between the ages of 14 to 75 (mean age: 45 ± 19). Their main clinical features are presented in Table I.

The pathogenesis of the cases of VT comprising the study is diverse, including: 9 cases of arrhythmogenic ventricular dysplasia; 7 cases of VT following myocar-

* Supported in part by grants from: Le Centre de Recherche sur les Maladies Cardiovasculaires de l'Association Claude Bernard.

Table I.

| | Age | SX | Path | LOC | FC | EF | IVT | NbMOR | NB | SI | LI | NCL | IF | Nb | ENERG | EPS | DRUG | IDT | IOD | RES | FLWUP |
|---|---|---|---|---|---|---|---|---|---|---|---|---|---|---|---|---|---|---|---|---|---|
| 1 CORM | 60 | M | MI | ANTSEP | 2 | <30% | 1 | 2 | >20 | <D | I | 0 | INCES | II | 260*1 | NI | AMIO | PRO | NP | OK | 23M |
| 2 BANT | 29 | M | | INF | 1 | 42% | 24 | 2 | 4 | M | M | 0 | PAROX | III | 160*6 | MC | A+Pr | TH | NP | OK | 11M |
| 3 BEC | 75 | M | | ANTSEP | 2 | <30% | 1 | 1 | 20 | <D | I | 1 | INCES | II | 160*1 | NP | AMIO | PRO | NP | OK | 15M |
| 4 GALI | 65 | M | | ANTSEP | 2 | – | 1 | 1 | 2 | D | W | 2 | MP | IV | 160*5 | NI | AMIO | PRO | NI | OK | 14M |
| 5 HOUS | 55 | M | | DIAPHR | 1 | – | 12 | 1 | 10 | M | M | 2 | PAROX | II | 240*2 | NI | AMIO | TH | NI | FAIL | 8M |
| 6 ZAIE | 60 | M | | ANTSEP | 3 | 25% | 24 | 1 | 10 | M | M | 1 | PAROX | ? | 240*2 | NP | ? | ? | ? | DC | DC4D |
| 7 FORT | 67 | M | | ANTSEP | 3 | <25% | 1 | 1 | 2 | <D | M | 0 | MP | ? | 240*2 | NP | AMIO | PRO | NP | OK | DC1M |
| 8 POLC | 18 | M | IDCM | ANTSEP | 2 | <30% | 12 | 1 | >20 | M | I | 0 | INCES | II | 260*5 | 0 | AMIO | TH | NI | OK | DC14M |
| 9 MANI | 14 | F | | SEPTLV | 3 | <20% | 168 | 1 | >20 | I | I | 0 | INCES | III | 160*3 | 0 | 0 | 0 | NP | OK | DC2M |
| 10 LECA | 56 | M | | LV | 2 | 20% | 36 | 1 | 6 | Y | M | 2 | PAROX | II | 240*3 | NI | AMIO | PRO | NI | OK | 11M |
| 11 DROU | 22 | M | IDIO | POSTSEP | 1 | – | 60 | 1 | >20 | M | W | 0 | PAROX | ? | 240*2 | ? | 0 | 0 | NP | OK | 11M |
| 12 RAGA | 53 | F | IDIO | INFUN | 1 | 59% | 96 | 1 | >20 | M | D | 0 | INCES | II | 240*2 | NI | 0 | 0 | NI | OK | 11M |
| 13 DUVA | 35 | M | ARVD | DIAPH | 1 | – | >20 | 1 | <2 | M | – | 1 | PAROX | I | 240*1 | ? | ? | ? | NP | DC | DCOD |
| 14 CARO | 62 | F | | DIAPH | 2 | – | 36 | 1 | >20 | M | W | 1 | PAROX | I | 160*5 | MC | 0 | 0 | MC | OK | 17M |
| 15 GENS | 74 | M | | INFUN | 2 | 52% | 12 | 1 | 3 | M | M | 0 | PAROX | I | 160*1 | NI | AMIO | PRO | NI | OK | 16M |
| 16 NAIT | 37 | M | | DIAPH | 1 | 58% | 6 | 1 | 3 | <D | M | 0 | PAROX | II | 240*6 | M | 0 | 0 | NI | OK | 13M |
| 17 MICH | 27 | M | | DIAPH | 5 | 25% | 20 | 5 | 6 | Y | I | 0 | INCES | IV | 160*17 | MC | – | – | NP | OK | DC8D |
| 18 GELI | 56 | M | | ANTSEP | 1 | 45% | 84 | 3 | >20 | Y | M | 2 | PAROX | II | 240*4 | MC | A+Pr | TH | IN | FAIL | 4M |
| 19 MORA | 41 | F | | INFUN | 1 | 59% | 48 | 2 | 10 | M | M | 1 | PAROX | II | 240*1 | TL | 0 | 0 | MC | OK | 7M |
| 20 BARB | 32 | M | | INFUN | 1 | – | 4 | 1 | 2 | <D | W | 0 | PAROX | I | 210*4 | TL | AMIO | PRO | NI | OK | 10M |
| 21 CORA | 30 | M | | FR WA | 1 | 28% | 12 | 1 | 2 | M | M | 0 | MP | I | 240*3 | TL | A+Fl | PRO | IN | FAIL | 10M |
| 22 MOIR | 21 | M | CONG | INFUN | 1 | 61% | 120 | 2 | >20 | M | D | 2 | ESV | I | 240*4 | NI | 0 | 0 | NP | OK | 16M |

545

dial infarction (with a minimum 3 weeks, maximum 20 years after initial event); 3 cases of non obstructive cardiomyopathy; 1 case of VT after correction of a congenital anomaly; 2 cases of idiopathic VT (right-sided in one case, left-sided in the other).

*Patient selection*

Patients were high risk cases referred for evaluation mainly in the scope of antiarrhythmic cardiovascular surgery.

The vast majority of these patients were restudied with investigationnal drugs before considering a fulguration procedure. It occurred that about one third of these patients were in fact appropriately managed by drugs including amiodarone given alone or in combination with class I antiarrhythmic agents. The most extensively studied drugs of this latter category being flecainide and propafenone.

Fulguration was finally decided: when drug management was ineffective (study included a mean value of at least four antiarrhythmic drugs), when effective drugs had unacceptable side effects, when effective drugs were not available in the country of patient origin and finally in case of noncompliance.

*VT features*

The first episode of VT varied in a wide range extending from 1 to 168 months (mean $40 \pm 48$ months). The number of attacks varied largely, some patients having only two, others having experienced inummerable episodes. The shortest and the longest interval between two consecutive episodes were also considered (Table I).

Clinical VT morphologies varied from one to five. Non-clinical VT were observed in some patients, these tachycardias were not always considered for fulguration.

The follow-up period ranged from 4 to 23 months (mean: $12 \pm 4,5$ months).

*Methods*

Class I anti-arrhythmic therapy was discontinued 48 hours before the procedure. Fulguration was performed under general anesthesia, since it is usually necessary to perform several consecutive fulgurations during the same procedure.

The main hemodynamic parameters were monitored by radial blood pressure. Pulmonary capillary blood pressure was also monitored with a Swan-Ganz catheter permitting simultaneous measurement of blood gases and cardiac output using thermodilution techniques.

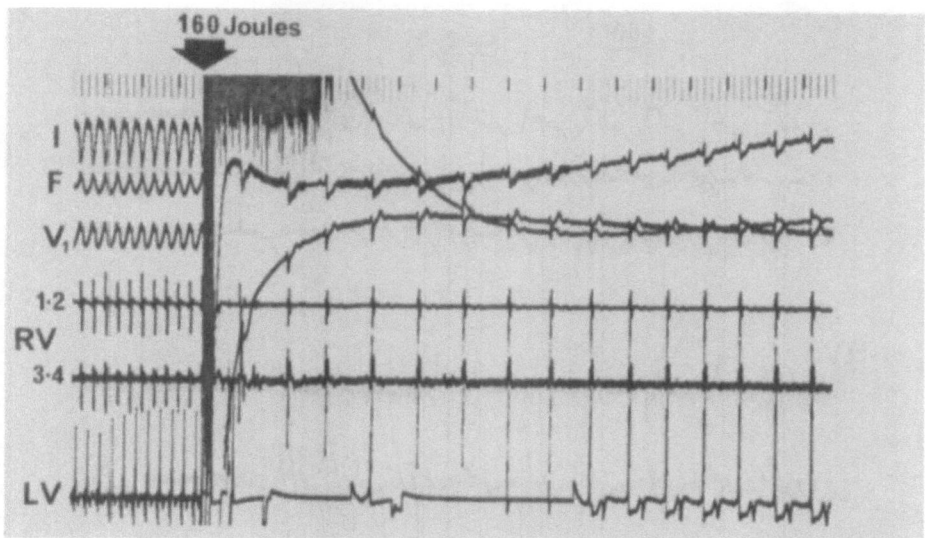

*Figure 1.* Endocardial shock of 160 Joules delivered inside the left ventricle in the area of ventricular tachycardia, origin. After the shock, sinus rhythm resumes with a transient ST segment elevation. From top to bottom: Surface leads (I, aVF, V1); endocardial quadripolar lead in the right ventricle (1–2, 3–4); LV, left ventricular lead also used for fulguration.

When non spontaneously present (incessant VT was observed in 6 cases), VT was induced by programmed pacing. Endocardial mapping was effected to localize the presumed origin of VT. Generally, we attempted to confirm the site of VT origin by pacemapping in sinus rhythm and during VT by single stimulus programmed pacing to duplicate the VT morphology [8].

The shock was synchronised on QRS complexes, either in sinus rhythm or during VT (Fig. 1). The shock was in all of the cases delivered between the distal electrode (being the anode) of the same catheter used for endocardial mapping and a back plate covered with conductive jelly (being the cathode). Pre-selected from experimental laboratory data, the energy is provided by discharges of 160 to 320 delivered Joules (mean 215 ± 40 SD) obtained with a modified defibrillator (ODAM, Defigard 5, Wissembourg, France).

After a 10-minute rest period, programmed stimulation was resumed to reinduce VT. The procedure was terminated when one of the following conditions occurred: (a) it was no longer possible to reinduce VT with programmed pacing; (b) VT was non sustained (lasting no more than 30 seconds) (Fig. 2); (c) a nonclinical VT (VT different from the spontaneous documented episodes) was observed [7].

A left subclavian endocardial catheter positionned at the apex of the right ventricle was left in place for the performance of a new series of programmed pacing tests 10 days following the procedure.

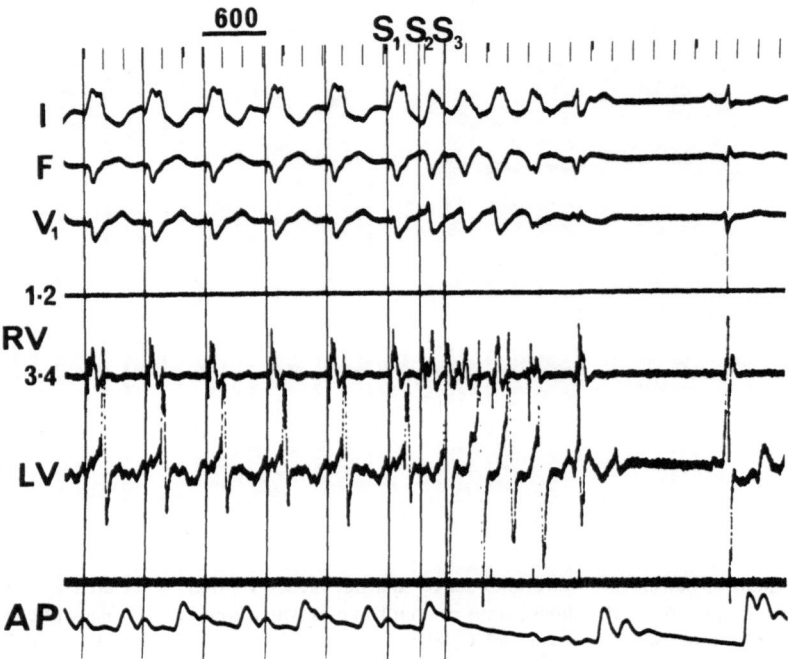

*Figure 2.* Programmed pacing stimulation performed at the end of the fulguration procedure. It is delivered at the tip of the right ventricular catheter 1–2, on the basic cycle length of 600 ms (100 bpm). Two premature stimulations S2–S3 are introduced, leading to a run of non sustained ventricular tachycardia. The bottom tracing (AP) represents a radial blood pressure measurement.

In cases where clinical VT reoccurred or was induced by programmed pacing, class I anti-arrhythmic treatment was readministered; when the latter proved ineffective, a new session of fulguration was advocated. Most of these patients had been treated by amiodarone therapy prior to the procedure, and this treatment was generally continued for a minimum period, particularly in cases where the VT were life-threatening. Table I indicates the anti-arrhythmic treatment given at the last follow-up.

## Results

The overall results are dramatic. Satisfactory prevention of VT was obtained in 85% of cases (17/20): (a) by means of the fulguration procedure alone in 7 cases; (b) followed up by prophylactic anti-arrhythmic treatment in 8 cases and therapeutic in 4 cases. However, one or several additional procedures were needed during the same hospital stay in 8 out of 20 cases. Rehospitalisation was required in 2 additional cases. It should be noted that 3 patients were moribond and 2 were unconscious when the last attempt was decided.

*Mortality*

No arrhythmia provoked death was observed. Three early deaths (death before 1 month) were observed at the beginning of our experience. One (N° 13) related to low cardiac output due to lack of blood pressure monitoring during endocardial mapping of VT in a patient with arrhythmogenic right ventricular dysplasia successfully operated 7 years previously. The patient had recently presented new episodes of life-threatening sustained recurrent VT at 240 b/mn. The second early death was also related to an inappropriate instant modification of the ana-esthesiologic protocol. This patient (N° 6) presenting with VT following myocar-dial infarction, had been previously rejected as a surgical candidate because of a very low ejection fraction. Cardiac arrest with a long period of low cardiac output led to irreversible brain damage and death 4 days after the fulguration procedure.

The third case (N° 17) presenting with a major form of arrhythmogenic right ventricular dysplasia was referred after multiple episodes of rapid VT occurring after angiography. This patient was unconscious and in permanent VT at the time of admission in our department. A series of 17 low-energy shocks (160 Joules) made it possible to slow down the cardiac rhythm, subsequently followed by disappearance of the VT. Although pulmonary complications of unknown origin already present before fulguration led to the death of the patient 8 days later, there was no recurrence of VT.

The anatomical and histological studies available in the first and the last case only showed modifications of the endocardium similar to those observed follow-ing endocavitary shocks in experimental studies (Fig. 3) superimposed on the particular pattern of arrhythmogenic right ventricular dysplasia.

Three late deaths were observed. In the first case (N° 7), death occurred one month after discharge and was due to pulmonary oedema. This patient, beyond operability, had a three-vessel disease and a low ejection fraction after myocar-dial infarction. Prior to fulguration, he had presented numerous episodes of cardiac failure and pulmonary oedema, two of them resulting in VT. Although both conditions reappeared after the fulguration procedure, they were not ac-companied by VT.

The second case of late death (N° 9) was a patient with non-obstructive cardiomyopathy who died of pulmonary oedema without recurrence of VT two months after the fulguration procedure.

The third case of late death (N° 8) was a patient presenting with familial congestive cardiomyopathy, and manifesting permanent intractable mono-morphic VT upon admission. Fulguration, followed by amiodarone treatment (recurrence of nondocumented VT one month after fulguration), succeeded in preventing VT for a 14 month period; death finally ensued, however, due to heart failure (low cardiac output).

In none of the cases did fulguration appear to be a precipitating factor but seemed to be the final deterioration of a preexisting precarious underlying heart condition.

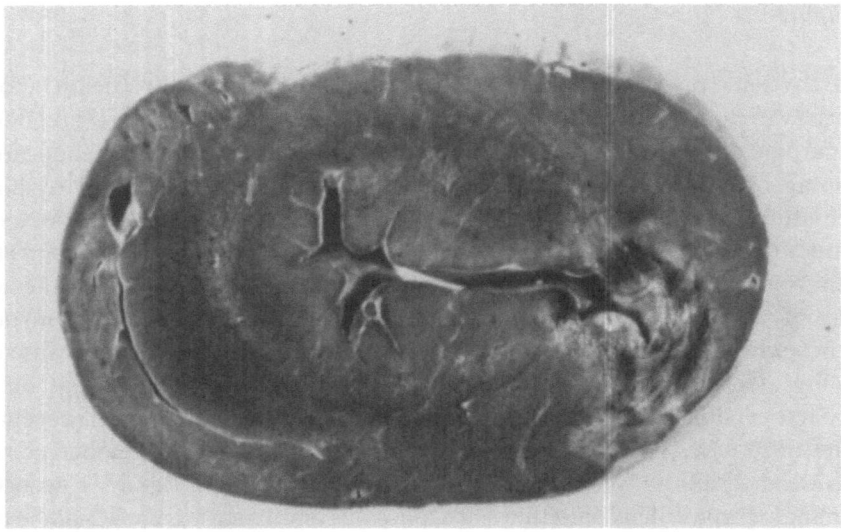

*Figure 3.* Experimental study showing the result of one shock of 320 Joules and one of 240 Joules, delivered in the left ventricle of a pig of 80 Kg. Heart weights 357 gr. Note the transmural scar of the lateral part of the left ventricle. Despite the fact that the specimen was obtained one month after fulguration, it remains still unstabilised signs of hemorrage.

## Recurrences

Recurrent episodes of VT having the same morphology, rhythm and duration as those of the documented recordings were observed in 9/20 cases (45%). A second fulguration procedure was performed in 9 cases; three procedures were carried out in 1 patient, and four in 2 patients.

Although the last-performed procedure was unsuccessful in 3 patients (N° 5, 18, 21), the arrhythmia in one of these patients (N° 5) has since been brought under control despite several further episodes and after 5 months no recurrence of VT has been recorded.

The two remaining patients partially controlled by anti-arrhythmic drugs are scheduled for a new fulguration procedure in case of worsening of their arrhythmias. Two others (N° 2, 8) have been successfully brought under control by previously ineffective anti-arrhythmic therapy.

## Complications

Besides the previously mentioned two cases of low output failure due to inappropriate protocols, pulmonary oedema was observed in two patients (N° 3, 5). It occurred in both cases ten minutes after the fulguration procedure; the oedema was however successfully brought under control using routine methods.

In one case (N° 18) precordial chest pain was observed during the second fulguration session, with ST segment modification and transient right bundle branch block during manipulation of the catheter in the cross of the aorta. In this patient, the increase in the CPK and CPK MB fraction was higher than the value recorded in the other cases.

A transient high grade atrioventricular block was observed in some cases (N° 1, 3) but disappeared after merely a 2-hour rest in the most difficult of these cases (N° 3). Transient intraventricular conduction defects were also observed in other patients. Ventricular arrhythmia in the form of VT acceleration or fibrillation was also observed in some cases immediately following the shock. They were easily corrected by external shock applied with the help of an anteriorly located patch defibrillating electrode, the back paddle being the same as the indifferent electrode used for fulguration.

The evolution of each patient was computer-monitored following fulguration. During the 10-day re-evaluation period, no case of severe arrhythmia were observed, and in particular, no case of VT aggravation nor ventricular fibrillation.

## Discussion

The first reported VT catheter ablation was practised in the infundibular area in a patient having undergone unsuccessful antiarrhythmic surgical attempts, and in two cases of VT complicating the chronic phase of myocardial infarction [4].

An additional case of resistant VT, complicating an arrhythmogenic right ventricular dysplasia successfully treated by fulguration, was also reported by PUECH [9].

### Successful results

In case of permanent VT, as well as VT occurring several times daily, the result of fulguration is easily evaluated. The evaluation becomes more difficult however, when the attacks are less frequent. For this reason, our study is limited to the 22 cases (out of the 31 patients having undergone fulguration procedure in our department) with a minimum follow-up of 4 months since the last fulguration procedure; the latter being equal to or exceeding the longest interval between episodes recorded during the months preceding to referral.

Although our study is limited to a small number of cases with only a short follow-up to date, it is clear from the above results that the fulguration technique may represent a definite contribution to the treatment of resistant cases of VT. It is interesting to note that in at least 3 cases (N° 1, 3, 15) a single shock with an amplitude extending from 160 to 240 Joules was enough to prevent on the long run, life-threatening VT.

The risks of the fulguration procedure appear minimal. Three of the patients fulgurated (N° 6, 7, 17) had been rejected as candidates for a surgical intervention. Moreover, three patients (N° 1, 3, 17) were moribond at the time an effective fulguration procedure was performed and at least 8 cases had an ejection fraction below 30%.

*Mortality*

In two patients (N° 6, 13) we believe that the outcome could have been avoided. In three other cases (N° 7, 9, 17) death was the result of the evolution of the underlying disease. In one of the latter the patient (N° 17) was unconscious at the arrival and death was due to a major hypoxia of unknown mechanism; in the two remaining latter cases (N° 7, 9), the deterioration of the clinical condition was already clinically observed in the period preceding the fulguration procedure.

*Recurrences*

In some patients, the ineffectiveness of the procedure was the result of technical failures: it has been observed that some catheters fail to transmit the full voltage and current necessary for the procedure [10] (N° 1, 20, 21). In the other cases, we could suggest that the endocavitary mapping during VT and sinus rhythm was not sufficiently precise to permit ablation of the arrhythmogenic site. Thus the main drawback of the fulguration technique appears to be due to the technical weaknesses of available equipment, and the difficulty encountered in mapping the endocardium with adequate precision. Also, it may be argued that in certain cases the area modified by the shock was not large enough to alter the arrhythmogenic substrate in such a way that propagation of the abnormal activation was prevented. The low values of CPK and CPK MB are an indication that, as already suggested by experimental studies, the fulguration procedure produces only minor myocardial injury. Consequently, it would appear indicated to reattempt fulguration after one or more previous unsuccessful sessions.

In cases where anti-arrhythmic treatment had previously proven ineffective, even a fulguration with only partial success is capable of rendering anti-arrhythmic therapy at last effective, thus leading to satisfactory control of the arrhythmia (N° 2, 5, 8).

However, many basic points remain to be clarified: the precise mechanism involved in the fulguration process; positioning of the indifferent electrode; selection of optimal electric parameters; size and shape of the fulgurating electrodes, criteria for locating the point of origin of VT.

*Side effects*

Possible secondary effects of the fulguration procedure include a brief but severe dilatation of the ventricular cavity during the blast occurring at the tip of the distal electrode. Some recent data provided by the experimental laboratory suggest that after the endocavitary fulguration applied in sinus rhythm to a normal heart (pig of 80 kg). it is possible to observe a drop in cardiac output of approximately 15%, requiring a recovery period of about 10 minutes. The latter phenomenon probably explains the pulmonary oedema observed in two patients, notably in one of them (N° 3) where for technical reasons the first fulguration attempt was performed in an almost normal myocardium.

Episodes of ventricular fibrillation or acceleration of VT were in some cases observed immediately after the fulguration procedure. Successfully converted by external shocks, they demonstrate the necessity of pre-connecting an independant defibrillator to an adhesive anterior patch electrodes, avoiding the time lost in moving the sterile surgical fields and X-Ray equipment.

No aggravation of the arrhythmia was however observed during the early follow-up period. This suggests that fulguration practised according to the technique described above is not of itself arrhythmogenic, contrary to the results obtained in certain experimental studies [11]. The myocardial infarction observed in one of our cases (N° 18) was not a consequence of the fulguration procedure per se, but resulted from difficulties encountered in manipulating the catheter in the cross of the aorta. Our technique has been modified to eliminate this difficulty.

The pacemaker of one patient needed to be replaced. The high voltage endocavitary shock, delivered in proximity to the pacemaker electrode, possibly either destroyed the pacemaker circuits or modified the interface between the pacemaker electrode tip and the myocardium [12].

*Technical difficulties*

This series does not afford conclusive evidence that the fulguration procedure succeeded in focusing exclusively upon the arrhythmogenic site since no last resort surgical intervention permitting such verification was ulteriorly attempted.

According to our study, it would appear that potentials recorded during VT at the onset of the QR complexes or after, are not reliable markers. Presystolic potential (recorded several tenths of ms. before the onset of the QRS complexes during VT) appears to be a better indicator; even the latter technique, however, is not totally statisfactory.

One case (N° 5) of spontaneously favorable evolution of the arrhythmogenic substratum following the fulguration procedure was observed. A possible late effect of fulguration in this case is still debated. Therefore, it remains to be determined whether, for optimal reevaluation, it is appropriate to control the

554

results immediately upon termination of the procedure or wait ten days or more.

As stated by others, the present pacemapping technique has certain limitations [13]. Pacemapping did nevertheless allow, in one case (N° 11), duplication of the morphology of the VT in a patient in whom arrhythmia could not be induced at the time of the procedure and the following fulgurations proved to be effective with a follow-up of eleven months.

## References

1. Scheinman MM, Morady F, Hess DS, Gonzalez R (1982) Catheter-induced ablation of the atrioventricular junction to control refractory supraventricular arrhythmias. JAMA 248: 851–855
2. Gallagher JJ, Svenson RH, Kasell JH, German LD, Bardy GH, Broughton A, Critelli G (1982) Catheter technique for closed-chest ablation of the atrioventricular conduction system. New Engl J Med 306: 194–200
3. Bardy GH, Ideker RE, Kasell J, Worley SJ, Smith WM, German LD, Gallagher JJ (1983) Transvenous ablation of the atrioventricular conduction system in dogs: electrophysiologic and histologic observations. Amer J Cardiol 51: 1775–1782
4. Hartzler GO (1983) Electrode catheter ablation of focal ventricular tachycardia. J Amer Coll Cardiol 1: 595
5. Hartzler GO (1983) Electrode catheter ablation of refractory focal ventricular tachycardia. J Amer Coll Cardiol 2: 1107–1113
6. Scheinman M, Morady F, Shen E (1983) Interventional electrophysiology: Catheter ablation technique. Clin. Prog. in Pacing and Electrophysiol 1: 375–381
7. Fontaine G, Tonet JL, Frank R, Gallais Y, Shqueir S, Grosgogeat Y (1984) La fulguration endocavitaire. Une nouvelle methode de traitement des troubles du rythme? Ann Cardiol Angeiol 33: 543–561
8. O'Keeffe DB, Curry PVL, Prior AL, Yates JK, Deverall PB, Sowton E (1980) Surgery for ventricular tachycardia using operative pace mapping. Brit Heart J 43: 116
9. Puech P, Gallay P, Grolleau R, Koliopoulos N (1984) Traitement par electrofulguration endocavitaire d'une tachycardie ventriculaire recidivante par dysplasie ventriculaire droite. Arch Mal Coeur 77: 826–835
10. Fontaine G, Cansell A, Lechat PH, Frank R, Tonet JL, Grosgogeat Y (1984) Les chocs electriques endocavitaires. Problemes lies au materiel. Arch Mal Coeur 77: 1307–1314
11. Lerman BB, Weiss JL, Bulkley BH, Becker LC, Weisfeldt ML (1984) Myocardial injury and induction of arrhythmia by direct current shock delivered via endocardial catheters in dogs. Circulation 69: 1006–1012
12. Fontaine G, Touil F, Frank R, Cansell A, Gorins D, Tonet JL, Grosgogeat Y (1984) Defibrillation, fulguration et cardioversion: effets sur les pacemakers. Stimucoeur 12: 91–1
13. Josephson ME, Waxman HL, Marchlinski FE, Buxton AE, Doherty JU, Kienzle MG Electrocardiographic features of ectopic impulse formation. Specificity of ventricular activation patterns. In: Josephon ME, Wellens HJJ (eds) (1984) Tachycardias. Mechanisms, diagnosis, treatment. Philadelphia. Lea & Febiger Pub P 363–386

# Surgical therapy of ventricular tachycardia*

A.E. BUXTON* *, J.M. MILLER, W.C. HARGROVE, III,
F.E. MARCHLINSKI* *, J.U.DOHERTY, A.H. HARKEN,
and M.E. JOSEPHSON

Two-thirds of deaths in patients with heart disease occur suddenly, and the majority of these events result from ventricular tachyarrhythmias. Approximately one-half of patients with potentially lethal (i.e. sustained) ventricular tachycardia or fibrillation respond to pharmacologic therapy. Therefore, a large number of patients are potential candidates for more aggressive therapy of these arrhythmias, and this has led to a variety of surgical approaches to this problem. Techniques developed for control of sustained ventricular arrhythmias may be divided into specific and non-specific approaches. Initial experiences with non-specific techniques including aorto-coronary bypass and dorsal sympathectomy, were associated with high failure rates and unacceptable operative mortality because they were based on the assumption that ventricular tachyarrhythmias resulted from the general disease state (e.g. coronary artery disease) rather than the specific mechanisms underlying these arrhythmias [1–5]. The one exception to this has been success of myocardial revascularization in the prevention of ventricular fibrillation and tachycardia precipitated by acute myocardial ischemia [6]. However, most sustained ventricular tachycardias do not appear to be precipitated by acute ischemia or other transient metabolic alterations. The association between sustained ventricular tachycardia and left ventricular aneurysms led to attempts at more specific therapy. Initially, non-directed left ventricular aneurysmectomy was performed [1, 7–9]. Unfortunately, the simple aneurysmectomy was associated with operative mortality rates ranging from 20–40% (with most deaths due to recurrent ventricular tachyarrhythmias), and arrhythmia recurrence rates ranging from 50–80%. The failure of standard aneurysmectomy stems from the fact that the arrhythmogenic areas are usually located in the border area between fibrous aneurysm and more normal muscle (vide infra); this border is

* Supported in part by grants from the American Heart Association, Southeastern Pennsylvania Chapter, Philadelphia, Pennsylvania, and National Heart, Lung, and Blood Institute, Bethesda, MD (HL2800093, HL00361, HL24278).
* * Supported by the University of Pennsylvania Department of Medicine Measey Foundation.

usually not resected in order to facilitate a reliable repair of the ventriculotomy (Fig. 1A).

A number of experimental and clinical studies performed over the past 15 years have suggested that most sustained ventricular tachycardias arise from a fairly stable electrophysiologic abnormality present in the myocardium. The development of techniques for activation mapping during ventricular tachycardia over the past decade has given us insight into the mechanisms underlying these arrhythmias, and has helped localize the sites of circuits giving rise to the arrhythmias. This understanding has paved the way to more effective surgical therapy for these arrhythmias. Two types of directed surgical procedures have been developed based on activation mapping: procedures which isolate the tachycardia sites (right ventricular exclusion for arrhythmogenic right ventricular dysplasia and encircling endocardial ventriculotomy or cryoablation for tachycardias arising in the left ventricle), and ablative procedures, including endocardial excision and cryoablation.

**Mechanisms of sustained ventricular tachycardia**

Although a number of potential mechanisms may give rise to ventricular tachycardia including automaticity, triggered activity and reentry, most evidence at present supports reentry as the basis for sustained ventricular tachycardia arising in patients with chronic coronary artery disease. Since coronary artery disease with previous myocardial infarction is the most common clinical setting associated with sustained ventricular tachycardia, most data is based on studies in patients with this condition. This information may not be directly applicable to ventricular arrhythmias arising in association with other types of cardiac disease. A hallmark of reentrant arrhythmias is the ability of programmed stimulation to reproducibly initiate, and in many cases, terminate them. The ability to reproducibly initiate and terminate reentrant sustained ventricular tachycardia in the catheterization laboratory using pacing techniques permits the study of these arrhythmias under safe, controlled conditions. The results of electrophysiologic studies of induced and spontaneous ventricular tachycardia suggest that most circuits in ischemic heart disease are micro-reentrant, i.e. occur within a small area of perhaps 4–6 cm$^2$ [10, 11]. However, in a small number of cases, macro-reentrant loops that appear to circulate around an aneurysm border have been mapped. Activation mapping has demonstrated that in the setting of chronic ischemic heart disease earliest electrical activity during ventricular tachycardia uniformly appears in the left ventricle or inter-ventricular septum [12]. This is true regardless of the surface QRS appearance (i.e. bundle branch block pattern) during tachycardia. Of great importance, endocardial activation during ventricular tachycardia uniformly precedes the earliest site of epicardial breakthrough, and the earliest endocardial site of activity (site of tachycardia 'origin') may be

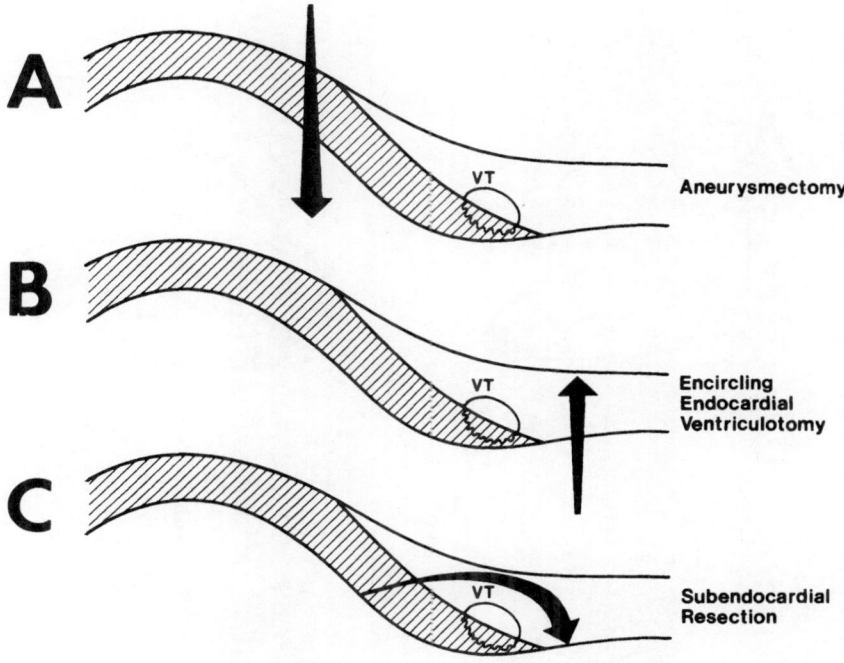

*Figure 1.* Diagramatic representation of procedures for cure of ventricular tachycardia associated with ventricular aneurysm. In each figure the hatched area represents scar tissue and aneurysm, and the clear area represents remaining normal myocardium. VT represents location of the ventricular tachycardia circuit. Arrows represent sites of incision and/or dissection with each surgical procedure. A = conventional aneurysmectomy, B = encircling endocardial ventriculotomy, C = subendocardial resection.

several centimeters removed from the epicardial breakthrough site [13–15]. (Fig. 2). Finally, these studies demonstrated that ventricular tachycardia arises at the junction between aneurysmal tissue and more normal myocardium (the area which is not removed by a conventional aneurysmectomy) (Figs. 1, 2). A pathologic correlate of the results of these mapping studies has been the discovery that a rim of surviving myocardial tissue is commonly found along the endocardial border of ventricular aneurysms. Histologic studies of this tissue demonstrate surviving myocardial fibers separated by ingrowth of connective tissue resulting in a marked decrease in the normal interconnections between muscle bundles [16, 17]. This disruption of the normal anatomy may give rise to asynchronous, anisotropic activation resulting in slowed conduction, as well as block of impulse conduction, thus supplying the requisite substrate for the establishment of re-entrant excitation.

558

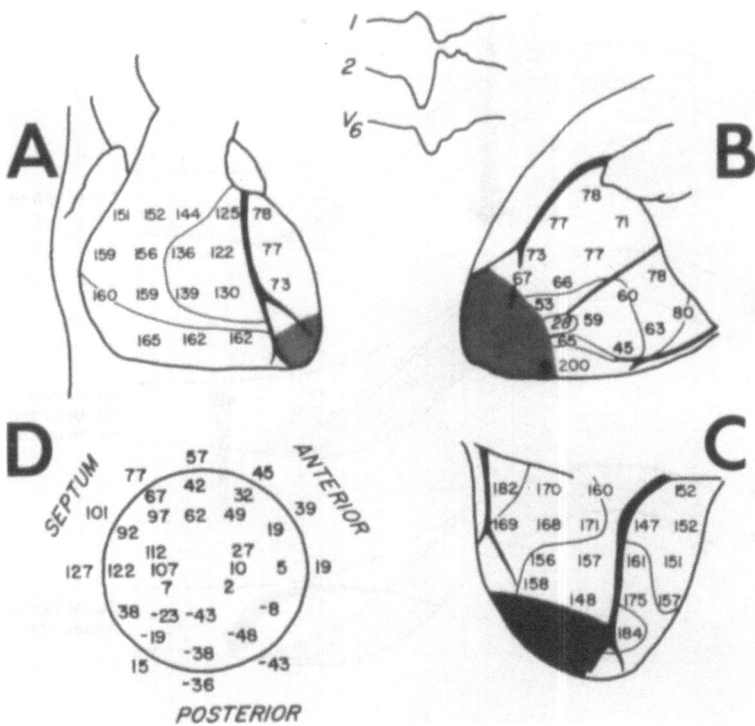

*Figure 2.* Comparison of endocardial and epicardial intraoperative activation mapping during ventricular tachycardia. At the top center portion of the figure is one complex of ventricular tachycardia having a right bundle branch block configuration. A, B and C represent anterior, lateral and posterior views of the epicardial surface of the heart. The stippled area represents that area encompassed by an aneurysm. Numbers represent epicardial activation times during each cycle of ventricular tachycardia. The dot in Figure B represents the earliest corresponding site of endocardial activation. In Figure D are endocardial activation times. Numbers with minus sign represent activation preceding the onset of the surface QRS complex. The solid line represents the proximal borders of the aneurysm and the center of Figure D represents the apical center of the aneurysm. Note: 1) Endocardial activation precedes epicardial activation. 2) Earliest activation occurs on the border of the aneurysm. 3) The earliest site of epicardial breakthrough is 3 cm from the endocardial origin (reproduced by permission from Horowitz et al, Circulation 61: 1227–1238, 1980).

## Directed surgical techniques

### Endocardial resection

Based on the above findings, a surgical technique was developed in which specific, localized areas of endocardium and subendocardium are resected [18, 19]. The areas to be resected are determined from the results of extensive activation mapping during tachycardia, both preoperatively using catheter techniques and intraoperatively (Fig. 3). The aim of mapping studies is to localize the 'site of origin' (site of earliest diastolic electrical activity during the tachycardia) of all tachycardias a patient has manifested. At least 24 hours prior to surgery all antiarrhythmic medications are discontinued. Prior to surgery a quadripolar electrode catheter is inserted percutaneously and advanced to the right ventricular apex for use as a reference recording and for pacing to induce ventricular tachycardia during surgery. After exposure of the heart through a median sternotomy, an intramyocardial plunge electrode is inserted into the left ventricular free wall as a second reference electrode. Cardiopulmonary bypass is then initiated and the aneurysm or myocardial scar incised. Programmed stimulation via the right ventricular endocardial catheter is then used to initiate ventricular tachycardia, and direct endocardial activation mapping is performed using a bipolar electrode (1 mm inter-electrode distance) mounted on a ring or stick. Mapping is performed circumferentially around the aneurysm in rows progressing away from the cut edge of the aneurysm back to normal myocardial tissue. If the patient has had more than one morphology of ventricular tachycardia (spontaneously or induced in the catheterization laboratory), attempts are made to induce and map each discrete morphology. In order to perform mapping, normothermic cardiopulmonary bypass must be maintained. After completion of the mapping procedure, cold cardioplegia is instituted with a decrease in perfusion temperature to 26°C. A 1–2 mm thick layer of subendocardium is then peeled back starting at the cut edge of the aneurysm to include all 'sites of origin' and a 2–3 cm surrounding margin of tissue. The ventriculotomy is then repaired in the standard fashion.

## Results of endocardial resection

We have performed subendocardial resection in 148 patients for ventricular tachycardia associated with chronic coronary artery disease. Preoperatively these patients had a mean left ventricular ejection fraction of 28 ± 9%. The mean left ventricular end diastolic pressure was 17 ± 8 mm Hg. There have been 16 operative deaths (deaths within 30 days of surgery), resulting from refractory heart failure, perioperative myocardial infarction, and in 2 cases sudden unexpected electromechanical disassociation one week following surgery. Over a mean follow-up period of 35 months, 87 patients have been complete surgical successes, without spontaneous or inducible VT off all antiarrhythmic drugs and 34 are partial successes, without spontaneous VT on antiarrhythmic drugs. Sudden cardiac death has occurred in 6 of the operative survivors and 5 patients have continued to have recurrent ventricular tachycardia in spite of antiarrhythmic medication, resulting in an overall success rate of 92% in the operative survivors. There have been 27 late non-sudden deaths: 15 patients died of progressive congestive heart failure, 7 patients died of recurrent myocardial infarction, 1 died of a ruptured left ventricular pseudoaneurysm and 4 patients died of miscellaneous non-cardiac causes (Fig. 4).

560

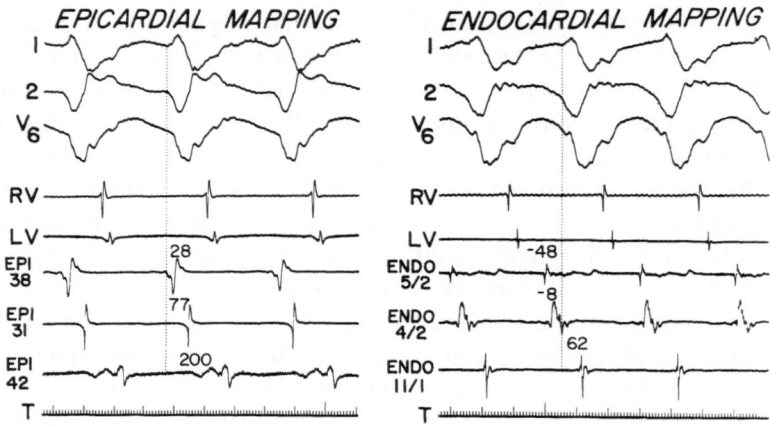

*Fig. 3.* Selected analog records of epicardial and endocardial activation during ventricular tachycardia which were used to construct the composite activation maps shown in Figure 2. Key: 1, 2 V₆ are surface electrocardiographic leads, RV and LV are right and left ventricular reference bipolar recordings and Epi 38, 31, and 42 are electrograms recorded at the site of epicardial breakthrough. Endo 5/2, 4/2, and 11/1 are endocardial electrograms. Endo 5/2 was the earliest site of activation. T refers to 10 and 100 msec time lines (reproduced by permission from Horowitz et al, Circulation 61: 1227–1238, 1980).

Postoperative electrophysiologic studies were performed before hospital discharge off antiarrhythmic medications, in order to assess the effects of endocardial resection on inducibility of ventricular tachycardia. Ninety-five patients had no inducible ventricular tachycardia, while 37 had inducible VT. The 37 patients with inducible VT underwent serial drug studies using programmed ventricular stimulation and in 23 patients, ventricular tachycardia remained inducible at hospital discharge in spite of antiarrhythmic medication. Five of these 23 patients have had spontaneous recurrences of ventricular tachycardia on drugs, and one died suddenly. None of the 14 patients whose VT was rendered non-inducible by antiarrhythmic drugs had a spontaneous recurrence but one suffered late sudden death. Of the 95 patients without inducible ventricular tachycardia at the postoperative electrophysiologic study, 4 suffered late (>1 year) postoperative cardiac arrests (1 during an episode of exertional angina, 1 of quinidine-induced polymorphic ventricular tachycardia, and the other 2 after 3 years free from ventricular tachycardia that had occurred many times yearly before surgery). Four patients had late spontaneous recurrences of a well-tolerated ventricular tachycardia. The latter 4 patients all underwent serial drug testing with programmed stimulation and following these none have had spontaneous recurrences of ventricular tachycardia on antiarrhythmic medication.

In the operative survivors the subendocardial resection has been well tolerated hemodynamically with a consistent increase in the postoperative left ventricular

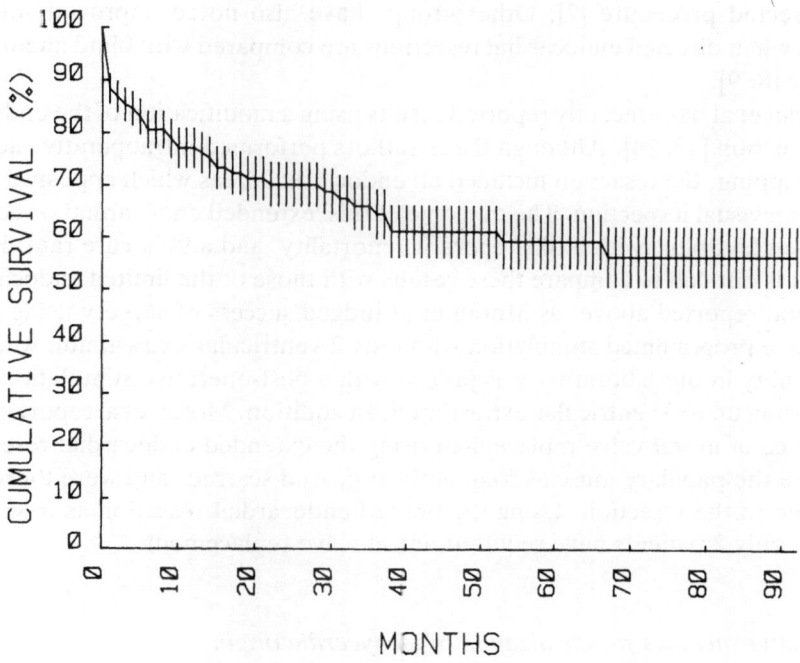

*Figure 4.* Actuarial survival curve of patients with coronary artery disease undergoing map-guided subendocardial resection and aneurysmectomy for ventricular tachyarrhythmias. Vertical bars represent one standard deviation.

ejection fraction and decrease in postoperative left ventricular end diastolic pressure compared to preoperative values [20]. Comparison of pre and postoperative ambulatory electrocardiograms has failed to reveal any consistent changes in the level of spontaneous ventricular ectopy, and the results of ambulatory monitoring do not correlate with results of programmed stimulation postoperatively or with clinical outcome [21].

Several factors have been identified which correlate with a lower surgical success rate, including the presence of multiple distinct morphologies of spontaneous ventricular tachycardias and the presence of tachycardias arising from widely separated areas in the heart ('disparate sites of origin') [22]. The location of the tachycardia site of origin also influences results, with lower success rates for tachycardias originating from the inferior wall of the left ventricle in comparison to the septum or anterior wall. This difference appears to result from the greater technical difficulty in performing an adequate resection of tachycardias located on the inferior wall, and the frequent involvement of the papillary muscle in the site of origin. While these results are far from optimal, a comparison of results using the directed endocardial resection with those following standard, nondirected aneurysmectomy shows a clear improvement in survival and cure with the directed procedure [7]. Other groups have also noted improved surgical results when directed endocardial resections are compared with blind aneurysmectomy [8, 9].

Moran et al have recently reported results using a modification of the endocardial resection [23, 24]. Although these authors performed intraoperative activation mapping, the resection included all endocardial areas which appeared scarred upon visual inspection. The outcome of this 'extended endocardial resection' has been favorable with a 10% operative mortality, and a 91% cure rate. However, it is difficult to compare these results with those of the limited endocardial resection reported above, as Moran et al judged success of surgery using post-operative programmed stimulation with only 2 ventricular extrastimuli whereas inducibility in our laboratory was judged with a post-operative stimulation protocol using up to 3 ventricular extrastimuli. In addition, Moran et al report a 13% incidence of mitral valve replacement using the extended endocardial resection because the papillary muscles frequently appeared scarred, and were therefore included in the resection. Using the limited endocardial resection as described above, only 2 patients have required mitral valve replacement.

*Alternative methods for localization of tachycardia origin*

Activation mapping during VT is difficult, time consuming, and not possible in every patient. In the catheterization laboratory, endocardial tachycardia activation mapping requires that the patient remain hemodynamically stable in a tachycardia having a constant, uniform morphology. A second limitation is the inability to achieve intraoperative induction of 10–20% of tachycardias previously inducible in the catheterization laboratory. In order to circumvent these difficulties, several alternatives have been proposed. O'Keeffe et al [25] utilized epicardial and intramural pacing in the operating room while recording multiple electrocardiographic leads in an attempt to produce a QRS morphology during pacing mimicking the tachycardia. The limitations of epicardial mapping, primarily the disparity between epicardial activation patterns, and endocardial and intramural sites of tachycardia origin, have been noted above. Further difficulties with the technique of pacemapping include the fact that tachycardias having similar morphologies may originate from disparate sites. We performed endocardial pacemapping in the catheterization laboratory but have not found this technique to be as accurate for the localization of tachycardia origin as activation mapping, nor does it take significantly less time to perform [26, 27].

A second approach to localization of tachycardia origin is sinus rhythm mapping. The frequent appearance of markedly abnormal endocardial electrograms in patients with ventricular tachycardia following myocardial infarction suggested that the presence of these abnormalities during sinus rhythm might correlate with sites of tachycardia origin. It was postulated that this technique could be used to

563

localize tachycardia origins in patients who were hemodynamically unstable during tachycardias induced in the electrophysiology laboratory, and might also be used to guide surgical resection in patients whose tachycardias could not be induced in the operating room. Unfortunately, abnormal electrograms during sinus rhythm are frequently widely distributed on the endocardium of patients with VT following infarction, and therefore are not sufficiently specific to guide limited resection [28, 29]. Thus directing surgery by sinus mapping alone would result in more extensive resection than is necessary to cure ventricular tachycardia. In addition, we have found that 14% of the time, normal electrograms are found at the site of tachycardia origin using catheter mapping [29]. Thus, no type of sinus rhythm electrogram is sufficiently specific or sensitive to guide limited endocardial resection.

*Encircling endocardial ventriculotomy*

Guiraudon and others have reported an alternative directed approach to therapy of ventricular tachycardia following myocardial infarction [30, 31]. The encircling endocardial ventriculotomy is an attempt to exclude the tachycardia circuit from the remaining normal myocardium in addition to ablating the site of origin. A transmural ventriculotomy perpendicular to the ventricular wall is performed from the endocardial aspect of the left ventricle after the aneurysm has been opened (Fig. 1C). The incision is carried along the limits of endocardial fibrosis separating the diseased from the healthy tissue. Only a narrow bridge of sub-epicardium and epicardial tissue including coronary arteries is spared. This procedure may also be performed on a more limited basis, for example, to isolate tachycardias originating at the base of papillary muscles, in combination with endocardial resection. Extensive encircling endocardial ventriculotomy has been associated with higher operative mortality than localized endocardial resection, apparently because of ischemia-induced ventricular failure [32]. However, when performed on a more limited basis it appears to be well tolerated hemodynamically, and is frequently successful in controlling ventricular tachycardia.

*Surgery for ventricular tachycardias unrelated to ischemic heart disease*

Activation mapping has permitted the extension of surgical techniques for the cure of ventricular tachycardias unrelated to chronic ischemic heart disease. We have employed localized endocardial resection in the treatment of 2 patients with ventricular tachycardia originating in the right ventricular outflow tract without associated structural heart disease. Both patients survived the procedure without adverse effects and have been cured of their arrhythmia. Procedures involving exclusion of tachycardia sites of origin have been developed by Guiraudon [33] and Cox [34] for therapy of ventricular tachycardia associated with arrhythmo-genic right ventricular dysplasia. This entity involves degeneration of the right ventricular free wall myocardium and is frequently associated with recurrent sustained ventricular tachycardia [35, 36]. Disarticulation of the right ventricular free wall at the junction with the interventricular septum in addition to cryoabla-tion where the free wall joins the tricuspid valve ring has been performed in patients with right ventricular dysplasia with good results.

## Perspective

Studies elucidating the mechanisms underlying ventricular arrhythmias over the past decade have led to more rational approaches to surgical therapy of ventricu-lar tachycardia than older, empiric techniques. These newer techniques based on defining and localizing the tachycardia circuits, have resulted in significantly higher operative survival and increased rates of cure. However, many limitations remain. More precise and automated techniques to enable rapid identification of the sites from which tachycardias originate are needed. The most critical un-solved problem is the need for techniques to improve myocardial function, as the greatest operative and postoperative mortality still results from refractory and progressive left ventricular failure.

## References

1. Buda AJ, Stinson EB, Harrison DC (1979) Surgery for life-threatening ventricular tachyar-rhythmias. Am J Cardiol 44: 1171–1177
2. Estes EH, Izlar HL (1961) Recurrent ventricular tachycardia. A case successfully treated by bilateral cardiac sympathectomy. Am J Med 31: 493–7
3. Lloyd R, Okada R, Stagg J, Anderson R, Hattler B, Marcus F (1974) The treatment of recurrent ventricular tachycardia with bilateral cervico-thoracic sympathetic-ganglionectomy. Circulation 50: 382–8
4. Schoonmaker FW, Carey T, Grow JB Sr (1975) Treatment of tachyarrhythmias and bradyar-rhythmias by cardiac sympathectomy and permanent ventricular pacing. Ann Thorac Surg 19: 80–7
5. Zipes DB, Festoff B, Schaal SF, Cox C, Sealy WC, Wallace AG (1968) Treatment of ventricular arrhythmia by permanent atrial pacemaker and cardiac sympathectomy. Ann Intern Med 68: 591–7
6. Tommaso C, Kehoe R, Zheutlin T (1982) Survivors of ischemic mediated sudden death – clinical angiographic and electrophysiologic features and response to therapy. Circulation (abstr)66 (Supp II): 25
7. Harken AH, Horowitz LN, Josephson ME (1980) Comparison of standard aneurysmectomy and aneurysmectomy with directed endocardial resection for the treatment of recurrent sustained ventricular tachycardia. J Thorac Cardiovasc Surg 80: 527–534
8. Mason JW, Stinson EB, Winkle RA, Griffin JC, Oyer PE, Ross DL, Derby G (1982) Surgery for ventricular tachycardia: Efficacy of left ventricular aneurysm resection compared with operation

guided by electrical activation mapping. Circulation 65: 1148–1155

9. Ostermeyer J, Breithardt G, Kolvenbach R, Borggrefe M, Seipel L, Schulte HD, Bircks W, Kirklin JW (1982) The surgical treatment of ventricular tachycardias. Simple anerysmectomy versus electrophysiologically guided procedures. J Thorac Cardiovasc Surgery 84: 704–715

10. Josephson ME, Horowitz LN, Farshidi A, Kastor JA (1976) Recurrent sustained ventricular tachycardia. 1. Mechanisms. Circulation 57: 431–439

11. Josephson ME, Horowitz LN, Farshidi A (1978) Continuous electrical activity. A mechanism of recurrent ventricular tachycardia. Circulation 57: 659–665

12. Josephson ME, Horowitz LN, Farshidi A, Spear JF, Kastor JA, Moore EN (1978) Recurrent sustained ventricular tachycardia. 2. Endocardial mapping. Circulation 57: 440–447

13. Spielman SR, Michelson EL, Horowitz LN. Spear JF, Moore EN (1978) The limitations of epicardial mapping as a guide to the surgical therapy of ventricular tachycardia. Circulation 57: 666–670

14. Horowitz LN, Josephson ME, Harken AH (1980) Epicardial and endocardial activation during sustained ventricular tachycardia in man. Circulation 61: 1227–1238

15. Josephson ME, Horowitz LN, Spielman SR, Greenspan AM, VandePol C, Harken AH (1980) Comparison of endocardial catheter mapping with intraoperative mapping of ventricular tachycardia. Circulation 61: 385–404

16. Fenoglio JJ Jr, Pham TD, Harken AH, Horowitz LN, Josephson ME, Wit AL (1983) Recurrent sustained ventricular tachycardia: structure and ultrastructure of subendocardial regions in which tachycardia originates. Circulation 68: III, 518–533

17. Gardner PI, Ursell PC, Pham TD, Fenoglio JJ Jr, Wit AL (1984) Experimental chronic ventricular tachycardia: anatomic and electrophysiologic substrates. In: Josephson ME & Wellens JJ (eds) Tachycardias: Mechanisms, diagnosis, and treatment. Philadelphia: p 29–60. Lea & Febiger

18. Horowitz LN, Harken AH, Kastor JA, Josephson ME (1980) Ventricular resection guided by epicardial and endocardial mapping to treatment of recurrent ventricular tachycardia. N Engl J 302: 589–93

19. Josephson ME, Harken AH, Horowitz LN (1979) Endocardial excision: a new surgical technique for the treatment of recurrent ventricular tachycardia. Circulation 60: 1430–1439

20. Martin JL, Untereker WJ, Harken AH, Horowitz LN, Josephson ME (1982) Aneurysmectomy and endocardial resection for ventricular tachycardia: favorable hemodynamic and anti-arrhythmic results in patients with global left ventricular dysfunction. Am Heart J 103: 960–965

21. Kienzle MG, Doherty JU, Roy D, Waxman HL, Harken AH, Josephson ME (1983) Subendocardial resection for refractory ventricular tachycardia: effects on ambulatory electrocardiogram, programmed stimulation and ejection fraction, and relation to outcome. JACC 2: 853–858

22. Miller JM, Kienzle MG, Harken AH, Josephson ME (1984) Subendocardial resection for ventricular tachycardia: predictors of surgical success. Circulation 70: 624–631

23. Moran JM, Kehoe RF, Loeb JM, Lichtenthal PR, Sanders JH Jr, Michaelis LL (1982) Extended endocardial resection for the treatment of ventricular tachycardia and ventricular fabrillation. Ann of Thorac Surg 34: 538–552

24. Moran JM, Kehoe RF, Loeb JM, Frederickson JW, Zheutlin TA, Sanders JH Jr, Michaelis LL (1983) The role of papillary muscle resection and mitral valve replacement in the control of refractory ventricular arrhythmia. Circulation 68 (Suppl II), II-154-160

25. O'Keeffe DB, Curry PVL, Prior AL, Yates AK, Deverall PB, Sowton E (1980) Surgery for ventricular tachycardia using operative pace mapping. Br Heart J 43: 116

26. Waxman HL, Josephson ME (1982) Ventricular activation during ventricular endocardial pacing: 1. Electrocardiographic patterns related to the site of pacing. Am J Cardiol 50: 1–10

27. Josephson ME, Waxman HL, Cain ME, Gardner MJ, Buxton AE (1982) Ventricular activation during ventricular endocardial pacing. II. Role of pace-mapping to localize origin of ventricular tachycardia. Am J of Cardiol 50: 11–22

28. Kienzle MG, Miller J, Falcone RA, Harken A, Josephson ME (1984) Intraoperative endocardial

mapping during sinus rhythm: relationship to site of origin of ventricular tachycardia. Circulation 70: 957–965

29. Cassidy DM, Vassallo JA, Buxton AE, Doherty JU, Marchlinski FE, Josephson ME (1984) The value of catheter mapping during sinus rhythm to localize site of origin of ventricular tachycardia. Circulation 69: 1103–1110

30. Guiraudon G, Fontaine G, Frank R, Escande G, Etievent P, Cabrol C (1978) Encircling endocardial ventriculotomy: a new surgical treatment for life-threatening ventricular tachycardias resistant to medical treatment following myocardial infarction. Ann Thorac Surg 26: 438

31. Cox JL, Gallagher JJ, Ungerleider RM (1982) Encircling endocardial ventriculotomy for refractory ischemic ventricular tachycardia. IV. Clinical indications, surgical technique, mechanism of action, and results. J Thorac Cardiovasc Surg 83: 865–872

32. Ungerleider RM, Stanley TE, Williams JM, Lofland GK, Cox JL (1980) Physiologic effects of the encircling endocardial ventriculotomy (EEV) for refractory ischemic ventricular tachycardia. Circulation (abstr) 62 (Suppl IV): IV–215

33. Guiraudon GM, Klein GJ, Gulamhusein SS, Painvin GA, DelCampo C, Gonzales JC, Ko PT (1983) Total disconnection of the right ventricular free wall: surgical treatment of right ventricular tachycardia associated with right ventricular dysplasia. Circulation 67: 463–470

34. Boineau JP, Cox JL (1982) Rationale for a direct surgical approach to control ventricular arrhythmias. Am J Cardiol 49: 381–394

35. Fontaine G, Guiraudon G, Frank R, Vedel J, Grosgogeat Y, Cabrol C, Facquet J (1977) Stimulation studies and epicardial mapping in ventricular tachycardia: study of mechanisms and selection for surgery. In: Kulbertus HE (ed) Re-entrant arrhythmias. Baltimore: University Park Press, p 334–350

36. Marcus FI, Fontaine GH, Guiraudon G, Frank R, Laurenceau JL, Malergue C, Grosgogeat Y (1982) Right ventricular dysplasia. A report of 24 cases. Circulation 65: 384–398

# Index of subjects